New Therapies in Advanced Cutaneous Malignancies

Piotr Rutkowski • Mario Mandalà

Editors

New Therapies in Advanced Cutaneous Malignancies

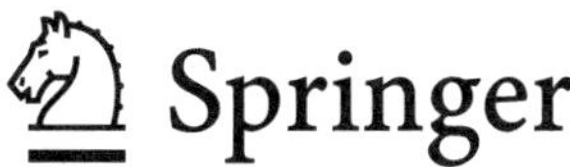 Springer

Editors
Piotr Rutkowski
Department of Soft Tissue/Bone Sarcoma
and Melanoma
Maria Sklodowska-Curie National Research
Institute of Oncology
Warsaw
Poland

Mario Mandalà
Department of Medicine and Surgery
Unit of Medical Oncology
University of Perugia
Perugia
Italy

ISBN 978-3-030-64011-8   ISBN 978-3-030-64009-5 (eBook)
https://doi.org/10.1007/978-3-030-64009-5

This Springer imprint is published by the registered company Springer Nature Switzerland AG
The registered company address is: Gewerbestrasse 11, 6330 Cham, Switzerland

Contents

Part I
Pathological, Molecular and Immunological Background of Cutaneous Malignancies

Chapter 1
Pathology of Melanoma and Skin Carcinomas

Anna Szumera-Ciećkiewicz and Daniela Massi

Melanoma

The fourth edition of the WHO Classification of Skin Tumors concerns two basic types of melanoma with a radial phase and those that develop vertically [1]. The first group includes superficial spreading melanoma (SMM) and lentigo maligna melanoma (LMM). In contrast, nodular melanoma (NM) has only a vertical growth phase, and also naevoid melanoma usually does not have a radial phase. Both types of melanoma growth differ in the clinical picture, genetic profile, and mechanism of oncogenesis, in which the most critical role is played by ultraviolet radiation, both naturally associated with sun exposure and artificial [2]. In the latest WHO classification of skin tumors, it is proposed to divide skin melanomas into the following categories: those with a high degree of solar damage resulting from high cumulative skin damage (high-CSD)/superficial spreading melanoma (SMM)—and those that develop in skin exposed to low UV exposure (low-CSD)—lentigo maligna melanoma (LMM) and desmoplastic melanoma (DM) [1, 3]. The high-CSD melanoma group outlines many point mutations, including the *NF1, NRAS, BRAF* (other than *p.V600E*), *KIT* (*MAPK* activation pathway), and *TP53* genes. In low-CSD melanomas, the dominant molecular signature is the mutation in codon 600 of the *BRAF*

A. Szumera-Ciećkiewicz (✉)
Department of Pathology and Laboratory Diagnostics, Maria Sklodowska-Curie National Research Institute of Oncology, Warsaw, Poland

Department of Diagnostic Hematology, Institute of Hematology and Transfusion Medicine, Warsaw, Poland
e-mail: Anna.Szumera-Cieckiewicz@pib-nio.pl

D. Massi
Department of Health Sciences, Section of Pathological Anatomy, University of Florence, Florence, Italy
e-mail: daniela.massi@unifi.it

© The Author(s), under exclusive license to Springer Nature Switzerland AG 2021
P. Rutkowski, M. Mandalà (eds.), *New Therapies in Advanced Cutaneous Malignancies*, https://doi.org/10.1007/978-3-030-64009-5_1

gene (*BRAF p.V600E*) [4–8]. A group of melanomas that are not associated with UV radiation exposure was also distinguished and included acral melanoma (AM), malignant Spitz tumor/Spitz melanoma, mucosal melanoma (genital, oral, sinonasal), and uveal melanoma. In all the above types, different genetic change profiles are detected, for example, mutations in the *HRAS* (Spitz melanoma), *KIT, NRAS, BRAF, HRAS, KRAS, ALK, NTRK3* (acral melanoma), *KIT, NRAS, KRAS* (mucosal melanoma); *GNAQ, GNA11, CYSLTR2* (uveal melanoma) [9]. The classification based on the nine molecular pathways is presented later in the chapter.

The differentiation of melanocytic lesions into benign or malignant is clear, but, still, some of them manifest uncertain malignant potential. In these cases, morphological features, immunohistochemical profile, and the status of genetic changes cannot determine the clinical prognosis. The fourth edition of the WHO classification provides definitions of terms used to describe atypical melanocytic proliferation, that is, Melanocytic Tumors of Uncertain Malignant Potential (MELTUMP) —atypical melanocytic proliferation in the dermis, which means that it has a "tumorigenic" phase in the absence of specific criteria needed to distinguish benign from a malignant lesion. Furthermore, the superficial atypical melanocytic proliferation of uncertain significance (SAMPUS) was also defined as atypical melanocytic proliferation located only in the epidermis and upper layer of the skin with insufficient features for a conclusive diagnosis, lacking the vertical growth phase but without the possibility of radial growth exclusion [1, 10–12]. Practically, the therapeutic procedure is identical and consists of widening the surgical margin (so-called scar cutting) and observing the patient. Differential diagnosis of SAMPUS is challenging and subjective, especially if the only available material is biopsy or regression is severe. The concept of "uncertain significance" in SAMPUS means the possibility of recurrence or progression, while "uncertain malignant potential" in MELTUMP strengthens the risk of malignant progression. Differential diagnosis of MELTUMP always includes melanoma, and the histopathological report must contain a detailed description and so-called "provisional" diagnosis. The pathologist should always try to determine the most precise and unambiguous result of the histopathological examination, and the borderline results should not exceed 1% of all diagnoses.

The melanocytic neoplasm of low malignant potential (provisional category) and melanocytoma were introduced to WHO classification as well. Both changes are included in the evolution pathway from benign naevus to melanoma [13–15]. Melanocytic neoplasm of low malignant potential is the proliferation that fulfills the traditional criteria of invasive melanoma. However, clinically, it is not associated with melanoma-related deaths (lesions thinner than 1 mm, without vertical growth, mitotic activity, and regression, diagnosed among patients >55 years of age). Melanocytoma was provided for tumorigenic lesions with increased cellularity and/or atypia and an increased risk of progression [1]. The above "intermediate" lesions still require further investigation and long-term clinical observation.

Pathology of Melanoma According to Molecular Pathways

Pathway I. Low-CSD Melanoma/Superficial Spreading Melanoma (SMM)

Low-CSD melanoma is characterized by the absence of marked solar elastosis and frequent *BRAF V600E* mutation (>50% of cases) [16]. According to the fourth ed. of the WHO classification, SMM is included in that category. It comprises approximately 60% of all melanoma types among people with lighter skinned people. Usually, it is found in locations with intermittent sun exposure with a predilection to legs in females and back or shoulders in males.

Macroscopically, low-CSD/SMM begins with a radial growth phase, and lesions in situ present as patches of pigmentation on the skin that progress into elevated plaques. Initially, the borders are sharply delimited and that lesions are indistinguishable from benign junctional nevi. The pigmentation is variable, from tan to black with white areas that represent regression areas. Some tumors are amelanocytic and may be misdiagnosed with keratinocytic neoplasms. The dermal invasion may present as a papule, usually without ulceration. As the lesion gradually develops, the distinctive "ABCDE" clinical characteristics are seen [17].

Microscopically, the pagetoid pattern of growth is seen in in situ lesions. The intraepidermal melanoma cells may form nests that can be prominent (buck-shot pagetoid spread). The extension along epidermal adnexes may be found. There is also a lentiginous pattern of low-CSD/SMM with the reduced pagetoid spread. The invasive usually starts with the single, scattered cells within the papillary dermis (invasive RGP) and may progress into large, expansive nests with brisk mitotic activity (VGP) (Fig. 1.1a). In the dermis, the diffuse fibroplasia and areas of regression may be found. The differentiation between low- vs. high-CSD requires evaluation of solar elastosis. The grading system includes mild (grade 1) single elastic fibers in the dermis visible at ×20 magnification; moderate (grade 2) altered fibers in bunches or fascicles; severe (grade 3) homogeneous clumps of elastotic material without that texture of individual fibrils [18]. Usually, most cases of SSM/low-CSD melanoma show some degree of mild-to-moderate solar elastosis. Melanomas on non-glabrous skin with no, mild, or moderate solar elastosis should be classified as low CSD. Lesions with histological features of SMM (pagetoid scatter, a predominance of large epithelioid melanocytes with powdery melanin pigmentation, or a contiguous melanocytic nevus as a precursor) despite severe solar elastosis should also be described as low-CSD/SSM.

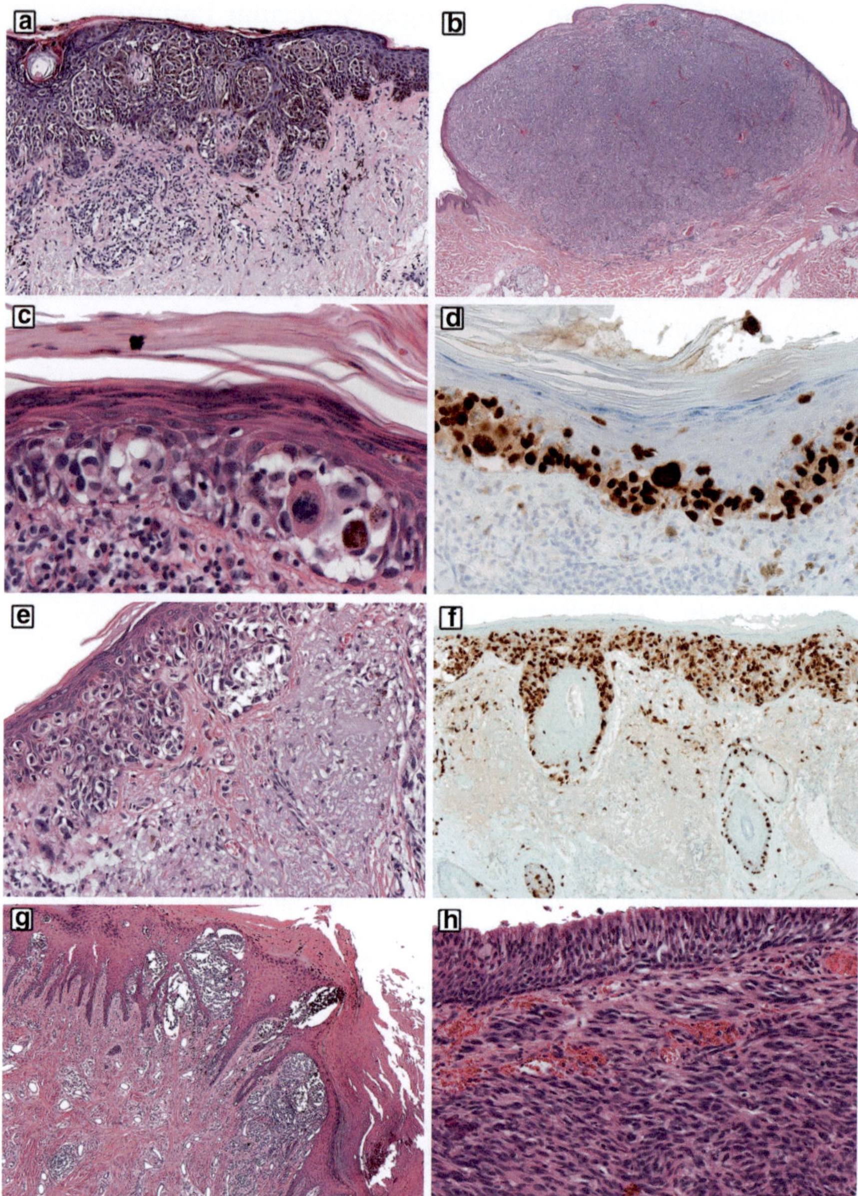

Fig. 1.1 (**a**) Low CSD/superficial spreading melanoma (200×), melanoma cells and nests present at all levels of the epidermis; (**b**) Nodular melanoma (HE, 10×), epidermis adjacent to melanoma lacks RGP component; (**c**, **d**) Lentigo maligna (HE, 600×) and in SOX10 immunostaining (400×), respectively; (**e**, **f**) Lentigo maligna melanoma (HE, 200×) and in SOX10 immunostaining (100×), respectively, severe solar elastosis is seen as an extension of melanoma along skin adnexes; (**g**) Acral melanoma (HE, 20×), atypical melanocytes present as nests and pagetoid spread; (**h**) Mucosal melanoma (HE, 200×), infiltration of the sinonasal tract

Pathway II: High-CSD Melanoma/Lentigo Maligna Melanoma (LMM)

High-CSD melanomas are less common than low-CSD/SMM and occur more frequently among older people who were chronically exposed to the sun [18]. That population includes particular outdoor professions as well as high daily exposure related to recreation.

Macroscopically, LMM presents as a patch or plaque, usually with a less circumscribed border. The lesions may extend a marked distance beyond the clinically visible border; thus, the local recurrence is found more frequently. The LMM evolve from RGP to VGP and subsequently fulfill the ABCDE criteria. The VGP progression (region of thickening, palpable or visible nodule, plaque-like area, desmoplastic) seems to be slower than in SMM [19]. Pigmentation is less expressed than in SSM; some lesions are amelanotic, and primarily may be diagnosed as an inflammatory skin disorder.

Microscopically, high-CSD melanomas/LMMs demonstrate severe (grade 3) solar elastosis. The RGP presents two types of growth: classic lentigo maligna (continuous proliferation of atypical naevoid to epithelioid melanocytes along dermo-epidermal junction) and dysplastic naevus-like lentigo maligna (nest formation tendency, with bridging adjacent elongated rete ridges) (Fig. 1.1c, d). The differentiation with dysplastic naevus can be challenging; LMM shows asymmetry and continuous growth [20]. On the contrary to solar and other lentigines, in LMM the rete ridges tend to be effaced rather than elongated, the epidermis is thinned, and the proliferation is at least focally continuous rather than intermittent. The so-called "skipped" regions with evident fibroplasia are the regression evidence. High-CSD melanomas are not derived from a precursor nevus (unlike low-CSD melanomas) [21]. The VGP of LMM is constituted from small-to-moderate, atypical ovoid melanocytes, which may resemble naevoid or spindle to desmoplastic melanocytes (Fig. 1.1e, f).

Pathway III: Desmoplastic Melanoma

Desmoplastic melanoma is a variant of spindle cell melanoma, which accounts for 1–4% of all cases. There is a slight predilection to females and older patients (median age at diagnosis approximately 65 years). Desmoplastic melanoma involves severely sun-damaged skin with a high mutation load.

Macroscopically, desmoplastic melanoma usually presents as a firm, painless scar-like tumor. The lesions are commonly localized at the head and neck region (nose, lip, ears, scalp) and are amelanotic or sparsely pigmented. The clinical differential diagnosis is difficult; only a few tumors rise below a preexisting pigmented patch. The lesions are typically endophytic and rarely form a nodule [22].

Microscopically, in most cases, there is an in situ/invasive RGP component, with general characteristics of LMM. Pigmentation is usually sparse or absent. In some cases, there is an inconspicuous junctional proliferation that does not meet the melanoma in situ criteria; limited cases present no junctional component. The VGP is composed of spindle cells that resemble schwannian differentiation pattern [23]. Melanoma cells are separated by delicate collagen fibers, which are synthesized by the tumor (Fig. 1.2a, b). A distinctive feature is the presence of lymphocytes aggregated into nodular clusters. The desmoplastic component is highly infiltrative and extend into the subcutis (diffusely or in fibrous bands) and may involve fascia and interlobular septa. The cytological atypia is generally mild, but typically a few larger cells with hyperchromatic nuclei are seen [24]. In the majority of cases, desmoplastic melanoma lacks HMB-45 and Melan A immunohistochemical expression; spindle cells are usually at least focally positive for SOX10 and pS100 [25, 26]. The differential diagnosis includes not only lesions with melanocytic origin (desmoplastic naevus, desmoplastic Spitz naevus, sclerosing blue naevus) but also immature scars and other spindle cell neoplasms (dermatofibroma, atypical fibroxantoma/pleomorphic dermal sarcoma, sarcomatoid carcinoma, leiomyosarcoma).

Pathway IV: Spitz Melanoma

Malignant Spitz tumor/Spitz melanoma is a rare variant of melanoma derived from Spitz naevus. The diagnosis criteria are based on clinical features, histopathological and cytological image, immunohistochemical pattern, genetic alterations profile, and clinical evolution [27]. The spectrum from Spitz naevus to Spitz melanoma is morphologically characterized by the distinctive large spindle and/or epithelioid melanocytes and genetically by a different set of driver mutations and fusion kinases. Lesions "in-between" are categorized as atypical Spitz tumors.

Macroscopically, Spitz melanoma presents as enlarging, asymmetrical, and changing plaque or nodule, which occurs in any age but more often among patients over 40 years of age, usually located on extremities and trunk. The features suggesting melanoma include larger size (>6 mm), irregular borders, color variegation, ulceration, or bleeding [28].

Microscopically, Spitz melanoma is defined by the presence of large spindle and/or epithelioid melanocytes with high-grade cytological atypia (Fig. 1.2c, d). The features supporting histopathological diagnosis in the epidermal component are size (often >10 mm), asymmetry, poor circumscription, ulceration, irregular and confluent nesting, extensive pagetoid spread, effacement of the epidermis, lack of maturation, high mitotic index (>6 and >3 mitoses/mm^2 in the dermal component in children and adults, respectively), deep or atypical mitoses and necrosis. Immunohistochemically, Spitz melanoma shows HMB-45 and Ki-67 expression in

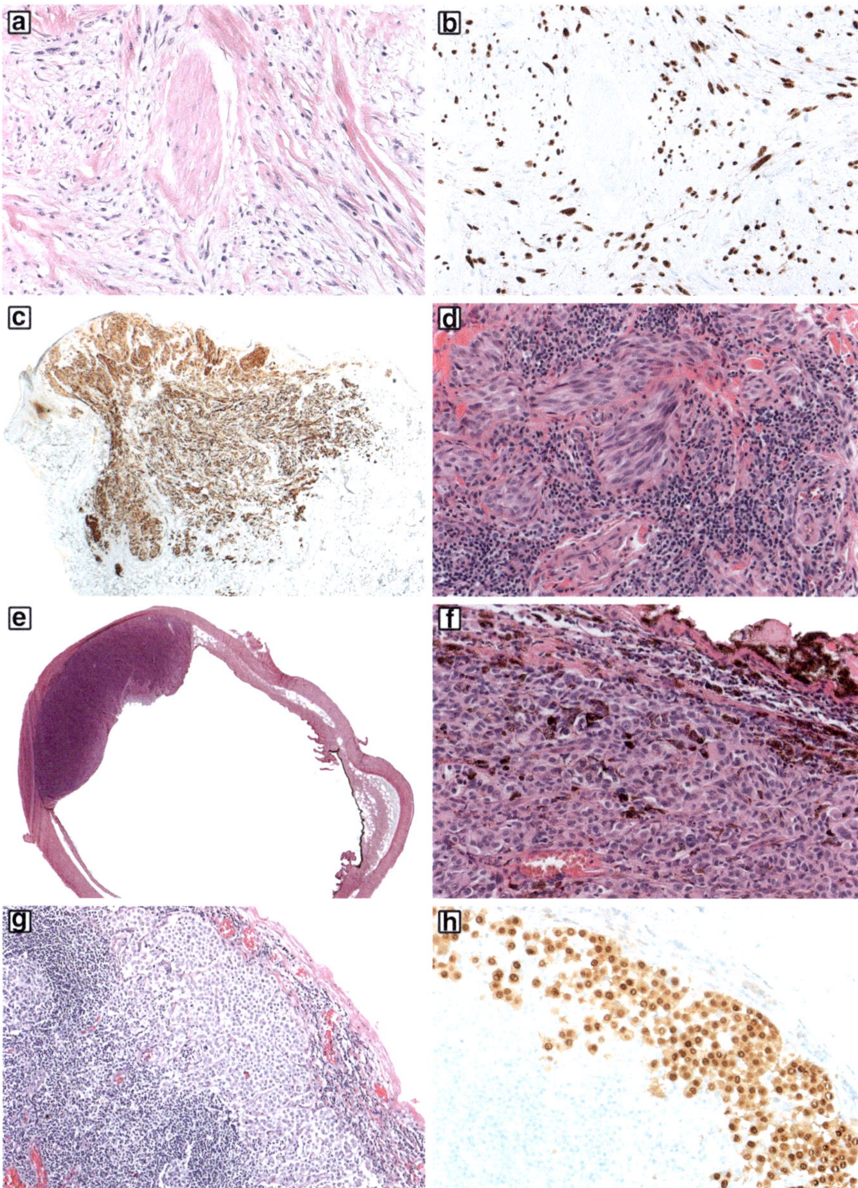

Fig. 1.2 (**a**, **b**) Desmoplastic melanoma (HE, 200×) and in SOX10 immunostaining (200×), respectively, malignant melanoma cells with elongated nuclei and cytological atypia are found within abundant collagen fibers; (**c**, **d**) Spitz melanoma in S100 immunostaining (20×) and HE (400×), respectively, asymmetrical, poorly circumscribed lesion with effacement of the epidermis and lack of maturation; (**e**, **f**) Uveal melanoma (10× and 400×); (**g**, **h**) lymph node metastasis of melanoma (HE and SOX10, 200× respectively)

more profound parts of a lesion; elevated Ki-67 (in a hot-spots >20%) and p16 staining loss are common findings [29–31]. The genomic landscape is also specific, but comprehensive molecular testing is not always accessible [32].

Pathway V: Acral Melanoma

Acral melanoma refers to melanoma occurring in the glabrous acral skin, including palms, soles, and nail beds. The non-hair-bearing volar surface of the skin has a thick stratum corneum, which is a natural barrier against UV radiation. The risk factors may be associated with mechanical or physical stress. The total incidence rate of acral melanomas is similar, but in some populations (Asian, Hispanic, African), it is the most frequent melanoma subtype [33, 34].

Macroscopically, acral melanoma begins with a patch lesion that enlarges into asymmetrical, black, pigmented irregular plaque. The RGP may be prolonged (several months to years) before progression to VGP. Advanced lesions usually become ulcerated nodules. Subungual melanoma often presents as longitudinal melanonychia, and Hutchinson's sign (pigmented patch spreads over the nail plate, beyond the proximal nail fold and hyponychium). Rare amelanocytic acral melanomas can be misdiagnosed with other, nonmalignant conditions. The dermoscopy is very supportive in making the diagnosis, while many features differentiating naevus and melanoma can be easily found [33].

Microscopically, acral melanomas most commonly present with a lentiginous pattern of proliferation (acral lentiginous melanomas). The pagetoid growth is less conventional, and both histologically and genetically resembles low-CSD/SSM (Fig. 1.1g). The VGP may be composed of spindle cells with or without a desmoplastic pattern of growth, which corresponds with increased neurotropism. The subungual melanomas show frequent bone invasion due to its superficial location. The differential diagnosis with acral naevi may be challenging also because of problems with proper biopsy of the nail [35, 36].

Pathway VI: Mucosal Melanoma

Melanoma occurring in a mucous membrane is most commonly found in genital sites, oral and nasal cavities, and conjunctiva. These lesions are not specific epidemiologically, and risk factors are largely unknown. Mucosal melanomas are not associated with UV exposure or other factors (chemical substances, viruses, or trauma) [37, 38].

Macroscopically, the pigmentation change is seen in the majority of cases. The difficulties in visualizing lesions located in nasal sinuses and visceral organs result in a bulky tumor presentation. These advanced tumors sometimes present with pain, bleeding, epistaxis, nasal stuffiness, proptosis, and diplopia [39, 40].

Microscopically, mucosal melanomas mostly show a lentiginous or nodular pattern of growth. Both epithelioid and spindle cell morphology is seen (Fig. 1.1h). The ulceration and lymphovascular invasion are typical.

Pathway VII: Melanoma Arising in a Congenital Nevus

Melanomas occur in giant congenital nevi; a lifetime incidence of melanoma is estimated at 2–5%. Most melanomas are located on the scalp or back and occur during childhood (first 5 years of life) within the epicenter of the intradermal or subcutaneous lesion [41, 42].

Macroscopically, rapidly growing nodules or plaques with ulceration are found. The differences in color and texture between melanoma and surrounding nevus are apparent. At the time of initial diagnosis, the lymph node metastatic spread is often found [43–45].

Microscopically, three main histological subtypes are epithelioid, spindled, or "small round blue" cells; rarely melanoma arising in congenital nevus may exhibit malignant schwannoma, rhabdomyosarcoma, or liposarcoma morphology. The developing melanoma may be clinically masked by the heavily pigmented nevus. Moreover, cellular and proliferative nodules in congenital nevi, which are benign lesions, need to be excluded [41, 45–47].

Pathway VIII: Melanoma Arising in Blue Nevus

That type of melanoma is rare and usually occurs on the scalp among adult individuals (usually >45 years). The risk factors remain unknown.

Macroscopically, it presents as a rapidly growing nodule; the residual cellular blue nevus may be found [48].

Microscopically, melanoma arising in a blue nevus is a tumorigenic proliferation. The diagnosis is usually late due to overlay with the presence of the precursor lesions. Ulceration may occur; however, some melanomas are deeply growing lesions, which are recognized only because of an increase in the size of the preexisting nevus. Melanoma consists of large, anaplastic cells with brisk mitotic activity. Loss of nuclear BAP1 expression favors the melanoma diagnosis as well [49, 50].

IX Uveal melanoma

Uveal melanoma is a malignant ocular melanocytic tumor that originates in the iris, ciliary body, or choroid (the most frequent localization constituting 90% of all cases). It occurs mainly within adults (median age 60 years) with an estimated incidence of 2–8 million cases per year.

Clinically, patients have visual problems. Large necrotic melanomas may manifest as painful uveitis or glaucoma.

Macroscopically, uveal melanomas grow like a dome- or mushroom-shaped tumors. The typical changes related to choroidal melanoma are retinal pigment epithelium disruption, lipofuscin accumulation, and serous retinal detachment. The invasive spread of melanoma along nerves (small nerves into orbit and optic nerve) and blood and lymphatic vessels is described [51, 52].

Microscopically, uveal melanomas may be epithelioid or spindle cells. The typical melanoma features such as mitotic figures, necrosis, lymphocytic infiltration, and melanophages are seen (Fig. 1.2e, f). In differential diagnosis, the panel of melanocytic markers should be used. Genetically, uveal melanomas show frequent loss-of-function mutations in *GNA11, GNAQ, BAP1, EIF11AX, SF3B11, PLCB4,* and *CYSLTR2* [46].

The conjunctival melanomas are included in ocular melanomas but genetically do not belong to the IX pathway (harbor *BRAF p.V600* mutations/low-CSD melanoma vs. *NRAS* or *KIT* mutations/high-CSD melanoma). Histologically, conjunctival melanoma is *the novo* malignancy; in the majority of cases, it can be associated with a precursor naevus or primary melanosis. The microscopical features are the same as in cutaneous melanoma, and all morphological variants can be found [53].

Nodular Melanoma

Nodular melanomas can occur in any of the pathways discussed above, and therefore the epidemiologic and genomic features are likely to be heterogeneous.

Macroscopically, nodular melanomas present as a rapidly growing papular or nodular lesion with a wide range of pigmentation. Typically, nodular melanomas are elevated above the epidermis, demonstrating the growth in an upward direction. They can be heavily melanized (dark nodules), but also amelanotic (pink papulonodular lesions) cases are seen. Nodular melanomas have a worse prognosis on average than other melanomas, but this difference diminishes in multivariable analyses [54].

Microscopically, nodular melanoma shows tumorigenic, vertical growth phase with generally high Breslow thickness. The lesions are usually ulcerated. The surrounding epidermis is normal (Fig. 1.1b). The melanoma cells are mostly epithelioid, but also spindle cell or a mixture of cells can be found (patchwork or clonal pattern). The pseudo-maturation (superficial cells are larger than cells located deeply) may lead to misdiagnosis with nevi of naevoid melanomas. The differential diagnosis includes metastatic melanoma and a wide range of non-melanocytic tumors (i.e., carcinomas, sarcomas, and lymphomas). Nodular melanomas are typically devoid of melanin, and additional immunohistochemistry needs to support the diagnosis [54, 55].

Reporting of Melanoma

The eighth edition of the American Joint Committee on Cancer (AJCC) staging system keeps microscopic infiltration depth of melanoma and ulceration as the most important prognostic parameters [56, 57]. Currently, the mitotic activity has not been included in the stratification of pT1 and does not change influence categorization from pT1a to pT1b. However, it remains an important prognostic factor and should be a component of histopathological diagnosis. Thin melanomas are lesions with a depth of up to 0.8 mm without ulceration. Clinically, these changes are treated as locally advanced and do not require a sentinel lymph node removal procedure. However, pT1 melanomas are characterized by the variable risk of recurrence (from 1% to 12%) [58, 59]. Still, there is a strong need for the identification of additional robust prognostic factors to support decision-making processes.

Moreover, the combination of the T and N categories led to the redefinition of stage III (Fig. 1.2g, h). Long-term observation under the AJCC database proved that the 10-year survival among patients with T1, T2, T3, and T4 melanomas were 92%, 80%, 63%, and 50%, respectively [67]. The most important prognostic factors in patients with extra-regional metastases are the localization of metastases and LDH activity. Patients with central nervous system metastases have the worst prognosis in this group. The detailed definitions, according to the eighth edition of the AJCC melanoma staging, are depicted in Table 1.1 [64].

Histopathological Prognostic Markers

Breslow Thickness

Breslow thickness is the most reproducible measurement (in millimeters) of the melanoma vertical growth phase. It should be assessed from the granular layer or, in ulcerated lesions, from the bottom of ulceration, up to the deepest part of infiltration [3, 65]. Adnexal involvement by melanoma is currently considered as in situ disease [66]. However, the classification and measurement of periadnexal extension melanoma remain ambiguous. If it is the only focus of invasion, it is recommended to measure Breslow thickness from the inner layer of the outer root sheath epithelium or inner luminal surface of sweat glands, to the furthest extent of infiltration into the

Table 1.1 pTNM for melanoma, according to the eighth edition of the AJCC staging [64]

T category		
	Breslow thickness (mm)	Ulceration
TX: primary tumor thickness cannot be assessed (e.g., fragmented biopsy)		
T0: no evidence of primary tumor (e.g., unknown primary or completely regressed primary melanoma		
T is (melanoma in situ)		
T1	*≤1.0*	Unknown or unspecified
T1a	<0.8	Without
T1b	<0.8	With
	0.8–1.0	Without or With
T2	*>1.0–2.0*	Unknown or unspecified
T2a		Without
T2b		With
T3	*>2.0–4.0*	Unknown or unspecified
T3a		Without
T3b		With
T4	*>4.0*	Unknown or unspecified
T4a		Without
T4b		With

N category		
	Extent of regional lymph node and/or lymphatic metastasis	Presence of in-transit, satellite, and/or microsatellite metastases
NX: Regional nodes not assessed (e.g., SLN biopsy not performed, regional nodes previously removed for another reason)		
Exception: pathological N category is not required for T1 melanomas, use cN, if regional lymph nodes not assessed for patient with T1 melanoma		
N0	0	No
N1	One tumor-involved node or any number of in-transit, satellite, and/or microsatellite metastases with no tumor-involved nodes	
N1a	Clinically occult (i.e., detected by SLN biopsy)	No
N1b	Clinically detected	No
N1c	No regional lymph node disease	Yes
N2	Two or three tumor-involved nodes or any number of in-transit, satellite, and/or microsatellite metastases with one tumor-involved node	
N2a	Clinically occult (i.e., detected by SLN biopsy)	No
N2b	At least one clinically detected	No
N2c	One clinically occult or clinically detected	Yes

Table 1.1 (continued)

N3	Four or more tumor-involved nodes or any number of in-transit, satellite, and/or microsatellite metastases with two or more tumor-involved nodes, or any number of matted nodes without or with in-transit, satellite, and/or microsatellite metastases	
N3a	Clinically occult (i.e., detected by SLN biopsy)	No
N3b	At least one of which was clinically detected, or presence of any number of matted nodes	No
N3c	Two or more clinically occult or clinically detected and/or presence of any number of matted nodes	Yes
M category		
	Anatomic site	LDH level
M0 No evidence of distant metastasis Not applicable		
M1	Evidence of distant metastasis	
M1a	Distant metastasis to skin, soft tissue including muscle, and/or nonregional lymph node	Not recorded or unspecified
M1a(0)		Not elevated
M1a(1)		Elevated
M1b	Distant metastasis to lung with or without M1a sites of disease	Not recorded or unspecified
M1b(0)		Not elevated
M1b(1)		Elevated
M1c	Distant metastasis to non-CNS visceral sites with or without M1a or M1b sites of disease	Not recorded or unspecified
M1c(0)		Not elevated
M1c(1)		Elevated
M1d	Distant metastasis to CNS with or without M1a, M1b, or M1c sites of disease	Not recorded or unspecified
M1d(0)		Not elevated
M1d(1)		Elevated

periadnexal dermis [66]. The interpretation problems of Breslow thickness include cases with a preexisting nevus, severe regression, or exophytic melanoma with verruciform architecture.

Nevertheless, Breslow's thickness is a highly reliable and accepted prognostic factor that shows an excellent correlation with mortality. The prognosis is worsening logarithmically with increasing thickness to 8 mm, then it achieves a plateau, but 100% mortality is never accomplished [56]. Long-term observation in the AJCC database proved that the 10-year survivals among patients with T1, T2, T3, and T4 melanomas were 92%, 80%,63%, and 50%, respectively [67].

Ulceration

Microscopical assessment of the presence of ulceration must be performed in each primary melanoma. The criteria of ulceration are well established and include full-thickness epidermal defect (including the absence of stratum corneum and basement membrane), evidence of reactive changes (fibrin deposition and neutrophils), thinning, effacement, or reactive hyperplasia of the surrounding epidermis in the absence of trauma or a recent surgical procedure. Recently, the extension of ulceration has shown substantial prognostic value; it may be reported as a diameter or percentage of tumor width [68]. Increasing melanoma thickness is correlated with more frequent ulceration (for thin vs. thick melanomas, ulceration is found in 6% vs. 63% of cases, respectively), but those two factors are independent prognostic factors [67]. The analysis of the eighth edition of the AJCC staging system showed that patients with ulcerated melanomas had a twofold higher estimated risk of dying due to melanoma in comparison to non-ulcerated tumors. Moreover, the presence of ulceration is reducing survival rates—these cases may be matched to the one level thicker non-ulcerated melanomas —5-year survival for T2b ulcerated vs. T3a non-ulcerated melanomas was 82% vs. 79%, T3b ulcerated vs. T4a non-ulcerated melanomas was 68% vs. 71%, respectively [56].

Mitotic Rate

In the previous AJCC staging system, the mitotic count was crucial in the pathological separation pT1a from pT1b melanoma [56]. The multivariate analysis presented the mitotic count as the strong prognostic factor, especially for thin melanomas. Currently, the number of mitoses per 1 mm^2 in the invasive dermal component, including "hot spots," should be reported [59]. Measurement of mitoses per mm^2 instead of per high-power field (HPF) is recommended because the HPF diameters vary between microscopes. Moreover, the reproducibility is high only when the scaling per 1 mm^2 and hot-spot method are used [69].

Tumor-Infiltrating Lymphocytes

The cross-talk between melanoma and microenvironment cells is still not fully understood. A significantly better prognosis among patients with a marked lymphocytic infiltrate within primary cutaneous melanoma than among those with absent TILs was found [70]. The TILs were classified according to their distribution and intensity as brisk (the lymphocytes present throughout the substance of the vertical growth phase or present and infiltrating across the entire base of the vertical growth phase), non-brisk (the lymphocytes in one focus or more foci of the vertical growth phase, either dispersed throughout or situated focally in the periphery), and absent (no lymphocytes or if the lymphocytes present but did not infiltrate the melanoma) [71]. The conflicting results of several studies under the role of TILs as prognostic factors were presented as well as modifications of TILs classification [72–74]. Regardless, the authors of the current AJCC system support the "classical" methods of TILs evaluation [59].

Clark's Level

Clark's level is based on the histopathological evaluation of the melanoma invasion related to the anatomical level of the skin [75]. Melanoma limited to the epidermis (in situ) is described as level I and characterizes excellent prognosis with low risk of distant metastases. Level II (superficial extension to the papillary dermis), III (infiltration of the papillary dermis up to the reticular dermis), IV (invasion of the reticular dermis), and V (invasion of subcutaneous fat) should be additionally reported, but they cannot replace Breslow thickness anymore [56].

Tumor Growth Phase

The radial (the proliferation of melanocytes in the epidermis and/or in the papillary dermis, without the formation of tumor nodule) and vertical phases (presence of an expansive nodule larger than the intraepidermal aggregates and/or by the presence of mitotic figures in the invasive melanoma component) are described. The evolution from radial to vertical growth is correlated with increased metastatic potential.

Tumor Regression

Regression is defined as a replacement of the melanoma by fibrosis. The increased vascularity, presence of scattered melanophages, and lymphocytes are also seen. The residual epidermal component can be identified. Regression is classified as partial (early to the intermediate stage; <75% of the melanoma) or extensive (late-stage; ≥75% of the melanoma) [76]. In the majority of studies, regression is indicated as an inferior prognostic factor. Lack of standardized diagnostic criteria and reduced interobserver reproducibility place regression among features that are assessed electively [77].

Lymphovascular Invasion

Melanoma cells within the blood vessels or lymphatics lumina are called lymphovascular invasion. Surprisingly, it is found in less than 10% of primary cutaneous melanoma [78]. The detectability rises when the immunohistochemical staining is applied. However, in routine diagnostics, it is not recommended. The presence of lymphovascular invasion is related to a worse prognosis [79, 80].

Microsatellites

Microsatellites are described as microscopic and discontinuous cutaneous and/or subcutaneous metastases >0.05 mm in diameter found adjacent to a primary melanoma (but separated from the main invasive component by a distance of at least 0.3 mm). Microsatellites are cutaneous or subcutaneous deposits of melanoma trapped within the lymphatics between the primary tumor and the regional lymph node basin. Microsatellitosis defines a subgroup of patients with a higher risk for regional and systemic recurrence [59, 64].

Melanoma Histotype

The melanoma histotypes (according to the fourth ed. of the WHO classification) have minor independent prognostic significance [1]. The interpretation is not objective, and the interobserver variability rate is high. Currently, the correlation of melanoma histotype with molecular signatures is emphasized [24, 81, 82].

The synoptic report for primary cutaneous melanoma, including the histopathological prognostic factors, is shown in Table 1.2 [3].

Keratinocytic/Epidermal Tumors

Keratinocytic neoplasms are the most frequent cancers from all other human malignancies. The spectrum of epidermal tumors includes benign lesions (i.e., verrucae, acanthomas, and seborrhoeic keratoses), premalignant lesions (i.e., actinic, arsenical and PUVA keratoses), and malignant lesions (squamous cell carcinoma and basal cell carcinoma). Merkel cell carcinoma, which originates from neuroendocrine skin cells, is incorporated into epidermal tumors according to the fourth edition of the World Health Organization (WHO) classification. Another significant change concerns keratoacanthoma, which should now be categorized as a variant of squamous cell carcinoma. High-risk variants of basal cell carcinoma were revised, and the pathological criteria were specified [1].

Table 1.2 Histopathological synoptic report for primary cutaneous melanoma [3]

Pathologic feature	
Site/localization	Right, left/anatomic site
Diagnosis	According to fourth ed. of the WHO classification
Breslow thickness	Value in mm
Clark level	I–V
Ulceration	Present/Absent
Dermal mitotic rate	Value per mm^2
Melanoma subtype	According to 4th ed. of the WHO classification
Vascular or lymphatic invasion	Present/Absent
Neurotropism	Present/Absent
TILs	Present [brisk/non-brisk]/ Absent
Microsatellites	Present/Absent
Regression	Present/Absent
Predominant cell type	Epithelioid/
Associated nevus	Description
Solar elastosis	Present/Absent
Margins of excision for invasive and in situ components (in mm)	Description
Comments	Description

Basal Cell Carcinoma

Basal cell carcinoma (BCC) is the most common skin cancer, accounting for about 75% of all skin cancers. It is characterized by slow growth and local malignancy, and distant metastases are extremely rare. BCC occurs in sun-exposed skin, primarily in the face (skin above the line connecting the corners of the mouth with external auditory ducts), especially nose, forehead, cheeks, eyelids, corner of the eye, and auricle. The superficial variant of BCC is located more frequently on the trunk [83–86]. The risk factors of BCC are similar to those of the squamous cell carcinoma. Gorlin syndrome or nevoid basal cell carcinoma syndrome is defined by numerous basal cell carcinomas occurring in young adults (below 30 years old), cysts within the jaw, and skeletal abnormalities. The disease is inherited autosomally dominant and is characterized by the loss of function PTCH1 suppressor gene mutation (9q22.1-q31) [87–89].

Macroscopically, basal cell carcinoma presents with one of the three most common appearances: nodular, ulcerative, or superficial.

The most common histological types of basal cell carcinoma, along with their characteristics, are presented in Table 1.3.

Microscopically, cell aggregates are derived from the basal layer of the epidermis. Cancer cells have scant cytoplasm and hyperchromatic nuclei. Fibromyxoid

Table 1.3 Morphological variants of basal cell carcinoma, including recurrence risk stratification grouping [1, 90]

BCC variant	Macroscopic presentation and the most important characteristics
Nodular	The most common variant (45–60%) Usually located on head and neck A slowly growing pearly flesh-colored flesh Well demarcated from the skin With numerous telangiectasias In the late phase, ulcers often have well-delimited, cylindrical margins ("nonhealing ulcer") It can grow as a primary ulcerative (previously called "rodent ulcer"): particularly dangerous in the medial corner of the eye, characterized by significant tissue destruction and high bone infiltration potential
Superficial	10–30% of all BCC The least aggressive, often numerous It is more common on the trunk and arms Slow course for months or years Flatly elevated lesions surrounded by an embankment, well-demarcated, pink to erythematous and scaly patches, non-ulcerative
Micronodular	The flat or slightly elevated lesion, not clearly defined Cancer cells appear as small, discrete nests or cysts that can deeply infiltrate and exhibit neuroinvasive features More aggressive course
Infiltrating	It resembles a scar Frequent recurrences after surgical treatment Usually infiltrates perineural spaces In later stages, stromal fibrosis occurs, and the image may overlap with the sclerosing/morpheic variant
Sclerosing/ morpheic	A flat, not clearly defined change resembles a scar Stroma highly collagenized Often, nerve invasion Frequent recurrences after surgical treatment
Pigmented	Contains melanin deposits Dermoscopic specific features: large blue-gray ovoid nests, blue-gray globules, leaf-like areas Nodular or superficial morphological variant It may resemble melanoma
Other morphological variants	
Basosquamous carcinoma Basal cell carcinoma with sarcomatoid differentiation Basal cell carcinoma with adnexal differentiation Fibroepithelial BCC (Pinkus tumor)	
BCC grouping according to recurrence risk stratification	
Higher risk	Location: nose, nasolabial fold, inner corner of the eye, lip, ear ≥20 mm Variants: Basosquamous carcinoma, Sclerosing/morpheic BCC, Infiltrating BCC, BCC with sarcomatoid differentiation, Micronodular BCC
Lower risk	Location: other than those listed for the higher risk type <20 mm Variants: Nodular BCC, Superficial BCC, Pigmented BCC, Infundibulocystic BCC, Fibroepithelial BCC

stromal change impacts on tumor retraction from the stroma. The different patterns, including solid, trabecular, cystic, adenoid, cribriform, are described. Additionally, within the BCC infiltrate, focal keratinization, desmoplasia, and scarring may be seen (Fig. 1.3b–d). A common feature is the peripheral palisading of neoplastic cells arranged as nests. On the contrary to squamous cell carcinoma, no intercellular bridges are visible; however, high mitotic activity and apoptosis can be found. BCC containing large amounts of melanin must be differentiated with melanoma. In the differential diagnosis, immunohistochemistry is used rarely. Combination of

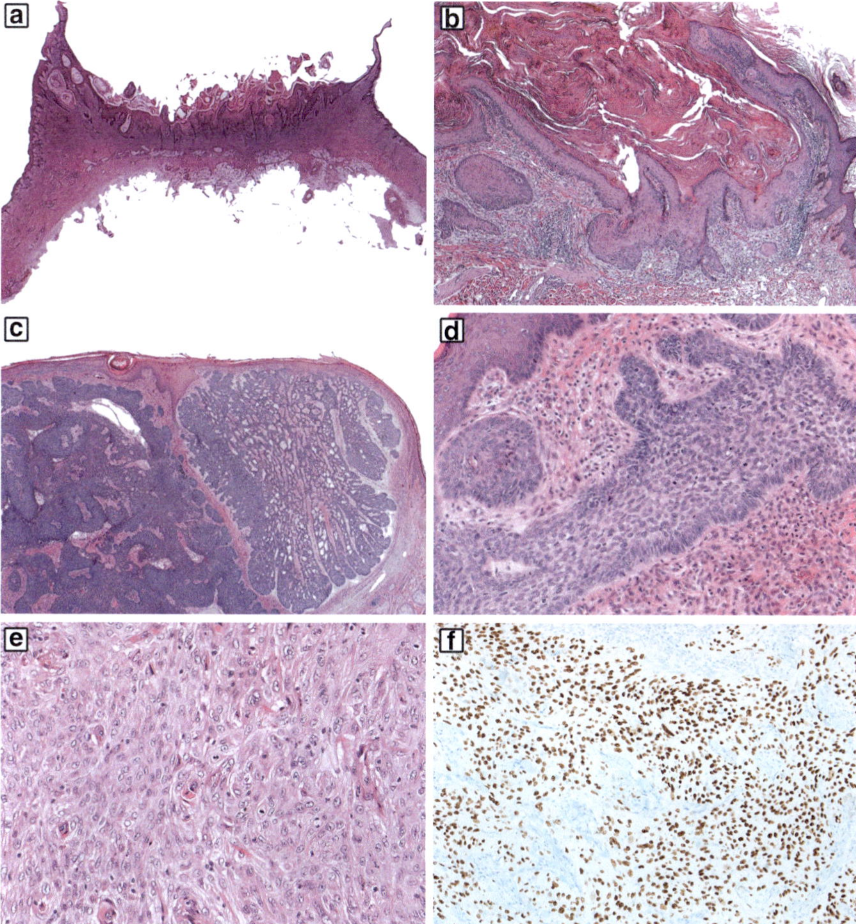

Fig. 1.3 Keratoacanthoma. (**a**) Mature stage of keratoacanthoma, characteristic crateriform architecture with central keratin masses (HE, 10×), peripheral epidermal lipping is seen; (**b**) keratin debris and proliferative squamous cells (HE, 40×). Basal cell carcinoma. (**c**) The nodular type of basal cell carcinoma (HE, 20×); (**d**) Characteristic peripheral palisading (HE, 200×); Squamous cell carcinoma. (**e**) Moderately differentiated squamous cell carcinoma with prominent cytological atypia, mitotic figures, and intercellular bridges (HE, 200×); (**f**) Squamous cell carcinoma is typically positive for p40 (200×)

BerEP4 and EMA is useful in distinguishing BCC from squamous cell carcinoma [BCC: BerEP4(+)/EMA(−); SCC: BerEP4(−)/EMA(+)] [1].

The TNM classification is not routinely used to determine the prognosis of BCC. The histopathological variant and the largest dimension of cancer infiltration, together with the depth of infiltration, and location are of significant importance for patient follow-up and risk stratification of local recurrence (see Table 1.3) [90]. The histopathological report requires the status of surgical margins [91].

Squamous Cell Carcinoma

Squamous cell carcinoma (SCC) is the second most common type of skin cancer. It usually occurs in elderly individuals on the skin exposed to sunlight (head and neck, auricles, dorsal parts of hands). Risk factors that are associated with SCC also include immunosuppressive treatment, human papillomavirus infection, burn scars, chronic inflammation, arsenic, and coal tar [92–95].

Macroscopically, SCC in situ may present as roughened hyperkeratotic lesions similar to benign keratoses, dermatoses, or lichen simplex chronicus. An invasive SCC can be described as exo- or endophytic lesion. The first occurs mainly on the face, auricles, and lips, and the second one develops on both sun-exposed skin and skin covered from UV radiation. The keratoacanthoma, which is a well-differentiated variant of SCC, shows a crateriform lesion with central keratin plugs (see also below).

Microscopically, the following variants of SCC are distinguished: acantholytic, spindle cell, verrucous, adenosquamous carcinoma, clear cell, and other (uncommon) rare variants, that is, SCS with sarcomatoid differentiation, lymphoepithelioma-like carcinoma, pseudovascular SCC, SCC with osteoclast-like giant cells. Regardless of the histological variant, the assessment of the histological grade is based on the establishment of the shape of cells with cellular atypia, mitotic activity, presence of necrosis, intercellular bridges, and keratin pearls (Fig. 1.3e, f). The well- (G1), medium- (G2), and low-differentiated (G3) SCC are distinguished. The histological grading system refers to the least differentiated part of SCC; even it is only a small part of the entire tumor. Well-differentiated SCC is characterized by the presence of large, polygonal cells with abundant acidophilic cytoplasm, with clearly visible intercellular bridges and the presence of keratin pearls, while the mitotic index is low. In low-differentiated SCC, the cells are often spindle-like or round with a medium abundant or scant cytoplasm; high atypia and brisk mitotic activity are found. Keratinization may be visible only in single cells. These lesions often present no apparent features of squamous cell differentiation and require immuno-histochemical confirmation of the diagnosis. Positive reactions with p40, p63, and CK5/6 antibodies are typical for SCC. The SCC, G2, is characterized by an intermediate differentiation between G1 and G3 [1, 96, 97].

The histopathological report of SCC should include macroscopic description: location of the lesion; type of diagnostic material (biopsy, surgical excision); dimensions of the material, and examined lesion; type of tumor growth; and margins of resection. A microscopic evaluation obligatorily present diagnosis with a morphological variant of SCC; histological grading; the largest dimension of carcinoma and the depth of the infiltrate (measured from the granular layer of the epidermis; does not apply to the "in situ" lesions); clinical staging (pTNM) [98, 99]; assessment of vessels and nerves infiltration; margins assessment [100]. Besides, in advanced SCC, bone and bone marrow infiltration may need to be described. In the case of SCC metastases to the lymph node/nodes, reporting of the number of lymph nodes, the largest dimension of the metastasis and extranodal metastasis extension is required [101, 102]. It is worth noting that the TNM classification of SCC is distinct for the following locations: conjunctiva, head and neck, perianal region, vagina, and penis [103].

Keratoacanthoma

Keratoacanthoma (KA) is a frequent change characterized by rapid growth and spontaneous regression. Histologically, it has a morphology that corresponds to well-differentiated SCC with a benign clinical course. Most often, these changes occur on sun-exposed skin on the face, dorsal part of hands, forearms, and legs among people over 50 years of age [104]. Multiple lesions are found in rare disease syndromes, that is, multiple familial keratoacanthomas or the Ferguson–Smith type or Muir–Torre syndrome. Exposure to UV radiation, effect of HPV, point mutations in the *TP53* gene, and *MAP 3K8* (*TPL2*) oncogene changes play a crucial role in pathogenesis [105, 106].

Macroscopically, it is a well-limited dome-shaped lesion with raised edges and a central "crater"—an ulcerative depression. Lesions are usually single, and their size does not exceed 3 cm.

Microscopically, the keratoacanthoma is symmetrical: in the central part (crater), keratin masses predominate, the lateral parts are composed of squamous epithelium forming nests and elongated bands (Fig. 1.3a). A characteristic feature is epidermal lipping on both sides of the keratin core. At the base of the lesion, usually dense, mixed inflammatory infiltrates and fibrosis are visible. Due to the macroscopic presentation in the fourth edition of the WHO classification, the following KA subtypes were distinguished: solitary KA, multiple KA, multiple familial KA of Ferguson–Smith type, centrifugum marginatum KA, generalized eruptive KA of Grzybowski, subungual KA. KAs undergo spontaneous regression and rarely recur, especially central facial giant KA and subungual KA [1, 107]. The clinical picture of KA may overlap with other SCC variants as well. The recent recommendations indicate that KA should be qualified for total surgical excision.

Merkel Cell Carcinoma

Merkel cell carcinoma (MCC) is a rare primary skin neuroendocrine tumor that occurs mainly in elderly patients (over the age of 70), usually in the scalp and neck (especially the eyelids and orbital area) and limbs [108]. It is characterized by an aggressive course with the presence of lymph node metastases in about 50% of cases at the time of diagnosis; local and distant metastases are found in 35–40% of patients [109–111].

Macroscopically, MCC presents itself as a hard, painless tumor with a smooth surface, usually covered with intact epidermis.

Microscopically, MCC is composed of small, oval cells with characteristic cell nuclei with granular chromatin described as "salt with pepper" (Fig. 1.4a, b). Cancer cells form solid infiltrates or alveolar, trabecular, or rosette-like structures. Merkel

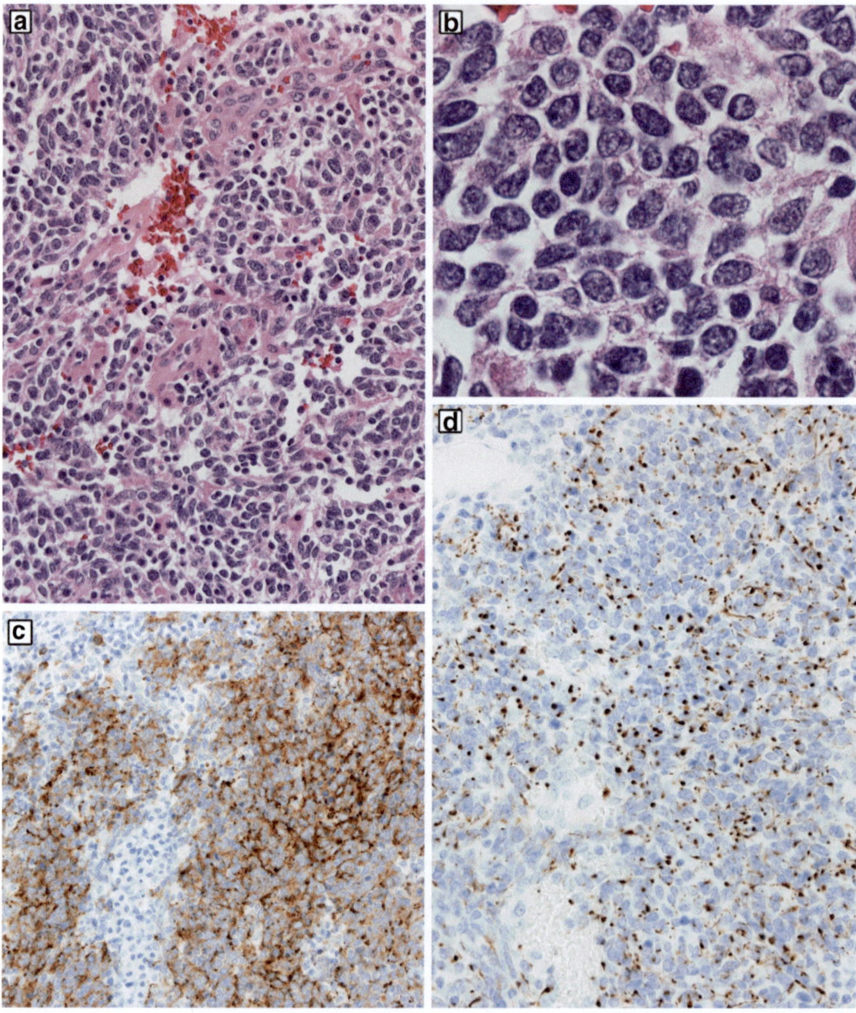

Fig. 1.4 Merkel cell carcinoma. (**a, b**) The intermediate cell type with nuclear salt-and-pepper chromatin pattern (200×, 600×); (**c**) Neuroendocrine markers include positive reaction with chromogranin (200×); (**d**) CK20 immunoreaction presents characteristic) perinuclear dot-like pattern (200×)

cell carcinoma resembles low-differentiated round cell neoplasm, which must be differentiated with small cell lung cancer (SCLC), melanoma, lymphoma, and Ewing's sarcoma [112–114]. The final diagnosis requires confirmation in immuno-histochemistry. The characteristic immunoprofile includes positive reactions with neuroendocrine markers, that is, synaptophysin, chromogranin A and CD56 and dot-like, perinuclear reaction with CK20 (Fig. 1.4c, d). Lack of S100, HMB-45, SOX-10, LCA/CD45, TTF-1 expression supports the exclusion of melanoma, lymphoma, and SCLC [115].

MCC high-risk factors in the adverse clinical course include lymph node metastases at the time of diagnosis, tumor size >2 cm, primary lesion location on the limbs, and male gender [110, 111, 114, 116]. The histopathological report additionally should include information about lymph node and in-transit metastases. The pTNM for MCC has been separated in the WHO classification [117, 118].

References

1. Elder DE, Massi D, Scolyer RA, Willemze R, editors. WHO classification of skin tumours. 4th ed. Lyon: International Agency for Research on Cancer (IARC); 2018.
2. World Health Organization. Skin cancers. 2013. http://www.who.int/uv/faq/skincancer/en/index1.html. Accessed 28 June 2013.
3. Scolyer RA, Rawson RV, Gershenwald JE, Ferguson PM, Prieto VG. Melanoma pathology reporting and staging. Mod Pathol. 2020;33(1):15–24.
4. Davies H, Bignell GR, Cox C, Stephens P, Edkins S, Clegg S, et al. Mutations of the BRAF gene in human cancer. Nature. 2002;417:949–54.
5. Edlundh-Rose E, Egyházi S, Omholt K, Månsson-Brahme E, Platz A, Hansson J, et al. BRAF mutations in melanoma tumours in relation to clinical characteristics: a study based on mutation screening by pyrosequencing. Melanoma Res. 2006;16(6):471–8.
6. Ellerhorst JA, Greene VR, Ekmekcioglu S, Warneke CL, Johnson MM, Cooke CP, et al. Clinical correlates of NRAS and BRAF mutations in primary human melanoma. Clin Cancer Res. 2011;17:229–35.
7. Long GV, Menzies AM, Nagrial AM, Haydu LE, Hamilton AL, Mann GJ, et al. Prognostic and clinicopathologic associations of oncogenic BRAF in metastatic melanoma. J Clin Oncol. 2011;29:1239–46.
8. Mann GJ, Pupo GM, Campain AE, Carter CD, Schramm SJ, Pianova S, et al. BRAF mutation, NRAS mutation, and the absence of an immune-related expressed gene profile predict poor outcome in patients with stage III melanoma. J Invest Dermatol. 2013;133:509–17.
9. Elder DE, Bastian BC, Cree IA, Massi D, Scolyer RA. The 2018 World Health Organization Classification of cutaneous, mucosal, and uveal melanoma: detailed analysis of 9 distinct subtypes defined by their evolutionary pathway. Arch Pathol Lab Med. 2020;144(4):500–22.
10. Roncati L, Piscioli F, Pusiol T. SAMPUS, MELTUMP and THIMUMP - diagnostic categories characterized by uncertain biological behavior. Klin Onkol. 2017;30(3):221–3.
11. Pusiol T, Morichetti D, Piscioli F, Zorzi MG. Theory and practical application of superficial atypical melanocytic proliferations of uncertain significance (SAMPUS) and melanocytic tumours of uncertain malignant potential (MELTUMP) terminology: experience with second opinion consultation. Pathologica. 2012;104(2):70–7.
12. Pusiol T, Piscioli F, Speziali L, Zorzi MG, Morichetti D, Roncati L. Clinical features, dermoscopic patterns, and histological diagnostic model for melanocytic tumors of uncertain malignant potential (MELTUMP). Acta Dermatovenerol Croat. 2015;23(3):185–94.

13. Zembowicz A, Scolyer RA. Nevus/Melanocytoma/Melanoma: an emerging paradigm for classification of melanocytic neoplasms? Arch Pathol Lab Med. 2011;135(3):300–6.
14. Yeh I. New and evolving concepts of melanocytic nevi and melanocytomas. Mod Pathol. 2020;33(Suppl 1):1–14.
15. Urso C. Melanocytic skin neoplasms: what lesson from genomic aberrations? Am J Dermatopathol. 2019;41(9):623–9.
16. Maldonado JL, Fridlyand J, Patel H, Jain AN, Busam K, Kageshita T, et al. Determinants of BRAF mutations in primary melanomas. J Natl Cancer Inst. 2003;95(24):1878–90.
17. Rigel DS, Friedman RJ, Kopf AW, Polsky D. ABCDE--an evolving concept in the early detection of melanoma. Arch Dermatol. 2005;141(8):1032–4.
18. Lee EY, Williamson R, Watt P, Hughes MC, Green AC, Whiteman DC. Sun exposure and host phenotype as predictors of cutaneous melanoma associated with neval remnants or dermal elastosis. Int J Cancer. 2006;119(3):636–42.
19. Viros A, Fridlyand J, Bauer J, Lasithiotakis K, Garbe C, Pinkel D, et al. Improving melanoma classification by integrating genetic and morphologic features. PLoS Med. 2008;5(6):e120.
20. Farrahi F, Egbert BM, Swetter SM. Histologic similarities between lentigo maligna and dysplastic nevus: importance of clinicopathologic distinction. J Cutan Pathol. 2005;32(6):405–12.
21. King R, Page RN, Googe PB, Mihm MC Jr. Lentiginous melanoma: a histologic pattern of melanoma to be distinguished from lentiginous nevus. Mod Pathol. 2005;18(10):1397–401.
22. Lens MB, Newton-Bishop JA, Boon AP. Desmoplastic malignant melanoma: a systematic review. Br J Dermatol. 2005;152(4):673–8.
23. Chen JY, Hruby G, Scolyer RA, Murali R, Hong A, Fitzgerald P. Desmoplastic neurotropic melanoma: a clinicopathologic analysis of 128 cases. Cancer. 2008;113:2770–8.
24. Busam KJ, Mujumdar U, Hummer AJ, Nobrega J, Hawkins WG, Coit DG. Cutaneous desmoplastic melanoma: reappraisal of morphologic heterogeneity and prognostic factors. Am J Surg Pathol. 2004;28:1518–25.
25. Plaza JA, Bonneau P, Prieto V, Sangueza M, Mackinnon A, Suster D, et al. Desmoplastic melanoma: an updated immunohistochemical analysis of 40 cases with a proposal for an additional panel of stains for diagnosis. J Cutan Pathol. 2016;43(4):313–23.
26. Kooper-Johnson S, Mahalingam M, Loo DS. SOX-10 and S100 negative desmoplastic melanoma: apropos a diagnostically challenging case. Am J Dermatopathol. 2020;42(9):697–9.
27. Newman S, Fan L, Pribnow A, Silkov A, Rice SV, Lee S, et al. Clinical genome sequencing uncovers potentially targetable truncations and fusions of MAP3K8 in spitzoid and other melanomas. Nat Med. 2019;25(4):597–602.
28. Cerrato F, Wallins JS, Webb ML, McCarty ER, Schmidt BA, Labow BI. Outcomes in pediatric atypical spitz tumors treated without sentinel lymph node biopsy. Pediatr Dermatol. 2012;29(4):448–53.
29. Requena C, Botella R, Nagore E, Sanmartín O, Llombart B, Serra-Guillén C, et al. Characteristics of spitzoid melanoma and clues for differential diagnosis with spitz nevus. Am J Dermatopathol. 2012;34(5):478–86.
30. Garrido-Ruiz MC, Requena L, Ortiz P, Pérez-Gómez B, Alonso SR, Peralto JL. The immunohistochemical profile of Spitz nevi and conventional (non-Spitzoid) melanomas: a baseline study. Mod Pathol. 2010;23(9):1215–24.
31. Crotty KA, Scolyer RA, Li L, Palmer AA, Wang L, McCarthy SW. Spitz naevus versus Spitzoid melanoma: when and how can they be distinguished? Pathology. 2002;34(1):6–12.
32. Indsto JO, Kumar S, Wang L, Crotty KA, Arbuckle SM, Mann GJ. Low prevalence of RAS-RAF-activating mutations in Spitz melanocytic nevi compared with other melanocytic lesions. J Cutan Pathol. 2007;34(6):448–55.
33. Durbec F, Martin L, Derancourt C, Grange F. Melanoma of the hand and foot: epidemiological, prognostic and genetic features. A systematic review. Br J Dermatol. 2012;166(4):727–39.
34. Basurto-Lozada P, Molina-Aguilar C, Castaneda-Garcia C, Vázquez-Cruz ME, Garcia-Salinas OI, Álvarez-Cano A, et al. Acral lentiginous melanoma: basic facts, biological characteristics and research perspectives of an understudied disease. Pigment Cell Melanoma Res. 2020; https://doi.org/10.1111/pcmr.12885.

35. Nakamura Y, Fujisawa Y. Diagnosis and management of acral lentiginous melanoma. Curr Treat Options in Oncol. 2018;19(8):42.
36. Darmawan CC, Jo G, Montenegro SE, Kwak Y, Cheol L, Cho KH, et al. Early detection of acral melanoma: A review of clinical, dermoscopic, histopathologic, and molecular characteristics. J Am Acad Dermatol. 2019;81(3):805–12.
37. Chen F, Zhang Q, Wang Y, Wang S, Feng S, Qi L, et al. KIT, NRAS, BRAF and FMNL2 mutations in oral mucosal melanoma and a systematic review of the literature. Oncol Lett. 2018;15(6):9786–92.
38. Lazarev S, Gupta V, Hu K, Harrison LB, Bakst R. Mucosal melanoma of the head and neck: a systematic review of the literature. Int J Radiat Oncol Biol Phys. 2014;90(5):1108–18.
39. Jarrom D, Paleri V, Kerawala C, Roques T, Bhide S, Newman L, et al. Mucosal melanoma of the upper airways tract mucosal melanoma: a systematic review with meta-analyses of treatment. Head Neck. 2017;39(4):819–25.
40. Kottschade LA, Grotz TE, Dronca RS, Salomao DR, Pulido JS, Wasif N, et al. Rare presentations of primary melanoma and special populations: a systematic review. Am J Clin Oncol. 2014;37(6):635–41.
41. Lim Y, Shin HT, Choi Y, Lee DY. Evolutionary processes of melanomas from giant congenital melanocytic nevi. Pigment Cell Melanoma Res. 2020;33(2):318–25.
42. Chopra A, Sharma R, Rao UNM. Pathology of melanoma. Surg Clin North Am. 2020;100(1):43–59.
43. Kiuru M, Tartar DM, Qi L, Chen D, Yu L, Konia T, et al. Improving classification of melanocytic nevi: association of BRAF V600E expression with distinct histomorphologic features. J Am Acad Dermatol. 2018;79(2):221–9.
44. Alendar T, Kittler H. Morphologic characteristics of nevi associated with melanoma: a clinical, dermatoscopic and histopathologic analysis. Dermatol Pract Concept. 2018;8(2):104–8.
45. Vergier B, Laharanne E, Prochazkova-Carlotti M, de la Fouchardière A, Merlio JP, Kadlub N, et al. Proliferative nodules vs melanoma arising in giant congenital melanocytic nevi during childhood. JAMA Dermatol. 2016;152(10):1147–51.
46. Toomey CB, Fraser K, Thorson JA, Goldbaum MH, Lin JH. GNAQ and PMS1 mutations associated with uveal melanoma, ocular surface melanosis, and nevus of ota. Ocular Oncol Pathol. 2019;5(4):267–72.
47. Oaxaca G, Billings SD, Ko JS. p16 Range of expression in dermal predominant benign epithelioid and spindled nevi and melanoma. J Cutan Pathol. 2020;47(9):815–23.
48. Borgenvik TL, Karlsvik TM, Ray S, Fawzy M, James N. Blue nevus-like and blue nevus-associated melanoma: a comprehensive review of the literature. ANZ J Surg. 2017;87(5):345–9.
49. Murali R, McCarthy SW, Scolyer RA. Blue nevi and related lesions: a review highlighting atypical and newly described variants, distinguishing features and diagnostic pitfalls. Adv Anat Pathol. 2009;16(6):365–82.
50. Loghavi S, Curry JL, Torres-Cabala CA, Ivan D, Patel KP, Mehrotra M, et al. Melanoma arising in association with blue nevus: a clinical and pathologic study of 24 cases and comprehensive review of the literature. Mod Pathol. 2014;27(11):1468–78.
51. Zhao M, Mu Y, Dang Y, Zhu Y. Secondary glaucoma as initial manifestation of ring melanoma: a case report and review of literature. Int J Clin Exp Pathol. 2014;7(11):8163–9.
52. Nayman T, Bostan C, Logan P, Burnier MN Jr. Uveal melanoma risk factors: a systematic review of meta-analyses. Curr Eye Res. 2017;42(8):1085–93.
53. Zhang HG, Moser JC, Dalvin LA. Characterization of uveal melanoma clinical trial design: a systematic review to establish an elusive standard of care. Acta Oncol (Stockholm, Sweden). 2020;59(11):1401–8.
54. Corneli P, Zalaudek I, Magaton Rizzi G, di Meo N. Improving the early diagnosis of early nodular melanoma: can we do better? Expert Rev Anticancer Ther. 2018;18(10):1007–12.
55. Greenwald HS, Friedman EB, Osman I. Superficial spreading and nodular melanoma are distinct biological entities: a challenge to the linear progression model. Melanoma Res. 2012;22(1):1–8.

56. Balch CM, Gershenwald JE, Soong SJ, Thompson JF, Atkins MB, Byrd DR, et al. Final version of 2009 AJCC melanoma staging and classification. J Clin Oncol. 2009;27(36):6199–206.
57. Gershenwald JE, Scolyer RA, Hess KR, Sondak VK, Long GV, Ross MI, et al. In: Amin MB, Edge SB, Greene FL, Carducci MA, Compton CA, editors. AJCC cancer staging manual. 8th ed. Springer International Publishing: New York; 2017. p. 563–85.
58. Gimotty PA, Guerry D, Ming ME, Elenitsas R, Xu X, Czerniecki B, et al. Thin primary cutaneous malignant melanoma: a prognostic tree for 10-year metastasis is more accurate than American Joint Committee on Cancer staging. J Clin Oncol. 2004;22(18):3668–76.
59. Gershenwald JE, Scolyer RA, Hess KR, Sondak VK, Long GV, Ross MI. Melanoma staging: evidence-based changes in the American Joint Committee on Cancer eighth edition cancer staging manual. CA Cancer J Clin. 2017;67:472–92.
60. Eggermont AMM, Blank CU, Mandala M, Long GV, Atkinson V, Dalle S. Adjuvant pembrolizumab versus placebo in resected stage III melanoma. N Engl J Med. 2018;378:1789–801.
61. Weber J, Mandala M, Vecchio M, Gogas HJ, Arance AM, Cowey CL. Adjuvant nivolumab versus ipilimumab in resected stage III or IV melanoma. N Engl J Med. 2017;377:1824–35.
62. Long GV, Hauschild A, Santinami M, Atkinson V, Mandala M, Chiarion-Sileni V. Adjuvant dabrafenib plus trametinib in stage III BRAF-mutated melanoma. N Engl J Med. 2017;377:1813–23.
63. Balch CM, Gershenwald JE, Soong SJ, Thompson JF, Ding S, Byrd DR, et al. Multivariate analysis of prognostic factors among 2,313 patients with stage III melanoma: comparison of nodal micrometastases versus macrometastases. J Clin Oncol. 2010;28:2452–9.
64. Gershenwald JE, Scolyer RA. Melanoma staging: American Joint Committee on Cancer (AJCC) 8th Edition and beyond. Ann Surg Oncol. 2018;25:2105–10.
65. Breslow A. Thickness, cross-sectional areas and depth of invasion in the prognosis of cutaneous melanoma. Ann Surg. 1970;172:902–8.
66. Dodds TJ, Lo S, Jackett L, Nieweg O, Thompson JF, Scolyer RA. Prognostic significance of periadnexal extension in cutaneous melanoma and its implications for pathologic reporting and staging. Am J Surg Pathol. 2018;42:359–66.
67. Barnhill RL, Fine JA, Roush GC, Berwick M. Predicting five-year outcome for patients with cutaneous melanoma in a population-based study. Cancer. 1996;78:427–32.
68. In 't Hout FE, Haydu LE, Murali R, Bonenkamp JJ, Thompson JF, Scolyer RA. Prognostic importance of the extent of ulceration in patients with clinically localized cutaneous melanoma. Ann Surg. 2012;255:1165–70.
69. Scolyer RA, Shaw HM, Thompson JF, Li LX, Colman MH, Lo SK. Interobserver reproducibility of histopathologic prognostic variables in primary cutaneous melanomas. Am J Surg Pathol. 2003;27:1571–6.
70. Klein G, Klein E. Surveillance against tumors: Is it mainly immunological? Immunol Lett. 2005;100:29–33.
71. Clark WH, Elder DE, Guerry D, Braitman LE, Trock BJ, Schultz D, et al. Model predicting survival in stage I melanoma based on progression. J Natl Cancer Inst. 1989;81:1893–904.
72. Taylor RC, Patel A, Panageas KS, Busam KJ, Brady MS. Tumor-infiltrating lymphocytes predict sentinel lymph node positivity in patients with cutaneous melanoma. J Clin Oncol. 2007;25:869–75.
73. Mandalà M, Imberti GL, Piazzalunga D, Belfiglio M, Labianca R, Barberis M, et al. Clinical and histopathological risk factors to predict sentinel lymph node positivity, disease-free and overall survival in clinical stages I–II AJCC skin melanoma: outcome analysis from a single-institution prospectively collected database. Eur J Cancer. 2009;45:2537–45.
74. Azimi F, Scolyer RA, Rumcheva P, Moncrieff M, Murali R, McCarthy SW. Tumor-infiltrating lymphocyte grade is an independent predictor of sentinel lymph node status and survival in patients with cutaneous melanoma. J Clin Oncol. 2012;30:2678–83.
75. Clark WH, From L, Bernardino EA, Mihm MC. The histogenesis and biologic behavior of primary human malignant melanomas of the skin. Cancer Res. 1969;29:705–27.
76. Morris KT, Busam KJ, Bero S, Patel A, Brady MS. Primary cutaneous melanoma with regression does not require a lower threshold for sentinel lymph node biopsy. Ann Surg Oncol. 2008;15:316–22.

77. Gualano MR, Osella-Abate S, Scaioli G, Marra E, Bert F, Faure E, et al. Prognostic role of histological regression in primary cutaneous melanoma: a systematic review and meta-analysis. Br J Dermatol. 2018;178(2):357–62.
78. Storr SJ, Safuan S, Mitra A, Elliott F, Walker C, Vasko MJ, et al. Objective assessment of blood and lymphatic vessel invasion and association with macrophage infiltration in cutaneous melanoma. Mod Pathol. 2012;25:493–504.
79. Massi D, Puig S, Franchi A, Malvehy J, Vidal-Sicart S, González-Cao M, et al. Tumour lymphangiogenesis is a possible predictor of sentinel lymph node status in cutaneous melanoma: a case–control study. J Clin Pathol. 2006;59:166–73.
80. Xu X, Chen L, Guerry D, Dawson PR, Hwang WT, VanBelle P, et al. Lymphatic invasion is independently prognostic of metastasis in primary cutaneous melanoma. Clin Cancer Res. 2012;18:229–37.
81. Murali R, Shaw HM, Lai K, McCarthy SW, Quinn MJ, Stretch JR. Prognostic factors in cutaneous desmoplastic melanoma: a study of 252 patients. Cancer. 2010;116:4130–8.
82. Eroglu Z, Zaretsky JM, Hu-Lieskovan S, Kim DW, Algazi A, Johnson DB, et al. High response rate to PD-1 blockade in desmoplastic melanomas. Nature. 2018;553:347–50.
83. Cives M, Mannavola F, Lospalluti L, Sergi MC, Cazzato G, Filoni E, et al. Non-melanoma skin cancers: biological and clinical features. Int J Mol Sci. 2020;21(15):5394.
84. Dika E, Scarfi F, Ferracin M, Broseghini E, Marcelli E, Bortolani B, et al. Basal cell carcinoma: a comprehensive review. Int J Mol Sci. 2020;21(15):5572.
85. McDaniel B, Badri T. Basal cell carcinoma. StatPearls. Treasure Island FL: © 2020, StatPearls Publishing LLC; 2020.
86. Nikolouzakis TK, Falzone L, Lasithiotakis K, Krüger-Krasagakis S, Kalogeraki A, Sifaki M, et al. Current and future trends in molecular biomarkers for diagnostic, prognostic, and predictive purposes in non-melanoma skin cancer. J Clin Med. 2020;9(9):2868.
87. Campione E, Di Prete M, Lozzi F, Lanna C, Spallone G, Mazzeo M, et al. High-risk recurrence basal cell carcinoma: focus on hedgehog pathway inhibitors and review of the literature. Chemotherapy. 2020;65:2–10.
88. Spiker AM, Troxell T, Ramsey ML. Gorlin syndrome (Basal Cell Nevus). StatPearls. Treasure Island FL: © 2020, StatPearls Publishing LLC; 2020.
89. Evans DG, Farndon PA. Nevoid basal cell carcinoma syndrome. In: Adam MP, Ardinger HH, Pagon RA, Wallace SE, Bean LJH, Stephens K, et al., editors. GeneReviews(®). Seattle WA: © 1993-2020, University of Washington, Seattle. GeneReviews is a registered trademark of the University of Washington, Seattle; 1993.
90. Bichakjian CK, Olencki T, Aasi SZ, Alam M, Andersen JS, Berg D, et al. Basal cell skin cancer, version 1.2016, NCCN clinical practice guidelines in oncology. J Natl Compr Canc Netw. 2016;14(5):574–97.
91. Quazi SJ, Aslam N, Saleem H, Rahman J, Khan S. Surgical margin of excision in basal cell carcinoma: a systematic review of literature. Cureus. 2020;12(7):e9211.
92. Azimi A, Kaufman KL, Kim J, Ali M, Mann GJ, Fernandez-Penas P. Proteomics: an emerging approach for the diagnosis and classification of cutaneous squamous cell carcinoma and its precursors. J Dermatol Sci. 2020;99(1):9–16.
93. Campos MA, Lopes JM, Soares P. The genetics of cutaneous squamous cell carcinogenesis. Eur J Dermatol. 2018;28(5):597–605.
94. Collins L, Quinn A, Stasko T. Skin cancer and immunosuppression. Dermatol Clin. 2019;37(1):83–94.
95. Wang J, Aldabagh B, Yu J, Arron ST. Role of human papillomavirus in cutaneous squamous cell carcinoma: a meta-analysis. J Am Acad Dermatol. 2014;70(4):621–9.
96. Alferraly IT, Munir D, Putra IB, Sembiring RJ. Correlation of Ki-67 expression as tumor cell proliferation activity marker with cutaneous squamous cell carcinoma grading. Open Access Maced J Med Sci. 2019;7(20):3384–6.
97. Yantsos VA, Conrad N, Zabawski E, Cockerell CJ. Incipient intraepidermal cutaneous squamous cell carcinoma: a proposal for reclassifying and grading solar (actinic) keratoses. Semin Cutan Med Surg. 1999;18(1):3–14.

98. Keohane SG, Proby CM, Newlands C, Motley RJ, Nasr I, Mohd Mustapa MF, et al. New 8th edition of TNM staging and implications for skin cancer. Br J Dermatol. 2018;179(4):824–8.
99. Brierley JD, Gospodarowicz MK, Wittekind CH. TNM classification of malignant tumours, Eighth Edition. Oxford: WILEY Blackwell; 2017. Union for International Cancer Control.
100. Heppt MV, Steeb T, Berking C, Nast A. Comparison of guidelines for the management of patients with high-risk and advanced cutaneous squamous cell carcinoma - a systematic review. J Eur Acad Dermatol Venereol. 2019;33(Suppl 8):25–32.
101. Claveau J, Archambault J, Ernst DS, Giacomantonio C, Limacher JJ, Murray C, et al. Multidisciplinary management of locally advanced and metastatic cutaneous squamous cell carcinoma. Curr Oncol (Toronto, Ont). 2020;27(4):e399–407.
102. Thompson AK, Kelley BF, Prokop LJ, Murad MH, Baum CL. Risk factors for cutaneous squamous cell carcinoma recurrence, metastasis, and disease-specific death: a systematic review and meta-analysis. JAMA Dermatol. 2016;152(4):419–28.
103. Nägeli MC, Ramelyte E, Dummer R. Cutaneous squamous cell carcinomas on special locations: perioral, periocular and genital area. J Eur Acad Dermatol Venereol. 2019;33(Suppl 8):21–4.
104. Savage JA, Maize JC Sr. Keratoacanthoma clinical behavior: a systematic review. Am J Dermatopathol. 2014;36(5):422–9.
105. Le S, Ansari U, Mumtaz A, Malik K, Patel P, Doyle A, et al. Lynch Syndrome and Muir-Torre Syndrome: an update and review on the genetics, epidemiology, and management of two related disorders. Dermatol Online J. 2017;23(11)
106. Lai V, Cranwell W, Sinclair R. Epidemiology of skin cancer in the mature patient. Clin Dermatol. 2018;36(2):167–76.
107. Paolino G, Donati M, Didona D, Mercuri SR, Cantisani C. Histology of non-melanoma skin cancers: an update. Biomedicines. 2017;5(4):71.
108. Calder KB, Smoller BR. New insights into merkel cell carcinoma. Adv Anat Pathol. 2010;17(3):155–61.
109. Cornejo C, Miller CJ. Merkel cell carcinoma: updates on staging and management. Dermatol Clin. 2019;37(3):269–77.
110. Keohane SG, Proby CM, Newlands C, Motley RJ, Nasr I, Mohd Mustapa MF, et al. The new 8th edition of TNM staging and its implications for skin cancer: a review by the British Association of Dermatologists and the Royal College of Pathologists, U.K. Br J Dermatol. 2018;179(4):824–8.
111. Portilla N, Alzate JP, Sierra FA, Parra-Medina R. A systematic review and meta-analysis of the survival and clinicopathological features of p63 expression in Merkel cell carcinoma. Australas J Dermatol. 2020;61(3):e276–e82.
112. Barksdale SK. Advances in Merkel cell carcinoma from a pathologist's perspective. Pathology. 2017;49(6):568–74.
113. Kervarrec T, Samimi M, Guyétant S, Sarma B, Chéret J, Blanchard E, et al. Histogenesis of Merkel cell carcinoma: a comprehensive review. Front Oncol. 2019;9:451.
114. Pulitzer M. Merkel cell carcinoma. Surg Pathol Clin. 2017;10(2):399–408.
115. Pasternak S, Carter MD, Ly TY, Doucette S, Walsh NM. Immunohistochemical profiles of different subsets of Merkel cell carcinoma. Hum Pathol. 2018;82:232–8.
116. Karunaratne YG, Gunaratne DA, Veness MJ. Systematic review of sentinel lymph node biopsy in Merkel cell carcinoma of the head and neck. Head Neck. 2018;40(12):2704–13.
117. Amin MB, Edge SB, Greene FL. AJCC cancer staging manual. 8th edn. Merkel cell carcinoma (Chapter 46). Springer; 2017.
118. Trinidad CM, Torres-Cabala CA, Prieto VG, Aung PP. Update on eighth edition American Joint Committee on Cancer classification for Merkel cell carcinoma and histopathological parameters that determine prognosis. J Clin Pathol. 2019;72(5):337.

Chapter 2
Molecular Landscape Profile of Melanoma

Giuseppe Palmieri, Maria Colombino, Milena Casula, Maria Cristina Sini, Antonella Manca, Marina Pisano, Panagiotis Paliogiannis, and Antonio Cossu

Abbreviations

AKT	RAC-alpha serine/threonine-protein kinase
ARAF	A-Raf proto-oncogene, serine/threonine kinase
ARID2	AT-rich interaction domain 2
ATM	ATM serine/threonine kinase
BAP1	BRCA1 associated protein 1
BRAF	B-Raf proto-oncogene, serine/threonine kinase
BRCA1–2	BRCA1–2, DNA repair associated
CCND1	cyclin D1
CDH1	cadherin 1
CDK4	cyclin-dependent kinase 4
CDKN2A	cyclin-dependent kinase inhibitor 2A
CHEK2	checkpoint kinase 2
CRAF	Raf-1 proto-oncogene, serine/threonine kinase
CSD	cumulative solar damage
CTNNB1	catenin beta 1
DDX3X	DEAD-box helicase 3, X-linked
EGFR	epidermal growth factor receptor
ERBB1–4	erb-b2 receptor tyrosine kinase 1–4

G. Palmieri (✉) · M. Colombino · M. Casula · M. C. Sini · A. Manca · M. Pisano
Unit of Cancer Genetics, Institute of Genetic and Biomedical Research (IRGB),
National Research Council (CNR), Sassari, Italy
e-mail: mariacristina.sini@cnr.it; antonella.manca@icb.cnr.it; marina.pisano@cnr.it

P. Paliogiannis · A. Cossu
Department of Medical, Surgical and Experimental Sciences, University of Sassari,
Sassari, Italy
e-mail: cossu@uniss.it

P. Rutkowski, M. Mandalà (eds.), *New Therapies in Advanced Cutaneous Malignancies*, https://doi.org/10.1007/978-3-030-64009-5_2

ERK	extracellular signal-regulated kinase
EZH2	enhancer of zeste 2 polycomb repressive complex 2 subunit
FISH	fluorescent in situ hybridization
GDP	guanosine diphosphate
GNA11	G protein subunit alpha 11
GNAQ	G protein subunit alpha q
GTP	guanosine triphosphate
HER2	human epidermal growth factor receptor 2
HRAS	HRas proto-oncogene, GTPase
IDH1	isocitrate dehydrogenase (NADP+) 1, cytosolic
KDR	kinase insert domain receptor
KIT	KIT proto-oncogene receptor tyrosine kinase
KRAS	KRAS proto-oncogene, GTPase
MAPK	mitogen-activated protein kinase
MC1R	melanocortin-1 receptor membrane receptor
MEK	MAPK/ERK kinase
MET	MET proto-oncogene, receptor tyrosine kinase
MITF	microphthalmia-associated transcription factor
mTOR	mechanistic target of rapamycin kinase
NF1	neurofibromin 1
NF-κB	nuclear factor kappa-light-chain-enhancer of activated B cells
NGS	next-generation sequencing
NRAS	NRAS proto-oncogene, GTPase
PALB2	partner and localizer of BRCA2
PD-L1	programmed death ligand 1
PDGFRA	platelet-derived growth factor receptor alpha
PI3K	phosphatidylinositol 3-kinase
PIK3CA	phosphatidylinositol 4,5-bisphosphate 3-kinase catalytic subunit alpha
POT1	protection of telomeres 1
PPP6C	protein phosphatase 6 catalytic subunit
PREX2	phosphatidylinositol-3,4,5-trisphosphate-dependent Rac exchange factor 2
PTEN	phosphatase and tensin homolog
RAC1	Rac family small GTPase 1
RAF1	Raf-1 proto-oncogene, serine/threonine kinase
RB1	RB transcriptional corepressor 1
RET	ret proto-oncogene
ROS	reactive oxygen species
RTK	receptor tyrosine kinase
SF3B1	splicing factor 3b subunit 1
SNX31	sorting nexin 31
SOS1	SOS Ras/Rac guanine nucleotide exchange factor 1
SPRED1	sprouty-related EVH1 domain containing 1
STK19	serine/threonine kinase 19
TERT	telomerase reverse transcriptase

TET   tet methylcytosine dioxygenase
TME   tumor microenvironment
TP53   tumor protein p53
UV   ultraviolet
VEGFR2   vascular endothelial growth factor receptor 2

Introduction

Cutaneous melanoma is mostly diagnosed at an early stage of disease and, although its incidence is continuously increasing in the population from western countries, it can be effectively treated by surgical excision [1]. Conversely, a large fraction of advanced stages remains refractory to systemic therapies [2]. Despite the impressive advancements into the treatment of the disease during the recent past years, clinical outcomes are still hardly predictable in melanoma patients due to the marked heterogeneity of the disease from the biological and molecular point of view [3, 4]. Therefore, the need to obtain a classification of the various tumor subtypes with distinct genetic and molecular characteristics becomes mandatory, definitively overcoming the concept according to which melanoma—as for all cancer subtypes—can be considered a single disease.

Given the central role of protein kinases in mediating different cell pathways, it is not surprising that aberrant kinase activity is a common feature of cancer cells and that kinase inhibitors are used and researched as anticancer therapies, including melanoma [5]. When constitutively activated, some kinases can be oncogenic and directly drive tumor growth, while other kinases can play an indirect role, acting as regulators of oncogenic intracellular signals or promoting extracellular effects into the tumor microenvironment such as the induction of angiogenesis or mechanisms for invasion and immune escape [6, 7].

From the genetic point of view, the pathogenesis of melanoma—like all other forms of malignant neoplasms—is based on the acquisition of sequential alterations affecting specific chromosome loci and genes involved in metabolic and molecular pathways controlling all such cellular homeostasis mechanisms [8, 9]. In other words, melanoma pathogenesis and, more in general, tumorigenesis may be actually considered as due to a process of sequential accumulation of mutations and changes in specific genes and DNA regions [8, 9].

Molecular Complexity of Melanoma

Cutaneous melanoma (CM) has a high prevalence of somatic mutations, both in primary lesions and—to a greater extent—in metastatic lesions, with an average mutation rate estimated to be much greater than 20 mutations per megabase of genomic DNA [10, 11]. Considering data from studies on CM with NGS-based mutation analysis, majority (up to 70–80%) of DNA sequence variations is represented by C > T substitutions (including a small fraction of <5% cases constituted by CC > TT transitions). These variants are due to the mutagenic effects of the ultraviolet (UV) radiations on exposed skin, and the entire set of them is usually indicated as the UV mutation signature [12, 13]. The UV effects on mutagenesis may thus contribute to determine that CM displays one of the highest mutation load compared to that from other cancer types [14]. On this regard, it appears clear that the threshold of the tumor mutation burden (TMB) may vary across cancer types, probably modified by the intervention of multiple factors linked to distinct tumor microenvironments (such as immune cell infiltration or exclusion, expression levels of cytokines and/or checkpoint molecules, and clonality rates) [11]. All these factors are involved into the different response rates and clinical benefits to immune checkpoint inhibitors across all cancer types [11, 14]. Although TMB assessment is not a standardized biomarker that affects treatment decisions, efforts are being conducted to implement TMB measurement assays and uniform the interpretation of the data [15].

As a confirmation of the UV impact on the increase of the TMB levels in the skin, noncutaneous (i.e., ocular and mucosal) melanomas present a markedly lower mutational load and lack the UV signature [16, 17]. Moreover, the mutation rate in melanomas occurring on chronically sun-exposed skin was found to be at least five times higher than those on the skin not subject to sun damage (ratio of >20 mutations per megabase vs. ≤5 mutations per megabase, respectively) [8, 18]. Finally, there is clear epidemiological evidence of a relationship between nevus number, sun exposure, and C > T mutations [19].

Over the past few years, specific oncogenic mutations have been identified in genes encoding for RAS/RAF/MEK/ERK kinases belonging to the so-called mitogen-activated protein kinase (MAPK) signal transduction cascade, which regulate the main processes of cell proliferation and cell survival [10, 16, 20]. On the basis of in-depth mutational analyses through several next-generation sequencing (NGS) approaches [10, 12, 16, 21, 22], CM patients are currently classified into the following distinct molecular subtypes according to their mutational status:

- Cases with mutations activating the *BRAF* oncogene
- Cases with mutations activating the *RAS* oncogenes (including the three isoforms: *HRAS*, *KRAS* and, mainly, *NRAS*)
- Cases without mutations in these two oncogenes (with occurrence of activating mutations in *KIT* and increased frequency of mutations inactivating the *NF1* gene)

However, additional genes may be mutated at different prevalence within such CM subtypes, contributing to the molecular heterogeneity of the disease at somatic level. According to the mutation frequency reported in studies with NGS-based mutation analysis in CM samples, the mutated driver genes associated with these three melanoma subtypes could be divided into three groups: one (*TP53*, *NF1*, *CDKN2A*, and *ARID2*), with mutation frequency between 10% and 20%; the second (*PTEN*, *PPP6C*, *RAC1*, and *DDX3X*), with mutation frequency ≥5% and <10%; and the third one (up to 20 genes), with mutation frequency <5% [12, 23]. In

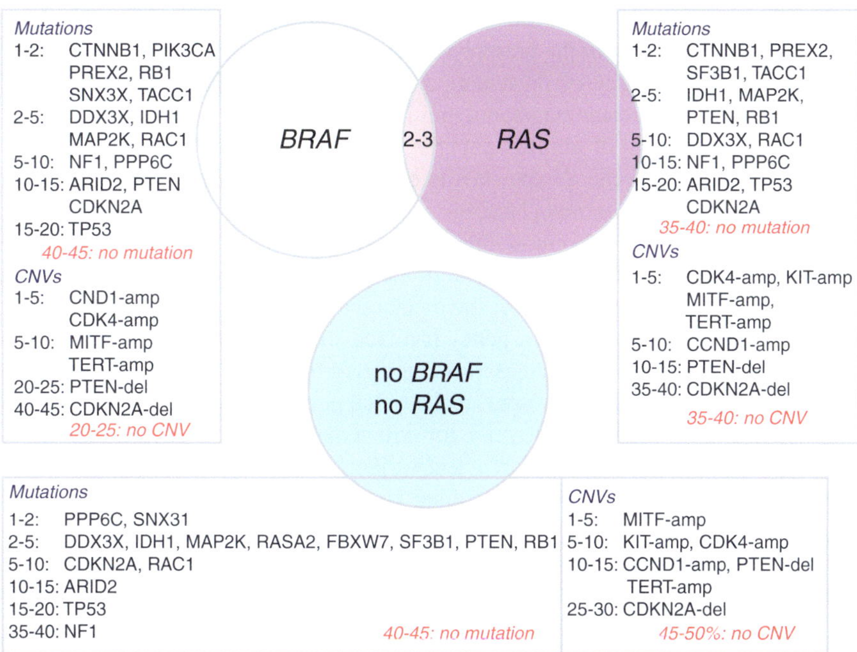

Fig. 2.1 The three main (BRAF[mut], RAS[mut], and non-BRAF[mut]/non-RAS[mut]) melanoma subtypes. Additional altered genes are reported for each subgroup. Numbers indicate the mutation frequency. *CNVs* copy number variations, *ampl* amplification, *del* deletion

Fig. 2.1, the three main mutational subtypes of melanoma and the frequencies of the coexisting mutated genes are summarized.

Overall, a complex model of tight interactions between such candidate genes and their signaling cascades whose alterations are important for the development of melanoma is emerging, including pathways mediating protection against ultraviolet-induced DNA damage and DNA repair, telomere maintenance, immunity, melanocyte differentiation, and cell adhesion. Some of them are involved in melanoma susceptibility and, therefore, in the increase of the risk for disease onset.

Genetic Integrity and Melanoma Susceptibility

The CM induction and development are extremely complex involving genetic and environmental factors, such as specific predisposing germline mutations, skin color, number and type of nevi, and sun exposure [24, 25]. About one tenth of melanomas occurs in patients with disease recurrence in family and less than half of these familial cases have been attributed to inheritance of a mutation in a highly penetrant predisposition gene [26]. In the majority of familial melanomas, a pattern of sequence variations in low- or very-low-penetrance predisposition genes are thought to contribute to the melanoma inheritance [27]. In other words, mutations in multiple high-penetrant genes or the presence of several moderate-to-low risk alleles may explain the heterogeneity of presentation of the various melanoma pedigrees, as well as the multiple melanoma phenotypes [27, 28]. In a more general view, a combination of inheritance of familial patterns of variants/polymorphisms in multiple genes and different levels of exposures to environmental mutagens participate into the development of melanoma [28, 29].

In addition to a "melanoma-dominant" pattern of inheritance, melanoma can also occur as a "subordinate" neoplasm in the context of mixed cancer syndromes [27–29]. The significant increase of the melanoma risk in mixed cancer syndromes is often caused by mutations in genes involved in DNA repair by homologous-recombination mechanisms such as those regulated by *BAP1*, *BRCA1*, *BRCA2*, and *TP53* genes [29, 30]. This represents a clear clue pointing at the importance of the maintenance of the genome integrity for cutaneous melanoma susceptibility. An association between multiple independent variants in the *TP53* gene and cutaneous melanoma has been described for a long time [31]. *TP53* responds to cellular stresses and early cancerogenic events by inducing DNA repair mechanisms, cell cycle arrest, apoptosis, and cellular senescence toward the elimination of extensively damaged cells [32]. Mutations/deletions enhancing dysfunction of TP53 or inducing up-regulation of HDM2 (mouse double minute 2, human homolog), whose gene product is the natural inhibitor of p53, may inactivate the p53—the so-called Guardian of the Genome [33]. In the skin, this results in clonal expansion of cells that carry accumulated mutations with an induced increase in both nevus density and cutaneous melanoma risk [29, 30]. A growing body of evidence is supporting a key role for telomere maintenance in cutaneous melanoma susceptibility, with partial involvement of *POT1* and *TERT* genes, as well as *CCND1* and *ATM* loci [29, 34, 35]. These genes play established roles not only in telomere maintenance but also in DNA repair and regulation of senescence [29]. As a further indication that controlling the telomere function/maintenance is somehow important in melanoma pathogenesis, predisposing mutations have been observed in *POT1* and *TERT* genes among few melanoma families with high recurrence of the disease [34, 35]. Among others, mutations in the *TERT* promoter (*TERTp*) represent a common mechanism for reactivating the telomerase reverse transcriptase protein and, thus, maintaining the telomere length in cancer cells among many solid tumors [36, 37]. The occurrence of such activating mutations may contribute to increase TERT expression levels, alterations into target transcription factor binding sites, telomere stabilization, and cell immortalization and proliferation [37]. Finally, inherited mutations in the *BAP1* gene, which were firstly reported as an inherited cause of uveal melanoma, have been associated with a risk of lung cancer and meningioma and now recognized to also increase the risk of cutaneous melanoma [38, 39].

Overall, the above-mentioned genes and other genes involved in melanocyte proliferation or differentiation (such as *CDK4*, *MITF*, *MC1R*, *PTEN*, *RB1*) are very rarely mutated in families with melanoma recurrence (altogether, less than 3% mutated cases in more than 2500 pedigrees) compared to the *CDKN2A* high-risk susceptibility gene, which remains the only most prevalent familial melanoma gene (about 20% mutated cases within the same large pedigrees' series) [40].

The *CDKN2A* tumor suppressor gene encodes two proteins: p16[CDKN2A] and p14[CDKN2A]; inactivation of both alleles is necessary for the development of melanoma [41]. In melanoma families, about one fifth of probands may carry germline mutations in *CDKN2A*, whereas about two-thirds of melanoma patients present a *CDKN2A* gene inactivation (by genetic or epigenetic mechanisms) at the somatic level [9, 29, 42]. Significant discrepancies in *CDKN2A* mutation frequency are reported in melanoma pedigrees from different geographical areas [43], including northern and the southern parts of Italy [44, 45]. This suggests that additional genetic factors tightly linked to the patients' origin (contributing to the so-called genetic background) may account for differences in the prevalence of germline mutations in *CDKN2A* gene [20, 29, 46]. Activation of the downstream CDK4-RB effectors through inactivation of p16[CDKN2A] has been reported to promote melanoma progression; indeed, prevalence of this activation significantly increases during transition from primary to metastatic melanomas and achieves the maximal level in melanoma cell lines [20]. Similarly, the inactivation of p14[CDKN2A] causes the reduction of the p53 protein levels, with consequent impairment of the cell-cycle progression control and inhibition of the apoptosis, contributing to increase the survival of melanoma cells [20]. Activation of the CDKN2A-dependent pathways may also be associated with the amplification of the *CyclinD1* (*CCND1*) gene, which is generally found in melanomas negative for *BRAF* and *RAS* mutations [12].

Finally, the *CDH1* gene, encoding E-cadherin, is specifically upregulated in both normal melanocytes and keratinocytes, playing a crucial role in cell-cell adhesion between these two cell types [47]. In melanoma, the expression levels of E-cadherin are markedly reduced or quite absent, promoting a concurrent switch into the type of cell-cell adhesion and a preferential association with fibroblasts and vascular endothelial cells [47, 48]. This loss of E-cadherin expression thus results in enhanced invasion and constitutes an independent factor of poor prognosis in melanoma patients [48]. Interestingly, germline variations leading to upregulation of the *CDH1* expression in melanocytes seem to act as a protective mechanism, limiting reactive oxygen-mediated apoptosis and allowing cells damaged by oxidative stress to survive in the skin [49].

Molecular Heterogeneity and Melanoma Pathogenesis

At somatic level, a specific core of genes and pathways has been shown to play a crucial role in the pathogenesis of melanoma: RAS-dependent BRAF-ERK pathway, RAS-dependent PI3K-AKT pathway, RAS-regulating NF1 and KIT genes (Fig. 2.2). Overall, less than one tenth of CMs has been found to be negative for any genetic alteration, including both deleterious mutation and copy number variation (CNV), as ascertained by NGS-based analyzes carried out in recent past years [12]. These findings further confirm that melanoma is a highly mutated malignancy.

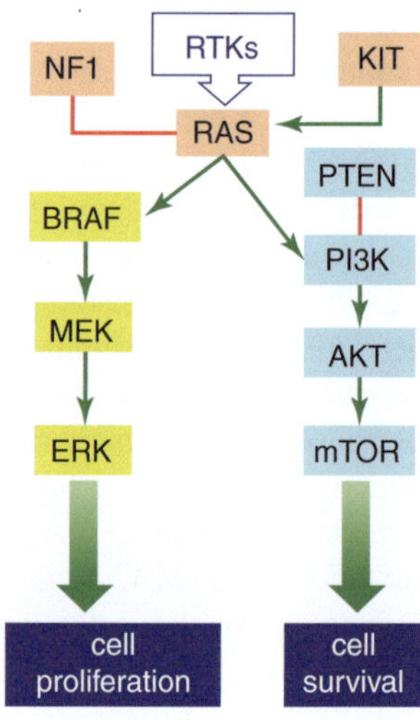

Fig. 2.2 Core signal transduction pathways involved in melanomagenesis. Green arrow, activating signals; red lines, inhibiting signals. *RTKs* receptor tyrosine kinases

Among the CNVs (Fig. 2.1), inactivation by deletion of *CDKN2A* and *PTEN* tumor suppressor genes has been confirmed to represent the structural rearrangement most frequently implicated in pathogenesis of all molecular subtypes of melanoma [12].

BRAF

The RAF kinase family consists of three proteins (ARAF, BRAF, and CRAF), all of which are part of the MAPK pathway; the formation of complexes by these different isoforms plays an important role in their activation [50]. In melanoma, the *BRAF* gene is mutated in 45–50% of cases; the most prevalent mutation (about 90% of cases) is represented by a substitution of a valine with glutamic acid at codon 600 (BRAF[V600E]) [10, 12]. The remaining *BRAF* mutations mostly occur at the same codon: V600K (the most frequent; <10% of cases), V600D, and V600R; mutations in codons other than V600 are not common (among them, K601 is the most prevalently affected codon) [51]. The constitutive oncogenic activation of BRAF promotes a continuous, uncontrolled stimulation of cell proliferation [52]. There is an inverse relationship between the prevalence of the *BRAF* mutation and the age of melanoma onset: >50% of patients <30 years and only 25% ≥70 years harbor a BRAF[V600E] mutation. Inversely, non-V600E mutations (including V600K) are reported to steadily raise with the increase of the diagnosis age: <20% of patients <50 years and >40% in those ≥70 years [8]. The demonstration that *BRAF* is mutated in the majority (>50%) of common nevi suggests that its oncogenic activation is a necessary but not sufficient condition for the development of melanoma, being considered as an initiation event in the neoplastic transformation of melanocytes [18, 53]. The precise pathogenesis of *BRAF* mutations remains as yet unclear, but these observations suggest a complex relationship between intermittent sun exposure and nevus formation [8, 31]. It has been questioned whether *BRAF* mutations might actually result from DNA damage consequent upon UV exposure. However, it is of note that neither *BRAF* nor *NRAS* mutations have the classical genetic signature of mutagenesis as a result of UV light exposure, which instead is associated with the BRAF/NRAS wild-type status [54].

Since common nevi are mutated in *BRAF*, alterations in other genes are therefore thought to cooperate with the *BRAF* mutations in inducing transformation and neoplastic progression of the melanocytic cells [10, 18, 31, 53]. On this regard, melanomas carrying a *BRAF* mutation are characterized by coexistence of additional specific gene alterations, mainly loss of PTEN and inactivation of *CDKN2A* or *TP53* (Fig. 2.1).

The NGS analyzes have clearly indicated that oncogenic mutations in *BRAF*, *RAS*, and *KIT*—within the core gene pathways involved in melanomagenesis reported in Fig. 2.2—are mutually exclusive ($\leq 3\%$ of patients presents with coexistence of mutations in such oncogenes at the time of diagnosis) [12]. The proportion of coexisting mutations in these genes is deeply modified by the use of the combination of BRAF and MEK inhibitors for the treatment of the patients with a BRAF-mutant melanoma, as consequence of the acquisition of resistance to the target therapy [55]. Patients with advanced melanoma (American Joint Committee on Cancer [AJCC] stage IV or III inoperable [56]), as well as those with radically operated AJCC stage III melanoma, both carrying a BRAF-V600 mutation, may be addressed to the therapy with BRAF and MEK inhibitors [57–65]. Although with lower efficacy, even patients with rare (V600 and non-V600) *BRAF* mutations can respond to targeted therapy [66]. The assessment of the BRAF mutational status has become mandatory for molecular classification of patients with stage III or IV melanomas [67].

From the practical point of view, the evaluation of the *BRAF* mutational status in stage IV melanoma patients should be carried out on tissue biopsy from the metastasis, as it represents the most recently developed tumor lesion and consists of a preponderant population of neoplastic cells. When this is not possible and in stage III melanomas, the mutational investigation may be performed on the tissue sample from primary melanoma. In this sense, a good agreement has been demonstrated in the *BRAF* mutational patterns between metastatic lesions (mainly, lymph node sites) and primary melanomas [68, 69]. In consideration of a certain rate of intertumoral heterogeneity [68, 70], a *BRAF* mutation analysis providing a wild-type result on the primary tumor among advanced melanoma patients should be however repeated on tissue biopsy from an accessible metastasis.

The *BRAF* mutational status can be assessed using methodologies presenting different degrees of sensitivity and specificity, though the complexity of the genes and pathways involved in melanomagenesis strongly suggest to move toward innovative approaches using a multigenic screening based on NGS assays [71]. The enrichment of the tissue sample is thus fundamental and the percentage of neoplastic cells present in the tissue to be sent for molecular analysis should be really representative (never be less than 50%) [72]. In the case of melanoma associated with nevus, it is crucial that the sample enrichment is focused on the isolation of a pure population of melanoma cells, as melanocytic nevi can be carriers of *BRAF* mutations at the same frequency found in melanomas (see above and [53]).

The recently increased importance of achieving the classification of the *BRAF* mutational status for other cancer types—mainly, lung [73, 74] and colorectal [75, 76] adenocarcinomas—have been demonstrated to be highly sensitive to the response to the treatment with combined BRAF and MEK inhibitors. According to recent publications [77–80], it has been suggested to define a sort of functional classification for the various BRAF variants:

- Class I *BRAF* mutations include V600 mutations, which are able to induce a constitutive activation of the MAPK signaling cascade without the need of dimerization and an upstream RAS activation.
- Class II *BRAF* mutations include variants in codons different from the V600 one (mainly, G464, G469, L597, and V601), which are still independent from the upstream RAS activation but require the protein dimerization to activate the signal transduction pathway.
- Class III *BRAF* mutations include variants in codons located outside the core kinase domains, which require either upstream activation and protein dimerization with CRAF or, in minimal part, with ARAF (see below).

RAS

The RAS family is composed of three tissue-specific gene isoforms: *HRAS*, *KRAS*, and *NRAS*. The latter gene is the one mostly mutated in melanoma [10]. *NRAS* mutations are found in about 25% of melanoma patients; they occur almost exclusively in a single gene codon (Q61, about 90% of cases); in the remaining 10% of cases, the mutated codon is G12 or G13 (31–33) [10, 81].

The oncogenic stimulation of RAS is able to activate specific cytoplasmic downstream proteins with kinase function: RAF and PI3K [81]. As previously mentioned, *RAS* mutations have been demonstrated to be mutually exclusive with *BRAF* mutations in nearly all cases (coexistence of the two genes mutated in a constitutive manner is reported in 2–3% of melanomas) [12]. Occurrence of RAS activation—both for the acquisition of mutations or functional oncogenic induction—may cause that the translation of the mitogenic signal in the MAPK pathway can be switched to dimerization of wild-type CRAF or, to a lesser extent, wild-type ARAF, which therefore acquires a key role in maintaining cell proliferation stimulation in this subset of melanomas [50, 82]. Interestingly, an increased activation of the NRAS-CRAF axis has been described as responsible for the acquired resistance to BRAF inhibitors [55]. On this regard, enhanced RAS-dependent RAF dimerization has also been involved into the pathogenesis of squamous cell carcinomas, as a side effect in subsets of patients treated with BRAF inhibitors [83]. These agents have been demonstrated to indeed activate MAPK pathway by inducing RAF dimerization in cells lacking *BRAF* mutations, leading to increased keratinocyte proliferation [84]. More in general, the enhanced RAF dimerization represents a process that may be constitutively promoted by any form of activation—through genetic (mutations) or functional mechanisms—in any of the three isoforms of *RAS* [84].

To date, there are no clinical studies that support the use of specific target therapy for melanoma with *NRAS* mutation. Two clinical studies (a phase II trial and a randomized phase III trial) have shown only a minimal therapeutic efficacy of the MEK inhibitor binimetinib in patients with advanced melanoma carrying an NRAS mutation [85, 86]. Therefore, detection of the *NRAS* mutation is not actually required in clinical practice, but it can be useful for the insertion of patients in further clinical studies only.

KIT

A limited fraction of melanomas that are not mutated in *BRAF* and *RAS* may carry activating mutations in *KIT* [10, 12] encoding a tyrosine kinase receptor of the cell membrane and resulting in a continuous induction of cell proliferation, through functional stimulation, mainly of the MAPK pathway (Fig. 2.2). Among the *KIT* mutations, those most frequently associated with melanoma are represented by the L576P mutation in exon 11 and the K642E mutation in exon 13 (other mutations of the KIT gene reported in melanoma are V599A, D816H, D820Y) [87]. The frequency of KIT mutations has been reported in 1–3% of total melanomas, but it may deeply vary among the different melanoma subtypes: 15–20% mucosal melanomas (the highest prevalence is observed in anal melanoma); 10–15% acral melanomas, 3% melanomas on chronically photo-exposed skin, almost total absence in melanomas in unexposed skin areas) [87–90].

The evaluation of the KIT mutational status is thus strongly indicated in the acral and mucosal melanomas, though after the evaluation of the BRAF mutational status (again, mutations in both genes are mutually exclusive; see above). In advanced melanomas with KIT mutation, treatment with immunotherapy is actually indicated. Albeit limited, some clinical experiences with phase II studies have shown objective responses with the use of KIT inhibitors in melanomas harboring mutations in exon 9, 11, or 13 [87, 91–93].

NF1

The NF1 mutations cause an inherited multisystem genetic disorder, neurofibromatosis type 1, at germline level and promote cell proliferation mainly through activation of the MAPK pathway at somatic level [94]. As reported by The Cancer Genome Atlas, inactivating mutations of the NF1 gene occur in a subset of melanomas (approximately 15% of cases) [10]. Physiologically, NF1 encodes for neurofibromin, a RAS-GTPase-activating protein, which negatively regulates RAS signaling by stabilizing the RAS-GDP-inactive form; mutations functionally silencing the NF1 gene result in RAS activation and enhancement of the malignant transformation in melanocytes [94]. These data demonstrate that inactivation of NF1 may contribute to increase the activity of several RASopathy genes—such as SOS1, PTPN11, RAF1, and SPRED1—in melanomagenesis [95, 96]. Tumors with mutations in NF1 and constitutive activation of RASopathy genes are often associated with a higher mutational load and, consequently, a greater probability of generating neoantigens [97]. Therefore, NF1-mutated tumors—including the desmoplastic melanoma subtype, which is characterized by a high mutational load and frequent NF1 mutations—are thought to be more sensitive to immunotherapy and, in particular, to treatment with immune checkpoint inhibitors [98].

Although the *NF1* mutations are the most prevalent alterations in the group of melanomas with both wild-type *BRAF* and wild-type *RAS* (about 35% of these cases), they are also present in *BRAF*- and *RAS*-mutated melanomas (about 5% and 15% of such cases, respectively) [12]. Melanomas with *NF1* mutations generally occur on chronically sun-exposed skin or in elder individuals and, as previously affirmed, show a higher mutation burden (to this latter, the UV-induced mutagenesis also contributes) [94, 96, 98]. Finally, an increase in frequency of *NF1* mutations is observed among BRAF-mutant tumors intrinsically resistant to BRAF inhibitors, as well as in melanomas of patients acquiring resistance to BRAF inhibitors [55].

PI3K-PTEN

The PTEN-PI3K-AKT-mTOR kinase cascade represents the core pathway—mainly dependent on RAS activation—involved in regulation of cell survival (Fig. 2.2). Oncogenic activation of the PI3K/AKT pathway, including that underlying the acquired resistance to treatment with BRAF and MEK inhibitors, can occur through several mechanisms: mutation and/or amplification of RTK genes (i.e., the four ERB-B receptor tyrosine kinase family members: *ERBB1*/EGFR, *ERBB2*/HER2, *ERBB3*/HER3, and *ERBB4*/HER4) [99, 100], deletion of PTEN [101, 102], somatic alterations of *AKT* [103, 104], or activating isoforms of RAS [94–96]. The *ERBB* genes encode transmembrane proteins that are activated by either homo- or heterodimerization with other *ERBB* family members, resulting in activation of both PI3K/AKT and MAPK signal transduction pathways [18, 100]. As a confirmation about the tight interaction between the *ERBB* genes and the PI3K/AKT pathway, mutations in the *ERBB* family members are targetable with PI3K inhibitors [100]. In melanoma, the PTEN gene is deleted in about a third of cases, with complete loss of expression of the corresponding protein in 10–20% of primary melanomas; the level of this loss increases during neoplastic progression, up to 40–50% in melanoma cell lines [10, 12]. The activation of the PI3K pathway results in aberrant growth of melanoma cells and increased survival capacity with the acquisition of resistance to apoptosis, as well as to acquired resistance to the treatment with targeted therapies in various tumor types (in melanoma, to the combination of BRAF and MEK inhibitors) [29]. Loss of PTEN in melanoma has been associated with poor or absent T-cell-inflamed tumor microenvironment, thus affecting the response to immune checkpoint inhibitors [105] and correlated with poor prognosis (a decreased overall survival and higher tendency to develop brain metastasis) in stage III melanoma patients carrying a BRAF mutation [106].

Molecular Classification of Melanoma Subtypes

As summarized in Fig. 2.3, the findings from the multigenic mutation analyses of the NGS-based studies indicate that CMM patients may be divided in at least six main distinct molecular subgroups [12]. Starting from the definition of the BRAF mutational status at baseline of any diagnostic and therapeutic path among AJCC stage III and IV patients, the molecular classification of the melanoma can identify molecular subtypes according to the coexistence of pathogenic mutations in other genes associated or not to the mutated and wild-type BRAF/NRAS (Fig. 2.3). From a practical point of view, the characterization of these subtypes becomes extremely important for a more appropriate assessment of clinical and biological features of patients with melanoma, as well as for programming the most correct therapeutic approach in each patient's subgroup.

Moving toward the use of the NGS-based assays for multigenic mutation testing in clinical practice, the following additional genes demonstrated markedly implied in melanomagenesis are required to be incorporated in mutational screening at somatic level. In recent past, several aspects have been clarified in order to more easily conduct the NGS analyses in hospital laboratories and, thus, to transfer the use of NGS assays in clinical practice [72, 107]. In particular, melanoma-specific gene panels have become commercially available for detecting somatic mutations through their use on the two most common NGS platforms [Illumina Inc. (San Diego, CA, USA) and Life Technologies-Thermo Fisher Scientific (Waltham, MA, USA)]. They include the following additional genes involved in melanoma pathogenesis:

- ARID2, CDK4, CDKN2A, CTNNB1, ERBB4, EZH2, GNA11, GNAQ, GRIN2A, HRAS, IDH1, KIT, KRAS, MAP 2 K1, MITF, PREX2, RAC1, RB1, TERT, TP53, TYR (Oncomine Melanoma extended panel; Life Technologies-Thermo Fisher Scientific)

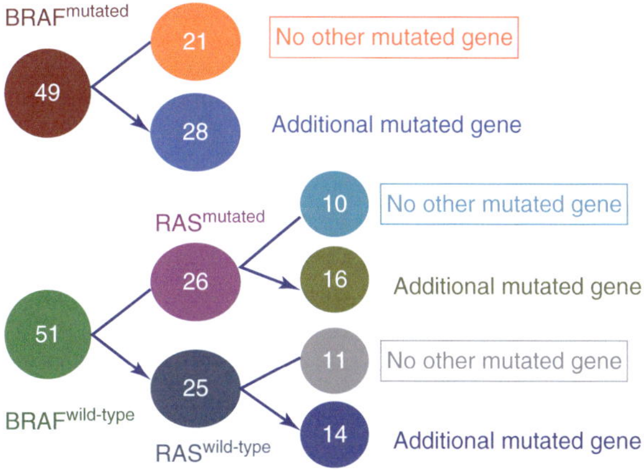

Fig. 2.3 Classification of 100 melanoma patients according to the gene mutation status distribution

- AKT, BRAF, CCND1, CDK4, CDK6, CTNNB1, ERBB2, ERBB3, ERBB4, GNA11, GNAQ, IDH1, KIT, KRAS, HRAS, MAP 2K1, MTOR, NRAS, PIK3CA, RAF1 (Focus Ampliseq panel, Illumina)

Here, we briefly summarize the characteristics of the main additional genes contributing to melanomagenesis.

CTNNB1

The *CTNNB1* gene encodes β-catenin, a scaffold protein interacting with components of the WNT signaling pathway, adhesion molecules (such as cadherin proteins and α-catenin), and epigenetic-transcriptional regulators (such as EZH2 and SMARCA) [108]. Among others, EZH2 positively regulates the WNT/CTNNB1 signaling in some cancer types, being essential for acquisition of cell motility [109]. On this regard, EZH2 has been found to positively regulate genes involved in cytoskeletal modifications underlying cell invasiveness and promotes CM motility and metastasis [109]. Coexistence of *BRAF*^{V600E} mutation and *EZH2* activation is rather prevalent in melanoma by enhancing proliferation and survival of melanoma cells [110]. Activating *CTNNB1* mutations, as well as inactivating mutations in negative regulators of the β-catenin pathway, may determine effect into the tumor microenvironment by interfering with the T-cell priming and infiltration, favoring immune evasive mechanisms (including the suppression of chemokines and cytokine gene expression by tumor cells) [111–114].

PREX2—GRIN2A

Activating mutations in *PREX2*, a guanine nucleotide exchange factor involved in regulating the activity of the *PTEN* gene product [23, 115, 116], and in *GRIN2A*, a glutamate receptor participating to the control of cell proliferation [23, 116], have been reported in about 15% and 33% of melanoma samples, respectively. Oncogenic activation of both genes contributes to facilitate survival, growth, and invasion of melanoma cells. Patients with GRIN2A mutations may have a more aggressive disease and a poorer clinical outcome, though further studies are needed to confirm a role for such alterations as a prognostic marker [117].

RAC1

In CM, activating mutations occur in a specific dipyrimidine site of the RAC1 gene, representing a typical UV signature [21]. Unlike common *RAS* oncogenic mutations that impair or abolish intrinsic GTP hydrolysis ability and render the kinase constitutively active in terms of signaling, the RAC1 mutant protein abnormally accelerates the exchange from inactive GDP- to active GTP-isoform [118]. In melanoma,

mutated *RAC1* is often found in combination with additional gain-of-function mutations of other oncogenes (*BRAF* or *NRAS*) and/or loss of function mutations in
tumor suppressor genes (*NF1*, *TP53*, or *PTEN*), suggesting that *RAC1* is not generally sufficient on its own to drive tumor formation [21, 119]. It has been suggested
that coexistence of BRAF mutation and *RAC1* mutation in primary CM may be
associated with thinner melanomas [120].

ARID2—IDH1

Somatic mutations in *ARID2* and *IDH1* genes, both involved in chromatin remodeling, have been found to be significantly associated with elevated levels of global
DNA methylation in several malignancies, including melanoma [121, 122]. In particular, mutations in these two genes may cause important epigenetic dysfunction
and hypermethylation of several target genomic loci, thus leading to aberrant gene
expression in both primary tumor and metastases [123]. *ARID2* and *IDH1* somatic
mutations have been found at a relatively high frequency (approximately 30%) in
melanoma [10, 12].

MITF

The *MITF* gene acts as a master regulator of melanocyte development, function, and
survival, by modulating various differentiation and cell-cycle progression genes
[124]. The levels of expression of *MITF* are demonstrated to determine two different behavior profiles for melanoma cells. A proliferative profile, which is based on
upregulation of *MITF* and other melanocytic genes (such as *TYR* and *DCT*), is associated with high rates of proliferation and low motility. Conversely, the invasive
signature, which is based on downregulation of these same genes and upregulation
of others ones (such as *INHBA* and *COL5A1*) involved in modifying the extracellular environment, is associated with lower rates of proliferation and high motility.
MITF is amplified in a fraction of human melanomas, and its amplification rates
increase in metastatic disease [124]. Coexistence of high MITF expression levels
and *BRAF* mutations is able to transform human melanocytes; thus, MITF can function as a melanoma oncogene [124, 125]. Moreover, a reduction of *MITF* activity
sensitizes melanoma cells to chemotherapeutic agents [125].

Conclusive Remarks

All these findings are strongly indicative of the existence of complex molecular
regulatory mechanisms, which ensure the integrity and regularity of the various cellular functions in normal melanocytes. As melanoma progresses from benign nevi
to invasive tumors, there are several changes into the genome, and molecular

pathways accumulate in cells and contribute to determine different biological features. In recent past years, concurrent intracellular alterations in molecular pathways have been found to even interfere with the homeostasis of the tumor microenvironment and interact with various extracellular factors participating in immune activity against the tumor. In the era of the precision medicine, an extensive mutation profile of the tumor becomes the first step toward the most accurate diagnostic classification of the patients, before taking the most appropriate therapeutic decision. More in general, the combination of multiple intracellular signaling pathways and extracellular modifications clearly indicates the need to evaluate more extensively the different molecular events underlying the biological and clinical behavior of the disease and the various actors playing a role in this complex scenario. An additional, practice changing advancement would be represented by characterization of the genetic and molecular assets not only at baseline but also during the course of treatment or follow-up in order to register any biological change of the disease due to its intrinsic and acquired intratumor heterogeneity. This will provide important clues to the clinician, dramatically improving the management of the melanoma patients.

Author Contributions GP, writing and draft preparation; MCo, Mca, MCS, AM, and MP, critical discussion of the manuscript; PP, review and editing; AC, supervision. All authors read and approved the final manuscript.

Conflict of Interest Giuseppe Palmieri has/had advisory role for Bristol Myers Squibb (BMS), Incyte, Merck Sharp & Dohme (MSD), Novartis, Pierre Fabre, and Roche-Genetech. All the remaining authors declare no conflict of interest.

Funding
Work was partially founded by the Associazione Italiana per la Ricerca sul Cancro (AIRC) "Programma di ricerca 5 per Mille 2018—Id.21073."

References

1. Elder DE, Massi D, Scolyer RA, Willemze R. WHO classification of skin tumours. Eds International Agency for Research on Cancer (IARC), Lyon Cedex 08 (France) 2018.
2. Ascierto PA, Agarwala SS, Botti G, Budillon A, Davies MA, Dummer R, Ernstoff M, Ferrone S, Formenti S, Gajewski TF, Garbe C, Hamid O, Lo RS, Luke JJ, Michielin O, Palmieri G, Zitvogel L, Marincola FM, Masucci G, Caracò C, Thurin M, Puzanov I. Perspectives in melanoma: meeting report from the Melanoma Bridge (November 29th-1 December 1st, 2018, Naples, Italy). J Transl Med. 2019;17:234.
3. Shannan B, Perego M, Somasundaram R, Herlyn M. Heterogeneity in melanoma. Cancer Treat Res. 2016;167:1–15.
4. Knackstedt RW, Knackstedt T, Gastman B. Gene expression profiling in melanoma: past results and future potential. Future Oncol. 2019;15(7):791–800.
5. Turner J, Couts K, Sheren J, Saichaemchan S, Ariyawutyakorn W, Avolio I, et al. Kinase gene fusions in defined subsets of melanoma. Pigment Cell Melanoma Res. 2017;30:53–62.
6. Hodis E, Watson IR, Kryukov GV, Arold ST, Imielinski M, Theurillat JP, et al. A landscape of driver mutations in melanoma. Cell. 2012;150:251–63.

7. Spranger S, Gajewski TF. Impact of oncogenic pathways on evasion of antitumour immune responses. Nat Rev Cancer. 2018;18(3):139–47.
8. Shain AH, Yeh I, Kovalyshyn I, Sriharan A, Talevich E, Gagnon A, Dummer R, North J, Pincus L, Ruben B, Rickaby W, D'Arrigo C, Robson A, Bastian BC. The genetic evolution of melanoma from precursor lesions. N Engl J Med. 2015;373:1926–36.
9. Sini MC, Manca A, Cossu A, Budroni M, Botti G, Ascierto PA, Cremona F, Muggiano A, D'Atri S, Casula M, Baldinu P, Palomba G, Lissia A, Tanda F, Palmieri G. Molecular alterations at chromosome 9p21 in melanocytic naevi and melanoma. Br J Dermatol. 2008;158(2):243–50.
10. The Cancer Genome Atlas Network. Genomic classification of cutaneous melanoma. Cell. 2015;161(7):1681–96.
11. Samstein RM, Lee CH, Shoushtari AN, Hellmann MD, Shen R, Janjigian YY, Barron DA, Zehir A, Jordan EJ, Omuro A, Kaley TJ, Kendall SM, Motzer RJ, Hakimi AA, Voss MH, Russo P, Rosenberg J, Iyer G, Bochner BH, Bajorin DF, Al-Ahmadie HA, Chaft JE, Rudin CM, Riely GJ, Baxi S, Ho AL, Wong RJ, Pfister DG, Wolchok JD, Barker CA, Gutin PH, Brennan CW, Tabar V, Mellinghoff IK, DeAngelis LM, Ariyan CE, Lee N, Tap WD, Gounder MM, D'Angelo SP, Saltz L, Stadler ZK, Scher HI, Baselga J, Razavi P, Klebanoff CA, Yaeger R, Segal NH, Ku GY, DeMatteo RP, Ladanyi M, Rizvi NA, Berger MF, Riaz N, Solit DB, Chan TA, Morris LGT. Tumor mutational load predicts survival after immunotherapy across multiple cancer types. Nat Genet. 2019;51(2):202–6.
12. Palmieri G, Colombino M, Casula M, et al. Italian Melanoma Intergroup (IMI). Molecular pathways in melanomagenesis: what we learned from next-generation sequencing approaches. Curr Oncol Rep. 2018;20:86.
13. Craig S, Earnshaw CH, Virós A. Ultraviolet light and melanoma. J Pathol. 2018;244:578–85.
14. Goodman AM, Kato S, Bazhenova L, Patel SP, Frampton GM, Miller V, Stephens PJ, Daniels GA, Kurzrock R. Tumor mutational burden as an independent predictor of response to immunotherapy in diverse cancers. Mol Cancer Ther. 2017;16:2598–608.
15. Büttner R, Longshore JW, López-Ríos F, Merkelbach-Bruse S, Normanno N, Rouleau E, Penault-Llorca F. Implementing TMB measurement in clinical practice: considerations on assay requirements. ESMO Open. 2019;4(1):e000442.
16. Hayward NK, Wilmott JS, Waddell N, Johansson PA, Field MA, Nones K, Patch AM, Kakavand H, Alexandrov LB, Burke H, Jakrot V, Kazakoff S, Holmes O, Leonard C, Sabarinathan R, Mularoni L, Wood S, Xu Q, Waddell N, Tembe V, Pupo GM, De Paoli-Iseppi R, Vilain RE, Shang P, Lau LMS, Dagg RA, Schramm SJ, Pritchard A, Dutton-Regester K, Newell F, Fitzgerald A, Shang CA, Grimmond SM, Pickett HA, Yang JY, Stretch JR, Behren A, Kefford RF, Hersey P, Long GV, Cebon J, Shackleton M, Spillane AJ, Saw RPM, López-Bigas N, Pearson JV, Thompson JF, Scolyer RA, Mann GJ. Whole-genome landscapes of major melanoma subtypes. Nature. 2017;545:175–80.
17. Newell F, Kong Y, Wilmott JS, Johansson PA, Ferguson PM, Cui C, Li Z, Kazakoff SH, Burke H, Dodds TJ, Patch AM, Nones K, Tembe V, Shang P, van der Weyden L, Wong K, Holmes O, Lo S, Leonard C, Wood S, Xu Q, Rawson RV, Mukhopadhyay P, Dummer R, Levesque MP, Jönsson G, Wang X, Yeh I, Wu H, Joseph N, Bastian BC, Long GV, Spillane AJ, Shannon KF, Thompson JF, Saw RPM, Adams DJ, Si L, Pearson JV, Hayward NK, Waddell N, Mann GJ, Guo J, Scolyer RA. Whole-genome landscape of mucosal melanoma reveals diverse drivers and therapeutic targets. Nat Commun. 2019;10(1):3163.
18. Shain AH, Bastian BC. From melanocytes to melanomas. Nat Rev Cancer. 2016;16(6):345–58.
19. Sun X, Zhang N, Yin C, Zhu B, Li X. Ultraviolet radiation and melanomagenesis: from mechanism to immunotherapy. Front Oncol. 2020;10:951.
20. Sini MC, Doneddu V, Paliogiannis P, Casula M, Colombino M, Manca A, Botti G, Ascierto PA, Lissia A, Cossu A, Palmieri G for the Italian Melanoma Intergroup. Genetic alterations in main candidate genes during melanoma progression. Oncotarget. 2018;9:8531–41.

21. Krauthammer M, Kong Y, Ha BH, Evans P, Bacchiocchi A, McCusker JP, Cheng E, Davis MJ, Goh G, Choi M, Ariyan S, Narayan D, Dutton-Regester K, Capatana A, Holman EC, Bosenberg M, Sznol M, Kluger HM, Brash DE, Stern DF, Materin MA, Lo RS, Mane S, Ma S, Kidd KK, Hayward NK, Lifton RP, Schlessinger J, Boggon TJ, Halaban R. Exome sequencing identifies recurrent somatic RAC1 mutations in melanoma. Nat Genet. 2012;44:1006–14.
22. Hodis E, Watson IR, Kryukov GV, Arold ST, Imielinski M, Theurillat JP, Nickerson E, Auclair D, Li L, Place C, Dicara D, Ramos AH, Lawrence MS, Cibulskis K, Sivachenko A, Voet D, Saksena G, Stransky N, Onofrio RC, Winckler W, Ardlie K, Wagle N, Wargo J, Chong K, Morton DL, Stemke-Hale K, Chen G, Noble M, Meyerson M, Ladbury JE, Davies MA, Gershenwald JE, Wagner SN, Hoon DS, Schadendorf D, Lander ES, Gabriel SB, Getz G, Garraway LA, Chin L. A landscape of driver mutations in melanoma. Cell. 2012;150:251–63.
23. de Unamuno Bustos B, Murria Estal R, Pérez Simó G, de Juan Jimenez I, Escutia Muñoz B, Rodríguez Serna M, Alegre de Miquel V, Llavador Ros M, Ballester Sánchez R, Nagore Enguídanos E, Palanca Suela S, Botella Estrada R. Towards personalized medicine in melanoma: implementation of a clinical next-generation sequencing panel. Sci Rep. 2017;7(1):495.
24. Leiter U, Eigentler T, Garbe C. Epidemiology of skin cancer. Adv Exp Med Biol. 2014;810:120–40.
25. Gu F, Chen TH, Pfeiffer RM, Fargnoli MC, Calista D, Ghiorzo P, Peris K, Puig S, Menin C, De Nicolo A, Rodolfo M, Pellegrini C, Pastorino L, Evangelou E, Zhang T, Hua X, Della Valle CT, Timothy Bishop D, MacGregor S, Iles MI, Law MH, Cust A, Brown KM, Stratigos AJ, Nagore E, Chanock S, Shi J, Consortium MM, Consortium M, Landi MT. Combining common genetic variants and non-genetic risk factors to predict risk of cutaneous melanoma. Hum Mol Genet. 2018;27:4145–56.
26. Ransohoff KJ, Jaju PD, Tang JY, Carbone M, Leachman S, Sarin KY. Familial skin cancer syndromes increased melanoma risk. J Am Acad Dermatol. 2016;74:423–34.
27. Landi MT, Bishop DT, MacGregor S, Machiela MJ, Stratigos AJ, Ghiorzo P, Brossard M, Calista D, Choi J, Fargnoli MC, Zhang T, Rodolfo M, Trower AJ, Menin C, Martinez J, Hadjisavvas A, Song L, Stefanaki I, Scolyer R, Yang R, Goldstein AM, Potrony M, Kypreou KP, Pastorino L, Queirolo P, Pellegrini C, Cattaneo L, Zawistowski M, Gimenez-Xavier P, Rodriguez A, Elefanti L, Manoukian S, Rivoltini L, Smith BH, Loizidou MA, Del Regno L, Massi D, Mandala M, Khosrotehrani K, Akslen LA, Amos CI, Andresen PA, Avril MF, Azizi E, Soyer HP, Bataille V, Dalmasso B, Bowdler LM, Burdon KP, Chen WV, Codd V, Craig JE, Dębniak T, Falchi M, Fang S, Friedman E, Simi S, Galan P, Garcia-Casado Z, Gillanders EM, Gordon S, Green A, Gruis NA, Hansson J, Harland M, Harris J, Helsing P, Henders A, Hočevar M, Höiom V, Hunter D, Ingvar C, Kumar R, Lang J, Lathrop GM, Lee JE, Li X, Lubiński J, Mackie RM, Malt M, Malvehy J, McAloney K, Mohamdi H, Molven A, Moses EK, Neale RE, Novaković S, Nyholt DR, Olsson H, Orr N, Fritsche LG, Puig-Butille JA, Qureshi AA, Radford-Smith GL, Randerson-Moor J, Requena C, Rowe C, Samani NJ, Sanna M, Schadendorf D, Schulze HJ, Simms LA, Smithers M, Song F, Swerdlow AJ, van der Stoep N, Kukutsch NA, Visconti A, Wallace L, Ward SV, Wheeler L, Sturm RA, Hutchinson A, Jones K, Malasky M, Vogt A, Zhou W, Pooley KA, Elder DE, Han J, Hicks B, Hayward NK, Kanetsky PA, Brummett C, Montgomery GW, Olsen CM, Hayward C, Dunning AM, Martin NG, Evangelou E, Mann GJ, Long G, PDP P, Easton DF, Barrett JH, Cust AE, Abecasis G, Duffy DL, Whiteman DC, Gogas H, De Nicolo A, Tucker MA, Newton-Bishop JA, GenoMEL Consortium; Q-MEGA and QTWIN Investigators; ATHENS Melanoma Study Group; 23andMe; SDH Study Group; IBD Investigators; Essen-Heidelberg Investigators; AMFS Investigators; MelaNostrum Consortium, Peris K, Chanock SJ, Demenais F, Brown KM, Puig S, Nagore E, Shi J, Iles MM, Law MH. Genome-wide association meta-analyses combining multiple risk phenotypes provide insights into the genetic architecture of cutaneous melanoma susceptibility. Nat Genet. 2020;52(5):494–504.
28. Leachman SA, Lucero OM, Sampson JE, Cassidy P, Bruno W, Queirolo P, Ghiorzo P. Identification, genetic testing, and management of hereditary melanoma. Cancer Metastasis Rev. 2017;36:77–90.

29. Newton-Bishop J, Bishop DT, Harland M. Melanoma genomics. Acta Derm Venereol. 2020;100(11):adv00138.
30. Toussi A, Mans N, Welborn J, Kiuru M. Germline mutations predisposing to melanoma. J Cutan Pathol. 2020;47(7):606–16.
31. Viros A, Sanchez-Laorden B, Pedersen M, Furney SJ, Rae J, Hogan K, Ejiama S, Girotti MR, Cook M, Dhomen N, Marais R. Ultraviolet radiation accelerates BRAF-driven melanomagenesis by targeting TP53. Nature. 2014;511:478–82.
32. Khoo KH, Verma CS, Lane DP. Drugging the p53 pathway: understanding the route to clinical efficacy. Nat Rev Drug Discov. 2014;13:217–36.
33. Kocik J, Machula M, Wisniewska A, Surmiak E, Holak TA, Skalniak L. Helping the released guardian: drug combinations for supporting the anticancer activity of HDM2 (MDM2) antagonists. Cancers (Basel). 2019;11(7):1014.
34. Heidenreich B, Nagore E, Rachakonda PS, Garcia-Casado Z, Requena C, Traves V, Becker J, Soufir N, Hemminki K, Kumar R. Telomerase reverse transcriptase promoter mutations in primary cutaneous melanoma. Nat Commun. 2014;5:3401.
35. Shi J, Yang XR, Ballew B, Rotunno M, Calista D, Fargnoli MC, Ghiorzo P, Bressac-de Paillerets B, Nagore E, Avril MF, Caporaso NE, ML MM, Cullen M, Wang Z, Zhang X, NCI DCEG Cancer Sequencing Working Group; NCI DCEG Cancer Genomics Research Laboratory; French Familial Melanoma Study Group, Bruno W, Pastorino L, Queirolo P, Banuls-Roca J, Garcia-Casado Z, Vaysse A, Mohamdi H, Riazalhosseini Y, Foglio M, Jouenne F, Hua X, Hyland PL, Yin J, Vallabhaneni H, Chai W, Minghetti P, Pellegrini C, Ravichandran S, Eggermont A, Lathrop M, Peris K, Scarra GB, Landi G, Savage SA, Sampson JN, He J, Yeager M, Goldin LR, Demenais F, Chanock SJ, Tucker MA, Goldstein AM, Liu Y, Landi MT. Rare missense variants in POT1 predispose to familial cutaneous malignant melanoma. Nat Genet. 2014;46(5):482–6.
36. Heidenreich B, Kumar R. TERT promoter mutations in telomere biology. Mutat Res. 2017;771:15–31.
37. Hafezi F, Perez BD. The *solo* play of *TERT* promoter mutations. Cell. 2020;9(3):749.
38. Abdel-Rahman MH, Pilarski R, Cebulla CM, Massengill JB, Christopher BN, Boru G, Hovland P, Davidorf FH. Germline BAP1 mutation predisposes to uveal melanoma, lung adenocarcinoma, meningioma, and other cancers. J Med Genet. 2011;48(12):856–9.
39. Carbone M, Harbour JW, Brugarolas J, Bononi A, Pagano I, Dey A, Krausz T, Pass HI, Yang H, Gaudino G. Biological mechanisms and clinical significance of BAP1 mutations in human cancer. Cancer Discov. 2020;10(8):1103–20.
40. Potrony M, Badenas C, Aguilera P, Puig-Butille JA, Carrera C, Malvehy J, Puig S. Update in genetic susceptibility in melanoma. Ann Transl Med. 2015;3(15):210.
41. Sharpless E, Chin L. The INK4a/ARF locus and melanoma. Oncogene. 2003;22(20):3092–8.
42. Freedberg DE, Rigas SH, Russak J, Gai W, Kaplow M, Osman I, Turner F, Randerson-Moor JA, Houghton A, Busam K, Timothy Bishop D, Bastian BC, Newton-Bishop JA, Polsky D. Frequent p16-independent inactivation of p14ARF in human melanoma. J Natl Cancer Inst. 2008;100(11):784–95.
43. Begg CB, Orlow I, Hummer AJ, Armstrong BK, Kricker A, Marrett LD, Millikan RC, Gruber SB, Anton-Culver H, Zanetti R, Gallagher RP, Dwyer T, Rebbeck TR, Mitra N, Busam K, From L, Berwick M, Genes Environment and Melanoma Study Group. Lifetime risk of melanoma in CDKN2A mutation carriers in a population-based sample. J Natl Cancer Inst. 2005;97(20):1507–15.
44. Casula M, Colombino M, Satta MP, Cossu A, Lissia A, Budroni M, Simeone E, Calemma R, Loddo C, Caracò C, Mozzillo N, Daponte A, Comella G, Canzanella S, Guida M, Castello G, Ascierto PA, Palmieri G, Italian Melanoma Intergroup. Factors predicting the occurrence of germline mutations in candidate genes among patients with cutaneous malignant melanoma from South Italy. Eur J Cancer. 2007;43(1):137–43.
45. Cossu A, Casula M, Cesaraccio R, Lissia A, Colombino M, Sini MC, Budroni M, Tanda F, Paliogiannis P, Palmieri G. Epidemiology and genetic susceptibility of malignant melanoma in North Sardinia, Italy. Eur J Cancer Prev. 2017;26:263–7.

46. Palmieri G, Capone ME, Ascierto ML, Gentilcore G, Stroncek DF, Casula M, Sini MC, Palla M, Mozzillo N, Ascierto PA. Main roads to melanoma. J Transl Med. 2009;7:86.
47. Kim JE, Leung E, Baguley BC, Finlay GJ. Heterogeneity of expression of epithelial-mesenchymal transition markers in melanocytes and melanoma cell lines. Front Genet. 2013;4:97.
48. Wenzina J, Holzner S, Puujalka E, Cheng PF, Forsthuber A, Neumüller K, Schossleitner K, Lichtenberger BM, Levesque MP, Petzelbauer P. Inhibition of p38/MK2 signaling prevents vascular invasion of melanoma. J Invest Dermatol. 2020;140(4):878–890.e5.
49. Caramel J, Papadogeorgakis E, Hill L, Browne GJ, Richard G, Wierinckx A, Saldanha G, Osborne J, Hutchinson P, Tse G, Lachuer J, Puisieux A, Pringle JH, Ansieau S, Tulchinsky E. A switch in the expression of embryonic EMT-inducers drives the development of malignant melanoma. Cancer Cell. 2013;24(4):466–80.
50. Rebocho AP, Marais R. ARAF acts as a scaffold to stabilize BRAF:CRAF heterodimers. Oncogene. 2013;32(26):3207–12.
51. Ascierto PA, Kirkwood JM, Grob JJ, Simeone E, Grimaldi AM, Maio M, Palmieri G, Testori A, Marincola FM, Mozzillo N. The role of BRAF V600 mutation in melanoma. J Transl Med. 2012;10:85.
52. Davies H, Bignell G, Cox C, Stephens P, Edkins S, Clegg S, Teague J, Woffendin H, Garnett M, Bottomley W, Davis N, Dicks E, Ewing R, Floyd Y, Gray K, Hall S, Hawes R, Hughes J, Kosmidou V, Menzies A, Mould C, Parker A, Stevens C, Watt S, Hooper S, Wilson R, Jayatilake H, Gusterson B, Cooper C, Shipley J, Hargrave D, Pritchard-Jones K, Maitland N, Chenevix-Trench G, Riggins G, Bigner D, Palmieri G, Cossu A, Flanagan A, Nicholson A, Ho J, Leung S, Yuen S, Weber B, Seigler H, Darrow T, Paterson H, Marais R, Marshall C, Wooster R, Stratton M, Futreal P. Mutations of the BRAF gene in human cancer. Nature. 2002;417:949–54.
53. Pollock PM, Harper UL, Hansen KS, et al. High frequency of BRAF mutations in nevi. Nat Genet. 2003;33:19–20.
54. Mar VJ, Wong SQ, Li J, Scolyer RA, McLean C, Papenfuss AT, Tothill RW, Kakavand H, Mann GJ, Thompson JF, Behren A, Cebon JS, Wolfe R, Kelly JW, Dobrovic A, McArthur GA. BRAF/NRAS wild-type melanomas have a high mutation load correlating with histologic and molecular signatures of UV damage. Clin Cancer Res. 2013;19:4589–98.
55. Sullivan RJ, Flaherty KT. Resistance to braf-targeted therapy in melanoma. Eur J Cancer. 2013;49:1297–304.
56. Gershenwald JE, Scolyer RA, Hess KR, et al. Melanoma staging: evidence-based changes in the American Joint Committee on Cancer eighth edition cancer staging manual. CA Cancer J Clin. 2017;67(6):472–92.
57. Ascierto PA, McArthur GA, Dréno B, Atkinson V, Liszkay G, Di Giacomo AM, Mandalà M, Demidov L, Stroyakovskiy D, Thomas L, de la Cruz-Merino L, Dutriaux C, Garbe C, Yan Y, Wongchenko M, Chang I, Hsu JJ, Koralek DO, Rooney I, Ribas A, Larkin J. Cobimetinib combined with vemurafenib in advanced BRAF(V600)-mutant melanoma (coBRIM): updated efficacy results from a randomised, double-blind, phase 3 trial. Lancet Oncol. 2016;17(9):1248–60.
58. Long GV, Flaherty KT, Stroyakovskiy D, Gogas H, Levchenko E, de Braud F, Larkin J, Garbe C, Jouary T, Hauschild A, Chiarion-Sileni V, Lebbe C, Mandalà M, Millward M, Arance A, Bondarenko I, Haanen JBAG, Hansson J, Utikal J, Ferraresi V, Mohr P, Probachai V, Schadendorf D, Nathan P, Robert C, Ribas A, Davies MA, Lane SR, Legos JJ, Mookerjee B, Grob JJ. Dabrafenib plus trametinib versus dabrafenib monotherapy in patients with metastatic BRAF V600E/K-mutant melanoma: long-term survival and safety analysis of a phase 3 study. Ann Oncol. 2017;28(7):1631–9.
59. Long GV, Hauschild A, Santinami M, Atkinson V, Mandalà M, Chiarion-Sileni V, Larkin J, Nyakas M, Dutriaux C, Haydon A, Robert C, Mortier L, Schachter J, Schadendorf D, Lesimple T, Plummer R, Ji R, Zhang P, Mookerjee B, Legos J, Kefford R, Dummer R,

Kirkwood JM. Adjuvant Dabrafenib plus Trametinib in Stage III BRAF-mutated melanoma. N Engl J Med. 2017;377(19):1813–23.

60. Hauschild A, Dummer R, Schadendorf D, Santinami M, Atkinson V, Mandalà M, Chiarion-Sileni V, Larkin J, Nyakas M, Dutriaux C, Haydon A, Robert C, Mortier L, Schachter J, Lesimple T, Plummer R, Dasgupta K, Haas T, Shilkrut M, Gasal E, Kefford R, Kirkwood JM, Long GV. Longer follow-up confirms relapse-free survival benefit with adjuvant Dabrafenib plus Trametinib in patients with resected BRAF V600-mutant Stage III melanoma. J Clin Oncol. 2018;36(35):3441–9.

61. Long GV, Eroglu Z, Infante J, Patel S, Daud A, Johnson DB, Gonzalez R, Kefford R, Hamid O, Schuchter L, Cebon J, Sharfman W, McWilliams R, Sznol M, Redhu S, Gasal E, Mookerjee B, Weber J, Flaherty KT. Long-term outcomes in patients with BRAF V600-mutant metastatic melanoma who received Dabrafenib combined with Trametinib. J Clin Oncol. 2018;36:667–73.

62. Ascierto PA, Borgognoni L, Botti G, Guida M, Marchetti P, Mocellin S, Muto P, Palmieri G, Patuzzo R, Quaglino P, Stanganelli I, Caracò C. New paradigm for stage III melanoma: from surgery to adjuvant treatment. J Transl Med. 2019;17(1):266.

63. Ascierto PA, Ferrucci PF, Fisher R, Del Vecchio M, Atkinson V, Schmidt H, Schachter J, Queirolo P, Long GV, Di Giacomo AM, Svane IM, Lotem M, Bar-Sela G, Couture F, Mookerjee B, Ghori R, Ibrahim N, Moreno BH, Ribas A. Dabrafenib, trametinib and pembrolizumab or placebo in BRAF-mutant melanoma. Nat Med. 2019;25(6):941–6.

64. Robert C, Grob JJ, Stroyakovskiy D, Karaszewska B, Hauschild A, Levchenko E, Chiarion Sileni V, Schachter J, Garbe C, Bondarenko I, Gogas H, Mandalá M, Haanen JBAG, Lebbé C, Mackiewicz A, Rutkowski P, Nathan PD, Ribas A, Davies MA, Flaherty KT, Burgess P, Tan M, Gasal E, Voi M, Schadendorf D, Long GV. Five-year outcomes with Dabrafenib plus Trametinib in metastatic melanoma. N Engl J Med. 2019;381(7):626–36.

65. Ascierto PA, Dummer R, Gogas HJ, Flaherty KT, Arance A, Mandala M, Liszkay G, Garbe C, Schadendorf D, Krajsova I, Gutzmer R, de Groot JWB, Loquai C, Gollerkeri A, Pickard MD, Robert C. Update on tolerability and overall survival in COLUMBUS: landmark analysis of a randomised phase 3 trial of encorafenib plus binimetinib vs vemurafenib or encorafenib in patients with BRAF V600-mutant melanoma. Eur J Cancer. 2020;126:33–44.

66. Menzer C, Menzies AM, Carlino MS, Reijers I, Groen EJ, Eigentler T, de Groot JWB, van der Veldt AAM, Johnson DB, Meiss F, Schlaak M, Schilling B, Westgeest HM, Gutzmer R, Pföhler C, Meier F, Zimmer L, Suijkerbuijk KPM, Haalck T, Thoms KM, Herbschleb K, Leichsenring J, Menzer A, Kopp-Schneider A, Long GV, Kefford R, Enk A, Blank CU, Hassel JC. Targeted therapy in advanced melanoma with rare *BRAF* mutations. J Clin Oncol. 2019;37(33):3142–51.

67. Coit DG, Thompson JA, Albertini MR, Barker C, Carson WE, Contreras C, Daniels GA, DiMaio D, Fields RC, Fleming MD, Freeman M, Galan A, Gastman B, Guild V, Johnson D, Joseph RW, Lange JR, Nath S, Olszanski AJ, Ott P, Gupta AP, Ross MI, Salama AK, Skitzki J, Sosman J, Swetter SM, Tanabe KK, Wuthrick E, McMillian NR, Engh AM. Cutaneous melanoma, version 2.2019, NCCN clinical practice guidelines in oncology. J Natl Compr Cancer Netw. 2019;17:367–402.

68. Colombino M, Capone M, Lissia A, Cossu A, Rubino C, De Giorgi V, Massi D, Fonsatti E, Staibano S, Nappi O, Pagani E, Casula M, Manca A, Sini M, Franco R, Botti G, Caracò C, Mozzillo N, Ascierto PA, Palmieri G. BRAF/NRAS mutation frequencies among primary tumors and metastases in patients with melanoma. J Clin Oncol. 2012;30:2522–9.

69. Casula M, Colombino M, Manca A, et al. Italian Melanoma Intergroup (IMI). Low levels of genetic heterogeneity in matched lymph node metastases from melanoma patients. J Invest Dermatol. 2016;136:1917–20.

70. Yancovitz M, Litterman A, Yoon J, et al. Intra- and inter-tumor heterogeneity of BRAF(V600E) mutations in primary and metastatic melanoma. PLoS One. 2012;7(1):e29336.

71. Colombino M, Rozzo C, Paliogiannis P, Casula M, Manca A, Doneddu V, Fedeli MA, Sini MC, Palomba G, Pisano M, Ascierto PA, Caracò C, Lissia A, Cossu A, Palmieri G. Comparison of

BRAF mutation screening strategies in a large real-life series of advanced melanoma patients. J Clin Med. 2020;9(8):E2430.

72. Ascierto PA, Bifulco C, Palmieri G, Peters S, Sidiropoulos N. Pre-analytic variables and tissue steward-ship for reliable next-generation sequencing (NGS) clinical analysis. J Mol Diagnostics. 2019;21(5):756–67.

73. Planchard D, Besse B, Groen HJM, Souquet PJ, Quoix E, Baik CS, Barlesi F, Kim TM, Mazieres J, Novello S, Rigas JR, Upalawanna A, D'Amelio AM Jr, Zhang P, Mookerjee B, Johnson BE. Dabrafenib plus trametinib in patients with previously treated BRAF(V600E)-mutant metastatic non-small cell lung cancer: an open-label, multicentre phase 2 trial. Lancet Oncol. 2016;17:984–93.

74. Planchard D, Smit EF, Groen HJM, Mazieres J, Besse B, Helland Å, Giannone V, D'Amelio AM Jr, Zhang P, Mookerjee B, Johnson BE. Dabrafenib plus trametinib in patients with previously untreated BRAFV600E-mutant metastatic non-small-cell lung cancer: an open-label, phase 2 trial. Lancet Oncol. 2017;18:1307–16.

75. Kopetz S, Grothey A, Yaeger R, Van Cutsem E, Desai J, Yoshino T, Wasan H, Ciardiello F, Loupakis F, Hong YS, Steeghs N, Guren TK, Arkenau HT, Garcia-Alfonso P, Pfeiffer P, Orlov S, Lonardi S, Elez E, Kim TW, Schellens JHM, Guo C, Krishnan A, Dekervel J, Morris V, Calvo Ferrandiz A, Tarpgaard LS, Braun M, Gollerkeri A, Keir C, Maharry K, Pickard M, Christy-Bittel J, Anderson L, Sandor V, Tabernero J. Encorafenib, Binimetinib, and Cetuximab in BRAF V600E-mutated colorectal cancer. N Engl J Med. 2019;381(17):1632–43.

76. Van Cutsem E, Huijberts S, Grothey A, Yaeger R, Cuyle PJ, Elez E, Fakih M, Montagut C, Peeters M, Yoshino T, Wasan H, Desai J, Ciardiello F, Gollerkeri A, Christy-Bittel J, Maharry K, Sandor V, Schellens JM, Kopetz S, Tabernero J. Binimetinib, Encorafenib, and Cetuximab triplet therapy for patients with BRAF V600E-mutant metastatic colorectal cancer: safety lead-in results from the phase III BEACON colorectal cancer study. J Clin Oncol. 2019;37(17):1460–9.

77. Dankner M, Rose AAN, Rajkumar S, Siegel PM, Watson IR. Classifying BRAF alterations in cancer: new rational therapeutic strategies for actionable mutations. Oncogene. 2018;37:3183–99.

78. Bracht JWP, Karachaliou N, Bivona T, Lanman RB, Faull I, Nagy RJ, Drozdowskyj A, Berenguer J, Fernandez-Bruno M, Molina-Vila MA, Rosell R. BRAF Mutations classes I, II, and III in NSCLC patients included in the SLLIP trial: the need for a new pre-clinical treatment rationale. Cancers (Basel). 2019;11:1381.

79. Yaeger R, Corcoran RB. Targeting alterations in the RAF-MEK pathway. Cancer Discov. 2019;9:329–41.

80. Frisone D, Friedlaender A, Malapelle U, Banna G, Addeo A. A BRAF new world. Crit Rev Oncol Hematol. 2020;152:103008.

81. Jenkins RW, Sullivan RJ. NRAS mutant melanoma: an overview for the clinician for melanoma management. Melanoma Manag. 2016;3(1):47–59.

82. Mooz J, Oberoi-Khanuja TK, Harms GS, Wang W, Jaiswal BS, Seshagiri S, Tikkanen R, Rajalingam K. Dimerization of the kinase ARAF promotes MAPK pathway activation and cell migration. Sci Signal. 2014;7(337):ra73.

83. Poulikakos PI, Zhang C, Bollag G, Shokat KM, Rosen N. RAF inhibitors transactivate RAF dimers and ERK signalling in cells with wild-type BRAF. Nature. 2010;464:427–30.

84. Heidorn SJ, Milagre C, Whittaker S, Nourry A, Niculescu-Duvas I, Dhomen N, Hussain J, Reis-Filho JS, Springer CJ, Pritchard C, Marais R. Kinase-dead BRAF and oncogenic RAS cooperate to drive tumour progression through CRAF. Cell. 2010;140:209–21.

85. Ascierto PA, Schadendorf D, Berking C, et al. MEK162 for patients with advanced melanoma harbouring NRAS or Val600 BRAF mutations: a non-randomised, open-label phase 2 study. Lancet Oncol. 2013;14(3):249–56.

86. Dummer R, Schadendorf D, Ascierto PA, et al. Binimetinib versus dacarbazine in patients with advanced NRAS-mutant melanoma (NEMO): a multicentre, open-label, randomised, phase 3 trial. Lancet Oncol. 2017;18:435–45.

87. Meng D, Carvajal RD. KIT as an oncogenic driver in melanoma: an update on clinical development. Am J Clin Dermatol. 2019;20(3):315–23.
88. Curtin JA, Busam K, Pinkel D, Bastian BC. Somatic activation of KIT in distinct subtypes of melanoma. J Clin Oncol. 2006;24(26):4340–6.
89. Handolias D, Salemi R, Murray W, et al. Mutations in KIT occur at low frequency in melanomas arising from anatomical sites associated with chronic and intermittent sun exposure. Pigment Cell Melanoma Res. 2010;23(2):210–5.
90. Lyle M, Long GV. Diagnosis and treatment of KIT-mutant metastatic melanoma. J Clin Oncol. 2013;31(26):3176–81.
91. Kim KB, Eton O, Davis DW, et al. Phase II trial of imatinib mesylate in patients with metastatic melanoma. Br J Cancer. 2008;99(5):734–40.
92. Carvajal RD, Antonescu CR, Wolchok JD, et al. KIT as a therapeutic target in metastatic melanoma. JAMA. 2011;305(22):2327–34.
93. Hodi FS, Corless CL, Giobbie-Hurder A, et al. Imatinib for melanomas harboring mutationally activated or amplified KIT arising on mucosal, acral, and chronically sun-damaged skin. J Clin Oncol. 2013;31(26):3182–90.
94. Kiuru M, Busam KJ. The NF1 gene in tumor syndromes and melanoma. Lab Investig. 2017;97(2):146–57.
95. Nissan MH, Pratilas CA, Jones AM, Ramirez R, Won H, Liu C, Tiwari S, Kong L, Hanrahan AJ, Yao Z, Merghoub T, Ribas A, Chapman PB, Yaeger R, Taylor BS, Schultz N, Berger MF, Rosen N, Solit DB. Loss of NF1 in cutaneous melanoma is associated with RAS activation and MEK dependence. Cancer Res. 2014;74:2340–50.
96. Krauthammer M, Kong Y, Bacchiocchi A, Evans P, Pornputtapong N, Wu C, McCusker JP, Ma S, Cheng E, Straub R, Serin M, Bosenberg M, Ariyan S, Narayan D, Sznol M, Kluger HM, Mane S, Schlessinger J, Lifton RP, Halaban R. Exome sequencing identifies recurrent mutations in NF1 and RASopathy genes in sun-exposed melanomas. Nat Genet. 2015;47:996–1002.
97. Halaban R, Krauthammer M. RASopathy gene mutations in melanoma. J Invest Dermatol. 2016;136(9):1755–9.
98. Eroglu Z, Zaretsky JM, Hu-Lieskovan S, Kim DW, Algazi A, Johnson DB, Liniker E, Kong B, Munhoz R, Rapisuwon S, Gherardini PF, Chmielowski B, Wang X, Shintaku IP, Wei C, Sosman JA, Joseph RW, Postow MA, Carlino MS, Hwu WJ, Scolyer RA, Messina J, Cochran AJ, Long GV, Ribas A. High response rate to PD-1 blockade in desmoplastic melanomas. Nature. 2018;553(7688):347–50.
99. Manca A, Lissia A, Cossu A, Rubino C, Ascierto PA, Stanganelli I, Palmieri G. Mutations in ERBB4 may play a minor role in melanoma pathogenesis. J Invest Dermatol. 2013;133:1685–7.
100. Milewska M, Cremona M, Morgan C, O'Shea J, Carr A, Vellanki SH, Hopkins AM, Toomey S, Madden SF, Hennessy BT, Eustace AJ. Development of a personalized therapeutic strategy for ERBB-gene-mutated cancers. Ther Adv Med Oncol. 2018;10:1758834017746040.
101. Aguissa-Touré AH, Li G. Genetic alterations of PTEN in human melanoma. Cell Mol Life Sci. 2012;69(9):1475–91.
102. Conde-Perez A, Larue L. PTEN and melanomagenesis. Future Oncol. 2012;8(9):1109–20.
103. Perna D, Karreth FA, Rust AG, Perez-Mancera PA, Rashid M, Iorio F, Alifrangis C, Arends MJ, Bosenberg MW, Bollag G, Tuveson DA, Adams DJ. BRAF inhibitor resistance mediated by the AKT pathway in an oncogenic BRAF mouse melanoma model. Proc Natl Acad Sci U S A. 2015;112(6):E536–45.
104. Lim SY, Menzies AM, Rizos H. Mechanisms and strategies to overcome resistance to molecularly targeted therapy for melanoma. Cancer. 2017;123(S11):2118–29.
105. Cabrita R, Mitra S, Sanna A, Ekedahl H, Lövgren K, Olsson H, Ingvar C, Isaksson K, Lauss M, Carneiro A, Jönsson G. The role of PTEN loss in immune escape, melanoma prognosis and therapy response. Cancers (Basel). 2020;12(3):742.

106. Bucheit AD, Chen G, Siroy A, Tetzlaff M, Broaddus R, Milton D, Fox P, Bassett R, Hwu P, Gershenwald JE, Lazar AJ, Davies MA. Complete loss of PTEN protein expression correlates with shorter time to brain metastasis and survival in stage IIIB/C melanoma patients with BRAFV600 mutations. Clin Cancer Res. 2014;20(21):5527–36.

107. Siroy AE, Boland GM, Milton DR, Roszik J, Frankian S, Malke J, Haydu L, Prieto VG, Tetzlaff M, Ivan D, Wang WL, Torres-Cabala C, Curry J, Roy-Chowdhuri S, Broaddus R, Rashid A, Stewart J, Gershenwald JE, Amaria RN, Patel SP, Papadopoulos NE, Bedikian A, Hwu WJ, Hwu P, Diab A, Woodman SE, Aldape KD, Luthra R, Patel KP, Shaw KR, Mills GB, Mendelsohn J, Meric-Bernstam F, Kim KB, Routbort MJ, Lazar AJ, Davies MA. Beyond BRAF(V600): clinical mutation panel testing by next-generation sequencing in advanced melanoma. J Invest Dermatol. 2015;135:508–15.

108. Kim S, Jeong S. Mutation hotspots in the β-catenin gene: lessons from the human cancer genome databases. Mol Cells. 2019;42(1):8–16.

109. Gunawan M, Venkatesan N, Loh JT, Wong JF, Berger H, Neo WH, et al. The methyltransferase Ezh2 controls cell adhesion and migration through direct methylation of the extranuclear regulatory protein Talin. Nat Immunol. 2015;16:505–16.

110. Yu H, Ma M, Yan J, Xu L, Yu J, Dai J, Xu T, Tang H, Wu X, Li S, Lian B, Mao L, Chi Z, Cui C, Guo J, Kong Y. Identification of coexistence of BRAF V600E mutation and EZH2 gain specifically in melanoma as a promising target for combination therapy. J Transl Med. 2017;15(1):243.

111. Massi D, Romano E, Rulli E, Merelli B, Nassini R, De Logu F, Bieche I, Baroni G, Cattaneo L, Xue G, Mandalà M. Baseline β-catenin, programmed death-ligand 1 expression and tumour-infiltrating lymphocytes predict response and poor prognosis in BRAF inhibitor-treated melanoma patients. Eur J Cancer. 2017;78:70–81.

112. Nsengimana J, Laye J, Filia A, O'Shea S, Muralidhar S, Poźniak J, Droop A, Chan M, Walker C, Parkinson L, Gascoyne J, Mell T, Polso M, Jewell R, Randerson-Moor J, Cook GP, Bishop DT, Newton-Bishop J. β-Catenin-mediated immune evasion pathway frequently operates in primary cutaneous melanomas. J Clin Invest. 2018;128(5):2048–63.

113. Luke JJ, Bao R, Sweis RF, Spranger S, Gajewski T. WNT/β-catenin pathway activation correlates with immune exclusion across human cancers. Clin Cancer Res. 2019;25(10):3074–83.

114. Massi D, Rulli E, Cossa M, Valeri B, Rodolfo M, Merelli B, De Logu F, Nassini R, Del Vecchio M, Di Guardo L, De Penni R, Guida M, Sileni VC, Di Giacomo AM, Tucci M, Occelli M, Portelli F, Vallacchi V, Consoli F, Quaglino P, Queirolo P, Baroni G, Carnevale-Schianca F, Cattaneo L, Minisini A, Palmieri G, Rivoltini L, Mandalà M, Italian Melanoma Intergroup. The density and spatial tissue distribution of CD8(+) and CD163(+) immune cells predict response and outcome in melanoma patients receiving MAPK inhibitors. J Immunother Cancer. 2019;7(1):308.

115. Lissanu Deribe Y, Shi Y, Rai K, Nezi L, Amin SB, Wu CC, Akdemir KC, Mahdavi M, Peng Q, Chang QE, Hornigold K, Arold ST, Welch HC, Garraway LA, Chin L. Truncating PREX2 mutations activate its GEF activity and alter gene expression regulation in NRAS-mutant melanoma. Proc Natl Acad Sci U S A. 2016;113:E1296–305.

116. Wangari-Talbot J, Chen S. Genetics of melanoma. Front Genet. 2013;3:330.

117. D'mello SA, Flanagan JU, Green TN, Leung EY, Askarian-Amiri ME, Joseph WR, McCrystal MR, Isaacs RJ, Shaw JH, Furneaux CE, During MJ, Finlay GJ, Baguley BC, Kalev-Zylinska ML. Evidence that GRIN2A mutations in melanoma correlate with decreased survival. Front Oncol. 2014;3:333.

118. Cannon AC, Uribe-Alvarez C, Chernoff J. RAC1 as a therapeutic target in malignant melanoma. Trends Cancer. 2020;6(6):478–88.

119. Lionarons DA, Hancock DC, Rana S, East P, Moore C, Murillo MM, Carvalho J, Spencer-Dene B, Herbert E, Stamp G, Damry D, Calado DP, Rosewell I, Fritsch R, Neubig RR, Molina-Arcas M, Downward J. RAC1^{P29S} induces a mesenchymal phenotypic switch via serum response factor to promote melanoma development and therapy resistance. Cancer Cell. 2019;36(1):68–83.e9.

120. Mar VJ, Wong SQ, Logan A, Nguyen T, Cebon J, Kelly JW, Wolfe R, Dobrovic A, McLean C, McArthur GA. Clinical and pathological associations of the activating RAC1 P29S mutation in primary cutaneous melanoma. Pigment Cell Melanoma Res. 2014;27(6):1117–25.
121. Duan Y, Tian L, Gao Q, Liang L, Zhang W, Yang Y, Zheng Y, Pan E, Li S, Tang N. Chromatin remodeling gene ARID2 targets cyclin D1 and cyclin E1 to suppress hepatoma cell progression. Oncotarget. 2016;7:45863–75.
122. Cimino PJ, Kung Y, Warrick JI, Chang SH, Keene CD. Mutational status of IDH1 in uveal melanoma. Exp Mol Pathol. 2016;100(3):476–81.
123. Moran B, Silva R, Perry AS, Gallagher WM. Epigenetics of malignant melanoma. Semin Cancer Biol. 2018;51:80–8.
124. Garraway LA, Widlund HR, Rubin MA, Getz G, Berger AJ, Ramaswamy S, Beroukhim R, Milner DA, Granter SR, Du J, Lee C, Wagner SN, Li C, Golub TR, Rimm DL, Meyerson ML, Fisher DE, Sellers WR. Integrative genomic analyses identify MITF as a lineage survival oncogene amplified in malignant melanoma. Nature. 2005;436(7047):117–22.
125. Seberg HE, Van Otterloo E, Cornell RA. Beyond MITF: Multiple transcription factors directly regulate the cellular phenotype in melanocytes and melanoma. Pigment Cell Melanoma Res. 2017;30:454–66.

Chapter 3
Molecular Landscape of Skin Carcinomas

Anna M. Czarnecka and Karolina Stachyra

Introduction

Non-melanoma skin cancer (NMSC) refers to a large group of tumours which develop within the skin tissue. It comprises several types of skin cancers such as basal cell carcinoma (BCC), squamous cell carcinoma (SCC) and Merkel cell carcinoma (MCC). Basal cell carcinoma (BCC) and cutaneous squamous cell carcinoma (SCC) constitute more than 75% of all diagnosed malignant tumours, thereby comprising the most prevalent malignancies amongst the Caucasian population. BCCs and SCCs make up to 99% NMSCs, while 75–80% of all of them are BCCs. Over the last decade, the incidence rate of skin cancers has been increasing every year, with disproportionate growth in SCCs [1]. The risk of developing skin cancers exceeds 20% in Caucasians. BCCs originate from basal keratinocytes, while SCCs are derived from squamous cells as well as from cells in percutaneous lesions, actinic keratoses, actinic cheilitis, or chronic radiodermatitis [2]. The lesions occur mostly on photoexposed areas such as head or neck while the trunk and extremities are affected only in 4% of patients. However, over time, a shift of the anatomical distribution is observed in BCCs and SCCs to the torso and limbs, respectively [1, 3, 4]. BCC and SCC are rarely metastatic and fatal if diagnosed and treated early

A. M. Czarnecka (✉)
Department of Soft Tissue/Bone, Sarcoma and Melanoma, Maria Sklodowska-Curie National Research Institute of Oncology, Warsaw, Poland

Department of Experimental Pharmacology, Mossakowski Medical Research Institute, Polish Academy of Sciences, Warsaw, Poland
e-mail: am.czarnecka@pib-nio.pl

K. Stachyra
Department of Soft Tissue/Bone, Sarcoma and Melanoma, Maria Sklodowska-Curie National Research Institute of Oncology, Warsaw, Poland

Faculty of Medicine, Medical University of Warsaw, Warsaw, Poland

P. Rutkowski, M. Mandalà (eds.), *New Therapies in Advanced Cutaneous Malignancies*, https://doi.org/10.1007/978-3-030-64009-5_3

with wide surgical excision. Nevertheless, they infiltrate and destroy surrounding tissues causing aesthetic defects and result in deterioration of the patients' quality of life (QoL). The main risk factor for developing both carcinomas is UV exposure. Nevertheless, immunosuppression, genetic disorders as well as acquired viral infections also increase the BCC and SCC incidence rate [3, 5]. On the contrary, Merkel cell carcinoma (MCC) is a very rare, highly malignant and often lethal disease. MCC mortality rate reaches up 50% at 5 years after diagnosis. It affects mainly older white men and develops on sun-exposed areas (head, neck, extremities) in 80% of patients. It is derived from neuroendocrine tissue. Immunosuppression, excessive UV exposure, and Merkel cell polyomavirus (MCPyV) infection are the greatest risk factors of MCCs. At least 80% of MCC patients are infected by MCPyV [6–8]. Other skin carcinomas, such as cutaneous appendageal carcinomas (CACs), occur very rarely, hence the knowledge about them is limited. The majority of CACs results from excessive UV exposure, causing direct DNA damage and immunosuppression. Sebaceous carcinoma, porocarcinoma, spiradenocarcinoma, adenoid cystic carcinoma, as well as hidradenocarcinoma, apocrine carcinoma, digital papillary carcinoma, mucinous carcinoma and many others make up this diverse group [9, 10].

Risk Factors

Ultraviolet radiation (UV) is known to be the greatest environmental risk factor of skin malignancies. Excessive exposure to UV results in an increasing NMSC morbidity [3, 11]. UV light has pleiotropic effects depending on its type—UVB mostly acts directly on DNA, while UVA has more indirect effects triggered by cytotoxic and mutagenic reactive oxygen species (ROS) and 8-oxo-guanine production. ROS are responsible for generating oxidative stress which can be neutralize by dietary antioxidants. Thus, reduced intake of dietary antioxidants, as well as glutathione deficiency, could be the reason for increased UV-induced skin cancers. 8-oxo-guanine causes G to T transversions during replication. Moreover, UVA contributes to chromosomal aberrations and modification in proteins and lipids [12]. UVB exposure induces characteristic "UV signature" mutations: C to T or CC to TT transitions. On average, 90% BCCs contain single-nucleotide substitution mutations, whereas dinucleotide substitutions are detected only in 5%. Generated photoproducts such as pyrimidine (6–4)pyrimidine and cyclobutane dimers play an essential role in NMSC tumourigenesis. In BCCs, C to A mutations mainly result from guanine oxidation. In fact, it has been proven that sun-exposed skin is genetically a patchwork of thousands of evolving clones with more than 25% of cells carrying cancer-related mutations at a density of ~140 mutations per square centimetre [13]. Mutations were reported in oncogenes, suppressor genes and cell cycle regulatory genes [14–17]. "UV signature" is commonly detected in Merkel cell polyomavirus negative (MCPyV-) MCCs, whereas in the development of MCPyV+ MCCs, UV exposure could contribute to immunosuppression, but there is a lack of the characteristic UV-induced mutations [7, 18]. The rise of incidence of NMSCs is associated with age (the peak is observed in patients eighties) as well as sex. It is higher amongst men which is probably due to their greater genetic variation rate [3, 7, 19, 20]. However, lesions frequently develop in young women probably on account of excessive tanning [7, 15, 21]. Moreover, people with skin phenotype 1 (fair-skinned) and red hair are at vulnerable group [14, 22–24]. Higher BCC genetic susceptibility is also thought to result in increased skin ageing, greater wrinkling and pigmentation [25].

Personal history of keratinocyte carcinoma (KC) significantly increases the likelihood of renewed skin malignancies [19]. There is a strong association between developing MCC and previously diagnosed SCC, BCC, cutaneous malignant melanoma, chronic lymphocytic leukaemia and non-Hodgkin lymphoma. The risk of SCC and chronic lymphocytic leukaemia occurrence is significant in MCC-diagnosed patients [6].

Vitamin D is both exogenous, absorbed from the digestive system, and endogenous, produced in the skin where sunlight exposure is essential. It is known to regulate the anti-cancer response. Vitamin D controls the repair of damaged DNA, apoptosis of altered cells, proliferation, as well as angiogenesis. It also regulates the DDIT4-mTOR signalling pathway, which is involved in cell autophagy in SCC, meaning that its depletion is another risk factor of skin malignancies [26].

Repair capacity of DNA damage is strongly associated with the risk of BCCs and single and nonaggressive SCCs. Reduction of 16% in DNA repair capacity (DRC) has been observed in NMSC patients [27]. Decreased DRC, like nucleotide excision repair (NER), global genome repair, transcription-coupled or combination repair, is caused by deleterious mutations, as well as differences in polymorphisms, which are characteristic for particular populations and have an impact on the organism's response to environmental and genetic factors [16, 28].

The defects in genes responsible for NER have been associated with Xeroderma pigmentosum (XP) . It is an autosomal recessive disease caused by mutations in the following genes: *XPA* (Xeroderma Pigmentosum, Complementation Group A, DNA Damage Recognition And Repair Factor) to *XPG* (Xeroderma Pigmentosum, Complementation Group G) and *POLH* (DNA Polymerase Eta). The risk of NMSC is estimated to be up to 10,000 folds, primarily on sun-exposed skin, due to a reduction in the correction of UV-induced DNA damage. Clinically, XP is characterized by sunlight hypersensitivity, premature skin ageing and pigmentary changes. Reaction to sunlight exposure occurs in severe sunburns, which is often the first diagnostic clue [28–31].

The most characteristic autosomal-dominant genetic disorder, which highly increases the risk of developing multiple BCCs at an early age, is basal cell nevus syndrome (BCNS), also known as Gorlin syndrome (GS). Besides early BCC development, odontogenic keratinocytes of the jaws, palmar or plantar pitting, lamellar calcification of the falx cerebri, and medulloblastoma are other major diagnostic criteria. BS results from alterations in the SHH (Sonic Hedgehog) signalling pathway comprising patched 1 (*PTCH1*), patched 2 (*PTCH2*) and SUFU negative regulator of hedgehog signaling (suppressor of fused homolog, *SUFU*) genes [29–31].

The latest studies found *TP53* modifications in Li-Fraumeni syndrome (LFS) to correlate with a higher incidence of skin cancers in these patients [32]. Other disorders, which are risk factors of NMSC, are shown in Table 3.1 [29–31, 33].

NMSCs are reported to be considerably immunogenic so that the treatment frequently contains immunological medications. Immunosuppression, as a symptom of genetic disorders, as well as immunosuppressive post-transplant treatment, significantly increases the risk of NMSCs due to the disability of antigen-presenting cell response that conducts anti-tumour immunity. UV exposure brings on the alterations causing T-lymphocyte-mediated immunosuppression. The modifications in DNA and urocanic acid result in abnormal expression of cytokines, including TNFα, IL-10, IL-1α/β, IL-3, IL-6, IL-8, IL-10, GM-CSF and NGF, which determines dominance of suppressive response of T helper two over T helper one cells. Moreover, tumour necrosis factor (TNF), which is responsible for the aforementioned UV-induced immunosuppression, could differ in microsatellite polymorphisms amongst populations. TNF allele haplotypes d4, d6 and a2b4d5 are associated with a higher predisposition to multiple BCC [34]. Immunodeficiency is also one of the greatest risk factors in MCC, which often develops after organ transplantation or HIV infection, as well as during B-cell malignancy. Chronic inflammatory diseases also correlate with an increased incidence of MCC [7, 35].

Acquired immune deficiency syndrome (AIDS) caused by the human immunodeficiency virus (HIV) is a widespread disease which increases the risk of NMSC nearly 3-fold and results in 11-fold higher incidence of MCC in comparison with the general population due to a depletion of CD4 lymphocytes that dysregulates the anti-tumour immune response [6, 28]. Patients with HIV have a 44% increased risk of subsequent NMSCs [6, 36].

The association between oncogenic types of human papillomavirus (HPV) and NMSCs was considered to be positive, especially concerning the immunosuppressed population. In this group, different virus types were found in 60% of patients affected by NMSCs, whereas in immunocompetent cases, this number reached 36% [23, 28]. Another study indicated HPV-38 as a factor responsible for the immortalization of human keratinocytes. It was found in 13% of SCCs, 16% of BCCs and 50% of all skin carcinomas overall [28]. The altered cells maintain expression of cytokeratin 14 and HPV16 E6 and E7 oncogenes, which impair the cell cycle by inactivation of tumour suppressors—p53 and p105-Rb, respectively, and trigger upregulation of *p16INK4A* [12, 37].

Other viral infections caused by Epstein-Barr virus (EBV) or Merkel cell polyomavirus (MCPyV) are associated with carcinogenesis of SCC and MCC, respectively. Another environmental factor of NMSCs is arsenic exposure, which results in a miR-155 increase. miR-155 regulates the NF-AT1-mediated immunological dysfunction that is associated with altered secretion of interleukin-2 (IL-2) and interferon-γ (IFN-γ). For that reason, arsenic is considered cancerogenic [23, 38, 39]. Moreover, cosmetic tattooing, especially using yellow and green colours, is correlated with an increased probability of early onset of BCCs [40].

Table 3.1 Genetic diseases which predispose to skin carcinomas

Disease	Associated skin carcinomas	Inheritance	Altered genes	Function of gene	Clinical features
Signaling Pathways					
Gorlin Syndrome	BCC	AD	*PTCH1, PTCH2, SUFU*	SHH signalling	Jaw keratocysts, palmar/plantar pits, calcification of the falx cerebri
Bazex-Dupre-Chrisol syndrome	BCC	XLD	unknown	Cell cycle regulation, DNA repair	Hypotrichosis, hypohidrosis, atrophoderma follicularis
Rombo syndrome	BCC	AD	unknown	unknown	Atrophoderma vermiculatum, erythromatous lesion, hypotrichosis, vellus hair cysts, telangiectasias
Xeroderma Pigmentosum	NMSC	XR	*XPA-XPG, POLH*	Nucleotide excision repair	Freckling, photosensitivity, ocular abnormalities, intellectual disability, peripheral neuropathy
Dyskeratosis congenita	SCC	XLR, AD, AR	*TERC, TINF2, TERT, RTEL1, NHP2, NOP10, WRAP53, CTC1, ACD*	Telomere maintenance	Blood and lymphatic cancers, solid tumours, bone marrow failure, pulmonary and hepatic fibrosis
Generalized follicular basaloid hamartoma syndrome	BCC	AD	unknown	unknown	Comedones, hypohidrosis, hypotrichosis, milia
Epidermolysis bullosa	NMSC, melanoma	multiple	multiple	Cutaneous integrity	Skin fragility, blistering, infections, non-healing wounds

(continued)

Table 3.1 (continued)

Disease	Associated skin carcinomas	Inheritance	Altered genes	Function of gene	Clinical features
Immunodeficiency					
Cartilage-Hair Hypoplasia	BCC	AR	*PMRP*	Cell cycle regulation, rRNA processing, mtDNA replication	Metaphyseal dysplasia, short stature, short and pudgy extremities, femur bowing, long fibulae
Epidermodysplasia Verruciformis	NMSC	AR	*EVER1*, *EVER2*	Distribution of zinc in the cell nucleus	Multiple pre−/ cancerous skin lesions
Melanin biosynthesis					
Oculocutaneous Albinism	NMSC, melanoma	AR	*MATP, TYR, TYRP1*	Melanin production	Hypopigmentation of the skin and hair and eye structures, foveal hypoplasia, misrouting of the optic nerve

PTCH1 patched 1, *PTCH2* patched 2, *SUFU* SUFU negative regulator of hedgehog signaling, suppressor of fused homolog, *XPA* xeroderma pigmentosum, complementation group A, *DNA* damage recognition and repair factor, *XPG* Xeroderma Pigmentosum, Complementation Group G, *POLH* DNA polymerase eta, *TERC* telomerase RNA component, *TINF2* TERF1 interacting nuclear factor 2, *TERT* telomerase reverse transcriptase, *RTEL1* regulator of telomere elongation helicase 1, *NPH2* neurexophilin 2, *NOP10* NOP10 ribonucleoprotein, *WRAP53* WD repeat containing antisense to TP53, *CTC1* CST telomere replication complex component 1, *ACD* ACD shelterin complex subunit and telomerase recruitment factor, *PMRP* RNA component of mitochondrial RNA processing endoribonuclease, *EVER1* transmembrane channel like 6, *EVER2* transmembrane channel like 8, *MATP* solute carrier family 45 member 2, *TYR* tyrosinase, *TYRP1* tyrosinase related protein 1

Basal Cell Carcinoma

Basal cell carcinoma (BCC) is the most prevalent malignancy in the Caucasian population making up 75–80% of all NMSC. BCCs affect mainly sun-exposed areas of the body, including the head and neck. BCC is often benign and non-fatal; however, it infiltrates surrounding tissues. It originates from basal keratinocytes in the interfollicular epidermis—epidermal stem cells. Bulge stem cells (SCs) and their hair follicle (HF) progeny are not competent to initiate BCC formation upon smoothened genes overexpression [41]. Activation of genes described below in hair follicle bulge stem cells and their progenitor cells does not induce BCC. BCC arises from long-term resident progenitor cells of the interfollicular epidermis and the upper infundibulum [42]. The risk factors of developing BCC are immunosuppression, genetic disorders such as Gorlin syndrome (GS), and most of all, exposure to UV. Around 90% of detected single-nucleotide variants (SNVs) detected in BCC cells are C to T transitions, and 5% are dinucleotide substitutions that are a characteristic "UV signature". Mechanistically C to A transversions result from guanine oxidation, which distinguishes BCC from melanoma [15, 17, 23]. Furthermore, alterations in BCCs are observed in microsatellites, a modified number of repeats in comparison to normal tissues. These changes are defined as microsatellite instability, while the phenomenon of complete loss of microsatellites is called loss of heterozygosity (LOH) . Frequently, LOH is detected in tumour suppressors, *PTCH1* and *TP53*, or their regulatory elements [16, 17, 43]. In the karyotype of BCC, aneuploidy—including loss of chromosome 9, 13, 14, or X and gain in chromosome 6, 20 or Y have been reported [44]. Over the last decade, more and more significant mutations and gene transcription deregulation events in BCC cells are being reported. Transcriptomic study with paired tumour samples and the adjacent normal skin tissues reported 804 differentially expressed genes in BCC with 414 up-regulated, and 390 down-regulated, while another one identifies 1884 up-regulated and 1106 down-regulated genes [45, 46]. In general, the average number of mutations in sporadic BCC is 65 mutations/Mb, while in GS patients, it is 21 mutations/Mb. This classifies BCC as cancer with the highest mutation rate [17]. In a recent comparative study, the tumour mutational burden (TMB; mutations/MB) was 90 (3–103) for the BCC cases versus 4 (1–860) for 1637 other cancers ($P < 0.0001$) [47].

Hedgehog Signalling Pathway

The hedgehog (HH) signalling pathway is deregulated in 85% of BCC cases. In normal cells, the HH pathway regulates growth in embryos as well as enables maintenance of stem/progenitor cell population and controls of hair follicle and sebaceous gland development. HH signalling also controls cell proliferation by up-regulation of N-Myc, Cyclin D/E, and forkhead box protein M1(FOXM1). It is activated by HH ligands including Sonic HH, Indian HH and Desert HH as well as by alternative cascades triggered by V-Ki-Ras2 Kirsten rat sarcoma 2 viral oncogene homolog (KRAS), transforming growth factor beta 1 (TGF-β), phosphatidylinositol-4,5-bisphosphate 3-kinase (PI3K)/AKT (protein kinase B, PKB) and protein kinase C alpha (PKC-α) that stimulate glioma-associated oncogene (GLI) zinc finger transcription factor (TF). In the conventional pathway, HH ligand binds to transmembrane receptors—protein patched homolog 1(PTCH1) and protein patched homolog 2 (PTCH2), which sustain PTCH-SMO (smoothened, frizzled family receptor) inhibition. SMO, transmembrane G protein-coupled receptor, releases Glioma-Associated Oncogene Homolog (GLI) proteins (GLI1/2/3) from their repressor—cytoplasmatic suppressor of fused homolog (SUFU) protein. GLI TFs transmit the signal to the nucleus and depending on its type (GLI1—activation, GLI2/3—activation or suppression), they regulate transcription of target genes including: cell cycle regulators as E2F transcription factors, D-type cyclins (*CCND1*), cyclin A2 (*CCNA2*), Cyclin Dependent Kinase 1 (*CDK1*), and cyclin B1 (*CCNB1*), as well as proto-oncogene int-1 homolog (*WNT*), Transforming Growth Factor Beta 1 - TGF-β (*TGFB1*), forkhead transcription factor (*FOXE1*),

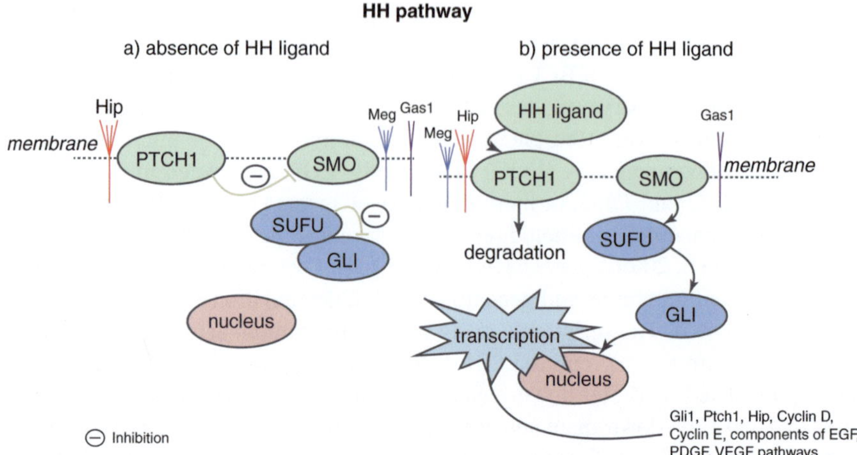

Fig. 3.1 Hedgehog signalling pathway. *PTCH1* protein patched homolog 1, *SMO* smoothened, *SUFU* suppressor of fused homolog, *GLI* glioma-associated oncogene transcription factor, *HH lignad* Hedgehog signaling pathway ligand, *Hip* Hedgehog-interacting protein, *Meg* megalin, *Gas1* growth arrest-specific gene 1, *EGF* epidermal growth factor, *PDGF* platelet-derived growth factor, *VEGF* vascular endothelial growth factor

zinc finger protein Snail1 (*SNAI1*), *PTCH1* and itself—*GLI1*. GLI1 protein creates a positive feedback loop, whereas proteins enocoded by *PTCH1*, *PTCH2* and Hsc70-interacting protein 1 (*HIP*) genes act as negative regulators (Fig. 3.1) [15, 17, 28, 48–50].

In BCC mutations most frequently localize in the *PTCH1* gene — in 11% to 75% of BCCs. The *PTCH1* locus is located on the long arm of chromosome 9 at position 22.32 (9q22.32). Protein patched homolog 1 (PTC) is a transmembrane glycoprotein with 12-membrane spanning domains and two large extracellular loops. Alterations found in *PTCH1* are point mutations, loss of heterozygosity (LOH) and uniparental disomy [15, 51]. Nonsense and splice site mutations make up the majority of mutations, but deleterious ones are also observed. These alterations contain C to T and CC to TT transitions, which are typical UV-induced mutations. However, oxidative stress could also be involved in *PTCH1* mutagenesis. LOH occurs between 24 and 92% of BCCs [15, 52]. Moreover, around 10–20% of BCCs carry missense or nonsense mutations in *SMO* and up to 8% in *SUFU* [53, 54]. Additionally, alterations in the *PTCH2* gene were reported in selected BCC cases [17]. SRY-Box Transcription Factor 9 (*SOX-9*), which is a downstream transcription factor of the HH pathway, is also known to be overexpressed in BCC. Three SOX-9-responsive motifs, that are located in the mechanistic target of rapamycin (mTOR) promoter region, activate its expression. In summary, due to the deregulation of an extensive network of genes induced by the up-regulation of the HH pathway, excessive BCC growth is observed [43, 47, 55].

As a result of HH signalling up-regulation, multiple downstream mediators contribute to skin carcinogenesis. Overexpression of apoptosis inhibitors B-cell CLL/lymphoma 2 (BCL-2), cellular caspase-8-like inhibitory protein (cFlip) and platelet-derived growth factor receptor-α (PDGFRα), as well as down-regulation of tumour necrosis factor receptor (FAS) and B lymphoma Mo-MLV insertion region 1 (BMI1), promote BCC development. The accumulation of GLI1 in the cell results in BCL-2 activity up-regulation, whereas GLI3 acts as an inhibitor of this process [56]. Forkhead box M1 (FOXM1) and forkhead box E (FOXE), which are also down-stream transducers of the HH pathway, are overexpressed and activate cell proliferation. Additionally, in a murine model, it was shown that mutated *TP53* activates the HH signalling pathway by up-regulation of *SMO* gene expression [15, 51, 57].

Moreover, overexpression of zinc finger protein GLI1 in pre-BCC cells causes a reduction of epithelial growth factor receptor (EGFR) expression and therefore repression of the extracellular signal-regulated kinase (ERK) in keratinocyte stem cells. This phenomenon enables keratinocytes to maintain the epithelial phenotype, form colonies, and develop into skin cancers. Cross-talk of HH and EGFR pathways is essential for BCC tumorigenesis due to EGFR-mediated activation of mitogen-activated protein kinase (MAPK) signalling [23, 58]. At the same time, the active PI3K-AKT pathway stimulates HH signalling by regulation of GLI transcription factor. Phosphatase and tensin homolog (PTEN) is an inhibitor of the PI3K-AKT pathway. Thus, loss-of-function mutations affecting PTEN result in the up-regulation of PI3K-AKT signalling and, in turn, activation of the HH pathway [23].

The Gorlin syndrome (GS) is an example of an autosomal dominant disorder that predisposes to the development of multiple BCCs. People with GS inherit a mutation of the HH pathway, including *PTCH1*, *PTCH2* and *SUFU* genes. Despite an increased risk of BCCs, other symptoms associated with GS are dyskeratotic palmar or plantar pitting and odontogenic keratinocytes [29–31]. Also, *xeroderma pigmentosum*-related BCC cases are reported to harbour *PTCH* mutations at a very high mutation frequency of 90%, as well as in the *TP53* gene in 38% of cases. In these patients, it was suggested that *PTCH* UV-specific C to T transitions represent an earlier event in the development of BCC than *TP53* mutations [59].

TP53 Gene

TP53, also known as the "guardian of the genome," is a well-known tumour suppressor gene. It is mapped on the short arm of chromosome 17 (17p13.1). Alterations of *TP53* are the most common mutations occurring in human cancers found in more than 50% of all neoplasms. It is involved in cell cycle regulation, apoptosis induction and DNA repair [15]. *TP53* is known to be the target of oncoviruses, such as HPV. The E6 protein of HPV-16/18 can bind to and induce the proteolytic breakdown of p53 protein so as to promote tumorigenesis. Arsenic exposure, which results in methylation of the components of the p53 pathway and *TP53* loss in BCC, leads to G2/M cell cycle arrest and DNA aneuploidy [23, 60]. Early reports have shown that *TP53* mutations are abundant in NMSCs, including BCCs. In 342 analysed patients, *TP53* mutations were detected in 66% BCCs, 38% of nonaggressive BCCs, 35% of aggressive SCCs, 50% of nonaggressive SCCs and 10% of samples of sun-exposed skin; among those up to 71% of mutations detected were UV signature mutations [61].

In general, 60% of all BCCs harbour aberrations in the *TP53* gene. Alterations of TP53 are predominantly missense mutations, which are mostly caused by UV exposure. Moreover, 45% of the point mutations are also accompanied by a second point mutation of the other allele [62]. In a study comparing the rate of *TP53* mutations in sunscreen users and non-users, it was found that the users had significantly fewer *TP53* mutations. These results confirmed the role of UV exposure in TP53 mutations in BCCs (and other NMSCs) [62, 63]. Characteristic C(C) to T(T) transitions were observed. General hot spots of *TP53* have been identified at codons 177, 196 and 245, while codon 177 mutations have been assumed to be specific for BCC. Presence of polymorphisms at codon 72 significantly increases the risk of BCC development. Also, tandem CC to TT mutations in codons 247 and 248 are associated with an increased risk of BCC development. *TP53* LOH was present in BCC samples [15, 17, 23, 64, 65]. Most recent studies confirm that Li-Fraumeni syndrome, which is caused by *TP53* germline mutations, increases the risk of developing skin cancers [32].

TP63 Gene

The tumour protein 63 gene (*TP63*) or keratinocyte transcription factor (*KET*), a member of the p53 family of proteins, is expressed in cells with high proliferation potential, and it is located in the basal compartment of the keratinocyte stem cell, maintaining the stem cell phenotype. In keratinocytes, p63 regulates the expression of adhesion proteins, including Bullous pemphigoid antigen 1 (BPAG1), hemidesmosome proteins (PREP), integrins: Integrin Subunit Alpha 6 (ITGA6) and Integrin Subunit Beta 4 (ITGB4) keratin intermediate filaments protein (KRT14) or P-cadherin (CDH3) and Fraser extracellular matrix complex subunit 1 (FRAS1). It also regulates chromatin remodelling proteins: special AT-rich sequence-binding protein-1 (SATB1) and SWI/SNF Related, Matrix Associated, Actin Dependent Regulator Of Chromatin, Subfamily A, Member 4 (SMARCA4), that regulate epidermal differentiation [66]. There are several isoforms which can bind to p53, activating it. Isoform TAp63γ is able to induce apoptosis, while a ΔN one has an antiapoptotic effect by inactivating p53. It was shown that the altered expression of p63 results in an impaired UVB-induced apoptotic pathway, which increases the risk of BCCs [28, 67]. Multiple studies report high expression of p63 in BCC cases, but pathological and physiological aspects of p63 function in BCC are still poorly described [66].

p16(INK4A) and p14(ARF) Proteins

The p16(INK4A) and p14(ARF) proteins are encoded by the cyclin-dependent kinase inhibitor 2A (*CDKN2A*) gene located at the short arm of chromosome 9 (9p21.3). p16 binds to CDK4 and suppresses phosphorylation of RB protein, which results in the cell remaining in the G1 phase and inhibition of its proliferation. Functional or structural alterations of p16 cause uncontrolled cell division and the development of malignant skin tumours. p16 is expressed at the high frequency in around 15% of BCC cases [23, 67, 68]. These mutations are also UV-dependent [69]. Some authors associated p16 expression with invasive BCCs with an infiltrative growth pattern. In superficial, nodular, and infiltrative histologic subtypes, p16 was overexpressed in 75.0%, 88.8% and 100.0% of cases, respectively. Other reports did not confirm the correlation of p16 with immunoreactivity [70, 71].

RB1 Gene

The RB transcriptional corepressor 1 (RB1) gene encodes a tumour suppressor protein called retinoblastoma protein (pRb), which acts by inhibiting cell cycle progression. It binds to and represses E2F transcription factor, maintaining the cell in the G1 phase. It prevents the replication of DNA by inhibiting progression from G1 to S phase of the cell cycle. It creates a complex with E2F binding to its transactivation domain. This complex binds to promoters of the genes essential for the transition to the S phase, repressing their transcription. pRb also remodels chromatin structure by interaction with the proteins (bHRM, BRG1, HDAC1) responsible for nucleosome remodelling, histone de-acetylation and methylation. *RB1* mutations occur in about 10% of BCCs, where 44% of them are LOH or loss-of-function ones [17, 72].

MYCN and FBXW7 Signalling

The *MYCN* (MYCN proto-oncogene, BHLH transcription factor) gene belongs to the MYC family of oncogenes and is found in the 2p24 locus [73]. It plays an important role in the growth of tissues and organs in embryos, whereas after birth, it controls cellular proliferation and apoptosis. In the first report, high Nmyc protein expression was detected in 72.7% (160/220) of all BCC specimens. Significantly higher N-myc expression was reported in infiltrative BCCs compared to nodular/ superficial BCCs, as well as in head BCCs in comparison to BCCs developing in the other anatomic sites. The prevalence of *MYCN gene* number gains was 17.5%, with nodular differentiation BCCs presenting numerous amplifications of the *MYCN* gene [74]. In general, missense mutations occur in 30% of BCCs, and most of them affect the sequence encoding the Myc box 1 (MB1) region. MB1 region alterations impair interaction between Myc and F-box/WD repeat-containing protein 7 (*FBXW7* gene), which is a substrate-binding component of the SCFFbxw7 E3 ubiquitin ligase. The binding complex ubiquitinates Myc resulting in its proteasome degradation. Moreover, deleterious mutations in *FBXW7* have been detected in 5% of BCCs, while LOH events overlapping *FBXW7* have been found in 8% of all cases. They are mainly located upstream of the WD40 domain, which is responsible for substrate binding. Myc accumulation, caused by a lack of interaction with ubiquitin ligase, leads to carcinogenesis [15, 17].

Hippo Pathway

The Hippo pathway is vital in embryogenesis and regulation of organ size as well as cell growth, apoptosis, migration and proliferation. It is known to be built by more than 30 proteins. While the Hippo pathway is inactivated, dephosphorylated Yes1-associated protein (YAP) and Tafazzin (TAZ) are in the cell nucleus where they interact with vestigial-like family member 4 (VGLL4) and TEA domain transcription factor 1–4 (TEAD1–4) inducing target gene transcription. Activated YAP and TAZ enhance progenitor cell phenotype, including self-renewal, epithelial–mesenchymal transition, proliferation and survival of epithelial skin cells.

The Hippo pathway is activated by mechanical forces—cell-to-cell contact, or energy status, as well as hormones. The majority of signals are transduced through G protein-coupled receptors of the cell membrane. It can also be activated by thousand and one amino acid protein kinase (TAOK), which phosphorylate macrophage stimulating 1 and 2 (MST1/2). MST1/2-activated scaffold proteins, Salvador family WW domain containing protein 1 (SAV1), Mps one binder kinase activator-like 1A or B (MOB1A/B) and neurofibromin 2 (NF2), phosphorylate large tumour

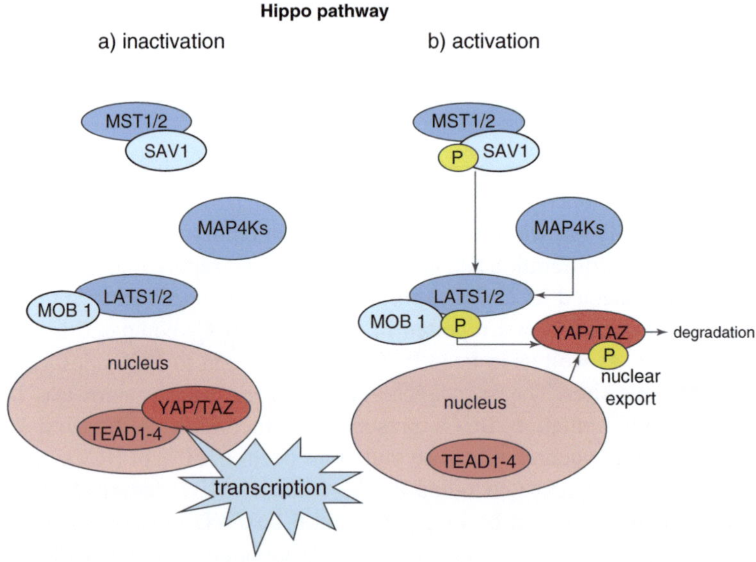

Fig. 3.2 Hippo signalling pathway. *MST1/2* mammalian Ste-20 like kinase 1 and 2, *SAV1* salvador family WW domain containing protein 1, *MAP4Ks* mitogen-activated protein kinase kinase kinase kinase, *LATS* 1/2 large tumor suppressor kinase 1 and 2, *MOB 1* monopolar spindle-one-binder protein 1, *YAP* yes-associated protein 1, *TAZ* tafazzin, *TEAD1*-4 transcriptional enhancer factor *TEF*-1-4 pathway

suppressor kinase 1 or 2 (LATS1/2), which finally phosphorylates YAP and TAZ. Phosphorylated transcription factors bind to 14-3-3 protein leading to their cytoplasmic retention and SCF-mediated degradation. LATS1/2 may also be activated by MAP4K1/2/3/5 and MAP4K4/6/7 (Mitogen-activated protein kinase kinase kinase kinase 2) (Fig. 3.2) [15, 75, 76].

The Hippo pathway dysregulation is often detected in BCC samples. Nuclear accumulation of YAP1 was observed in 26% assessed BCCs. *LATS1* deleterious mutations have been detected in around 16% of all BCC cases of which 24% are truncating ones. The *LATS2* gene is known to be altered in 12% of BCCs. Furthermore, mutations of tyrosine-protein phosphatase non-receptor type 14 gene (*PTPN14*), which normally promotes nuclear export of YAP/ZAP, are found in about 23% of BCCs, and 61% out of them are truncating alterations [17]. Moreover, YAP depletion in BCC tumours results in the deregulation of the c-*Jun* N-terminal kinases (JNK) signalling that regulates cell death by c-Jun and Fos, apoptosis by Bcl-2–interacting mediator of cell death (BIM), Bcl2-associated agonist of cell death (BAD) Bcl-2–associated X protein (BAX) and p53, as well as survival by signal transducer and activator of transcription (STAT) protein family and cyclic AMP response element-binding protein (CREB) [77]. Moreover, high expression of YAP induces CCN family member 1 (CCN1) and promotes proliferation and survival of BCC cells, while via CCN family member 2 (CCN2), it is responsible for tumour stroma cell activation (type I collagen, fibronectin and α-smooth muscle actin) and stroma remodelling [78].

NFκB Pathway

The nuclear factor kappa-light-chain-enhancer of activated B cells (NFκB) pathway plays an important role in inflammation and embryogenesis of epithelial appendages, as well as in the development of BCC. NFκB is activated through phosphorylation of NFκB inhibitor IκB kinase (IKK) by the IκB kinase complex. Phosphorylation of IκB results in its ubiquitination and degradation in proteasomes. NFκB essential modulator (NEMO), which is part of the IκB kinase complex, binds cylindromatosis (CYLD). The *CYLD* gene encodes a de-ubiquitinating enzyme which sustains the complex of NFκB and NFκB inhibitor IκB kinase. Hence, CYLD down-regulates the NFκB pathway. Furthermore, TNF receptor-associated factor 2 (TRAF2) and TNF receptor-associated factor 6 (TRAF6), which are auto-ubiquitinating proteins and require the ubiquitin tag for their function, activate the NFκB pathway. The interaction between NEMO and CYLD contributes to TRAF2 and TRAF6 deubiquitination, thereby suppressing the NFκB pathway [28]. The NF-kB signalling pathway, involved in inflammatory processes and embryogenesis of skin adnexal epithelium, is also important in the development of BCC. Deficiency in NF-κB, one of the signal pathway components was reported in BCC samples [79]. Activated forms of NFκBp65 and NFκBp50 were identified as highly expressed in superficial BCC [80]. It was also proven that nuclear IKKα binds to promoters of inflammation factors and a stem cell marker leucine-rich repeat-containing G-protein coupled receptor 5 (LGR5). As a result, overexpressed LGR5 activates the STAT3 signalling pathway and promotes BCC progression [81].

NOTCH1/2 Gene

Neurogenic locus notch homolog protein (*NOTCH*) family genes are considered to have a tumour suppressor role in BCCs. *NOTCH1* controls cell differentiation, proliferation, as well as apoptosis. *NOTCH2* is vital for the determination of cell destination in embryos, while after birth, it is involved in tissue repair, bone remodelling, and immune system regulation; 29% of BCCs carry *NOTCH1* mutations, of which 25% are loss-of-function ones. Alterations of the *NOTCH2* gene occur in 26% of BCCs, where 30% of them are loss-of-function mutations, and 22% affect neoplasms with paired loss-of-function ones [17]. Notch signalling pathway activity is suppressed in BCCs, while Notch signalling stimulation induces apoptosis of BCC cells [82]. Notch1 loss in the skin or in primary keratinocytes results in constant overexpression of zinc finger protein GLI2 and development of BCC [83].

Telomerase Reverse Transcriptase Gene

The telomerase reverse transcriptase (TERT) gene is located on the short arm of chromosome 5 (5p15.33) and encodes the catalytic reverse transcriptase subunit of telomerase. Telomerase maintains the length of the repeated segments of DNA, called telomeres, located at the end of every chromosome. In the majority of cells, the telomeres become shorter after every cell division. After many proliferations, telomeres are so reduced that the cell has to undergo apoptosis. *TERT* gene overexpression, resulting from gain-of-function UV-induced mutations, increases telomerase activity, which elongates telomeres. This event allows for an increased number of cell proliferations which significantly contribute to the development of NMSCs. Mutations of the *TERT* promoter are present in about 56–59% of all BCCs and show a UV signature (C to T or CC to TT). These mutations are found both in sporadic BCCs — even up to 78%; and in tumours from patients with nevoid basal cell carcinoma syndrome — in 68% [15, 84–86].

Brahma Gene

Brahma (BRM) is a catalytic subunit of the mammalian SWItch/sucrose non-fermentable (SWI/SNF) complex, which remodels chromatin transcription and DNA repair. GRM provides energy for remodelling. It is also a common mutation in NMSCs, which occurs in 33% of BCC cases. G to C and T to A transversions, which are characteristic for UV-induced mutations, are observed [23, 87]. *BRM* expression is down-regulated at the mRNA level in BCC [88].

Melanocortin-1 Receptor

Melanin, which occurs in two forms: photoprotective - black eumelanin, and photo-sensitive - red pheomelanin, is produced by melanocytes. Melanin synthesis results in different skin pigmentation and protection against UV. Melanocortin-1 receptor (MC1R) is a G-protein-coupled receptor that is expressed on the melanocyte surface. MC1R is activated by αmelanocyte-stimulating hormone (αMSH). MC1R stimulates the cAMP pathway, which loss of activation results in increased production of pheomelanin. More than 80 MC1R types have been discovered and associated with particular skin colours. Three main red hair colour (RHC) variants—R151C, R160W, and R294H—are responsible for 93% of all RHC cases. The "RHC phenotype" is associated with fair skin, freckles and photosensitivity, which occur due to increased production of pheomelanin or reduction of eumelanin in melanocytes. The particular *MC1R* variants (V60L, D84E, V92M, R151C, R160W, R163Q and D294H) are significant risk factors for NMSCs, including BCCs and SCCs. Moreover, melanocytes with loss-of-function *MC1R* variants have decreased ability to repair UV-induced mutations, which also contributes to increased risk of BCCs [23, 24]. Additionally, mutations in the agouti signalling protein (*ASIP*) and the tyrosinase (*TYR*) genes are also involved in BCC development. Agouti signalling protein acts as an inhibitor of the interaction between αMSH and MC1R. It impairs cAMP signalling causing pheomelanin overproduction [23].

DPH3 Gene

Diphthamide biosynthesis 3 (DPH3) is vital for the synthesis of diphthamide, which is a residue in eukaryotic translation elongation factor 2. This factor is responsible for maintaining translation fidelity so that its alterations may be significant in tumourigenesis. Mutations of the *DPH3* promoter, also known as the bidirectional promoter region of *DPH3-OXNAD1*, occur in 38–42% of BCCs. The most frequent alteration is observed at −8 and −9 bp, where 18.3% and 8.9% of them are C to T transition and CC to TT tandem mutations, respectively. These mutations again show a typical UV signature—C to T transitions at dipyrimidine sites [15, 84, 89].

Detoxifying Proteins

The detoxifying proteins, which are involved in the cell response to UV-induced oxidative stress, play a significant role in BCC development. Glutathione S-transferases (GTSs) are responsible for the detoxification of harmful substances by using reduced glutathione (GSH). Due to the oxidative stress, UV exposure leads to lipid peroxidation as well as DNA hydroperoxide formation. These altered products are mutagenic and are neutralized by GTSs. GTS isoenzymes are divided into five classes, including π, which is predominant in the human skin. The lack of GTS-π increases the risk of developing BCCs. Moreover, several polymorphisms of GSTs are identified to impair the process of detoxification. Both the GSTT1 genotype, connected with UV hypersensitivity, and the GSTM1 genotype, which acts against UV-induced oxidative stress, are risk factors of BCCs [14, 23, 28, 90]. Cytochrome P450 (CYP) is another enzyme that takes part in detoxification. The CYP family consists of over 30 isoforms, of which CYP2D6 is significantly associated with BCC carcinogenesis [14].

Gap Junctional Intercellular Communication

Gap junctions are essential for the maintenance of cell homeostasis. They are formed by proteins called connexins (Cxs). Generally, there is a reduction of Cxs in tumours which contributes to impairment of cellular communication and uncontrolled growth of lesions. An increased amount of Cx26 and a decreased amount of Cx43 are associated with the development of BCCs. Normally, Cx26 and Cx30 are detected in different areas of the cell, whereas in BCCs, they are concentrated in the basal parts. Moreover, there is an observed increase of Cx26 and Cx30 deep in the dermis compared to their small amount in epidermal areas [23].

Cyclooxygenase Gene

Cyclooxygenase (COX) synthesizes prostaglandins (PGs), which are vital for the development of acute and chronic skin inflammation triggered by exogenous (UV light, wounding) and endogenous stimuli. COX-1 isoform is expressed constitutively, whereas COX-2 is induced transiently. Both overexpression of *COX-2*, which is involved in the production of PGs, and down-regulation of the tumour suppressor gene 15-hydroxyprostaglandin dehydrogenase (*15-PGDH*), which in contrast inactivates PGs, result in increased levels of PGE2 and PGF2α in premalignant or malignant epithelial skin cancers. Altered *COX-2* up-regulation has been shown to contribute to tumour promotion and progression rather than its initiation. *COX-2* overexpression is significantly higher in recurrent BCCs than in the primary BCCs [91]. *COX-2* is involved in pre-invasive growth by delaying the onset of terminal differentiation and by stimulating cell hyperproliferation. *COX-2* overexpressing cells are mostly found on the infiltrating site of the tumour [92]. In BCCs, genetic alterations of *COX-1*, as well as *COX-2*, result in down-regulation of *PTCH1*. The lack of protein patched homolog 1 (PTC1), in turn, stimulates the Hedgehog pathway and leads to BCC development [93]. *COX-2* is up-regulated in BCC, and it is considered as a biomarker for the prognosis of BCC patients with a high risk of recurrence [94]. Moreover, the fibrosing BCC subtype, which is considered to present with a higher degree of inflammation, also expresses more COX-2 than nodular BCC [92].

IL-6/JAK/STAT3 Signalling

Interleukin 6 (IL-6) is a pleiotropic cytokine that plays direct and indirect roles in lesion growth. It acts in an autocrine or paracrine manner and also governs modifications of the tumour microenvironment. IL-6 stimulates different pathways, including IL-6/JAK/STAT3, which is overactive in BCCs. Normally, IL-6 is expressed in proliferating keratinocytes, but UV exposure also contributes to the excessive release of cytokines, including IL-1, IL-6, IL-10, IL-12 and tumor necrosis factor-α (TNF-α). IL-6 is known to stimulate DNA synthesis and angiogenesis as well as to inhibit apoptosis. This cytokine may act through activation of anti-apoptotic protein induced myeloid leukemia cell differentiation protein (Mcl-1), vascular endothelial growth factor (VEGF), and COX-2. Moreover, IL-6 may induce activation of the HH pathway. IL-6 enhances the tumorigenic activity of BCC cells by both suppressing apoptosis and actively promoting angiogenesis [95]. In fact, it is basic fibroblast growth factor (bFGF) and COX-2 that are downstream effectors of IL-6. These proteins are responsible for the angiogenic activity. The IL-6-mediated bFGF up-regulation in BCC is executed by the JAK/STAT3 and PI3-Kinase/Akt pathways [96]. The G/C polymorphism of the IL-6 promoter in position −174 is considered to significantly increase the risk of BCC development. *STAT3* is known to be involved in proliferation, invasion of malignant cells as well as angiogenesis and suppression of anti-tumour immunity. *STAT3* alterations are another risk factor for BCC and are caused by the prevalent single-nucleotide polymorphisms (SNPs), including rs4796793 (located in the promoter) and rs2293152 (located in intron 11) [97]. Signal integration of IL6 and HH pathways occurs at the level of *cis*-regulatory sequences by co-binding of GLI and STAT3 to HH and IL6 target gene promoters [98].

Programmed Cell Death-1 Gene and FAS Gene

Programmed cell death-1 (PD-1) protein plays a suppressive role in the immune response. It is located in the membrane of a variety of immune cells. Binding to its ligand - programmed cell death 1 ligand 1(PD-L1), PD-1 inhibits activation of the immune system. This process results in tolerance to self-antigens and thus prevents the development of autoimmune diseases. Up-regulation of the *PDCD-1* gene and overexpression of PDCD1L1 gene are detected in malignant cells, including BCCs, so that neoplasms protect themselves against an anti-tumour immune response. The high frequency of the G allele in *PD1.3* as well as the AC haplotype of the *PDCD1* gene is associated with BCCs [99].

The *FAS* gene encodes a transmembrane protein which is involved in the cell signalling. Three FAS proteins group together to form trimer which binds to FAS ligands (FASL), resulting in activation of caspase cascade and finally cell apoptosis. FAS/FASL is significantly decreased in BCCs [45].

Human Leukocyte Antigen Genes

Particular human leukocyte antigen (*HLA*) genes play a minor role in the development of BCCs. HLA composition on the tumour cell surface could be a significant clue for diagnosis. The presence of *HLA-DR7* and decrease in *HLA-DR4* is characteristic for BCCs [100], as well as *HLA-DR1* [101]. Moreover, there is a weak association between the development of multiple BCC and presence of *HLA-DR1* [28, 102]. A significant interaction between *HLA-C* and the activating gene *KIR2DS3*—belonging to the family of killer immunoglobulin-like receptors (KIR)—was described in BCC [103]. Natural killer (NK) cells are components of the innate immune system and take part in the first line of defence against viral infections and transformed cells. Killer-cell immunoglobulin-like receptors (KIR), which occur mainly in NK cells, exclusively bind to HLA class I. The NK cell phenotype is partially determined by the type of KIR-HLA interaction. Significant interactions in BCCs were observed between *HLA-C* and the activating gene *KIR2DS3* as well as between *HLA-B* and telomeric KIR B haplotype (containing the activating genes *KIR3DS1* and *KIR2DS1*) and *HLA-B* and the activating KIR gene *KIR2DS5*. Moreover, KIR centromeric B haplotype was correlated with significant risk of multiple BCCs [104].

Other Genes

Multiple genes have been reported as mutated in BCCs. Serine/threonine-protein phosphatase 6 catalytic subunit (PPP6C) controls the cell cycle through regulation of cyclin D1 and inactivation of RB1. It also takes part in LATS1 activation. *PPP6C* is altered in about 15% of BCCs, resulting in impaired phosphatase activity. Substitution mutations in another serine/threonine protein phosphatase—serine/threonine-protein kinase 19 (*STK19*) are observed in 10% of BCCs [15, 17]. The AT-rich interactive domain-containing protein 1A (*ARID1A*) gene encodes a protein which is a subunit of several different SWI/SNF protein complexes. The SWI/SNF complex is known to be responsible for chromatin remodelling so that *ARID1A* mutations, which occur in around 26% of BCCs, alter several essential cellular processes such as replication of DNA, controlling cell growth, division and differentiation [17]. The caspase 8 (*CASP8*) gene, also reported as mutated in BBC, encodes a cysteine-aspartic acid protease, called caspase. Activation of the caspase cascade is vital in the execution phase of cell apoptosis. Caspases are triggered by FAS and other apoptotic stimuli. Alterations in caspases result in an impaired process of programmed cell death. Mutations in the *CASP8* gene occur in 11% of BCCs, of which 14% are nonsense ones [17]. Also, cytoplasmic FMR1 interacting protein 2 (*CYFIP2*), homeobox B8 (*HOXB5*), epidermal growth factor receptor (*EGFR*), forkhead box N3 (*FOXN3*), protein tyrosine phosphatase non-receptor type 3 (*PTPN3*), cell division cycle 20 (*CDC20*), MARCKS like 1 (*MARCKSL1*) and *FAS* were shown to be essential in the initiation and progression of BCC. Four of these genes were shown to play a role in the cell cycle, of which *CYFIP2* and *MARCKSL1* were up-regulated. Hot spot mutations of signal transducer and activator of transcription 5B (*STAT5B*), crooked neck pre-mRNA splicing factor 1 (*CRNKL1*) and nebulette (*NEBL*) are also found in BCCs. Most alterations result from C to T transition, characteristic for UV exposure. STAT5B serves the functions of signal transducer and transcription factor. Triggered by cytokines and growth factors, STAT5B is phosphorylated, forms dimers and is translocated to the nucleus. It is involved in TCR signalling and apoptosis. CRNKL1 regulates pre-mRNA splicing [44]. The BRCA1-Associated Protein (*BAP1*) gene encodes a deubiquitinating enzyme which is known to be a tumour suppressor. Loss-of-function mutations are a common reason for frequent BCCs [105]. Basal keratin K5, especially the G138E variant, also results in BCC susceptibility [23]. Mutations of other genes, including kinetochore localized astrin (SPAG5) binding protein (*KNSTRN*) (2%), erb-b2 receptor tyrosine kinase 2 (*ERBB2*) (4%), *KRAS* (4%), *NRAS* (4%), *HRAS* (4%), phosphatidylinositol-4,5-bisphosphate 3-kinase catalytic subunit alpha (*PIK3CA*) (4%) and Rac family small GTPase 1 (*RAC1*) (1%), have also been identified in BCCs [17].

Squamous Cell Carcinoma

Cutaneous squamous cell carcinoma (SCC) is the second most prevalent NMSC, making up 20% of all skin malignancy cases. SCC is more aggressive than BCC and metastasizes more rapidly. About 8% of patients with skin SCC experience local relapse, and in 5% of cases, metastatic disease is diagnosed within 5 years, while the frequency of lymph node metastases is 4%. In patients with metastatic SCC, only 10–20% survive 10 years and prognosis is poor [3, 106, 107]. SCC originates from the altered squamous cells (SCs) of the skin—hair follicle bulge SCs as well as from nonhairy epidermis [41]. Nevertheless, SCCs can also be derived from percutaneous lesions such as Bowen's disease (BD), actinic keratoses (AK), actinic cheilitis or chronic radiodermatitis in contrast to BCCs which develop only "de novo" [2]. Primary SCCs are located in the sun-exposed areas of the skin on account of chronic exposure to UV radiation, especially UVB, which is a major risk factor for SCC development [16]. Development of SCCs results from genomic disruption, specific genetic mutations as well as altered expression of key molecules in the squamous cells. Moreover, underlying stromal cells, which built the SCC niche, also play an essential role in SCC initiation and progression by promoting escape from the immune surveillance [12]. Cutaneous SCC is considered to have a greater rate of mutations compared to other (internal) squamous cell carcinomas. Cutaneous SCC was reported to harbour the highest TMB among all cancers with 41.3% of cases demonstrating a very high TMB (≥ 50 mutations/Mb) [47]. The detailed transcriptomic analysis reported that 601 genes were up-regulated and 1382 down-regulated in SCCs [46].

TP53 Gene

The *TP53* is the main tumour suppressor gene which plays an essential role in DNA repair regulation, cell division as well as apoptosis, as described above. *TP53* mutations are the most frequent alterations in SCCs, occurring in about 64–90% of all cases and represent a UV signature. Nevertheless, mutations of *TP53* are rare in HPV+ SCCs where p53 function is impaired by degradation promoted by the viral E6 oncogene [12, 108, 109]. Missense hot spot mutations are the most common aberrations, of which most are loss-of-function. In SCC, high levels of mutant p53 accumulate in the cytoplasm [109], which is detected as overexpression [110]. Presence of any *TP53* mutation in SCC is associated with faster recurrence and decreased overall survival with most impact from disruptive mutations, that is, non-conservative mutations located inside the key DNA-binding domain (L2–L3 region), or stop codons in any region of *TP53* gene [110, 111]. Mutated p53 associated with other transcription factors can alter gene expression. Moreover, the tetramer complex of mutated p53 has altered ability of interaction with p63 and p73 so that it affects their normal functions [12]. The p53 pathway is significant in SCC with perineural invasion (PNI). Gene expression of SCC with PNI is characterized by activation of the p53 pathway and increased expression of p53-target genes, including cyclin dependent kinase inhibitor 1A (*CDKN1A*), BCL2 binding component 3 (*BBC3*) and tumor protein p53 inducible protein 3 (*TP53I3*). Among *TP53* mutations detected in the SCC samples with PNI, gain-of-function mutations (p.G245; p.P151; p.L194) were reported, as well as those directly adjacent to (p.P152; p.H193) these previous positions. At the same time, significant overexpression of *MDM2* proto-oncogene—p53 for ubiquitin ligase—was detected in cases with PNI; while the deubiquitinating enzymes encoded by ubiquitin specific peptidase 2 (USP2) and ubiquitin specific peptidase 7 (USP7) that target *MDM2* were significantly down-regulated [112].

TP63 Gene

The *TP63* gene encodes two main isoforms of the protein—Tap63 and ΔNp63—which result from alternative splicing. It is essential for epithelial cell development as well as in the maintenance of skin stem cells and transition from simple to stratified and glandular epithelia. p63 was shown to promote initial stages of tumour development, whereas it was suppressive at later stages. It regulates epithelial/keratinocyte proliferation. In SCC, p63 is of great importance, as the direct target of p63 is the fibroblast growth factor receptor 2 (FGFR2). Increased FGFR signalling promotes SCC development. What is more, ΔNp63α overexpression causes epidermal hyperplasia by interaction with Ras/MAP kinase signalling. Cells with deregulated ΔNp63α express high levels of Lsh and Sirt1 that enable overcoming of cellular senescence. These cells also present down-regulated p16INK4 and p19ARF protein levels. At the same time, overexpression of p63 in SCC results in repression of p73-dependent proapoptotic transcriptional program, as well as repression of p21/ cyclin-dependent kinase inhibitor 1A (CDKN1A) and the microRNA-34 family. Moreover, physical interaction has been detected between p63 and SOX2 in SCC cells. This interaction results in transcriptional coregulation of 93 target genes, including the oncogene *ETV4* [113]. In SCC, p63 and SOX2 interaction induces overexpression of facilitated glucose transporter member 1 (GLUT1) and promotes glucose influx and metabolism, as well as SCC cell survival [114]. SOX2 is a transcription factor and plays a key role in pluripotency of embryonic stem cells and cell fate determination. *SOX2*, *TP63*, and *PIK3CA* have adjacent chromosomal localization (3q26/28); hence, they are commonly co-amplified in SCCs [12, 67, 113, 115, 116].

CDKN2A Gene

The cyclin dependent kinase inhibitor 2A (*CDKN2A*) gene encodes several proteins, including the p16(INK4A) and the p14(ARF). Both proteins are the tumour suppressors. p16(INK4A) and p14(ARF) control the cell cycle and are involved in cell senescence. The p16(INK4A) protein inhibits CDK4 and CDK6, which normally take part in cell cycle progression. p14(ARF) prevents p53 from being degraded. Their functions actually prevent tumour formation. *CDKN2A*-derived proteins suppress p105-Rb activity so that *CDKN2A* loss-of-function mutations result in uncontrolled cell growth and divisions [12, 67]. In SCC, most of CDKN2A gene mutations are often not UV-dependent and are reported in 24–76% SCC cases [117]. In fact, inactivation of *CDKN2A* genes, via allelic loss and/or mutation, was reported as significant for SCC development [118]. In addition to mutations, also promoter methylation was reported as a mechanism of p16(INK4A) and p14(ARF) inactivation in SCC [119]. Finally, *CDKN2A* mutations have been reported in metastatic SCC as one of the top three recurrently mutated genes (with *TP53* and *NOTCH1/2/4*) [120].

CCDN1 and CCNE1 Genes

The *CCDN1* gene encodes cyclin D1, which forms a complex with cyclin-dependent kinase 4 (CDK4). The cyclin D1-CDK4 complex phosphorylates and inactivates pRb. This process allows dissociation of the transcription factor E2F and subsequently, transcription of the E2F target genes, which take part in progression through G1 to S phase. Moreover, the cyclin D1-CDK4 complex phosphorylates mothers against decapentaplegic homolog 3 (SMAD3) in a cell cycle-dependent manner repressing its transcriptional activity [12]. *CCNE1* codes for cyclin E1 which in contrast binds to cyclin-dependent kinase 2 (CDK2). This complex is also required for progression from G1 to S cell cycle phase. Additionally, cyclin E1 is involved in phosphorylation of the NPAT protein, which regulates histone gene expression and plays a pivotal role in the cell cycle progression in the absence of pRb. *CCDN1* and *CCNE1* genes are commonly amplificated in SCCs [12, 108]. In case series analysis of 24 SCC patients, cyclin D1 was found to be overexpressed in 70% of them [121]. *CCND1* gene overexpression is responsible for mTOR inhibitor resistance in SSCs [122].

MYC and FBXW7 Gene

The *MYC* (MYC proto-oncogene, bHLH transcription factor) gene is a protoonco-gene which encodes nuclear phosphoprotein. c-Myc interacts with transforming growth factor α (TGF-α), epidermal growth factor receptor (EGFR), Ras, PI3K, and NF-κB and regulates *cyclin D1* gene expression that is a common downstream target of multiple signalling pathways. *MYC* amplification is frequent in SCCs. It is indicated to promote SCC progression. At the same time, activation of c-Myc in adult suprabasal epidermis induces proliferation and inhibits differentiation of keratinocytes. *MYC* deregulation therefore drives SCC progression and promotes an aggressive phenotype [123, 124]. c-Myc also forms a heterodimer with transcription factor MAX, which binds to the E box DNA sequence, regulating the transcription of target genes. Amplification of this gene frequently occurs in SCCs and other human cancers. *FBXW7* encodes the subunit of SCFFbxw7 E3 ubiquitin ligase which is responsible for binding c-Myc as well as cyclin E and Notch 1, causing their degradation. Loss-of-function mutations in *FBXW7* are also common in SCCs [12]. In SCC cells, *MYC* is regulated upstream by miR-203 that suppresses *MYC* expression and transcriptional activity when overexpressed [125].

Notch Signalling

Notch signalling is involved in the maintenance of normal skin structure and functions. It is responsible for switching between proliferation and differentiation of keratinocytes. It also controls permeability barrier function and forms direct cell-to-cell communication. Out of the four family members, Notch1 protein plays an essential role in cell fate determination as well as tumour suppression. The *NOTCH1* gene is a target of p53 in keratinocytes [126]. *NOTCH2* and *NOTCH3* are also frequently deregulated in SCCs. Missense substitutions, as well as nonsense and frameshift alterations, were identified. Nevertheless, the combined loss of *NOTCH1* and *NOTCH2* has a more significant impact on the development of SCC compared with *NOTCH1* alone [12]. Moreover, *NOTCH1/2/4* mutations have been reported in metastatic SCC as one of the top three recurrently mutated genes (with *TP53* and *CDKN2A*) [120]. *NOTCH1* or *NOTCH2* mutations/loss of function have been reported in almost 75% of SCC cases. Missense loss-of-function mutations were found to localize in NECD EGF-like repeats, NECD HD domain and intracellular RAM domain. These mutations reduced ligand-mediated *NOTCH1* activation (D469G and R1594Q) and interfere with Notch transcription complex assembly (P1770S). Down-regulation of *NOTCH* and its target HES1 protein was reported in SCC. Loss or down-regulation of *NOTCH1* induces proliferation of basal epidermal cells and deregulation of differentiation markers. On the contrary, activated *NOTCH1* induces p21 expression and suppresses keratinocyte growth [127, 128]. Nuclear factor erythroid 2-related factor 2 (Nrf2) is a transcription factor and regulates transcription of enzymes which take part in a protective response against ROS and in metabolism. The self-renewal of basal epithelial stem cells is regulated by the dynamic variations in ROS levels, which are regulated by Nrf2-dependent Notch signalling. Both up-regulation of *NFE2L2*, coding for Nrf2, and loss-of-function mutation of the Nrf2-inactivating kelch like ECH associated protein 1 (*KEAP1*) gene are observed in SCCs. p21(CDKN1A) stabilization of Nrf2 results in increased ROS protection and resistance to the chemotherapy [12].

Tyrosine Kinase Receptors

Epidermal growth factor receptor (EGFR) is a receptor for multiple ligands and is a common target in SCC therapies. Amplifications, as well as mutations of tyrosine kinase receptor genes, such as *EGFR* and *ERBB2*, are prevalent in SCC cases. *EGFR* is overexpressed in about 30% of SCC cases. *EGFR* overexpression promotes a more aggressive SCC phenotype and correlates with short overall survival [129]. Biding of EGF, TGF-α, or IGF with EGFR promotes keratinocyte proliferation. EGFR activates Ras and therefore induces keratinocyte proliferation (by Raf/MEK/ERK) and inhibits their differentiation (by PI-3K/Akt). In fact, EGFR may activate not only PI3K/AKT/mTOR and RAS-RAF-MEK-MAP but also PLC-gamma/PKC and STAT or NF-kB signalling in SCC [128]. Leucine-rich repeats and immunoglobulin-like domains 2 (LRIG2) protein is a transmembrane protein involved in the feedback loop regulation of the ERBB receptor family. The ERBB receptor family is vital for skin development and homeostasis. Hence, *LRIG2* overexpression, which contributes to the activation of EGFR/ERBB4-MAKP signalling, is believed to be cancerogenic in SCCs [130]. *ERBB2* (*HER-2*) and *ERBB3* (*HER-3*) mutations have been reported in SCC [131]. SCC was also shown to present with c-erbB-2 protein overexpression with a trend to higher expression in metastatic foci [132].

Fibroblast growth factor receptor (*FGFR*) genes, especially *FGFR1*, are also frequently amplified in SCCs. *FGFR* gene activation is considered to be pro-oncogenic, whereas the up-regulation of *FGFR3* is the most frequent genetic alteration in the photo-aged keratinocytes as well as in normal human cells. *FGFR1* (P252R/S/T) mutations have been reported in SCC. The G380R *FGFR* mutation induces ligand-independent phosphorylation of the receptor, which results in constitutive activation of downstream signalling [133]. Moreover, *FGFR3* activation can result in dedifferentiation as well as an enhanced proliferation of keratinocytes [12]. In SCC, autocrine FGF10–FGFR2 signalling was found to result from PTEN loss and to activate mTOR [134].

RAS-RAF-MEK-ERK Signalling Pathway

RAS proteins, called small GTPases, which are activated by tyrosine kinases, are known to be one of the most common oncogenes in the human cells. In SCCs, *HRAS* (up to 20% of cases) is affected more frequently than *KRAS* and *NRAS* genes [135]. In the epidermis cells, Ras is activated by EGFR as well as integrins and inhibited by E-cadherins. RAF proto-oncogene serine/threonine-protein kinase (*RAF-1*) was reported as overexpressed in SCC. Mutations or overexpression of mitogen-activated protein kinase kinase (*MAP2K*) or mitogen-activated protein kinase (*MAPK)* in SCC has not been reported yet, but B-Raf proto-oncogene, serine/threonine kinase (*BRAF*) was shown to be down-regulated in SCC. At the same time, RKIP- Raf kinase inhibitory protein, a negative regulator of Raf-mediated MEK/ERK activation, was reported as lost in SCC [128, 136]. Moreover, *HRAS* alterations are found selectively in HPV tumours. This could be explained by transformation through the activation of surface TK receptors associated with Human Papillomavirus (HPV) E5 protein. Moreover, MAPK signalling is also commonly up-regulated in SCCs, and the MAP/ERK pathway promotes proliferation and inhibits differentiation of epidermis cells via CDK4 activation [12, 128, 136].

PI3K/AKT/mTOR Pathway

Phosphatidylinositol 3-kinase (PI3K), which p110α subunit, is encoded by the *PIK3CA* gene, takes part in cell growth, proliferation as well as migration and translation of new proteins. Thus, the PI3K/AKT pathway is essential for cell survival. Additionally, PTEN acts as a negative regulator of PI3K and is a tumour suppressor. Amplifications and mutations in the PI3K/AKT pathway, as well as loss-of-function mutations of *PTEN*, result in uncontrolled cell growth and are prevalent in SCC cases. As mentioned previously, *PIK3CA*, *TP63*, and *SOX2* genes are commonly co-amplified due to their adjacent chromosomal localization [12]. Genomic alterations in *PIK3CA* are found in about 6% of the SCC cases [137], also in metastatic SCC and SCC with lymph node metastases (*PIK3CAP471L* mutation) [120]. At the same time, down-regulation of AKT serine/threonine kinase 1 (*AKT1*) and up-regulation of AKT serine/threonine kinase 2 (*AKT2*) were found frequently in SCC. Hyperphosphorylation of Akt (Ser473) was reported [138].

Epigenetic Regulators

Epigenetic alterations are known to be potentially reversible and can maintain a balance between stem cell renewal and differentiation. Epigenetic regulators are usually enzymes involved in DNA methylation and histone modifications [12]. Moreover, DNA-methylation signature analysis can predict the further prognosis of SCC patients [139]. As Enhancer of Zeste Homolog 2 (EZH2) is the main component of polycomb repressive complex 2, it regulates proliferative potential of self-renewing keratinocytes due to repressing the INK4A-INK4B locus as well as suppressing the AP1 transcription factor, which normally promotes transcription of differentiation marker genes. Elevated expression of *EZH2* is essential for the survival of cancer stem cells. Increased expression of *EZH2* is associated with SCC progression and differentiation. Additionally, EZH2 impairs tumour immunosurveillance; thus, its up-regulation correlates with a higher risk of metastases [12, 140, 141]. Mixed lineage leukaemia (*MLL*) genes, including *MLL2*, *MLL3*, lysine methyltransferase 2D (*KMT2D*) and lysine methyltransferase 2C (*KMT2C*), code for H3K4 methyltransferases. Truncating and missense mutations of these genes have been detected in SCCs [12]. Mediator complex subunit 1 (MED1) is involved in transcription regulation of almost all RNA polymerase II-dependent genes. Furthermore, it is a subunit of a cofactor required for the SP1 activation (CRSP) complex, which promotes activation of SP1 by interaction with TFIID. It also controls p53-dependent apoptosis. MED1 plays a key role in keratinocyte differentiation, and its mutations are frequently observed in SCCs [12]. The p300 protein, encoded by the E1A binding protein p300 (*EP300*) gene, is critical for the normal development before and after birth, by regulation of cell growth and division as well as differentiation. p300 is responsible for histone acetylation, hence in turn for making target genes available for transcription. Together with CREB binding protein (*CREBBP*) gene, p300 regulates transition from the G1 to S cell cycle phase and controls DNA repair. Loss-of-function mutations in *EP300* and *CREBBP* are also commonly identified in SCCs [12, 142].

Nuclear IKKα and PS-IκBα

Component of inhibitor of nuclear factor kappa B kinase complex (IKKα) is one of the catalytic subunits of the IκB kinase (IKK) complex which is responsible for IκB degradation, in turn activating NFκB. Nevertheless, nuclear IKKα plays a major role in epidermal differentiation, also Ca2+-induced, and proliferation. A murine model without *IKKα* expression showed a lack of terminally differentiated keratinocytes and epidermal hyperplasia [143]. Moreover, IKKα interacts with the TGFβ-Smad2/3 pathway, which is involved in the cell cycle arrest in the keratinocyte terminal differentiation [144]. Furthermore, nuclear IKKα in cooperation with the transforming growth factor β (TGFβ) pathway inhibits Myc. Additionally, it binds and inhibits the promoter of the epidermal growth factor (EGF), suppressing the EGFR/RAS/ERK pathway. Nuclear IKKα also binds to histone H3 at the 14-3-3 sigma locus, preventing its hypermethylation so that 14-3-3 sigma can be expressed. 14-3-3 sigma regulates the nuclear export of CDC25, which plays a major role in the cell cycle. Thus, the lack of IKKα results in excess of CDC25 and uncontrolled growth and proliferation of altered cells. IKKα also supports activation of antiproliferative Myc antagonists, including mitotic arrest deficient 1/2 (Mad1, Mad2) and putative transcription factor Ovo-like 1 (Ovol1), through Smad2/3, inducing keratinocyte differentiation [145, 146]. Changed localization and decreased level of IKKα, often occurring in SCCs, cause increased cell vulnerability to chemical and UVB-induced tumorigenesis. Moreover, deleterious and loss of heterozygosity mutations affecting the *IKKα* gene, which is located at 10q24.31, are a significant risk factor for spontaneous skin SCC development [143]. However, other studies considered *IKKα* to be oncogenic. SCCs with an accumulation of nuclear IKKα have been shown to have a higher risk of metastasizing. IKKα inactivates phospho-SUMO-IκBα (PS-IκBα) which is responsible for the regulation of multiple developmental- and stemness-related genes, such as homeobox genes (*HOX*) and iroquois homeobox (*IRX*), which bind histones H2A and H4, promoting keratinocyte transformation [147]. Additionally, the nuclear IKKα level was inversely correlated with the level of the metastasis suppressor mammary serine protease inhibitor (Maspin) [145, 148].

PS-IκBα binds histone deacetylases (HDACs) and the polycomb repressive complex 2 (PRC2) so as to regulate expression of the genes involved in development and differentiation in the TNFα-dependent, but NF-κB-independent, manner. These genes are essential for the maintenance of skin homeostasis. Cytoplasmatic accumulation of IκBα with overactivation of the *HOX* gene was associated with SCC development [147]. In aggressive SCCs, the level of nuclear PS-IκBα is significantly reduced or totally lost [145].

Other Genes

In a study of exome profiling of 39 SCCs paired with normal tissues (lymphocytes) of the patients, driver genes were identified, including *TP53*, *CDKN2A*, *NOTCH1/2* as well as ajuba LIM protein (*AJUBA*), HRas proto-oncogene, GTPase (*HRAS*), Caspase 8 (CASP8), FAT atypical cadherin 1, cadherin-related tumour suppressor homolog (*FAT1*), and *KMT2C* (*MLL3*; histone-lysine N-methyltransferase 2C), Par-3 family cell polarity regulator, protein phosphatase 1, regulatory subunit 118 (*PARD3*) and Ras GTPase-activating protein 1 (*RASA1*). Moreover, mutations in *KMT2C* were associated with shorter overall survival [149]. A more recent report confirmed mutations in *TP53, CDKN2A, NOTCH1/2, HRAS* in cSCCs and also added mutations in calcium voltage-gated channel subunit alpha1 C (*CACNA1C*), *GPR98* (ADGRV1, also known as G protein-coupled receptor 98), *KRAS* (V-Ki-Ras2 Kirsten rat sarcoma 2 viral oncogene homolog), *PAPPA2* (Pappalysin 2), and *PTCH1* to the spectrum [150]. These data confirm previous reports indicating that 70% of SCC cases present with abnormalities in the RB1/p16 and/or p53 pathway, either genetic or epigenetic [151]. Functionally validated activating mutations in metastatic cSCC include *BRAFG464R, BRAFG469R, KRASG12C, FGFR3G380R, KITE562D, HRASG13D, EGFRS720F, ERBB4E563K, EZH2Y641S, MTORS2215F, PIK3CAP471L, HGFE199K, CARD11E24K* and *CARD11D199N* [120].

Fanconi anaemia (FA) is a rare autosomal recessive genetic disorder that affects bone marrow, causing its early life-threatening failure. Furthermore, it is associated with an increased risk of developing leukaemias and solid tumours, including cutaneous SCCs. Mutations were reported in the FA pathway, which is triggered by DNA replication or DNA damage. The FA pathway alterations result in the accumulation of damaged DNA and in turn increase the risk of tumorigenesis. Table 3.2 presents mutated genes from the FA pathway, which are involved in the development of SCCs [108]. *BCL-6* codes for zinc finger transcription factor with the N-terminal POZ domain. It acts as a transcriptional repressor and regulates the transcription of STAT-dependent IL-4 responses of B cells. *BLC-6* is mainly found in the lymphoid system. Nevertheless, *BCL-6* takes part in the differentiation of keratinocytes at the

Table 3.2 Fanconi anaemia DNA repair pathway genes

BRCA1	XRCC2
BRCA2	RFWD3
FANCM	FANCC
FANCB	FANCL
SLX4	RAD51C
FANCA	FANCG
BRIP1	MAD2L2
FANCI	FANCF
PALB2	RAD51
ERCC4	UBE2T
FANCD2	FANCE

BRCA1 BRCA1 DNA repair associated, *BRCA2* BRCA2 DNA repair associated, *BRIP1* BRCA1 interacting protein C-terminal helicase 1, *ERCC4* ERCC excision repair 4, endonuclease catalytic subunit, *FANCA* FA complementation group A, *FANCB* FA complementation group B, *FANCC* FA complementation group C, *FANCD2* FA complementation group D2, *FANCF* FA complementation group F, *FANCG* FA complementation group G, *FANCI* FA complementation group I, *FANCL* FA complementation group L, *FANCM* FA complementation group M, *MAD2L2* mitotic arrest deficient 2 like 2, *PALB2* partner and localizer of BRCA2, *RAD51* RAD51 recombinase, *RAD51C* RAD51 paralog C, *RFWD3* ring finger and WD repeat domain 3, *SLX4* SLX4 structure-specific endonuclease subunit, *UBE2T* ubiquitin conjugating enzyme E2, XRCC2

terminal stage. The overexpression of *BCL-6* occurs in about 18.2% of SCCs [12]. The melanocortin-1-receptor (*MC1R*) gene, which takes part in creating human pigmentation, binds to αmelanocyte-stimulating hormone (α-MSH). This interaction results in the synthesis of melanin-activating cyclase enzyme, thereby increasing the level of cyclic adenosine monophosphate (cAMP). *MCR1* has more than 100 identified polymorphisms where V60L, D84E, V92M, R151C, R160W, R163Q and D294H variants are significantly associated with an increased incidence of SCCs [24]. *FAT1* belongs to the cadherin family and probably functions as an adhesion molecule and signalling receptor. In Drosophila, it acts as a tumour suppressor and regulates planar cell polarity. In humans, protocadherin Fat 1 is known to interact with other major pathways, such as β-catenin and Hippo signalling. Aberrations in *FAT1*, as well as other genes encoding adherens junctions, and desmosomal proteins, including desmoglein 1-4 (DSG1–4), are identified in SCCs [12]. Cyclooxygenase (COX)-derived prostaglandins (PGs) are vital mediators of skin inflammation. Increased levels of PGE2 and PGF2α are commonly observed in premalignant and malignant skin carcinomas. Moreover, over-activated COX-2-dependent signalling results in pre-invasive growth by suppressing terminal differentiation or stimulation of hyperproliferation and survival. Overexpression of *COX-2* exclusively contributes to SCC development, whereas both *COX-2* and *COX-1* are essential in BCC development [93]. Finally, as in BCC, also in SCC, the phenotype of natural killer (NK) cells is dependent on an interaction between killer-cell immunoglobulin-like receptor (KIR) and HLA class I ligand. Both KIR centromeric B haplotype and *HLA-C* and the activating gene *KIR2DS3* are associated with a higher risk of multiple SCC tumours. Moreover, interactions between *HLA-B* and telomeric KIR B haplotype (containing *KIR3DS1* and *KIR2DS1* genes) as well as between *HLA-B* and *KIR2DS5* gene also increase the SCC incidence [104].

Merkel Carcinoma

Merkel cell carcinoma (MCC) is an uncommon and highly aggressive skin cancer developing within the dermis and subcutis. It has an immunophenotype (Cytokeratin 20—CK20) corresponding to sensory Merkel cells of the skin—mechanoreceptor cells of the basal layer of the epidermis. More detailed analysis accumulating over last years suggests that MCC cells (cytokeratin 20 - CK20+, neuron-specific enolase - NSE+, paired box protein PAX5+, neuroendocrine-specific protein - NSP+, terminal deoxynucleotidyl transferas -TdT+, thyroid transcription factor-1 -TTF-1−, leukocyte common antigen - LCA−, S100−) are not the progeny of mature Merkel cells (CK20+) and the true origin of MCC remains unknown [152]. It develops within chronically sun-exposed areas of the skin and mostly affects the fair-skinned population at an advanced age. Immunosuppression, excessive UV exposure, and Merkel cell polyomavirus (MCPyV) infection are the greatest risk factors for MCC. Immunological disorders, such as AIDS or haematological malignancies, as well as solid-organ transplantations and UV light, result in the impairment of the immune response, which plays a particularly important role in MCPyV+ MCC development. In the process of non-viral-mediated carcinogenesis, ultraviolet radiation damages DNA [6–8, 153]. MCPyV- MCCs contain numerous DNA mutations caused by UV damage, whereas MCPyV+ MCCs have an incorporated viral genome and few mutations with "UV signature". MCPyV- MCCs have between 25 and 90-fold increased rate of UV-induced mutations compared to MCPyV+ MCCs. Moreover, in the viral-mediated mechanism, the majority of genes are intact, and interaction between these wild-type genes and viral proteins results in the development of MCCs [7, 18, 154]. The median mutation burden in MCPyV- MCCs is estimated to be 1121 somatic single nucleotide variants (SSNVs) per exome with frequently down-regulated *RB1* and *TP53*. Mutations affect genes responsible for chromatin modifications (ASXL transcriptional regulator 1 - *ASXL1*, *MLL2/3*) and DNA-damage repair (*ATM, MSH2, BRCA2*). Aberrations of x-Jun N-terminal kinases (JNKs) (mitogen-activated protein kinase kinase kinase 1 - *MAP3K1*, TNF receptor associated factor 7 - *TRAF7*) were also identified. Activation of the PI3K pathway and suppression of the Notch pathway are present in MCCs [154].

Merkel Cell Polyomavirus

The recently discovered Merkel cell polyomavirus (MCPyV)—belonging to the Polyomaviridae family of small double-stranded DNA viruses—is detected in 60–80% of MCC cases as integrated within the genome [155, 156]. MCPyV has a circular, double-stranded DNA genome, which is divided into the early and late regions. The latter region consists of viral coat proteins—VP1 and VP2, as well as miRNA—which act on T antigen transcripts. In the early region, the large T antigen (LT) and the small T antigen (ST) are encoded. LT is responsible for viral replication. Acting like a helicase, LT unwinds viral DNA and additionally mobilises host cellular DNA polymerases. MCPyV was proven to enter many cell types, including keratinocytes and dermal fibroblasts. Once acquired, MCPyV becomes a lifelong resident of human skin flora [157]. In cells, the copy number of integrated viral genomes varies from cell to cell [158]. Initially MCPyV is latent, non-replicative after infection. Preliminary productive viral infection induces host cell death, not oncogenic transformation [159]. In fact, oncogenic transformation by MCPyV requires two molecular events: integration of the MCP genome into the human genome and truncation of LT that makes the virus non-replicating. MCPyV infection is facilitated by matrix metalloproteinase (MMP). The deregulation of MMPs is stimulated by growth factors inducing WNT/β-catenin signalling. The WNT signalling pathway is also induced by classical clinical MCC risk factors, such as UV radiation and ageing, which in this way facilitate MCC tumorigenesis [152]. In MCCs, mutations of MCPyV result in truncated LT, which preserves the LXCXE motif. LT is truncated by premature stop codons or deletions that lead to loss of the C-terminal origin binding (OBD) and helicase domains important for MCPyV replication [158]. The LXCXE motif binds the cellular tumour suppressors, including p53 (TP53 gene) and retinoblastoma-associated protein (RB1 gene) as well as the

DnaJ chaperone, which is critical for MCC carcinogenesis. ST is also expressed by MCPyV+ MCC. It binds to protein phosphatase 2A (PP2A), causing deregulation in phosphorylation of c-Myc, and therefore increasing the level of 4E-binding protein 1 (4E-BP1). It also promotes the induction of the proglycolytic genes. ST has an LT-stabilizing domain (LSD) which elevates the level of LT and enables it to disrupt the function of F-box/WD repeat-containing protein 7 (FBXW7) and cell division cycle protein 20 homolog (CDC20) [7, 153, 158].

RB1 Gene

The function of pRb protein is to inhibit cell cycle progression and maintain the cell in G1 phase by binding and repressing E2F, as described above. The copy loss of *RB1* is detected in most of MCPyV- MCC cases [160]. On the other hand, in MCPyV+ MCCs viral truncated large T antigen binds to pRb by the LXCXE motif—MCPyV-LT binds pRb potently. Inactivation of pRb by MCPyV-LT is sufficient for MCC tumour growth out of MCPyV-positive MCC cells [161]. An additional mechanism indicated as inducing pRb down-regulation in MCC are also *RB1* promoter hypermethylation and miRNA induced down-regulation of expression [160]. Despite the difference in the mechanisms, in both viral and non-viral MCC, a lack of functional pRb results in an uncontrollable proliferation of the altered cells. This pathologic process lies at the bottom of the MCC carcinogenesis [7, 18].

TP53 Gene

Another common dysfunction in MCCs involves tumour protein p53 (*TP53* gene) which is one of the most well-known suppressor proteins in human cells, as described above. The frequency of p53-inactivating mutations has been reported to be relatively low in MCC, between 10% and 27% [162–164]. MCPyV- MCCs frequently contain inactivating mutations of *TP53* or its deletions, while in MCPyV+ MCCs, *TP53* was reported mostly not to be mutated, but its activity is down-regulated [7, 18]. In fact, both in MCPyV-negative and in MCPyV-positive cases, *TP53* inactivating mutations were reported [164]. Very recently, a complicated loop of molecular interactions was discovered in MCC pathogenesis. MCV LT that binds to pRb induces accumulation of p14(ARF) that physiologically is an inhibitor of Mdm2 (p53 ubiquitin ligase). At the same time, expression of ST reduced p53 activity. MCPyV ST recruits the MYC homolog MYCL (L-Myc) to the E1A-binding protein p400 (*EP400*) chromatin remodeller complex that decreases p53 expression. MCPyV ST–MYCL–EP400 complex inactivates p53. EP400 targets Mdm2 and casein kinase 1 (CK1α)—activator of Mdm4. As an effect, high levels of Mdm4, which binds the p53 tumour suppressor protein and inhibits its activity, are accumulated [165].

NOTCH Genes

In MCCs mutations also occur in the *NOTCH* family which can function as either oncogenic or suppressing genes, depending on the type of cell. Both Notch1 signalling, which takes part in cell fate determination, proliferation, differentiation and apoptosis, and Notch2 signalling, which is responsible for determination of the cell destination in the embryo as well as for regulation of the immune system and tissue repair, are particularly affected in MCCs. The majority of mutations contain a typical "UV signature". Loss-of-function mutations occurring in MCPyV-MCCs indicate its suppressive role in MCCs and other neuroendocrine malignancies [7, 18, 154]. It was shown that the expression of *NOTCH3* is an independent predictor of MCC outcome [166].

PI3K-AKT-mTOR Pathway

The PI3K-AKT-mTOR pathway is known to be overactivated in MCCs. PI3K phosphorylates signalling molecules which transmit signals from the cytoplasm to the cell nucleus. It plays an important role in cell cycle regulation, movement of cells and is involved in the regulation of insulin and maturation of fat cells. Gain-of-function mutations in *AKT1*, *HRAS* and *KRAS* have also been reported. Moreover, activating mutations occur in phosphatidylinositol-3,4,5-trisphosphate dependent Rac exchange factor 2 (*PREX2*), which is an inhibitor of PTEN [7, 18, 154].

Other Genes

Single copy loss is detected in the *PTEN* gene, which acts as a tumour suppressor, preventing the cell from growing and dividing uncontrollably. Loss-of-function mutations occur in neurofibromin 1 (*NF1*), which inhibits cell growth and turns off the RAS protein (which has an adverse, stimulating effect) as well as in prune homolog 2 with BCH domain (*PRUNE2*), which is a proapoptotic factor. The glutamate ionotropic receptor NMDA type subunit 2A (*GRIN2A*) gene, which encodes a protein that forms a subunit of NMDA receptors, and *BRCA2*, which is involved in repairing damaged DNA, are also down-regulated in MCCs. The expression of the TSC complex subunit 1 (*TSC1*) gene is also decreased [7, 18].

Other Skin Carcinomas

Cutaneous appendageal carcinoma (CAC) refers to a rare group of neoplasms which arise "de novo" or derive from precursor lesions such as nevus sebaceous or pre-existing benign counterpart. Men have a higher incidence rate, while the peak occurs in the eighth decade of life. The face, scalp and neck are the most frequent localizations of CACs. Till 2010, there were only 62 reported cases of spiradenocarcinoma and adenoid cystic carcinoma and less than 100 cases of other apocrine-eccrine carcinomas, including hidradenocarcinoma, apocrine carcinoma, digital papillary carcinoma, and malignant mixed tumour, as well as around 200 cases of mucinous carcinomas and 300 of porocarcinomas. The rare prevalence of CACs results in limited knowledge concerning these diseases [9, 10, 167]. UV exposure was confirmed as a significant risk factor for spiradenocarcinoma, hidradenocarcinoma and microcystic adnexal carcinoma. Lesions are mainly located in the sun-exposed areas. UV radiation can act through direct DNA damage as well as supporting local immunosuppression. Moreover, CAC prevalence is higher in the immunosuppressed population [9].

Genetic disorders such as Muir–Torre syndrome (MTS) or Brooke–Spiegler syndrome can predispose to the development of CACs, sebaceous carcinoma (SeC) and spiradenocarcinoma, respectively. Muir–Torre syndrome (MTS) is an autosomal dominant disease, which is a subtype of Lynch disease. Inherited germline mutations occur in mutL homolog 1/2/6 (*MLH1*, *MSH2*, *MSH6*) or PMS1 homolog 2, mismatch repair system component (*PMS2*). These genes encode proteins responsible for mismatch DNA repair so that the loss of their functions results in increased sebaceous carcinogenesis. MTS patients often develop two or more malignancies besides SeCs. Brooke–Spiegler syndrome is caused by aberrations in the CYLD lysine 63 deubiquitinase (*CYLD*) gene, which regulates *NF-κB* and acts as a tumour suppressor. Generally, *NF-κB* controls the process of apoptosis, so the defect in *CYLD* causes uncontrolled growth of altered tissue [9, 168–170].

Mismatch repair-derived insertions and deletions or ultraviolet (UV) signature single-nucleotide mutations are shown to be dominant aberrations in SeCs. SeCs harbour somatic mutations in PI3K signalling components as well as in *TP53* and *RB1* genes. Moreover, impairments are detected in the process of DNA repair and in the chromatin remodelling pathway. SeCs carry a high level of microsatellite instability with alterations in mismatch-repair genes, *MLH1* and *MSH2*. Multiple point mutations which are identified in *NOTCH1*, *NOTCH2*, zinc finger protein 750 (*ZNF750*), ras responsive element binding protein 1 (*RREB1*), lysine methyltransferase 2D (*KMT2D*) and FAT atypical cadherin 3 (*FAT3*). Furthermore, SeCs acquire mutations which have been identified in cutaneous SCCs, including *TP53*, *KMT2D* and *NOTCH1/NOTCH2*. These tumours are considered to share epigenetic similarity and transcriptional patterns. There is an increased SCC incidence amongst CAC patients [169, 171].

Summary and Conclusions

Non-melanoma skin cancers (NMSCs) are considered to have one of the highest rates of mutations amongst all human tumours. The majority of alterations are caused by UV exposure which induces characteristic "UV signature" mutations, such as C to T and CC to TT transitions. Pyrimidine (6–4) pyrimidine and cyclobutane dimers are generated photoproducts which play a key role in the carcinogenesis.

The major hallmark of basal cell carcinomas are aberrations in the HH pathway. The *PTCH1* gene, the suppressing component of HH signalling, is altered in up to 75% of BCC cases. Other mutations affecting HH pathway mutations occur in *SMO* as well as less frequently in *SUFU* and *PTCH2* genes. Nevertheless, several proto-oncogenes and suppressor genes, including *TP53, TP63, RB1, MYCN, NOTCH1/2*, as well as Hippo pathway factors (*YAP1, LATS1/2* and *PTPN14*) are also significantly changed. Different variants of *MC1R* increase the risk of BCC development. Moreover, other aberrations affect *TERT* and *DPH3* promoter, detoxifying proteins, p16(INK4A) and p14(ARF), connexins, gap junctional intracellular communication, cyclooxygenase-dependent signalling, NFκB pathway as well as collagen genes. The immune system can also take part in the development of BCCs. Impairment of the IL-6/JAK/STAT3 signalling, up-regulation of *PD-1* gene, overexpression of PD-1 L and decreased FAS/FASL are common for the altered tumour cells. Presence of particular human leukocyte antigen genes, including the decrease of *HLA-DR4* and increase of *HLA-DR7*, also contributes to BCC carcinogenesis.

Alterations of the *TP53* gene, which is known as the "guardian of the genome", are the most frequent mutations in SCCs. Besides *TP53*, changes are observed in the other cell-cycle controlling genes, including *CDKN2A, RB1, CCDN1, CCNE1* and *MYC*. Impairment of signalling and cell adhesion genes (*EGFR, FGFR1, PIK3CA, FAT1, YAP1* and *PTEN*) also supports the development of SCCs. *TP63, SOX2* as well as *NOTCH1* genes are known to be responsible for keratinocyte differentiation, and their mutations increase tumourigenesis. Moreover, Fanconi anaemia is a genetic disease which alters the Fanconi DNA repair pathway, predisposing to SCC development. Other affected genes, including *NRF2, BCL-6*, and epigenetic regulators, are involved in SCC formation.

Mutations in MCCs are mainly caused by Merkel cell polyomavirus infection or UV exposure. High frequency of *TP53* and *RB1* mutations are characteristic for MCCs. *NOTCH* genes and the PI3K-AKT-mTOR pathway are also involved in tumourigenesis. Single copy loss of *PTEN*, loss-of-function mutations of *NF1* and modifications in *BRCA2* and *GRIN2A* genes are identified in SCCs. Furthermore, mutations affect genes responsible for chromatin modifications (*ASXL1, MLL2/3*) and DNA damage repair (*ATM, MSH2* and *BRCA2*).

CACs are very rare tumours so that the knowledge concerning these diseases is limited. Nevertheless, genetic aberrations mostly result from excess UV exposure as well as local immunosuppression. Genetic disorders, such as Muir–Torre syndrome or Brooke–Spiegler syndrome, can predispose to the development of CACs, sebaceous carcinoma (SeC) and spiradenocarcinoma, respectively. Mutations of *MLH1, MSH2, MSH6* and *PMS2* genes occur in Muir–Torre syndrome, whereas in Brooke–Spiegler syndrome, the *CYLD* gene is affected. Additionally, in SeCs aberrations of PI3K signalling, *TP53, RB1* as well as of *NOTCH1, NOTCH2, ZNF750, RREB1, KMT2D* and *FAT3* have been detected. Furthermore, a similar spectrum of mutations occurs in both SeCs and SCCs.

Acknowledgements The authors thank Prof. Ewa Bartnik for proofreading of the text.

References

1. Muzic JG, Wright AC, Alniemi DT, Zubair AS, Olazagasti Lourido JM, Sosa Seda IM, Weaver AL, Baum CL. Incidence and trends of basal cell carcinoma and cutaneous squamous cell carcinoma: a population-based study in Olmsted County, Minnesota, 2000 to 2010. Mayo Clin Proc. 2017;92(6):890–8.
2. Atasoy M, et al. HLA antigen profile differences in patients with SCC (squamous cell carcinoma) in-situ/actinic keratosis and invasive SCC: Is there a genetic succeptibility for invasive SCC development? Eurasian J Med. 2009;41(3):162–4.
3. Rutkowski P, Owczarek W. Skin carcinomas. Oncol Clin Pract. 2018;14(3):129–47.
4. Dourmishev LA, Rusinova D, Botev I. *Clinical variants, stages, and management of basal cell carcinoma*. Indian Dermatol Online J. 2013;4:12–7.
5. Clayman GL, et al. Mortality risk from squamous cell skin cancer. J Clin Oncol. 2005;23(4):759–65.
6. Kaae J, Hansen AV, Biggar RJ, Boyd HA, Moore PS, Wohlfahrt J, Melbye M. Merkel cell carcinoma: incidence, mortality, and risk of other cancer. J Natl Cancer Inst. 2010;102(11):793–801.
7. Becker JC, Stang A, DeCaprio JA, Cerroni L, Lebbé C, Veness M, Nghiem P. Merkel cell carcinoma. Nat Rev Dis Primers. 2017;3:17077.
8. Clarke CA, Robbins HA, Tatalovich Z, Lynch CF, Pawlish KS, Finch JL, Hernandez BY, Fraumeni JF Jr, Madeleine MM, Engels EA. Risk of merkel cell carcinoma after solid organ transplantation. J Natl Cancer Inst. 2015;107(2):dju382.
9. Blake PW, Bradford PT, Devesa SS, Toro JR. *Cutaneous appendageal carcinoma incidence and survival patterns in the United States*. Arch Dermatol Res. 2010;146(6):625–32.
10. Craig PJ. An overview of uncommon cutaneous malignancies, including skin appendageal (adnexal) tumours and sarcomas. Clin Oncol. 2019;31(11):769–78.
11. Kamińska-Winciorek G, et al. Principles of prophylactic and therapeutic management of skin toxicity during treatment with checkpoint inhibitors. Adv Dermatol Allergol/Postępy Dermatol Alergol. 2019;36(4):382–91.
12. Paolo Dotto G, Rustgi AK. *Squamous cell cancers: a unified perspective on biology and genetics*. Cancer Cell. 2016;29(5):622–37.
13. Martincorena I, et al. Tumor evolution. High burden and pervasive positive selection of somatic mutations in normal human skin. Science. 2015;348(6237):880–6.
14. Lear JT, Hoban P, Strange RC, Fryer AA. *Basal cell carcinoma: from host response and polymorphic variants to tumour suppressor genes*. Clin Exp Dermatol. 2005;30:49–55.
15. Pellegrini C, Maturo MG, Di Nardo L, Ciciarelli V, García-Rodrigo CG, Fargnoli MC. *Understanding the Molecular Genetics of Basal Cell Carcinoma*. Int J Mol Sci. 2017;18(11):2485.
16. Martinez MAR, Francisco G, Cabral LS, Ruiz IRG, Neto CF. Molecular genetics of non-melanoma skin cancer. Anais Brasileiros de Dermatologia. 2006;81(5):405–19.
17. Bonilla X, Parmentier L, King B, Bezrukov F, Kaya G, Zoete V, Seplyarskiy VB, Sharpe HJ, McKee T, Letourneau A, Ribaux PG, Popadin K, Basset-Seguin N, Chaabene RB, Santoni FA, Andrianova MA, Guipponi M, Garieri M, Verdan C, Grosdemange K, Sumara O, Eilers M, Aifantis I, Michielin O, de Sauvage FJ, Antonarakis SE, Nikolaev SI. Genomic analysis identifies new drivers and progression pathways in skin basal cell carcinoma. Nat Genet. 2016;48:398–406.
18. Harms PW, Vats P, Verhaegen ME, Robinson DR, Wu Y-M, Dhanasekaran SM, Palanisamy N, Siddiqui J, Cao X, Fengyun S, Wang R, Xiao H, Kunju LP, Mehra R, Tomlins SA, Fullen DR, Bichakjian CK, Johnson TM, Dlugosz AA, Chinnaiya AM. The distinctive mutational spectra of polyomavirus-negative merkel cell carcinoma. Cancer Res. 2015;75(18):3720–7.
19. Small J, Barton V, Peterson B, Alberg AJ. Keratinocyte carcinoma as a marker of a high cancer-risk phenotype. Adv Cancer Res. 2016;130:257–91.
20. Verkouteren JAC, Pardo LM, Uitterlinden AG, Nijste T. Non-genetic and genetic predictors of a superficial first basal cell carcinoma. J Eur Acad Dermatol Venereol. 2019;33(3):533–40.

21. Roberts MR, Sordillo JE, Kraft P, Asgari MM. Sex-stratified polygenic risk score identifies individuals at increased risk of basal cell carcinoma. J Invest Dermatol. 2020;140(5):971–5.
22. Nan H, Kraft P, Hunter DJ, Han J. Genetic variants in pigmentation genes, pigmentary phenotypes, and risk of skin cancer in Caucasians. Int J Cancer. 2009;125:909–17.
23. de Zwaan SE, Haass NK. Genetics of basal cell carcinoma. Australas J Dermatol. 2010;51:81–94.
24. Tagliabue E, Fargnoli MC, Gandini S, Maisonneuve P, Liu F, Kayser M, Nijsten T, Han J, Kumar R, Gruis NA, Ferrucci L, Branicki W, Dwyer T, Blizzard L, Helsing P, Autier P, García-Borrón JC, Kanetsky PA, Landi MT, Little J, Newton-Bishop J, Sera F, Raimondi S. MC1R gene variants and non-melanoma skin cancer: a pooled-analysis from the M-SKIP project. Br J Cancer. 2015;113:354–63.
25. van der Poort EKJ, Gunn DA, Beekman M, Griffiths CEM, Slagboom PE, van Heemst D, Noordam R. Basal cell carcinoma genetic susceptibility increases the rate of skin ageing: a Mendelian randomization study. Eur Acad Dermatol Venereol. 2020;34(1):97–100.
26. Vishlaghi N, Lisse TS. Exploring vitamin D signaling within skin cancer. Clin Endocrinol. 2020;92(4):273–81.
27. Wang L-E, Li C, Strom SS, Goldberg LH, Brewster A, Guo Z, Qiao Y, Clayman GL, Lee JJ, El-Naggar AK, Prieto VG, Duvic M, Lippman SM, Weber RS, Kripke ML, Wei Q. Repair capacity for UV light - induced DNA damage associated with risk of nonmelanoma skin cancer and tumor progression. Clin Cancer Res. 2007;13(21):6532–9.
28. Tilli CMLJ, Van Steensel MAM, Krekels GAM, Neumann HAM, Ramaekers FCS. Molecular aetiology and pathogenesis of basal cell carcinoma. Br J Dermatol. 2004;152:1108–24.
29. Castori M, Morrone A, Kanitakis J, Grammatico P. Genetic skin diseases predisposing to basal cell carcinoma. Eur J Dermatol. 2012;22(3):299–309.
30. Fogel AL, Sarin KY, Teng JMC. Genetic diseases associated with an increased risk of skin cancer development in childhood. Curr Opin Pediatr. 2017;29(4):426–33.
31. Schierbeck J, Vestergaard T, Bygum A. Skin cancer associated genodermatoses: a literature review. Acta Derm Venereol. 2019;99(4):360–9.
32. Nieuwenburg SA, Adan F, Ruijs MWG, Sonke GS, van Leerdam ME, Crijns MB. Cumulative risk of skin cancer in patients with Li-Fraumeni syndrome. Fam Cancer. 2020;19(4):347–51.
33. Kalińska-Bienias A, Kowalewski C, Majewski S. The EVER genes – the genetic etiology of carcinogenesis in epidermodysplasia verruciformis and a possible role in non-epidermodysplasia verruciformis patients. Adv Dermatol Allergol. 2016;33(2):75–80.
34. Hajeer AH, Lear JT, Ollier WE, Naves M, Worthington J, Bell DA, Smith AG, Bowers WP, Jones PW, Strange RC, Fryer AA. Preliminary evidence of an association of tumour necrosis factor microsatellites with increased risk of multiple basal cell carcinomas. Br J Dermatol. 2000;142(3):441–5.
35. Sahi H, Sihto H, Artama M, Koljonen V, Böhling T, Pukkala E. History of chronic inflammatory disorders increases the risk of Merkel cell carcinoma, but does not correlate with Merkel cell polyomavirus infection. Br J Cancer. 2017;116(2):260–4.
36. Fahradyan A, Howell AC, Wolfswinkel EM, Tsuha M, Sheth P, Wong AK. Updates on the management of non-melanoma skin cancer (NMSC). Healthcare. 2017;5(4):82.
37. Mestre VF, Medeiros-Fonseca B, Estêvão D, Casaca F, Silva S, Félixe A, Silva F, Colaço B, Seixas F, Bastos MMSM, Lopes C, Medeiros R, Oliveira PA, Gil da Costa RM. HPV16 is sufficient to induce squamous cell carcinoma specifically in the tongue base in transgenic mice. J Pathol. 2020;251(1):4–11.
38. Qibing Zeng AZ. Assessing potential mechanisms of arsenic-induced skin lesions and cancers: human and in vitro evidence. Environ Pollut. 2020;260:113919.
39. Ho S-Y, Tsai Y-C, Lee M-C, Guo H-R. Merkel cell carcinoma in patients with long-term ingestion of arsenic. J Occup Health. 2005;47(2):188–92.
40. Barton DT, Zens MS, Marmarelis EL, Gilbert-Diamond D, Karagas MR. Cosmetic tattooing and early onset basal cell carcinoma: a population-based case–control study from new hampshire. Epidemiology. 2020;31(3):448–50.

41. Lapouge G, et al. Identifying the cellular origin of squamous skin tumors. Proc Natl Acad Sci U S A. 2011;108(18):7431–6.
42. Youssef KK, et al. Identification of the cell lineage at the origin of basal cell carcinoma. Nat Cell Biol. 2010;12(3):299–305.
43. Pellegrini C, et al. Understanding the molecular genetics of basal cell carcinoma. Int J Mol Sci. 2017;18(11):2485.
44. Jayaraman SS, Rayhan DJ, Hazany S, Kolodney MS. Mutational landscape of basal cell carcinomas by whole-exome sequencing. J Invest Dermat. 2014;134:213–20.
45. Liu Y, Liu H, Bian Q. Identification of potential biomarkers associated with basal cell carcinoma. Hindawi BioMed Res Int. 2020;2020:2073690.
46. Jun Wan, Hongji Dai, Xiaoli Zhang, Sheng Liu, Yuan Lin, Ally-Khan Somani, Jingwu Xie, Jiali Han. Distinct transcriptomic landscapes of cutaneous basal cell carcinomas and squamous cell carcinomas. Genes Dis; 2019.
47. Goodman AM, et al. Genomic landscape of advanced basal cell carcinoma: implications for precision treatment with targeted and immune therapies. Onco Targets Ther. 2018;7(3):e1404217.
48. Katoh Y, Katoh M. Hedgehog target genes: mechanisms of carcinogenesis induced by aberrant hedgehog signaling activation. Curr Mol Med. 2009;9(7):873–86.
49. Huq AJ, Walsh M, Rajagopalan B, Finlay M, Trainer AH, Bonnet F, Sevenet N, Winship IM. Mutations in SUFU and PTCH1 genes may cause different cutaneous cancer predisposition syndromes: similar, but not the same. Fam Cancer. 2018;17:601–6.
50. Regl G, et al. The zinc-finger transcription factor GLI2 antagonizes contact inhibition and differentiation of human epidermal cells. Oncogene. 2004;23(6):1263–74.
51. Zhang H, et al. Role of PTCH and p53 genes in early-onset basal cell carcinoma. Am J Pathol. 2001;158(2):381–5.
52. Skodric-Trifunovic V, et al. Novel patched 1 mutations in patients with nevoid basal cell carcinoma syndrome--case report. Croat Med J. 2015;56(1):63–7.
53. Ogden T, et al. The relevance of a suppressor of fused (SUFU) mutation in the diagnosis and treatment of Gorlin syndrome. JAAD Case Rep. 2018;4(2):196–9.
54. Pricl S, et al. Smoothened (SMO) receptor mutations dictate resistance to vismodegib in basal cell carcinoma. Mol Oncol. 2015;9(2):389–97.
55. Kim AL, Back JH, Chaudhary SC, Zhu Y, Athar M, Bickers DR. SOX9 transcriptionally regulates mTOR-induced proliferation of basal cell carcinomas. J Invest Dermatol. 2018;138(8):1716–25.
56. Bigelow RL, Chari NS, Unden AB, Spurgers KB, Lee S, Roop DR, Toftgård R, McDonnel TJ. Transcriptional regulation of bcl-2 mediated by the sonic hedgehog signaling pathway through gli-1. J Biol Chem. 2003;279(9):1197–205.
57. Shea CR, et al. Overexpression of p53 protein in basal cell carcinomas of human skin. Am J Pathol. 1992;141(1):25–9.
58. Neill GW, Harrison WJ, Ikram MS, Williams TDL, Bianchi LS, Nadendla SK, Green JL, Ghali L, Frischauf A-M, O'Toole EA, Aberger F, Philpott MP. GLI1 repression of ERK activity correlates with colony formation and impaired migration in human epidermal keratinocytes. Carcinogenesis. 2008;29(4):738–46.
59. D'Errico M, et al. UV mutation signature in tumor suppressor genes involved in skin carcinogenesis in xeroderma pigmentosum patients. Oncogene. 2000;19(3):463–7.
60. Boonchai W, et al. Expression of p53 in arsenic-related and sporadic basal cell carcinoma. Arch Dermatol. 2000;136(2):195–8.
61. Bolshakov S, et al. p53 mutations in human aggressive and nonaggressive basal and squamous cell carcinomas. Clin Cancer Res. 2003;9(1):228–34.
62. Ziegler A, et al. Mutation hotspots due to sunlight in the p53 gene of nonmelanoma skin cancers. Proc Natl Acad Sci U S A. 1993;90(9):4216–20.
63. Rosenstein BS, et al. p53 mutations in basal cell carcinomas arising in routine users of sunscreens. Photochem Photobiol. 1999;70(5):798–806.

64. Ouhtit A, et al. UV-radiation-specific p53 mutation frequency in normal skin as a predictor of risk of basal cell carcinoma. J Natl Cancer Inst. 1998;90(7):523–31.
65. Giglia-Mari G, Sarasin A. TP53 mutations in human skin cancers. Hum Mutat. 2003;21(3):217–28.
66. Smirnov A, et al. p63 is a promising marker in the diagnosis of unusual skin cancer. Int J Mol Sci. 2019;20(22):5781.
67. Zheng Z, Kye Y, Zhang X, Kim A, Kim I. Expression of p63, bcl-2, bcl-6 and p16 in basal cell carcinoma and squamous cell carcinoma of the skin. Korean J Pathol. 2005;39:91–8.
68. Eshkoor SA, et al. p16 gene expression in basal cell carcinoma. Arch Med Res. 2008;39(7):668–73.
69. Soufir N, et al. P16 UV mutations in human skin epithelial tumors. Oncogene. 1999;18(39):5477–81.
70. Bartos V. Expression of p16 protein in cutaneous basal cell carcinoma: still far from being clearly understood. Acta Dermatovenerol Croat. 2020;28(1):43–4.
71. Villada G, et al. A limited immunohistochemical panel to distinguish basal cell carcinoma of cutaneous origin from basaloid squamous cell carcinoma of the head and neck. Appl Immunohistochem Mol Morphol. 2018;26(2):126–31.
72. Giacinti C, Giordano A. RB and cell cycle progression. Oncogene. 2006;25:5220–7.
73. Stacey SN, et al. New basal cell carcinoma susceptibility loci. Nat Commun. 2015;6:6825.
74. Freier K, et al. Recurrent NMYC copy number gain and high protein expression in basal cell carcinoma. Oncol Rep. 2006;15(5):1141–5.
75. Meng Z, Moroishi T, Guan K-L. Mechanisms of Hippo pathway regulation. Genes Dev. 2016;30(1):1–17.
76. Ma S, Meng Z, Chen R, Guan K-L. The hippo pathway: biology and pathophysiology. Annu Rev Biochem. 2019;88:577–604.
77. Maglic D, et al. YAP-TEAD signaling promotes basal cell carcinoma development via a c-JUN/AP1 axis. EMBO J. 2018;37(17):e98642.
78. Quan T, et al. Elevated YAP and its downstream targets CCN1 and CCN2 in basal cell carcinoma: impact on keratinocyte proliferation and stromal cell activation. Am J Pathol. 2014;184(4):937–43.
79. Miller SJ. Etiology and pathogenesis of basal cell carcinoma. Clin Dermatol. 1995;13(6):527–36.
80. Reyes O, et al. Mucina1 (MUC1) en los engrosamientos epidérmicos del carcinoma basocelular (CBC). Med Cutan Ibero Lat Am. 2019;47(3):178–87.
81. Jia J, et al. LGR5 expression is controlled by IKKalpha in basal cell carcinoma through activating STAT3 signaling pathway. Oncotarget. 2016;7(19):27280–94.
82. Shi FT, et al. Notch signaling is significantly suppressed in basal cell carcinomas and activation induces basal cell carcinoma cell apoptosis. Mol Med Rep. 2017;15(4):1441–54.
83. Nicolas M, et al. Notch1 functions as a tumor suppressor in mouse skin. Nat Genet. 2003;33(3):416–21.
84. Maturo MG, Rachakonda S, Heidenreich B, Pellegrini C, Srinivas N, Requena C, Serra-Guillen C, Llombart B, Sanmartin O, Guillen C, Di Nardo L, Peris K, Fargnoli MC, Nagore E, Kumar R. Coding and noncoding somatic mutations in candidate genes in basal cell carcinoma. Sci Rep. 2020;10:8005.
85. Griewank KG, et al. TERT promoter mutations are frequent in cutaneous basal cell carcinoma and squamous cell carcinoma. PLoS One. 2013;8(11):e80354.
86. Scott GA, Laughlin TS, Rothberg PG. Mutations of the TERT promoter are common in basal cell carcinoma and squamous cell carcinoma. Mod Pathol. 2014;27(4):516–23.
87. Moloney FJ, Lyons JG, Bock VL, Huang XX, Bugeja MJ, Halliday GM. Hotspot mutation of Brahma in non-melanoma skin cancer. J Invest Dermatol. 2009;129(4):1012–5.
88. Bock VL, et al. BRM and BRG1 subunits of the SWI/SNF chromatin remodelling complex are downregulated upon progression of benign skin lesions into invasive tumours. Br J Dermatol. 2011;164(6):1221–7.

89. Denisova E, et al. Frequent DPH3 promoter mutations in skin cancers. Oncotarget. 2015;6(34):35922–30.
90. Nebert DW, Vasiliou V. Analysis of the glutathione S-transferase (GST) gene family. Hum Genomics. 2004;1(6):460–4.
91. Karahan N, et al. Increased expression of COX-2 in recurrent basal cell carcinoma of the skin: a pilot study. Indian J Pathol Microbiol. 2011;54(3):526–31.
92. Kaiser U, et al. Polarization and distribution of tumor-associated macrophages and COX-2 expression in basal cell carcinoma of the ocular adnexae. Curr Eye Res. 2018;43(9):1126–35.
93. Müller-Decker K. Cyclooxygenase-dependent signaling is causally linked to non-melanoma skin carcinogenesis: pharmacological, genetic, and clinical evidence. Cancer Metastasis Rev. 2011;30:343–61.
94. Chen Y, Liu J. The prognostic roles of cyclooxygenase-2 for patients with basal cell carcinoma. Artif Cells Nanomed Biotechnol. 2019;47(1):3053–7.
95. Jee SH, et al. Overexpression of interleukin-6 in human basal cell carcinoma cell lines increases anti-apoptotic activity and tumorigenic potency. Oncogene. 2001;20(2):198–208.
96. Jee SH, et al. Interleukin-6 induced basic fibroblast growth factor-dependent angiogenesis in basal cell carcinoma cell line via JAK/STAT3 and PI3-kinase/Akt pathways. J Invest Dermatol. 2004;123(6):1169–75.
97. Sławińska M, Zabłotna M, Gleń J, Lakomy J, Nowicki RJ, Sobjanek M. STAT3 polymorphisms and IL-6 polymorphism are associated with the risk of basal cell carcinoma in patients from northern Poland. Arch Dermatol Res. 2019;311:697–704.
98. Sternberg C, et al. Synergistic cross-talk of hedgehog and interleukin-6 signaling drives growth of basal cell carcinoma. Int J Cancer. 2018;143(11):2943–54.
99. Fathi F, Ebrahimi M, Eslami A, Hafezi H, Eskandari N, Motedayyen H. Association of programmed death-1 gene polymorphisms with the risk of basal cell carcinoma. Int J Immunogenet. 2019;46:444–50.
100. Rompel R, Petres J, Kaupert K, Mueller-Eckhardt G. HLA phenotypes and multiple basal cell carcinomas. Dermatology. 1994;189(3):222–4.
101. de Carvalho AV, et al. Positivity for HLA DR1 is associated with basal cell carcinoma in renal transplant patients in southern Brazil. Int J Dermatol. 2012;51(12):1448–53.
102. Czarnecki D, et al. Multiple basal cell carcinomas and HLA frequencies in southern Australia. J Am Acad Dermatol. 1991;24(4):559–61.
103. Vineretsky KA, et al. Skin cancer risk is modified by KIR/HLA interactions that influence the activation of natural killer immune cells. Cancer Res. 2016;76(2):370–6.
104. Vineretsky KA, Karagas MR, Christensen BC, Kuriger-Laber JK, Perry AE, Storm CA, Nelson HH. Skin cancer risk is modified by KIR/HLA interactions that influence the activation of natural killer immune cells. Cancer Res. 2016;76(2):370–6.
105. de la Fouchardière A, Cabaret O, Savin L, Combemale P, Schvartz H, Penet C, Bonadona V, Soufir N, Bressac-de Paillerets B. Germline BAP1 mutations predispose also to multiple basal cell carcinomas. Clin Genet. 2015;88(3):273–7.
106. Alam M, Ratner D. Cutaneous squamous-cell carcinoma. N Engl J Med. 2001;344(13):975–83.
107. Schmults CD, et al. Factors predictive of recurrence and death from cutaneous squamous cell carcinoma: a 10-year, single-institution cohort study. JAMA Dermatol. 2013;149(5):541–7.
108. Corina Lorz, Carmen Segrelles, Ricardo Errazquin and Ramon Garcia-Escudero, Comprehensive molecular characterization of squamous cell carcinomas, in squamous cell carcinoma - hallmark and treatment modalities, H.E. Daaboul, Editor; 2019.
109. Black AP, Ogg GS. The role of p53 in the immunobiology of cutaneous squamous cell carcinoma. Clin Exp Immunol. 2003;132(3):379–84.
110. Campos MA, et al. Prognostic significance of RAS mutations and P53 expression in cutaneous squamous cell carcinomas. Genes (Basel). 2020;11(7):751.
111. Poeta ML, et al. TP53 mutations and survival in squamous-cell carcinoma of the head and neck. N Engl J Med. 2007;357(25):2552–61.

112. Warren TA, et al. Expression profiling of cutaneous squamous cell carcinoma with perineural invasion implicates the p53 pathway in the process. Sci Rep. 2016;6(1):34081.
113. Missero C, Antonini D. p63 in squamous cell carcinoma of the skin: more than a stem cell/progenitor marker. J Invest Dermatol. 2017;137(2):280–1.
114. Hsieh MH, et al. p63 and SOX2 dictate glucose reliance and metabolic vulnerabilities in squamous cell carcinomas. Cell Rep. 2019;28(7):1860–1878.e9.
115. Koh SP, Brasch HD, de Jongh J, Itinteang T, Tan ST. Cancer stem cell subpopulations in moderately differentiated head and neck cutaneous squamous cell carcinoma. Heliyon. 2019;5(8):e02257.
116. Watanabe H, et al. SOX2 and p63 colocalize at genetic loci in squamous cell carcinomas. J Clin Invest. 2014;124(4):1636–45.
117. Pacifico A, Leone G. Role of p53 and CDKN2A inactivation in human squamous cell carcinomas. J Biomed Biotechnol. 2007;2007(3):43418.
118. Saridaki Z, et al. Mutational analysis of CDKN2A genes in patients with squamous cell carcinoma of the skin. Br J Dermatol. 2003;148(4):638–48.
119. Brown VL, et al. p16INK4a and p14ARF tumor suppressor genes are commonly inactivated in cutaneous squamous cell carcinoma. J Invest Dermatol. 2004;122(5):1284–92.
120. Li YY, et al. Genomic analysis of metastatic cutaneous squamous cell carcinoma. Clin Cancer Res. 2015;21(6):1447–56.
121. Shen Y, et al. Cyclin D1 expression in Bowen's disease and cutaneous squamous cell carcinoma. Mol Clin Oncol. 2014;2(4):545–8.
122. Yu SL, et al. Identification of mTOR inhibitor-resistant genes in cutaneous squamous cell carcinoma. Cancer Manag Res. 2018;10:6379–89.
123. Pelengaris S, et al. Reversible activation of c-Myc in skin: induction of a complex neoplastic phenotype by a single oncogenic lesion. Mol Cell. 1999;3(5):565–77.
124. Toll A, et al. MYC gene numerical aberrations in actinic keratosis and cutaneous squamous cell carcinoma. Br J Dermatol. 2009;161(5):1112–8.
125. Lohcharoenkal W, et al. MicroRNA-203 inversely correlates with differentiation grade, targets c-MYC, and functions as a tumor suppressor in cSCC. J Invest Dermatol. 2016;136(12):2485–94.
126. Lefort K, et al. Notch1 is a p53 target gene involved in human keratinocyte tumor suppression through negative regulation of ROCK1/2 and MRCKalpha kinases. Genes Dev. 2007;21(5):562–77.
127. Zhang M, et al. Does Notch play a tumor suppressor role across diverse squamous cell carcinomas? Cancer Med. 2016;5(8):2048–60.
128. Corchado-Cobos R, et al. Cutaneous squamous cell carcinoma: from biology to therapy. Int J Mol Sci. 2020;21(8):2956.
129. Canueto J, et al. Epidermal growth factor receptor expression is associated with poor outcome in cutaneous squamous cell carcinoma. Br J Dermatol. 2017;176(5):1279–87.
130. Hoesl C, Fröhlich T, Hundt JE, Kneitz H, Goebeler M, Wolf R, Schneider MR, Dahlhoff M. The transmembrane protein LRIG2 increases tumor progression in skin carcinogenesis. Mol Oncol. 2019;13(11):2476–92.
131. Strickley JD, et al. Metastatic squamous cell carcinoma of the skin with clinical response to lapatinib. Exp Hematol Oncol. 2018;7:20.
132. Ahmed NU, Ueda M, Ichihashi M. Increased level of c-erbB-2/neu/HER-2 protein in cutaneous squamous cell carcinoma. Br J Dermatol. 1997;136(6):908–12.
133. Czyz M. Fibroblast growth factor receptor signaling in skin cancers. Cell. 2019;8(6):540.
134. Hertzler-Schaefer K, et al. Pten loss induces autocrine FGF signaling to promote skin tumorigenesis. Cell Rep. 2014;6(5):818–26.
135. Su F, et al. RAS mutations in cutaneous squamous-cell carcinomas in patients treated with BRAF inhibitors. N Engl J Med. 2012;366(3):207–15.
136. Kern F, Niault T, Baccarini M. Ras and Raf pathways in epidermis development and carcinogenesis. Br J Cancer. 2011;104(2):229–34.

137. Al-Rohil RN, et al. Evaluation of 122 advanced-stage cutaneous squamous cell carcinomas by comprehensive genomic profiling opens the door for new routes to targeted therapies. Cancer. 2016;122(2):249–57.

138. Chen SJ, et al. Activation of the mammalian target of rapamycin signalling pathway in epidermal tumours and its correlation with cyclin-dependent kinase 2. Br J Dermatol. 2009;160(2):442–5.

139. Hervás-Marín D, Higgings F, Sanmartín O, López-Guerrero JA, Carmen Bañó M, Carlos Igual J, Quilis I, Sandoval J. Genome wide DNA methylation profiling identifies specific epigenetic features in high-risk cutaneous squamous cell carcinoma. PLoS One. 2019;14(12):e0223341.

140. Hernández-Ruiz E, Toll A, García-Diez I, Andrades E, Ferrandiz-Pulido C, Masferrer E, Yébenes M, Jaka A, Gimeno J, Gimeno R, García-Patos V, Pujol RM, Hernández-Muñoz I. The Polycomb proteins RING1B and EZH2 repress the tumoral pro-inflammatory function in metastasizing primary cutaneous squamous cell carcinoma. Carcinogenesis. 2018;39(9):503–13.

141. Xie Q, Wang H, Heilman ER, Walsh MG, Haseeb MA, Gupta R. Increased expression of enhancer of Zeste Homolog 2 (EZH2) differentiates squamous cell carcinoma from normal skin and actinic keratosis. Eur J Dermatol. 2014;24(1):41–5.

142. Anastasi S, Alemà S, Segatto O. Making sense of Cbp/p300 loss of function mutations in skin tumorigenesis. J Pathol. 2019;249:39–51.

143. Park E, Liu B, Xia X, Zhu F, Jami W-B, Hu Y. Role of IKKα in skin squamous cell carcinomas. Future Oncol. 2011;7(1):123–34.

144. Descargues P, Sil AK, Karin M. IKKα, a critical regulator of epidermal differentiation and a suppressor of skin cancer. EMBO J. 2008;27(20):2639–47.

145. Colomer C, Marruecos L, Vert A, Bigas A, Espinosa L. NF-κB members left home: NF-κB-independent roles in cancer. Biomedicine. 2017;5:26.

146. Descargues P, Sik AK, Sano Y, Korchynskyi O, Han G, Owens P, Wang X-J, Karin M. IKKalpha is a critical coregulator of a Smad4-independent TGFbeta-Smad2/3 signalling pathway that controls keratinocyte differentiation. Proc Natl Acad Sci U S A. 2008;105(7):2487–92.

147. Mulero MC, Ferres-Marco D, Islam A, Margalef P, Pecoraro M, Toll A, Drechsel N, Charneco C, Davis S, Bellora N, Gallardo F, López-Arribillaga E, Asensio-Juan E, Rodilla V, González J, Iglesias M, Vincent S, Mar Albà M, Di Croce L, Hoffmann A, Miyamoto S, Villà-Freixa J, López-Bigas N, Keyes WM, Domínguez M, Bigas A, Espinosa L. Chromatin-bound IκBα regulates a subset of polycomb target genes in differentiation and cancer. Cancer Cell. 2013;24(2):151–66.

148. Toll A, Margalef P, Masferrer E, Ferrándiz-Pulido C, Gimeno J, Pujol RM, Bigas A, Espinosa L. Active nuclear IKK correlates with metastatic risk in cutaneous squamous cell carcinoma. Arch Dermatol Res. 2015;307(8):721–9.

149. Pickering CR, et al. Mutational landscape of aggressive cutaneous squamous cell carcinoma. Clin Cancer Res. 2014;20(24):6582–92.

150. Albibas AA, et al. Subclonal evolution of cancer-related gene mutations in p53 immunopositive patches in human skin. J Invest Dermatol. 2018;138(1):189–98.

151. Murao K, et al. Epigenetic abnormalities in cutaneous squamous cell carcinomas: frequent inactivation of the RB1/p16 and p53 pathways. Br J Dermatol. 2006;155(5):999–1005.

152. Liu W, MacDonald M, You J. Merkel cell polyomavirus infection and Merkel cell carcinoma. Curr Opin Virol. 2016;20:20–7.

153. Cheng J, Rozenblatt-Rosen O, Paulson KG, Nghiem P, DeCapri JA. Merkel cell polyomavirus large T antigen has growth-promoting and inhibitory activities. J Virol. 2013;87(11):6118–26.

154. Goh G, Walradt T, Markarov V, Blom A, Riaz N, Doumani R, Stafstrom K, Moshiri A, Yelistratova L, Levinsohn J, Chan TA, Nghiem P, Lifton RP, Choi J. Mutational landscape of MCPyV-positive and MCPyV-negative Merkel cell carcinomas with implications for immunotherapy. Oncotarget. 2015;7(3):3403–15.

155. Harms PW, et al. The biology and treatment of Merkel cell carcinoma: current understanding and research priorities. Nat Rev Clin Oncol. 2018;15(12):763–76.

156. Feng H, et al. Clonal integration of a polyomavirus in human Merkel cell carcinoma. Science. 2008;319(5866):1096–100.
157. Chen T, et al. Serological evidence of Merkel cell polyomavirus primary infections in childhood. J Clin Virol. 2011;50(2):125–9.
158. Velasquez C, et al. Characterization of a merkel cell polyomavirus-positive merkel cell carcinoma cell line CVG-1. Front Microbiol. 2018;9:713.
159. Kwun HJ, Chang Y, Moore PS. Protein-mediated viral latency is a novel mechanism for Merkel cell polyomavirus persistence. Proc Natl Acad Sci U S A. 2017;114(20):E4040–7.
160. Sahi H, et al. RB1 gene in Merkel cell carcinoma: hypermethylation in all tumors and concurrent heterozygous deletions in the polyomavirus-negative subgroup. APMIS. 2014;122(12):1157–66.
161. Hesbacher S, et al. RB1 is the crucial target of the Merkel cell polyomavirus Large T antigen in Merkel cell carcinoma cells. Oncotarget. 2016;7(22):32956–68.
162. Van Gele M, et al. Mutation analysis of P73 and TP53 in Merkel cell carcinoma. Br J Cancer. 2000;82(4):823–6.
163. Lassacher A, et al. p14ARF hypermethylation is common but INK4a-ARF locus or p53 mutations are rare in Merkel cell carcinoma. J Invest Dermatol. 2008;128(7):1788–96.
164. Houben R, et al. Mechanisms of p53 restriction in Merkel cell carcinoma cells are independent of the Merkel cell polyoma virus T antigens. J Invest Dermatol. 2013;133(10):2453–60.
165. Park DE, et al. Dual inhibition of MDM2 and MDM4 in virus-positive Merkel cell carcinoma enhances the p53 response. Proc Natl Acad Sci U S A. 2019;116(3):1027–32.
166. Wardhani LO, et al. Expression of notch 3 and jagged 1 Is associated with merkel cell polyomavirus status and prognosis in merkel cell carcinoma. Anticancer Res. 2019;39(1):319–29.
167. Dasgupta T, Wilson LD, Yu JB. A retrospective review of 1349 cases of sebaccous carcinoma. Cancer Metastasis Rev. 2008;115(1):158–65.
168. Dores GM, Curtis RE, Toro JR, Devesa SS, Fraumeni JF Jr. Incidence of cutaneous sebaceous carcinoma and risk of associated neoplasms: Insight into Muir-Torré syndrome. Cancer Metastasis Rev. 2008;113(12):3372–81.
169. North JP, Golovato J, Vaske CJ, Sanborn JZ, Nguyen A, Wu W, Goode B, Stevers M, McMullen K, Perez White BE, Collisson EA, Bloomer M, Solomon DA, Benz SC, Cho RJ. Cell of origin and mutation pattern define three clinically distinct classes of sebaceous carcinoma. Nat Commun. 2018;9:1894.
170. Roberts ME, Riegert-Johnson DL, Thomas BC, Rumilla KM, Thomas CS, Heckman MG, Purcell JU, Hanson NB, Leppig KA, Lim J, Cappel MA. A clinical scoring system to identify patients with sebaceous neoplasms at risk for the Muir–Torre variant of Lynch syndrome. Genet Med. 2014;16:711–6.
171. De Giorgi V, Salvati L, Barchielli A, Caldarella A, Gori A, Scarfi F, Savarese I, Pimpinelli N, Urso C, Massi D. The burden of cutaneous adnexal carcinomas and the risk of associated squamous cell carcinoma: a population-based study. Br J Dermatol. 2018;180(3):565–73.

Chapter 4
Immunological Features of Melanoma: Clinical Implications in the Era of New Therapies

Licia Rivoltini, Agata Cova, and Paola Squarcina

Background

The last decade has represented the crowning achievement of a long research path started back in the 1960 by scattered "believers" within the scientific community, and focused on proving that tumor immunity could provide effective tools for cancer therapy, particularly in melanoma [1]. The turning point in this path has been represented by the discovery of immune checkpoints and the clinical effects of antibodies antagonizing their blocking activity on T-cell antitumor function. Since then, detailed information about the pathways ruling the interaction between tumor and the immune system has been continuously emerging at amazing pace, thanks to novel technologies based on -omics and single-cell analyses. Most of these data confirmed or extended the mechanisms and pathways that have been hypothesized for long based on results obtained from murine models and pioneering clinical trials. This proves that the level of knowledge about the mechanisms underlying tumor-immune cross-talk has reached significant extent, revealing the complexity of the process and the potential routes to gain immune-mediated cancer control in clinical setting. Pivotal successes have been obtained, thanks to immune checkpoint inhibitors, with survival rising to unprecedented levels in metastatic melanoma patients. Still, the currently established evidence that a sizable subset of cases are refractory to treatment, together with the need for patient-tailored algorithms to sustain therapeutic choice, remains one of the top challenges to be addressed in cancer immunotherapy [2], requiring further efforts and the concerted work of

L. Rivoltini (✉) · A. Cova · P. Squarcina
Unit of Immunotherapy of Human Tumors, Fondazione IRCCS Istituto Nazionale Tumori, Milan, Italy
e-mail: licia.rivoltini@istitutotumori.mi.it; agata.cova@istitutotumori.mi.it; paola.squarcina@istitutotumori.mi.it

P. Rutkowski, M. Mandalà (eds.), *New Therapies in Advanced Cutaneous Malignancies*, https://doi.org/10.1007/978-3-030-64009-5_4

clinicians and researchers worldwide. A major goal is now to finally start transferring some of the acquired scientific knowledge into real-life clinical practice, for patients' benefit.

ABC Rules of Tumor Immunology

The immune system is composed of a complex network of cells and soluble factors that dynamically interact to protect the host from environmental dangers. Involving different organs and sites, such as bone marrow, lymph nodes, thymus, spleen, different peripheral tissues, and blood (the latter representing a conduit for most immune cells circulating in the body), the immune systems surveys the organism, ready to spike once foreign, non-self signals occur. Albeit showing significant inter-individual variability due to heritable and non-heritable factors, immune responses in humans are rather stable over time under physiological conditions [3]. In the presence of an acute challenge (usually represented by the so-called antigens), drastic changes take place, with selected immune populations expanding and serum protein concentrations starkly increasing. Protective responses usually involve the adaptive immunity, with a predominant role of T-lymphocytes or B cells, depending on the nature and structure of the stimulatory challenge. Innate immunity might also contribute to host defense in specific pathological conditions, including effectors such as natural killer (NK) cells, or unconventional T-lymphocytes (i.e., NKT cells, mucosal-associated invariant T cells, and $\gamma\delta$ T cells) [4].

Once the antigen has been eliminated, cellular and soluble immune components quickly return to baseline state. The mechanisms regulating this tightly controlled course are not fully understood, but they are part of the homeostatic process required to avoid auto-aggression and damage of normal tissues.

Over the last few years, it has been emerging that Immune balance is mainly conserved, thanks to coordinated and redundant mechanisms rapidly shutting down immune responses after acute variations. These pathways include a rich array of cell surface receptors (globally known as immune checkpoints) and diverse regulatory cells with immunosuppressive functions. Receptors and cells work concomitantly to finely tune immune responses, modulating the threshold for activation and contributing to its subsequent switch-off. To the maintenance of normal tissue, integrity also contributes a complex process known as "immune tolerance," which is in sum a functional state of immune unresponsiveness to host self components achieved through multiple central and peripheral mechanisms [5].

Cancer-Associated Immune Variations

Cancer represents a pathological condition heavily altering the immune balance. Although most, if not all, the cellular components of the immune system are somehow affected by the presence of a neoplastic process in the organism and might play a role in contrasting its development, preclinical studies in murine models have largely pointed to T-lymphocytes as the predominant mediators of cancer immuno-surveillance [6, 7].

Indeed, despite arising from host cellular components and having thus a "self" origin, neoplastic cells could be detected and effectively recognized by T-lymphocytes. As a matter of fact, genetic and epigenetic alterations characterizing malignant cells may produce aberrant protein repertoires that resemble foreign pathogens and act as antigenic stimuli. Largely depending on the histotype as well as the biological features of tumor cells, these immune responses can profoundly impact on disease course and response to therapy in most cancer patients [8]. Based on preclinical studies and clinical epidemiological evidence, it is believed that effective T-cell response might restrain carcinogenesis and represent a first filter of surveillance against neoplastic transformation [6]. Very recently, data are emerging about a potential protective role also of B cells in human cancer, particularly in terms of favorable outcome for melanoma patients treated with immunotherapy [9].

Nevertheless, tumors reaching clinical diagnosis have obviously overcome this filter, indicating that cancer cells can also acquire the ability to evade immune control and grow in an immunocompetent host. The process, globally defined as "tumor immune escape" [10], consists in a multifaceted phenomenon that involves different steps of tumor–immune interaction. However, the escape pathways often include the same mechanisms controlling immune homeostasis under physiological conditions, such as the upregulation of immune checkpoints or the accrual of immuno-suppressive cells. In sum, although the driving elements may differ in individual tumors and organs, most of the principal features are shared across cancers [11]. Getting insights into the molecular patterns regulating tumor immunity has provided over the last decade novel biomarkers and therapeutic targets that are drastically changing the clinical management of cancer patients.

Melanoma Immunogenicity, So Unique

Immunogenicity of melanoma, meaning the ability of this tumor to raise spontaneous T responses in bearing patients, has been known for long. Pioneering trials by the team of S.A. Rosenberg, showing that T cells isolated from metastatic melanoma (TIL, tumor-infiltrating lymphocytes), expanded in vitro by interleukin-2 and subsequently re-transferred into individual patients, could mediate impressive tumor regressions [12], paved the way to the use of adoptive cell therapy (ACT) in cancer treatment [13]. Clinical efficacy of ACT in that setting was associated with the ability of TIL to recognize and lyse autologous melanoma cells, indicating the presence of antigen-specific T-lymphocyte in tumor microenvironment [11]. Indeed, in line with the potential role of antitumor T-cell response in cancer immunosurveillance, the level of T-cell infiltrate (particularly of CD8+ T cells) in both primary and metastatic melanoma is a hallmark of patients with good prognosis, long survival, and positive response to therapy, including immunotherapy [14, 15]. The baseline level of T-cell infiltrate is so relevant that a specific algorithm comprehensively assessing the quantity and the topographic distribution of lymphocyte populations within the tumor lesion (the so-called Immunoscore) has been developed for clinical application [16]. The Immunoscore is based on the staining of lymphocyte populations, in particular CD3+ and CD8+ T cells, in formalin-fixed, paraffin-embedded slides through a digital pathology approach. This assay has been validated in colorectal carcinoma, but it represents a promising tool to define immune fitness in melanoma patients and predict their disease outcome [17].

The biological reasons underlying the marked ability of melanoma to trigger T-cell responses are complex and still not fully understood. T cells, as mentioned above, recognize antigenic determinants expressed by tumor cells, so one of the first mechanisms of melanoma immunogenicity could be related to a high antigenic expression [18]. However, a high level of antigenic expression might not be sufficient, as for being recognized by T cells, altered tumor proteins have to be efficiently processed and presented on cancer cell surface [6]. In addition, tumor cells are generally not equipped to directly activate T lymphocytes, but the intervention of professional "antigen-presenting cells" (such as dendritic cells, DC) in the adequate immunological milieu (lymph nodes, spleen, or peripheral lymphoid structures) is required. Finally, immunological contexture, that is, the presence of resident memory T cells already experienced in antigenic recognition may also remarkably contribute to the onset of full-fledged immune responses [6, 7]. In each of the different subsequent steps of this complex process, melanoma has been reported to be the best-performing cancer among human malignancies.

The Rich Repertoire of Melanoma T-Cell Antigens

Because of the easiness to grow them in vitro and their strong immunogenicity in vivo, melanoma cells provided in the early years of tumor immunology the optimal conditions to identify the nature of human tumor antigens and the mechanisms of their recognition by T cells [19]. This approach, which was also aimed at designing potential cancer vaccines as a strategy for melanoma immunotherapy, allowed to first identify molecules shared among different melanoma and patients. Proteins associated with melanogenesis and melanin synthesis (so-called differentiation antigens, such as gp100, MelanA/Mart-1, and tyrosinase) were found to be expressed in most melanoma at such high level to break immune tolerance toward self structures and trigger autoreactive T cells able to cross-recognize melanoma cells [20]. Molecules expressed selectively in embryonic cells and re-acquired by melanoma and other cancer (known as cancer-testis antigens), like proteins of the Mage, NY-Eso1, and Prame families, also escape immune tolerance and generate in patients melanoma-specific T-cell responses with significant antitumor activity [21].

However, fundamental rules of immunology dictate that the affinity of T cells for the cognate antigen is usually depending on how different is that antigen from the corresponding self structure, so that the originating immune response is not controlled by immune tolerance. According to this principle, tumor antigens stemming from aberrantly/ectopically expressed nonmutated proteins would generate weak immune responses, while mutated proteins are supposed to produce stronger T cells [22]. The latter antigens, resulting mostly from DNA alterations due to the intrinsic cancer genetic instability, represent in cancer novel structures with respect to the self-antigenic repertoire of the host; hence, they are defined as neo-antigens. Because usually stemming from random mutations unrelated to driver oncogenic pathways, they are individual and patient-specific. For capturing this concept, the so called tumor mutational burden (TMB) has been recently introduced to define tumor's ability to produce immunogenic neo-antigens. TMB evaluation, albeit in retrospective setting, revealed that T-cell frequency infiltrating melanoma correlates with the number of mutational antigens corresponding to nonsynonymous mutations. Most importantly, TMB has been associated with the baseline level of spontaneous immunity in melanoma patients and the sensitivity to immune checkpoint inhibitors particularly of the PD-1/PD-L1 axis [23].

Nevertheless, despite the remarkable efforts to exploit this information for generating reliable biomarkers of melanoma immunogenicity, ex vivo data from clinical setting are clearly depicting more complex immunological requirements. In fact, whole-exome and whole-transcriptome sequencing of pretreatment tumors in large case sets of melanoma patients has recently shown that TMB predictive value may not reproducibly predict clinical outcome, whereas other genomic and transcriptomic features, including those related to antigen processing and presentation, might be more relevant [24]. However, in this regard, it is worth mentioning that defined melanoma subtypes, such as, for instance, the desmoplastic variant, which is highly linked with ultraviolet light-induced DNA damage (as proved by the elevated rate of mutations in the neurofibromatosis—NF1—gene), is endowed with very high TMB and remarkable sensitivity to immunotherapy based on immune checkpoint inhibitors [25].

The Potential Role of Skin Origin in Melanoma Immunogenicity

The fact that melanoma arises from skin may not be irrelevant for the immunogenicity of this tumor. At first, the link of melanoma with UV light exposure is likely to play a role in promoting a rich antigenic repertoire. Indeed, recent studies have shown that UVs induce specific DNA mutations in genes known to drive the onset of melanoma in humans, and that melanoma cells do express these UV-associated DNA mutational signatures [26], which are then likely involved in generating the T cell-recognized antigenic determinants. In addition, a link between autoimmunity and enhanced antitumor immunity has long been recognized, particularly in melanoma. In this regard, preclinical studies have demonstrated that although the exact mechanistic relationship between these two phenomena remains unclear, the autoimmune destruction of melanocytes (i.e., vitiligo) produces self-antigens that can induce persistent and protective memory CD8[+] T-cell responses to melanoma. This evidence implies that melanocyte destruction may be a key determinant of persisting melanoma-reactive immunity, hence indicating how immune-mediated destruction of normal tissues can contribute to maintain adaptive immune responses to cancer [27]. A key role in this process might also be played by tissue-resident memory T cells, which are strategic effectors of adaptive immunity against infection in the periphery and could be involved in perpetuating local and systemic antitumor immunity in melanoma [28].

Optimal Antigenic Processing and Presentation by Melanoma Cells

To be recognized by T cells, antigens need to be processed from the inner compartment of the tumor cells and presented on the cell surface in a groove within the HLA molecules. This implies that the molecular mechanisms helping the antigenic proteins to reach the tumor cell surface might be crucial in the induction of antitumor T-cell responses. Recent studies based on high-resolution mass spectrometry of melanoma specimens have revealed that enrichment in proteins associated with antigen presentation, which are linked to oxidative phosphorylation and lipid metabolism, is associated with better disease course in clinical setting [29, 30]. In line with these findings, overexpression of different components of the immunoproteasome is predictive of improved survival and response to immune-checkpoint inhibitors in melanoma patients [31]. The immunoproteasome is a highly efficient proteolytic machinery playing a central role in degrading antigens to the structure that can be optimally recognized by immune cells. Of note, immunoproteasome expression levels have been recently reported in melanoma patients to be stronger predictors of tumor antigenicity than the tumor mutational burden, indicating the potential use of these proteins as biomarkers for patient stratification [31].

A very recent discovery confirming melanoma as an optimal "antigen processor and presenter" points to the ability of this tumor to promote local formation of tertiary lymphoid structures (TLS). TLS are ectopic lymphoid organs arising at the sites of chronic inflammation including tumors, where they support antigen presentation and activation of resident immune cells [32]. Because of their role, the enrichment in these secondary lymphoid organs containing mostly antigen-presenting cells such as B-lymphocytes has been recently reported to occur more frequently in tumor tissue from patients subsequently responding to immunotherapy [9]. B and TLS can thus be considered as novel and promising predicting factors and therapeutic target in melanoma

Not All Melanoma Are "Antigenically" Equal: The Role of Tumor and Host Heterogeneity

Despite the usually enriched repertoire by melanoma cells of altered proteins that might be recognized by T cells as non-self structures, not all these molecules may give rise to a sufficient level of antigenic determinants to trigger effective immune responses. One of the mechanisms of this process could stem from intratumor heterogeneity (ITH), a process characterizing most solid tumors and arising through complex genetic, epigenetic, and protein modifications that mold phenotypic selection in response to environmental pressures [33]. ITH may profoundly reduce the amount of antigenic structures that can engage T-cell clones, leading to suboptimal immune response or even T-cell ignorance. The relevance of ITH in protective antitumor immunity is proved by the evidence that melanoma patients with low levels of ITH have improved survival rates with respect to patients displaying instead high ITH [34]. When transferred into immunocompetent mice, melanomas with lower ITH are less aggressive, grow more slowly, and display higher immunogenicity, in terms of T-cell responses, than tumors with high ITH. Altogether, these findings underline the relevance of clonal mutations in mediating robust immune surveillance and the need to determine ITH at individual level to gain global hints on melanoma immunogenicity.

Individual level of cancer antigenicity might also depend on the differences occurring in others of the multiple steps required for T-cell activation. Worth mentioning is the recent evidence that patient-specific HLA class I germ line genotype can also influence melanoma clinical outcome and response to cancer immunotherapy [34]. Indeed, HLA class I heterozygosity has been found to associate with better prognosis and increased survival with respect to HLA homozygosity. This is most likely due to the fact that antigens are presented to T cells by HLA molecules expressed on the surface of antigen-presenting cells or target cells. So, the more heterogeneous is the repertoire of HLA in the different A, B, and C loci, the higher is the number of antigens exposed to T cells and the wider is the T-cell repertoire of the activated immune responses. This very relevant evidence indicates, for the first time, that individual predisposition related to the genetic background of the patient may influence the level of antitumor immunity, as it influences responses to environmental pathogens in healthy individuals [35].

Melanoma Evasion as a Consequence of Immune Recognition

In the cases reaching clinical diagnosis, melanoma cells have developed strategies to grow and progress despite the presence of an active and sometimes powerful immune response. As mentioned above, this process is defined as tumor immune escape, and represent among the hottest fields of research in cancer immunology and immunotherapy. Thanks to their genetic and epigenetic instability, tumor cells rapidly adapt to microenvironmental changes through a sort of Darwinian selection process, and modulate multiple pathways to allow their survival. Concomitantly, also immune responses dynamically regulate their activity because of the chronic stimulation, and react by setting up mechanisms aimed at maintaining immune homeostasis and preserve T-cell integrity. The final result is a paradoxical scenario where cancer cells and anti-cancer lymphocytes coexist in the same lesions, under a dynamic balance [6].

Melanoma has provided, once again, the opportunity to identify and characterize most of the mechanisms underlying T cell/tumor coexistence. The major finding consists in the discovery that infiltrating T cells enter a state of partial activity (known as immune exhaustion) [36] due to the onset of multiple regulatory mechanisms. Immune exhaustion allows some T-cell functions, such as production of IFNγ, but most or the antitumor activities, as well as metabolic processes, are reversibly interrupted. T-cell exhaustion came to the spotlights in melanoma a decade ago, because it is mainly mediated by immune checkpoints such as PD-1, CTLA4, LAG3, TIM3, and others, expressed by chronically stimulated T cells [37–39]. Concomitantly, through the residual IFNγ release, T cells induce the microenviromment, to upregulate the cognate immune checkpoint ligands (PD-L1, CD80/86, HLA-II, and galectin 9, respectively), so that the receptor–ligand interaction leads to the functional switching-off of T cells [40]. As extensively proven [41], the use of antibodies impeding this receptor–ligand contact can effectively reestablish full-fledged immune responses that, in turn, eliminate tumor cells and mediate significant clinical benefit in melanoma patients, as well as in other malignancies.

Preexisting Tumor Immunity as Biomarker of Favorable Disease Course and Response to Therapy

As for the preclinical studies, melanoma has been also the first setting that offered the opportunity to test the efficacy of immunotherapeutic approaches in human cancer. From adoptive cell transfer with TIL [12], to shared or individual cancer vaccines, and immune checkpoint inhibitors, melanoma has been for over three decades and is still the epicenter for the clinical development of cancer immunotherapeutics [38].

On the basis of the information depicted above, it comes easy to hypothesize that the predisposition of melanoma to respond to immunotherapy is related to its strong immunogenicity. According to large amount of data published so far, most of the biomarkers predicting clinical benefit to immune checkpoint inhibitors in melanoma patients are related to the presence of a preexisting T-cell response [38, 42, 43] (Fig. 4.1a). From the number of DNA mutations giving rise to tumor neoantigens, to the expression of immune checkpoints and cognate ligands at tumor site, or the level and activation state of tumor-infiltrating T cells, any biomarker that surrogates the presence of spontaneous immune response at tumor site identifies patients who will benefit from immune checkpoint inhibitors [44]. Notably, such a correlation (which has been confirmed at pan-cancer level) can be detected also when immunogenicity is measured through a genetic approach, that is, by combining tumor mutational burden (TMB) with an IFNγ-related transcriptional signature of

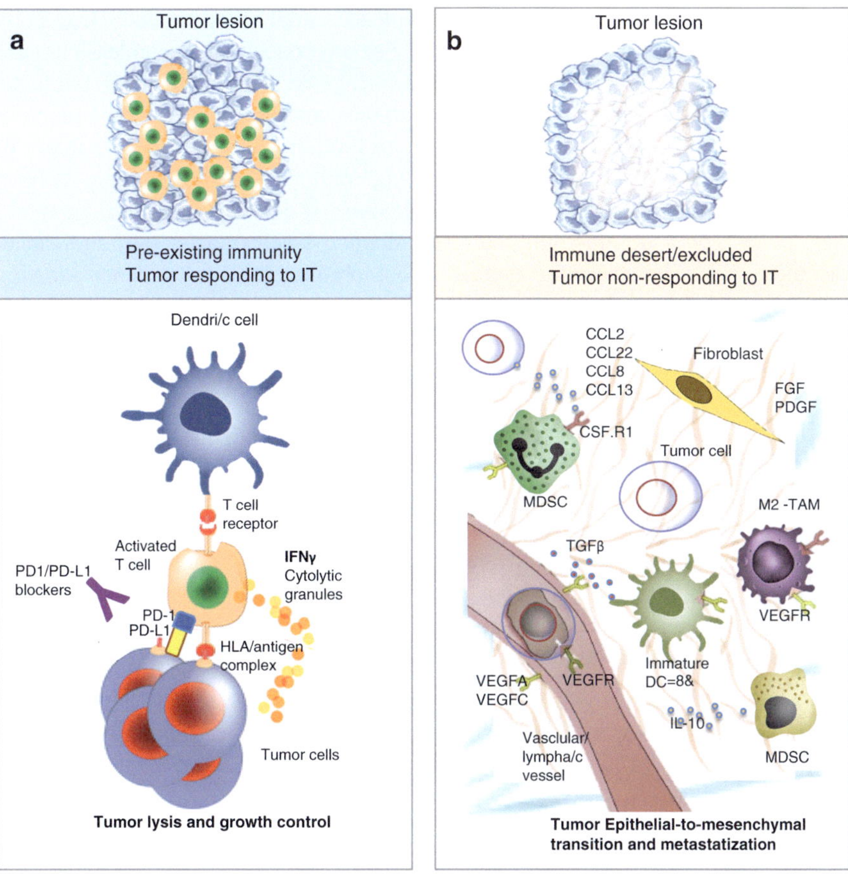

Fig. 4.1 Immune composition and interactions of melanoma lesions with pre-existing immunity vs immune desert/excluded microenvironment. Schematic composition of tumor microenviroment, in terms of soluble factors and immune cells, according to a dichotomized vision of immune responsive vs immune resistant tumors. (**a**) Optimized scenario of melanoma with pre-existing immunity and predispose to respond to immunotherapy, in which tumor antigens are properly processed and presented by dendritic cells (DC) to specific T-lymphocytes. T cells undergo full-fledged activation but eventually upregulate immune checkpoints (exemplified by the PD-1/PD-L1 axis) that switch-off their ability to destroy tumor cells and cause functional exhaustion. Antagonizing antibodies (immune checkpoint blockers, ICB) can revert T-cell functional paralysis and repristinate antitumor immunity. (**b**) Immune-desert or immune-excluded melanoma, unlikely to respond to immunotherapy. Lacking T cells, this tumor is enriched in immunosuppressive cells (myeloid-derived suppressor cells, MDSC; regulatory T cells, Treg; tumor-associated immunosuppressive macrophages, TAM-M2; immature DC), fibroblasts, fibrosis, angiogenesis, and multiple soluble factors sustaining the function and the accrual of all these cells, as well as tumor dedifferentiation (epithelial-to-mesenchymal transition)

T-cell activation [45]. Altogether, these evidences imply that immune checkpoint inhibitors (particularly for what PD-1/PD-L1 axis is concerned) can unleash a spontaneous immune response that the tumor has triggered and then escaped, but it can hardly induce immunity ex novo, at least with the current immune checkpoint inhibitors. This feature, which is obviously a major limitation as a remarkable subset of melanoma patients lack signs of preexisting immunity, does not apply only to checkpoint blockers, but it seems to involve most, if not all, cancer immunotherapies. Indeed, data are emerging that also adoptive T-cell transfer [46] and cancer vaccines [47] exert their therapeutic effect preferentially in patients showing already-established antitumor immunity at baseline either in peripheral circulation or at tumor site. Data generated in murine tumors showed that the inner memory T-cell responses present in hosts bearing immunogenic tumors display a trophic and helper effect on T cells newly generated by immunotherapy, expanding and sustaining them in tumor growth control [48]. Of note, also BRAF/MEK inhibitors display better efficacy in patients having preexistent immune response [49], which indicates that immunity can cooperate with other anti-cancer therapies through the immune-mediated tumor growth control.

On the other hand, the general view is that most current immunological strategies do work in immunogenic tumors but they may not be so efficient in rescuing nonimmunogenic cancers; this entails that others are the pathways of the immune system needing to be taken into account to deal with immune desert, cold tumors.

Why Not All Melanomas Are Immunogenic?

Studies of melanomas characterized within the Cancer Genome Atlas (TCGA) have recently suggested that the lack of immune infiltrate is not easily explained by a low antigen load of the tumor [50]. In fact, the rich repertoire detected in melanoma lesions in terms of differentiation, cancer-testis, and neo-antigens should be largely sufficient to give rise to protective immunity in most patients. In this regard, it is emerging that individual genetic background, in terms of polymorphisms and germline gene variations of immune-related pathways, such as the already-mentioned HLA-I genotype and the recently reported IFN and autoimmunity-related SNPs [51], do influence the onset of spontaneous immunity in bearing patients. Nevertheless, the lack of T-cell infiltrate (in the so-called immune-desert or cold tumors) or the maintenance of T cells at tumor periphery (in the immune-excluded tumors) may originate from quite complex and only partially understood processes. The dissection of the molecular pathways contributing to these scenarios currently represents one of the hottest and most promising research fields in the discovery of novel melanoma biomarkers and therapeutics.

Transformed cells are known to mold tumor immunity not only by expressing tumor antigens and triggering adaptive immunity but also by producing a series of immune modulating factors that can heavily shape immune microenvironment. By mostly exploiting the very same mechanisms that the immune system itself utilizes for maintaining immune homeostasis, or setting up novel strategies to overcome immune recognition, melanoma cells can create a very hostile milieu hardy accessible to tumor-specific T cells.

Immune-Desert/Cold Tumors Are Enriched in Other Immune Cells

Pan-cancer studies, involving also melanoma, have clearly revealed that, if T-cell infiltrate is associated with good prognosis and response to therapy, enrichment in regulatory and immunosuppressive immune cells is instead a major hallmark of bad disease course and aggressive disease [6, 52]. In melanoma, the tumor enrichment of myeloid cells, usually detected by the expression of CD163 and CD68 markers, is associated with poor prognosis in both primary and metastatic disease [53, 54]. In this regard, the density and the spatial distribution of myeloid cells with respect to T cells, expressed by the CD8+/CD163+ ratio, predict poor response of metastatic melanoma to target therapy [49], indicating that the local balance between anti- and pro-tumor immune responses represents a potential surrogate of immune-mediated cancer control at individual patient level.

The presence of myeloid cells in a tumor microenvironment is indeed part of a complex process that ultimately favors cancer progression and reduced response to therapy through a series of multiple and pleiotropic pathways. Pivotal studies on the transcriptome analysis of baseline metastatic melanoma biopsies revealed that innately resistant, cold tumors display a specific signature concomitantly including the up-regulation of multiple genes involved in immunosuppression and tumor aggressiveness [55, 56]. In cold/desert tumors, the lack of T-cell immunity is largely counterbalanced by a quite rich scenario in terms of protumor factors and cellular components, involving pathways of epithelial-to-mesenchymal transition, cell adhesion, extracellular matrix remodeling, angiogenesis, and wound healing (Fig. 4.1b). Fibrosis and fibroblasts are also enriched, together with a broad array of dysfunctional myeloid cells including myeloid-derived suppressor cells (MDSC), pro-tumor-associated macrophages (TAM-M2) and immature DC. In contrast with T-lymphocytes, myeloid cells are among potent allies of cancer. This symbiotic relationship is due to the unique ability of these cells to sustain tumor progression through inflammatory processes that would lead to tissue repair under physiological conditions but produce persistent inflammation in chronic diseases such as cancer [55]. Coadiuvated by cancer-associated fibroblasts and other immune regulatory elements like Treg, myeloid cells "colonize" tumor site and the host at systemic level. Hence, they progressively create a globally inflamed milieu that favors tumor progression and dissemination at the expense of protective antitumor T cells. Phenotypically, myeloid cells are present in tumor-bearing organism as a broad spectrum of immature monocyte- or granulocyte-like cells comprehensively defined as the already-mentioned MDSC (myeloid-derived suppressor cells) [57]. MDSC favor tumor growth by inhibiting antitumor T cells via immunosuppressive molecules such as TGFb, IDO, ROS, arginase I, IL-6, and others. Endowed with the plasticity of myeloid cells, MDSC sustain neoangiogenesis (by releasing VEGF and transdifferentiating into pericytes), stroma remodeling for local progression (mostly via TGFb) and epithelial-to-mesenchymal transition (EMT) in tumor cells (thus favoring metastatization). All the genes encoding these pathways, including TGFb and the EMT-related MITF/AXL pathway, are enriched in cold melanomas and in lesions nonresponding to immue checkpoint inhibitors [58].

Tumor Intrinsic Mechanisms of Immune Exclusion

The molecular mechanisms underlying tumor immune escape in preclinical and human settings have been extensively reviewed in the last years, with a large amount of detailed information on the cancer- and patient-specific pathways often affecting different arms of the immune system [10, 59]. Most of these studies involve melanoma, together with other human malignancies that are recently entering the therapeutic area of immuno-oncology.

Shaping of the immune landscape in melanomas lacking preexisting immunity may stem from cancer-cell-intrinsic pathways. Despite representing the oncogenic hallmark of this cancer, the driver *BRAF* mutations appear to be "silent" in term of immunological outcomes; indeed, immune-related biomarkers as well as response to immune checkpoint inhibitors cluster melanoma patients regardless of *BRAF* mutation status [60]. In contrast, activating *NRAS* mutations that are found in 15–20% of melanomas associate with improved sensitivity to immunotherapies including interleukin-2, anti-CTLA4, or anti-PD-1/PD-L1 mAbs [61]. The mechanism of these improved responses are currently unknown, albeit a higher PDL-1 expression, or more likely the lack of the immunosuppressive effects associated with the PTEN loss (mutually exclusive with *NRAS*mut) may play a role [61].

Indeed, the *PTEN* gene, which is frequently mutated in melanoma, is thought to promote immune evasion and is *PTEN* loss because of its association with poor prognosis, resistance to therapy, and immune escape [62]. Melanomas with *PTEN* alterations display decreased frequency of T-cell infiltration and transcriptional properties linked to defective immunogenicity and antigenicity. The same phenotype is displayed by related oncogenic mutations such as the loss of function of the melanoma lineage-specific gene *MITF*, or activating gain-of-function mutations of *CTNNB1* oncogene, which lead to beta-catenin protein production [62]. The fine mechanisms by which *PTEN* deletion and related oncogenic pathways might promote immune evasion are incompletely understood. However, mutations in *PTEN* activate the phosphoinositide 3-kinase (PI3K) and the mammalian target of rapamycin (mTOR) signaling, which confer strong immunosuppressive behavior to tumor cells along with more aggressive grow in the host. *PTEN* loss is globally associated with the release by melanoma cells of cytokines and chemokines involved in the bone marrow mobilization and accrual at tumor site of Treg and MDSC, such as

CCL2, CCL22, G-CSF, and GM-CSF [62]. Because PI3K activation has a prevalent role in melanoma cells and is a key transducer of MDSC immunosuppressive functions, clinical trials testing the synergistic effect of specific PI3K inhibitors in combination with ICB are currently ongoing [63, 64].

Melanoma Metabolism as an Emerging New Source of Immunosuppressive Pathways

Melanoma cells, to cope with their fast proliferative activity and the bio-energetic demands while evading immunosurveillance or therapeutic interventions, undergo rapid metabolic adaptations [65].

One of the first steps to face are hypoxic conditions, which melanoma cells cope by activating glycolysis and changing cell behavior through the remodeling extracellular matrix and increasing migratory and metastatic behavior. These effects are paired with potent immunosuppressive effects, including the upregulation of PD-L1 expression by tumor cells via HIF1a [66] and the release of the damage-associated molecular pattern high-mobility group box 1 protein (HMGB1) [67], both representing chronic inflammatory signals that cause accrual of immunosuppressive cells at tumor site. A further metabolic consequence of the hypoxic/glycolytic melanoma axis is the lowering of the local pH, which can reach levels of frank acidity that blocks T-cell proliferation and function [68]. This evidence points to the potential role of anti-acid drugs including proton pump inhibitors to overcome immune escape and potentiate the effects of melanoma immunotherapy [69].

Other targetable melanoma cell metabolic pathways to modulate immunosuppressive microenvironment are represented by enzymes involved in the lipid metabolism, which are rapidly emerging as major mediators of MDSC metabolic reprogramming [70]. In particular, recent data have depicted sphingosine kinase-1 (SK1) as a key regulator of melanoma immune suppression and MDSC accrual through the release of CCL1, IDO, and TGFb, while SK1 silencing reduces various immunosuppressive factors in the tumor microenvironment [71]. Coherently, patients with SK1+ melanoma have shorter survival upon treatment anti-PD-1 [71], which points to lipid kinase as an innovative target to enhance melanoma sensitivity to immunotherapy through the modulation of lipid metabolism.

Systemic Signs of Immunosuppression in Melanoma

Most of the cancer–immune interactions depicted so far involve tumor microenvironment and are assessed in tumor biopsies. Nevertheless, preclinical evidence proves that systemic immune responses are essential for the achievement of effective immune-mediated tumor eradication [72]. Similarly, also immunosuppressive pathways accumulating within melanoma microenvironment are the consequence of a systemic process involving the cross-talk with the host bone marrow that the tumor cells establish since the first stage of the oncogenic process [73, 74]. The process, recently reported to include also the spleen [75], leads to the release of MDSC into the peripheral blood, which are then accrued back to the tumor site by chemotactic factors, to feed the immunosuppressive microenvironment with proinflammatory signals [76]. This loop, including cells of both monocytic and granulocytic-lineage sharing immunosuppressive activity, is part of the physiological process of wound healing and immune homeostasis maintenance [77, 78]. MDSC accumulation in peripheral blood, quantifiable through complex myeloid markers panels and multiparametric flow cytometry [79], is a confirmed biomarker of negative prognosis in melanoma patients, according to recent meta-analyses [80]. The first report about MDSC in this clinical setting came from our laboratory, which described the increase frequency in patients receiving a GM-CSF-based tumor vaccine, of immunosuppressive CD14+ monocytes expressing low level of HLA-DR (as a sign of immature state) and suppressing T-cell proliferation and function by TGFb secretion [81]. The high blood frequency of CD14$^+$HLA-DR^{neg} cells at baseline, potentiated by the administration of the myeloid growth factor GM-CSF, predicted low clinical benefit of the vaccine and poor disease outcome in vaccinated patients [81].

Increased blood CD14$^+$HLA-DR^{neg} cells in melanoma patients have been then reported by several groups worldwide, always in association with bad prognosis and resistance to treatment [82, 83]. Nevertheless, MDSC have been recently depicted as "the most important cell you have never heard of" [84], to indicate the poor translation of this potent biomarker into real-life clinical practice thus far. To push the field forward, we recently developed a simplified flow cytometry test (defined as myeloid index score—MIS), according to which four markers (CD14, CD15, HLA-DR, and PD-L1) are sufficient to detect and quantify prognostic MDSC in peripheral circulation [85]. MIS, calculated on the above cut-off frequency of CD14+, CD15+, CD14-HLA-DRneg, or CD14 + PD-L1+ cells, clusters patients according to progressively worse prognosis, with patients with MIS = 0 showing the best disease course, and patients with MIS = 4 the worst. Prognostication according to MIS is independent of the type of therapy (BRAFi/MEKi vs Immune checkpoint blockers, ICB) and other standard clinical prognostic biomarkers, with HR > 10 when analyzed in multivariate analysis. To further prompt introduction of MDSC quantification into real-life clinical practice, a MIS for whole blood is presently under development within the EU-funded ERANET-PERMED Serpentine project [86], in line with work by others [87].

Recent studies in clinical setting are expanding the prognostic/predictive impact of MDSC to other forms of melanoma therapy. For instance, lymphodepleted chemotherapy administered to condition melanoma prior to TIL administration has been reported to cause an IL6-mediated reactive boost of blood MDSC that is associated with ACT-reduced clinical efficacy [88]. These results, besides reinforcing the role of MDSC in preventing clinical efficacy of immunotherapeutics, underlie how chemotherapy might play detrimental effects on tumor immunity by dysregulating myelopoiesis.

Myeloid Cell Counts in Blood as Potential Surrogates of Immunosuppressive Biomarkers

The alterations of blood monocyte and neutrophil cell counts have been known for long to be a cancer hallmark [89, 90]. In light of the above-mentioned information on MDSC and tumor–myeloid cross-talk, it could be hypothesized that the increased absolute and relative numbers of neutrophils and monocytes often reported to occur in cancer patients might be the result of the same process underlying MDSC genesis, as recently suggested in prostate cancer [91]. Because of the feasibility of blood cell count analysis, absolute myeloid cell counts and relative ratios with lymphocytes (i.e., neutrophil-to-lymphocyte ratio, NLR, and lymphocyte-to-monocyte ratio, LMR) have been recently introduced in melanoma clinical setting to assess prognosis and predict sensitivity to immunotherapy. A recent meta-analysis including 12 studies and 3207 patients showed that a high NLR was associated with poor OS and PFS, with HRs ranging from 1.6 to 3.04 for OS [92]. Of note, NLR appears to be a predictor of recurrence in stage II melanoma patients [93], in line with that reported for circulating MDSC [94]. Less popular but still promising is LMR, which results to be a positive prognostic factor and predict good response to immunotherapy [95, 96], in line with that observed with tumor infiltrate with the CD8$^+$/CD163$^+$ ratio [49]. Together with NLR, LMR could represent cost-effective and easy-to-perform prognostic biomarker to assess systemic immunosuppression in melanoma, although the prognostic value of this type of analyses is remarkably inferior to that achievable by MDSC blood profiling [85].

Extracellular Vesicles and Their Involvement in Melanoma MDSC Accrual

For sending conditioning messages to distant immune organs such as the bone marrow and spleen, melanoma cells must adopt an efficient delivery system allowing to concentrate relevant signals to the target site. A major pathway revealed again in melanoma is the shuttling of active molecules within extracellular vesicles (EVs) actively secreted by tumor cells [97]. EVs are one of the predominant tools of intracellular cross-talk used by eukaryotic cells. Exacerbated in tumor cells that exploit them for molecular discharge, EVs have been emerging over the last decades as mediators of different progression-associated cancer processes and a potential source of plasma cancer and immune biomarkers [98]. In preclinical studies based on murine and in vitro models, melanoma EVs were proved to promote local and systemic disease progression by instigating proinflammatory and immunosuppressive signals in the different cell components of the premetastatic niche [99].

With respect to soluble factors, EVs can carry a rich repertoire of proteins and genetic material that is transferred within the peripheral circulation in a protected form, to be then delivered at distance in a simultaneous and efficient manner. Tumor-shed EVs enable the "soil" at distant metastatic sites to sustain the outgrowth of incoming cancer cells [99]. EVs isolated from plasma of melanoma patients have been reported to mediate immunosuppressive activity on autologous T and NK cells when tested ex vivo [100, 101], while their phenotype profiling by multiplex microchips recently unraveled a possible application in monitoring melanoma drug resistance [102].

We and others have found that EVs isolated from melanoma cells in vitro or from plasma of melanoma patients can convert monocytes into bona fide MDSC [103, 104]. The process, which confers potent immunosuppressive activity to CD14[+] myeloid cells, is caused by the direct EV-mediated transfer of microRNAs that can regulate multiple MDSC-related transcriptional pathways. Most importantly, quantifying the level of the MDSC-associated miRNAs in plasma anticipates resistance to immune checkpoint blockers (but not to BRAF/MEK inhibitors) in advanced melanoma patients [103]. These latter data further strengthen the relevance of melanoma–myeloid cross-talk as a relevant source of immunosuppressive biomarkers in this specific cancer setting. The EV-mediated bone marrow conditioning, which results in the MDSC release in peripheral circulation and the following migration of these cells to the tumor site according a sort of self-perpetuating vicious immunosuppressive path, allowed the identification of multiple biomarkers to be assessed in blood and tumor site (Fig. 4.2).

How to Overcome Intrinsic Immune Resistance

Based on the current scenario, melanoma patients featured by preexisting antitumor immunity should benefit from some form of immunotherapy, including immune checkpoint inhibitors, adoptive T-cell transfer or other experimental immune therapeutics. This immunological background predisposes melanoma patients also to a better disease course, independently of the type of therapy. Interestingly, the recent data showing that even patients progressing after ICB can still have a significant disease control rate (in about 50%, depending on the type of ICB) [105] indicate that the predisposition to respond to immunotherapy may be an intrinsic feature of defined tumors and/or patients, and as such, it might not be easy to lose. In line with this hypothesis is the evidence that T cells isolated and expanded from melanoma lesions that progressed during or after PD-1 and CTLA4 blockade treatment, still display specific antitumor activity against melanoma cells and mediate clinical efficacy once reinjected in vivo in autologous patient setting [106].

In contrast, melanomas lacking T-cell recognition are unlikely to react to current immunotherapies, but they might gain a sufficient level of immunogenicity if appropriate conditions should be put in place. Strategies for attracting tumor-specific T cells are under intensive investigation at preclinical level, based on the specific targeting of immunosuppressive pathways within tumor microenvironment [107]. On the other site, to promptly rescue cold/desert tumors in clinical setting, the off-target immunomodulating effects of standard cancer therapies, as well as old and novel specific strategies to favor tumor T-cell infiltrate, are being tested through combinatorial treatment schedules [107, 108].

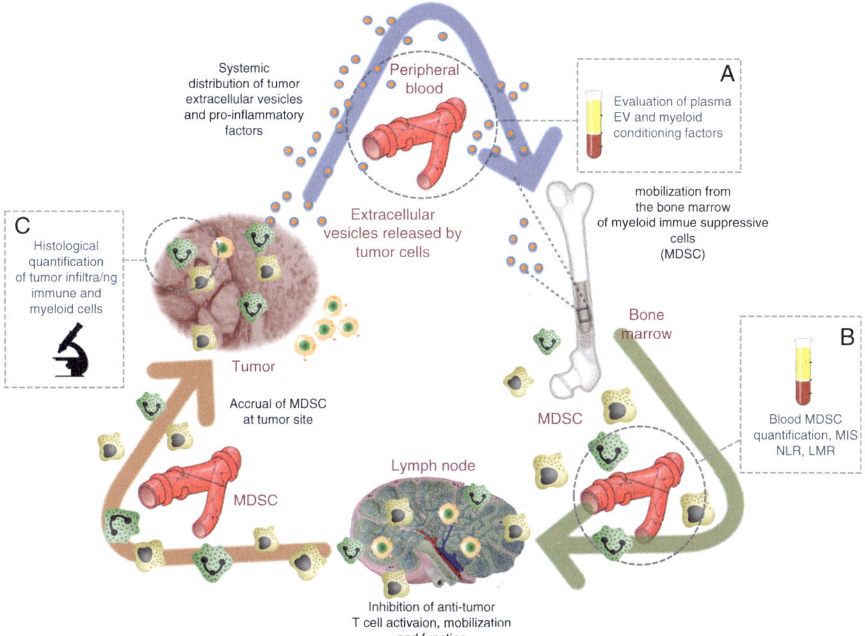

Fig. 4.2 The melanoma–bone marrow immunosuppressive triangle (with related blood and tumor biomarkers. Melanoma cells release into the peripheral circulation extracellular vesicles (EV) enriched in various genetic and protein content, including a selected panel of myeloid-conditioning microRNAs. These EV migrate to the bone marrow where they are internalized by myeloid cells and affect myelopoiesis, causing the egression of dysfunctional immunosuppressive myeloid cells, collectively known as myeloid-derived suppressor cells (MDSC). MDSC accumulate in peripheral circulation and colonize immune organs (including spleen and lymph nodes) where they impair T-cell activation. They are also attracted by tumor site via the production of chemotactic factors, and they infiltrate the tumor, causing a hostile microenviroment for antitumor T cells but favoring tumor progression. This path is a rich source of immunosuppressive biomarkers: tumor-released EVs and MDSC-related microRNAs in plasma (**a**); blood MDSC as well as their surrogate biomarkers (myeloid index score, Neutrophil-to-lymphocyte ratio—NLR, Monocyte-to-lymphocyte ratio—LMR) (**b**); tumor-infiltrating myeloid cells, and their ratio with lymphocytes (**c**)

Tumor Immunomodulating by Standard Melanoma Treatments

In addition to immunotherapy based on ICB, current standard treatments for metastatic melanoma include only BRAFi/MEKi (confined in theory to patients with BRAFmut melanoma); chemotherapy has been largely abandoned over the last decade, although tailored approaches for the treatment of ICB and BRAFi/MEKi-resistant patients are still under investigation [109].

BRAF inhibitors (BRAFi) and MEK inhibitors (MEKi) are reported to exert some level of immune modulation either thanks to the rapid disease control that relieves cancer-mediated immunosuppression, the induction of increased HLA levels in melanoma cells [110] or through direct effects on immune effectors still not fully understood [111]. The latter hypothesis is suggested by the evidence that

BRAFi/MEKi exerts effects in vivo also in BRAF-wild type melanomas, indicating a potential indirect antitumor activity likely passing through the immune system [112].

Chemotherapy has been also for long considered a potential immunomodulating strategy to boost antitumor immunity and synergize with ICB activity, as suggested by the potentiated clinical activity that the combination treatment has shown in NSCLC and other malignancies [113]. Specific chemotherapeutics are deemed to potentiate tumor immunity by causing "immunogeneic tumor cell death," that is, a form of tumor cell destruction that activates antitigen-presenting cells and favors the triggering of antigen-specific T cells [114]. Nevertheless, chemotherapy might also be beneficial to tumor immunity, thanks to the myelotoxicity that most of the drugs of this family mediate, which might lead to a reduced MDSC and TAM, with a consequent boost of antitumor T-cell responses [115].

Dacarbazine, representing the backbone of melanoma chemotherapy, has been reported to boost antitumor cytolytic and IFNγ-secreting effectors including CD8[+] T and NK cells [116]. Although data on the immunomodulating effects of melanoma chemotherapeutics are relatively limited, we observed that the combination of fotemustine and ipilimumab, leading to a significant clinical benefit in advanced pretreated melanoma patients [117], is linked to a reduction of blood myeloid cells, particularly in patients displaying better PFS and OS *(Rivoltini L., unpublished)*. These data point to the potential use of fotemustine as a myelo-conditioning treatment able to reduce immunosuppressive pressure and rescue sensitivity to ICB in patients lacking preexisting immunity.

Old and Novel Therapeutic Strategies to Counteract Cold/Desert Melanoma Microenvironment

As in most cancers, melanoma local progression relies on the support of neoangiogenesis, which is the formation of new vascular structures from existing blood vessels. Triggered by hypoxic conditions, a complex and tightly regulated network is indeed established within the melanoma microenvironment including the production of vascular endothelial growth factor (VEGF), fibroblast growth factor (FGF), platelet-derived growth factor (PDGF), interleukin 8 (IL-8), metalloproteinases (MMPs), and others, as well as the engagement of endothelial cells and pericytes [118]. Melanoma angiogenesis is not only aimed at supporting the nutrients and oxygen supply required for persistent tumor proliferation but also at contributing to the onset of the immunosuppression needed for allowing tissue repair without the onset of autoimmunity as dictated by the tissue repair process [119]. Indeed, several preclinical and clinical evidences demonstrated that VEGF and other angiogenic factors induce direct T-cell inhibition and recruit MDSC and Treg at tumor site. In contrast, the administration of anti-angiogenic drugs usually leads to a rapid drop in immunosuppressive cells and the recovery of immunosurveillance in blood and tumor site [120]. The effect could be mostly due to the blunting of VEGF-related immune suppressive effects, but the targeting of regulatory immune cells (expressing VEGFR and producing VEGF) or even to the known myelotoxicity linked particularly to anti-angiogenic TKIs, could be involved [121].

Treatment with single anti-angiogenics has not demonstrated sufficient clinical efficacy in melanoma patients to enter the current therapeutic algorithms of this disease; however, immunomonitoring of patients treated with bevacizumab + cisplatin showed higher CD8+ T-cell levels and reduced plasma IL-6 concentrations with respect to patients receiving cisplatin alone, indicating the immunomodulating effect of bevacizumab [122].

In this view, anti-angiogenics could be reconsidered in light of their remarkable immunomodulating properties, and introduced to promote T-cell infiltrate in cold/desert melanomas for possibly increased responsiveness to ICB. In this regard, it is worth here reporting that data obtained in RCC patients treated with pazopanib or cabozantinib suggest that the modulating activity of these drugs is remarkable but transitory [123, 124].This indicates that an intermitting alternate schedule of anti-angiogenics + ICB would maximize treatment synergy more than a concomitant and continuous drug combination. The latter strategy could be also penalized by the potential inhibitory activity that some anti-angiogenics might exert on T-cell proliferation [125].

Based on the huge amount of data unraveling the complexity of a cold/desert tumor microenvironment, multiple strategies are under evaluation to select pathways worth to be tested in clinical setting. Drugs to eliminate MDSC and TAM block their activity or convert them toward antitumor effectors are being considered, including CSF1R [126], Arginase I blockers, STAT3 inhibitors, and others [127].

Novel approaches relying on a pleiotropic modulation of tumor immunity are also under preclinical and clinical evaluation, based on interfering on immune metabolism by dietary intervention. The general idea behind this latter approach is that tumor immunosuppressive activity could be reduced and a reshape of systemic tumor immunity obtained by impacting on blood metabolites and growth factors through the change of dietary income (for instance, by fasting or fasting–mimicking diets, FMD). Preclinical models and studies in healthy subjects have demonstrated that anti-inflammatory and immunomodulating effects can be achieved with a remarkable tumor control [128, 129]. Based on this rational, in our Institution, we are intensively testing the metabolic and immunomodulating properties of FMD in different clinical settings including melanoma [130, 131]. This type of studies, echoing the efforts ongoing worldwide to test dietary intervention for cancer prevention and anti-inflammatory effects, points to the possibility of molding tumor immunity by drug-free strategies that might be applied to complement cancer immunotherapy.

Potential Practical Implications for Clinical Practice

The knowledge in the field of melanoma immunology has dramatically grown in the last years, with a present scenario depicting complex and often redundant information on the rules that govern tumor-immune cross-talk in vivo. Many of these mechanisms have been identified through elegant and solid works often paralleling preclinical analyses with clinical studies, which obviously strengthen the conclusions and make them pillars on the discovery path of novel biomarkers to guide therapeutic choice in melanoma. Table 4.1 lists the pillar immunological mechanisms that help in profiling patient immune state, their clinical implications, and the corresponding biomarkers that could be applied to patient's tumor tissue or blood.

Table 4.1 Key immune-related biomarkers for disease outcome and response to therapy in melanoma patients

Mechanism	Target	Biological implications	Clinical implications	Related biomarker for clinical practise	Effect of disease outcome
High DNA mutations and alterations	Melanoma cells	Generation of T cell antigens and T cell protective immune responses	Better clinical outcome and improved response to IT	TMB, NGS	Positive
Efficient recognition of antigenic determinants by T cells	Immune cells	Accrual of activated T cells at tumor site	Better clinical outcome and improved response to therapy, including IT	TIL (tumor infiltrating lymphocytes) Immunoscore (CD8+ quantification)	Positive
Prevalence of tumor infiltrating T cells with respect to myeloid cells	TME	Tumor microenvironment with a prevalence of antitumor preexisting immunity above immunosuppression	Better disease outcome and improved response to therapy, including IT	CD8+(CD3+)/CD163 ratio	Positive
High antigenic Intratumor heterogeneity (ITH)	Melanoma cells	Induction of insufficient level of tumor-specific T cells	Worse disease outcome and response to IT in patient with high ITH	NGS and computational analyses for T cell epitope prediction	Negative
Enrichment in tumor tertiary lymphoid structures (TLS)	TME	B cells located into TLS process and present tumor antigens for T cell priming	Better response to IT, including ICB	B cell infiltrate and TLS histological quantification	Positive
HLA-I germ line heterozygosous genotype	Host	In the presence of heterozygosis of A, B, C loci, the number of presented antigens is higher and the T cell repertoire is enriched	Better survival and response to IT in patient with HLA-I heterozygosis	HLA-I molecular typing	Positive

Table 4.1 (continued)

Mechanism	Target	Biological implications	Clinical implications	Related biomarker for clinical practise	Effect of disease outcome
High plasma soluble PD-1/PD-L1	Melanoma and immune cells	Soluble checkpoint (PD-1/PD-L1) bind to immune checkpoint inhibitors and act as decoy receptors	Less ICB bioavailability and lower clinical efficacy of ICB	sPD-1/sPD-L1 Elisa	Negative
High myeloid cell dysfunctions	Blood	Altered myeloid cells inhibit antitumor T cells and immune responses, promote tumor angiogenesis and EMT, stroma remodeling, distant metastases	Disease progression and dedifferentiation Poor response to therapies Resistance to IT	MDSC flow cytometry profile[a] Myeloid Index Score (MIS)[b] Neutrophil-to-lymphocyte ratio (NLR)[c]	Negative
Enriched lymphocytes vs to myeloid cells	Blood	Lower systemic myeloid dysfunctions	Less aggressive disease and better response to therapy	Lymphocyte-to-monocyte ratio (LMR)[d]	Positive

IT immunotherapy, *TMB* tumor mutational burden, *NGS* next generation sequencing, *TME* tumor microenvironment, *ICB* immune checkpoint blockers (PD-1), *EMT* eplthellal-to-mesenchymal transition
[a]For flow cutometry guidelines, see [79]
[b] [85]
[c] [91–93]
[d] [49]

Unfortunately, for reasons not fully understandable, only few (if any) of these biomarkers have made to be actually translated into real-life clinical practice. This implies that even in an immunogenic and well-studied tumor such as melanoma, there is still large room for improving patient management by tailoring treatment on the basis of some level of individual immune profile. Hence, we would like to conclude this review by going through the most promising and accessible of these biomarkers, summarizing their scientific relevance, the clinical implications, and the corresponding technical assays to evaluate them.

The **Immunoscore**, that is, the evaluation of quantitative and qualitative distribution of CD8+ T cells within tumor lesions, can be applied to assess preexisting immunity both in surgical specimens [15] and in tumor biopsy [132]. Based on the immunostaining of lymphocyte populations, in particular CD3$^+$ and CD8$^+$ T cells, in formalin-fixed paraffin-embedded slides through a digital pathology approach, represents a reliable tool to prove immune fitness in melanoma patients and predict their positive disease outcome [16]. Of note, a recent study by the same author who developed Immunoscore assessed the analytical performances of the Immunoscore, demonstrating that CD3$^+$ and CD8$^+$ cells could be quantified also by optical counts, with data highly concordant with those obtained by automatic evaluation [133].

Comparable and, in a way extended, information can be obtained by the **CD8/CD163 ratio** in tumor lesions or biopsies. Again using the immunostaining of T cell and myeloid infiltrate by a T cell (CD8) and a myeloid cell/macrophage marker (CD163), in formalin-fixed paraffin-embedded slides, it allows to evaluate the general balance between antitumor and pro-tumor/immunosuppressive cells within the tumor lesion, and helps in predicting response to both ICB and BRAFl/MEKi administration, as well as patient prognosis [49].

In blood, the tumor–bone marrow crosstalk leading to the accrual of immunosuppressive myeloid cells that so strongly impact on melanoma patients' prognosis can be reliably and relatively easily intercepted. Guidelines to define and quantify **myeloid-derived suppressor cells (MDSC)** by flow cytometry are available [79] and they can be applied on peripheral blood mononuclear cells (PBMC) isolated by Ficoll gradient. A surrogate of this measurement is represented by the myeloid index score, calculated on the **neutrophil-to-lymphocyte ratio** frequency of CD14$^+$, CD15$^+$, CD14$^+$HLA-DR^{neg} and CD14$^+$PDL-1$^+$ cells in frozen PBMC. The value above defined cut-offs of any of these four cell subsets is associated with poor prognosis and rapid progression upon ICB or BRAFi/MEKi treatment in metastatic melanoma patients [85].

Possibly assessing the same biological process underlying MDSC blood accrual is the evaluation of the ratio between the absolute counts of circulating myeloid and lymphoid cells obtained from standard blood tests. The **neutrophil-to-lymphocyte ratio (NLR)** [92] and the **lymphocyte-to-monocyte ratio (LMR)** [95] are ready-to-assess blood biomarkers of bad prognosis, and resistance to therapy the first (NLR) and good prognosis and response to treatment, the second (LMR). Their level above (NLR) or below (LMR) defined cut-offs can readily identify patients likely to display aggressive disease and resistance to diverse types of treatments, with significant HR that however do not reach the prognostication power of MDSC direct quantification.

Few words need to be finally spent of PD-L1 expression in melanoma cells and microenvironment. As for most human malignancies, this FDA-approved biomarker does not seem to reliably predict prognosis nor response to ICB [134–136]. More interesting are instead the recent data produced on soluble PD-L1 and PD-1, whose higher levels in plasma predict resistance to treatment with PD-1 blockade but not to BRAFi/MEKi in advanced melanoma patients. These latter results indicate that soluble immune checkpoints might antagonize ICB activity by exerting a decoy effect that limits the antibody availability to bind PD-1 expressed on exhausted T cells [137].

Conclusions

Melanoma immunology and immunotherapy have become a well-established field in cancer research and treatment. However, after the unprecedented effort of the last decade to dissect the mechanisms of tumor-immune interaction and generate innovative immunotherapy approaches, there is now an urgent need to concentrate on the remaining crucial issues that may lead to clinical progress. Several challenges have still to be faced to make immunotherapy an effective tool for most patients and not only for a selected subset. Gaining the confidence to translate preclinical findings into clinical setting, to personalize treatments on the immune profile of any given patient, and design scientifically sounded combination therapies that could overcome individual immune defects would definitively allow to move forward in cancer curability. The concerted effort of basic researchers and clinicians must be continued and even intensified, for producing true advances for real-life clinical practice and further broadening accessibility to immunotherapeutics in the near future.

Acknowledgments The authors are supported by funding to LR from TRANSCAN-ERANET (Project code ER-2017-2364968), Horizon2020 (PRECIOUS Project, Grant Agreement n° 686089), and AIRC IG 2017 n° 20752.

References

1. Zhang Y, Zhang Z. The history and advances in cancer immunotherapy: understanding the characteristics of tumor-infiltrating immune cells and their therapeutic implications. Cell Mol Immunol. 2020;17:807–21. https://doi.org/10.1038/s41423-020-0488-6.
2. Hegde PS, Chen DS. Top 10 challenges in cancer immunotherapy. Immunity. 2020;52(1):17–35. https://doi.org/10.1016/j.immuni.2019.12.011.
3. Brodin P, Davis MM. Human immune system variation. Nat Rev Immunol. 2017;17:21–9.
4. Godfrey DI, Le Nours J, Andrews DM, Uldrich AP, Rossjohn J. Unconventional T cell targets for cancer immunotherapy. Immunity. 2018;48(3):453–73. https://doi.org/10.1016/j.immuni.2018.03.009.
5. Nepom GT, St. Clair EW, Turka LA. Challenges in the pursuit of immune tolerance. Immunol Rev. 2011;241(1):49–62.
6. Finn OJ. A believer's overview of cancer immunosurveillance and immunotherapy. J Immunol. 2018;200(2):385–91. https://doi.org/10.4049/jimmunol.1701302.
7. Waldman AD, Fritz JM, Lenardo MJ. A guide to cancer immunotherapy: from T cell basic science to clinical practice. Nat Rev Immunol. 2020;20(11):651–68. https://doi.org/10.1038/s41577-020-0306-5.
8. Gentles A, Newman A, Liu C, et al. The prognostic landscape of genes and infiltrating immune cells across human cancers. Nat Med. 2015;21:938–45. https://doi.org/10.1038/nm.3909.
9. Bruno TC. New predictors for immunotherapy responses sharpen our view of the tumour microenvironment. Nature. 2020;577:474–6. https://doi.org/10.1038/d41586-019-03943-0.

10. Spranger S, Gajewski TF. Mechanisms of Tumor cell–intrinsic immune evasion. Annu Rev Cancer Biol. 2018;2(1):213–28.
11. Taube J, Galon J, Sholl L, et al. Implications of the tumor immune microenvironment for staging and therapeutics. Mod Pathol. 2018;31:214–34. https://doi.org/10.1038/modpathol.2017.156.
12. Rosenberg SA, Restifo NP, Yang JC, Morgan RA, Dudley ME. Adoptive cell transfer: a clinical path to effective cancer immunotherapy. Nat Rev Cancer. 2008;8(4):299–308. https://doi.org/10.1038/nrc2355.
13. Dafni U, Michielin O, Lluesma SM, et al. Efficacy of adoptive therapy with tumor-infiltrating lymphocytes and recombinant interleukin-2 in advanced cutaneous melanoma: a systematic review and meta-analysis. Ann Oncol. 2019;30(12):1902–13. https://doi.org/10.1093/annonc/mdz398.
14. Fu Q, Chen N, Ge C, et al. Prognostic value of tumor-infiltrating lymphocytes in melanoma: a systematic review and meta-analysis. Oncoimmunology. 2019;8(7):1593806. https://doi.org/10.1080/2162402X.2019.1593806.
15. Lee N, Zakka LR, Mihm MC, Schatton T. Tumour-infiltrating lymphocytes in melanoma prognosis and cancer immunotherapy. Pathology. 2016;48(2):177–87. https://doi.org/10.1016/j.pathol.2015.12.006.
16. Bruni D, Angell HK, Galon J. The immune contexture and Immunoscore in cancer prognosis and therapeutic efficacy. Nat Rev Cancer. 2020;20(11):662–80. https://doi.org/10.1038/s41568-020-0285-7.
17. Angell HK, Bruni D, Barrett JC, Herbst R, Galon J. The immunoscore: colon cancer and beyond. Clin Cancer Res. 2020;26(2):332–9. https://doi.org/10.1158/1078-0432.CCR-18-1851.
18. Zamora AE, Crawford JC, Thomas PG. Hitting the target: how T cells detect and eliminate tumors. J Immunol. 2018;200(2):392–9. https://doi.org/10.4049/jimmunol.1701413.
19. Parmiani G. Melanoma antigens and their recognition by T cells. Keio J Med. 2001;50(2):86–90. https://doi.org/10.2302/kjm.50.86.
20. Ramirez-Montagut T, Turk MJ, Wolchok JD, Guevara-Patino JA, Houghton AN. Immunity to melanoma: unraveling the relation of tumor immunity and autoimmunity. Oncogene. 2003;22(20):3180–7. https://doi.org/10.1038/sj.onc.1206462.
21. Faramarzi S, Ghafouri-Fard S. Melanoma: a prototype of cancer-testis antigen-expressing malignancies. Immunotherapy. 2017;9(13):1103–13. https://doi.org/10.2217/imt-2017-0091.
22. Parmiani G, De Filippo A, Novellino L, Castelli C. Unique human tumor antigens: immunobiology and use in clinical trials. J Immunol. 2007;178(4):1975–9. https://doi.org/10.4049/jimmunol.178.4.1975.
23. Krieger T, Pearson I, Bell J, et al. Targeted literature review on use of tumor mutational burden status and programmed cell death ligand 1 expression to predict outcomes of checkpoint inhibitor treatment. Diagn Pathol. 2020;15:6. https://doi.org/10.1186/s13000-020-0927-9.
24. Liu D, Schilling B, Liu D, et al. Integrative molecular and clinical modeling of clinical outcomes to PD1 blockade in patients with metastatic melanoma [published correction appears in Nat Med. 2020 Jul;26(7):1147]. Nat Med. 2019;25(12):1916–27. https://doi.org/10.1038/s41591-019-0654-5.
25. Eroglu Z, Zaretsky J, Hu-Lieskovan S, et al. High response rate to PD-1 blockade in desmoplastic melanomas. Nature. 2018;553:347–50. https://doi.org/10.1038/nature25187.
26. Mao P, Brown AJ, Esaki S, Lockwood S, Poon GMK, Smerdon MJ, Roberts SA, Wyrick JJ. ETS transcription factors induce a unique UV damage signature that drives recurrent mutagenesis in melanoma. Nat Commun. 2018;9(1):2626. https://doi.org/10.1038/s41467-018-05064-0.
27. Byrne KT, Côté AL, Zhang P, et al. Autoimmune melanocyte destruction is required for robust CD8+ memory T cell responses to mouse melanoma. J Clin Invest. 2011;121(5):1797–809. https://doi.org/10.1172/JCI44849.
28. Malik BT, Byrne KT, Vella JL, et al. Resident memory T cells in the skin mediate durable immunity to melanoma. Sci Immunol. 2017;2(10):eaam6346. https://doi.org/10.1126/sciimmunol.aam6346.

29. Harel M, Ortenberg R, Varanasi SK, et al. Proteomics of melanoma response to immunotherapy reveals mitochondrial dependence. Cell. 2019;179(1):236–250.e18. https://doi.org/10.1016/j.cell.2019.08.012.
30. Harjes U. Helping tumour antigens to the surface. Nat Rev Cancer. 2019;19:608. https://doi.org/10.1038/s41568-019-0212-y.
31. Kalaora S, Lee JS, Barnea E, et al. Immunoproteasome expression is associated with better prognosis and response to checkpoint therapies in melanoma. Nat Commun. 2020;11:896. https://doi.org/10.1038/s41467-020-14639-9.
32. Sautès-Fridman C, Petitprez F, Calderaro J, et al. Tertiary lymphoid structures in the era of cancer immunotherapy. Nat Rev Cancer. 2019;19:307–25. https://doi.org/10.1038/s41568-019-0144-6.
33. Ramón y Cajal S, Sesé M, Capdevila C, et al. Clinical implications of intratumor heterogeneity: challenges and opportunities. J Mol Med. 2020;98:161–77. https://doi.org/10.1007/s00109-020-01874-2.
34. Wolf Y, Bartok O, Patkar S, et al. UVB-induced tumor heterogeneity diminishes immune response in melanoma. Cell. 2019;179(1):219–235.e21. https://doi.org/10.1016/j.cell.2019.08.032.
35. Duffy D, Rouilly V, Libri V, Hasan M, Beitz B, David M, Urrutia A, Bisiaux A, Labrie ST, Dubois A, et al. Functional analysis via standardized whole-blood stimulation systems defines the boundaries of a healthy immune response to complex stimuli. Immunity. 2014;40:436–50. https://doi.org/10.1016/j.immuni.2014.03.002.
36. Thommen DS, Schumacher TN. T cell dysfunction in cancer. Cancer Cell. 2018;33(4):547–62. https://doi.org/10.1016/j.ccell.2018.03.012.
37. Gros A, Robbins PF, Yao X, et al. PD-1 identifies the patient-specific CD8$^+$ tumor-reactive repertoire infiltrating human tumors. J Clin Invest. 2014;124(5):2246–59. https://doi.org/10.1172/JCI73639;.
38. Havel JJ, Chowell D, Chan TA. The evolving landscape of biomarkers for checkpoint inhibitor immunotherapy. Nat Rev Cancer. 2019;19(3):133–50. https://doi.org/10.1038/s41568-019-0116-x.
39. Gorris MAJ, Halilovic A, Rabold K, et al. Eight-color multiplex immunohistochemistry for simultaneous detection of multiple immune checkpoint molecules within the tumor microenvironment. J Immunol. 2018;200(1):347–54. https://doi.org/10.4049/jimmunol.1701262.
40. Rotte A, Jin JY, Lemaire V. Mechanistic overview of immune checkpoints to support the rational design of their combinations in cancer immunotherapy. Ann Oncol. 2018;29(1):71–83. https://doi.org/10.1093/annonc/mdx686.
41. Wei SC, Duffy CR, Allison JP. Fundamental mechanisms of immune checkpoint blockade therapy. Cancer Discov. 2018;8(9):1069–86. https://doi.org/10.1158/2159-8290.CD-18-0367.
42. Tarhini A, Kudchadkar RR. Predictive and on-treatment monitoring biomarkers in advanced melanoma: moving toward personalized medicine. Cancer Treat Rev. 2018;71:8–18. https://doi.org/10.1016/j.ctrv.2018.09.005.
43. Gibney GT, Weiner LM, Atkins MB. Predictive biomarkers for checkpoint inhibitor-based immunotherapy. Lancet Oncol. 2016;17(12):e542–51. https://doi.org/10.1016/S1470-2045(16)30406-5.
44. Hegde PS, Karanikas V, Evers S. The where, the when, and the how of immune monitoring for cancer immunotherapies in the era of checkpoint inhibition. Clin Cancer Res. 2016;22(8):1865–74. https://doi.org/10.1158/1078-0432.CCR-15-1507.
45. Cristescu R, Mogg R, Ayers M, et al. Pan-tumor genomic biomarkers for PD-1 checkpoint blockade–based immunotherapy. Science. 2018;362(6411):eaar3593. https://doi.org/10.1126/science.aar3593.
46. van Belzen IAEM, Kesmir C. Immune biomarkers for predicting response to adoptive cell transfer as cancer treatment. Immunogenetics. 2019;71:71–86. https://doi.org/10.1007/s00251-018-1083-1.
47. van der Burg SH. Correlates of immune and clinical activity of novel cancer vaccines. Semin Immunol. 2018;39:119–36. https://doi.org/10.1016/j.smim.2018.04.001.

48. Chen P-H, Lipschitz M, Jason L. Weirather, et al. Activation of CAR and non-CAR T cells within the tumor microenvironment following CAR T cell therapy. JCI Insight. 2020;5(12):e134612. https://doi.org/10.1172/jci.insight.134612.
49. Massi D, Rulli E, Cossa M, et al. The density and spatial tissue distribution of CD8+ and CD163+ immune cells predict response and outcome in melanoma patients receiving MAPK inhibitors. J Immunother Cancer. 2019;7(1):308. https://doi.org/10.1186/s40425-019-0797-4.
50. Spranger S, Luke JJ, Bao R, et al. Antigen-density inflamed vs. non inflamed tumors. Proc Natl Acad Sci U S A. 2016;113(48):E7759–68. https://doi.org/10.1073/pnas.1609376113.
51. Sayaman RW, Saad M, Thorsson V, et al. Germline genetic contribution to the immune landscape of cancer. bioRxiv. 2020; https://doi.org/10.1101/2020.01.30.926527.
52. Duan Q, Zhang H, Zheng J, Zhang L. Turning cold into hot: firing up the tumor microenvironment. Trends Cancer. 2020;6(7):605–18. https://doi.org/10.1016/j.trecan.2020.02.02.
53. Jensen TO, Schmidt H, Møller HJ, Høyer M, Maniecki MB, Sjoegren P, Christensen IJ, Steiniche T. Macrophage markers in serum and tumor have prognostic impact in American joint committee on cancer stage I/II melanoma. J Clin Oncol. 2009;27(20):3330–7.
54. Salmi S, Siiskonen H, Sironen R, et al. The number and localization of CD68+ and CD163+ macrophages in different stages of cutaneous melanoma. Melanoma Res. 2019;29(3):237–47. https://doi.org/10.1097/CMR.0000000000000522.
55. Bu X, Mahoney KM, Freeman GJ. Learning from PD-1 resistance: new combination strategies. Trends Mol Med. 2016;22(6):448–51. https://doi.org/10.1016/j.molmed.2016.04.008.
56. Hugo W, Zaretsky JM, Sun L, et al. Genomic and transcriptomic features of response to anti-PD-1 therapy in metastatic melanoma. Cell. 2017;168(3):542. https://doi.org/10.1016/j.cell.2017.01.010.
57. Engblom C, Pfirschke C, Pittet M. The role of myeloid cells in cancer therapies. Nat Rev Cancer. 2016;16:447–62. https://doi.org/10.1038/nrc.2016.54.
58. Lee JH, Shklovskaya E, Lim SY, et al. Transcriptional downregulation of MHC class I and melanoma de- differentiation in resistance to PD-1 inhibition. Nat Commun. 2020;11:1897. https://doi.org/10.1038/s41467-020-15726-7.
59. Mahmoud F, Shields B, Makhoul I, et al. Immune surveillance in melanoma: from immune attack to melanoma escape and even counterattack. Cancer Biol Ther. 2017;18(7):451–69. https://doi.org/10.1080/15384047.2017.1323596.
60. Puzanov I, et al. Association of BRAF V600E/K mutation status and prior BRAF/MEK inhibition with pembrolizumab outcomes in advanced melanoma: pooled analysis of 3 clinical trials. JAMA Oncol. 2020;6(8):1256–64. https://doi.org/10.1001/jamaoncol.2020.2288.
61. Johnson DB, Lovly CM, Flavin M, et al. Impact of NRAS mutations for patients with advanced melanoma treated with immune therapies. Cancer Immunol Res. 2015;3(3):288–95. https://doi.org/10.1158/2326-6066.CIR-14-0207.
62. Vidotto T, Melo CM, Castelli E, et al. Emerging role of PTEN loss in evasion of the immune response to tumours. Br J Cancer. 2020;122:1732–43. https://doi.org/10.1038/s41416-020-0834-6.
63. Rizvi NA, Chan TA. Immunotherapy and oncogenic pathways: the PTEN connection. Cancer Discov. 2016;6(2):128–9. https://doi.org/10.1158/2159-8290.CD-15-1501.
64. Spranger S, Gajewski TF. Impact of oncogenic pathways on evasion of antitumor immune responses. Nat Rev. 2018;18:139–47. https://doi.org/10.1038/nrc.2017.117.
65. Li F, Simon MC. Cancer cells don't live alone: metabolic communication within tumor microenvironments. Dev Cell. 2020;54(2):183–95. https://doi.org/10.1016/j.devcel.2020.06.018.
66. Noman MZ, Hasmim M, Lequeux A, et al. Improving cancer immunotherapy by targeting the hypoxic tumor microenvironment: new opportunities and challenges. Cells. 2019;8(9):1083. https://doi.org/10.3390/cells8091083.
67. Huber R, Meier B, Otsuka A, et al. Tumour hypoxia promotes melanoma growth and metastasis via High Mobility Group Box-1 and M2-like macrophages. Sci Rep. 2016;6:29914. https://doi.org/10.1038/srep2991.
68. Calcinotto A, Filipazzi P, Grioni M, et al. Modulation of microenvironment acidity reverses anergy in human and murine tumor-infiltrating T lymphocytes. Cancer Res. 2012;72(11):2746–56. https://doi.org/10.1158/0008-5472.CAN-11-1272.

69. Bellone M, Calcinotto A, Filipazzi P, et al. The acidity of the tumor microenvironment is a mechanism of immune escape that can be overcome by proton pump inhibitors. Oncoimmunology. 2013;2(1):e22058. https://doi.org/10.4161/onci.22058.
70. Yan D, Adeshakin AO, Xu M, et al. Lipid metabolic pathways confer the immunosuppressive function of myeloid-derived suppressor cells in tumor. Front Immunol. 2019;10:1399. https://doi.org/10.3389/fimmu.2019.01399.
71. Imbert C, Montfort A, Fraisse M, et al. Resistance of melanoma to immune checkpoint inhibitors is overcome by targeting the sphingosine kinase-1. Nat Commun. 2020;11:437. https://doi.org/10.1038/s41467-019-14218-7.
72. Spitzer MH, Carmi Y, Reticker-Flynn NE, et al. Systemic immunity is required for effective cancer immunotherapy. Cell. 2017;168(3):487–502.e15. https://doi.org/10.1016/j.cell.2016.12.022.
73. Vanmeerbeek I, Sprooten J, De Ruysscher D, et al. Trial watch: chemotherapy-induced immunogenic cell death in immuno-oncology. Oncoimmunology. 2020;9(1):1703449. https://doi.org/10.1080/2162402X.2019.1703449.
74. Groth C, Hu X, Weber R, et al. Immunosuppression mediated by myeloid-derived suppressor cells (MDSCs) during tumour progression. Br J Cancer. 2019;120:16–25. https://doi.org/10.1038/s41416-018-0333-1.
75. Wu C, Hua Q, Zheng L. Generation of myeloid cells in cancer: the spleen matters. Front Immunol. 2020;11:1126. https://doi.org/10.3389/fimmu.2020.01126.
76. Ugel S, De Sanctis F, Mandruzzato S, Bronte V. Tumor-induced myeloid deviation: when myeloid-derived suppressor cells meet tumor-associated macrophages. J Clin Invest. 2015;125(9):3365–76. https://doi.org/10.1172/JCI80006.
77. Veglia F, Perego M, Gabrilovich D. Myeloid-derived suppressor cells coming of age. Nat Immunol. 2018;19(2):108–19. https://doi.org/10.1038/s41590-017-0022-x.
78. Ostrand-Rosenberg S, Fenselau C. Myeloid-derived suppressor cells: immune-suppressive cells that impair antitumor immunity and are sculpted by their environment. J Immunol. 2018;200(2):422–31. https://doi.org/10.4049/jimmunol.1701019.
79. Bronte V, Brandau S, Chen S, et al. Recommendations for myeloid-derived suppressor cell nomenclature and characterization standards. Nat Commun. 2016;7:12150. https://doi.org/10.1038/ncomms12150.
80. Ai L, Mu S, Wang Y, et al. Prognostic role of myeloid-derived suppressor cells in cancers: a systematic review and meta-analysis. BMC Cancer. 2018;18:1220. https://doi.org/10.1186/s12885-018-5086-y.
81. Filipazzi P, Valenti R, Huber V, et al. Identification of a new subset of myeloid suppressor cells in peripheral blood of melanoma patients with modulation by a granulocyte-macrophage colony-stimulation factor-based antitumor vaccine. J Clin Oncol. 2007;25(18):2546–53. https://doi.org/10.1200/JCO.2006.08.5829.
82. Weber R, Fleming V, Hu X, et al. Myeloid-derived suppressor cells hinder the anti-cancer activity of immune checkpoint inhibitors. Front Immunol. 2018;9:1310. https://doi.org/10.3389/fimmu.2018.01310.
83. Martens A, Wistuba-Hamprecht K, Geukes Foppen M, et al. Baseline peripheral blood biomarkers associated with clinical outcome of advanced melanoma patients treated with ipilimumab. Clin Cancer Res. 2016;22(12):2908–18. https://doi.org/10.1158/1078-0432.CCR-15-2412.
84. Tesi RJ. MDSC; the most important cell you have never heard of. Trends Pharmacol Sci. 2019;40(1):4–7. https://doi.org/10.1016/j.tips.2018.10.008.
85. Huber V, DI Guardo L, Lalli L. et al. Back to simplicity: a 4-marker blood cell score to quantify prognostically relevant myeloid cells in melanoma patients. JITC; 2020.
86. https://www.era-learn.eu/network-information/networks/era-permed/personalised-medicine-multidisciplinary-research-towards-implementation/quantifying-systemic-immunosuppression-to-personalize-cancer-therapy
87. Apodaca MC, Wright AE, Riggins AM, et al. Characterization of a whole blood assay for quantifying myeloid-derived suppressor cells. J Immunother Cancer. 2019;7:230. https://doi.org/10.1186/s40425-019-0674-1.

88. Patrick Innamarato, Krithika Kodumudi, Sarah Asby, et al. Reactive myelopoiesis triggered by lymphodepleting chemotherapy limits the efficacy of adoptive T cell therapy. Mol Ther; 2020. https://doi.org/10.1016/j.ymthe.2020.06.025.

89. Barret O'N Jr. Monocytosis in malignant disease. Ann Intern Med. 1970;73(6):991–2.

90. Schmidt H, Bastholt L, Geertsen P, et al. Elevated neutrophil and monocyte counts in peripheral blood are associated with poor survival in patients with metastatic melanoma: a prognostic model. Br J Cancer. 2005;93:273–8. https://doi.org/10.1038/sj.bjc.6602702.

91. Basu A, Kollengode KA, Rafatnia A, et al. Relationship between neutrophil lymphocyte ratio (NLR) and MDSC concentration in localized and metastatic castration resistant prostate cancer (mCRPC) patients. J Clin Oncol. 2018;36(6_suppl):338.

92. Ding Y, Zhang S, Qiao J. Prognostic value of neutrophil-to-lymphocyte ratio in melanoma: evidence from a PRISMA-compliant meta-analysis. Medicine (Baltimore). 2018;97(30):e11446. https://doi.org/10.1097/MD.0000000000011446.

93. Ma J, Kuzman J, Ray A, et al. Neutrophil-to-lymphocyte Ratio (NLR) as a predictor for recurrence in patients with stage III melanoma. Sci Rep. 2018;8(1):4044. https://doi.org/10.1038/s41598-018-22425-3.

94. Filipazzi P, Pilla L, Mariani L, et al. Limited induction of tumor cross-reactive T cells without a measurable clinical benefit in early melanoma patients vaccinated with human leukocyte antigen class I-modified peptides. Clin Cancer Res. 2012;18(23):6485–96. https://doi.org/10.1158/1078-0432.CCR-12-1516.

95. Iacono D, Basile D, Gerratana L, et al. Prognostic role of disease extent and lymphocyte–monocyte ratio in advanced melanoma. Melanoma Res. 2019;29(5):510–5. https://doi.org/10.1097/CMR.0000000000000584.

96. Failing JJ, Yan Y, Porrata LF, Markovic SN. Lymphocyte-to-monocyte ratio is associated with survival in pembrolizumab-treated metastatic melanoma patients. Melanoma Res. 2017;27(6):596–600. https://doi.org/10.1097/CMR.0000000000000404.

97. Gowda R, Robertson BM, Iyer S, et al. The role of exosomes in metastasis and progression of melanoma. Cancer Treat Rev. 2020;85:101975. https://doi.org/10.1016/j.ctrv.2020.101975.

98. Gener Lahav T, Adler O, Zait Y, Shani O, Amer M, Doron H, Abramovitz L, Yofe I, Cohen N, Erez N. Melanoma-derived extracellular vesicles instigate proinflammatory signaling in the metastatic microenvironment. Int J Cancer. 2019;145:2521–34. https://doi.org/10.1002/ijc.32521.

99. Peinado H, Zhang H, Matei IR, et al. Pre-metastatic niches: organ-specific homes for metastases. Nat Rev Cancer. 2017;17(5):302–17. https://doi.org/10.1038/nrc.2017.6.

100. Sharma P, Diergaarde B, Ferrone S, et al. Melanoma cell-derived exosomes in plasma of melanoma patients suppress functions of immune effector cells. Sci Rep. 2020;10:92. https://doi.org/10.1038/s41598-019-56542-4.

101. Andreola G, Rivoltini L, Castelli C, et al. Induction of lymphocyte apoptosis by tumor cell secretion of FasL-bearing microvesicles. J Exp Med. 2002;195(10):1303–16. https://doi.org/10.1084/jem.20011624.

102. Wang J, Wuethrich A, Ibn Sina AA, et al. Tracking extracellular vesicle phenotypic changes enables treatment monitoring in melanoma. Sci Adv. 2020;6(9):eaax3223. https://doi.org/10.1126/sciadv.aax3223.

103. Huber V, Vallacchi V, Fleming V, et al. Tumor-derived microRNAs induce myeloid suppressor cells and predict immunotherapy resistance in melanoma. J Clin Invest. 2018;128(12):5505–16. https://doi.org/10.1172/JCI98060.

104. Fleming V, Hu X, Weller C, et al. Melanoma extracellular vesicles generate immunosuppressive myeloid cells by upregulating PD-L1 via TLR4 signaling. Cancer Res. 2019;79(18):4715–28. https://doi.org/10.1158/0008-5472.CAN-19-0053.

105. Reschke R, Ziemer M. Rechallenge with checkpoint inhibitors in metastatic melanoma. Journal der Deutschen Dermatologischen Gesellschaft. 2020;18:429–36. https://doi.org/10.1111/ddg.14091.

106. Andersen R, Borch TH, Draghi A, et al. T cells isolated from patients with checkpoint inhibitor-resistant melanoma are functional and can mediate tumor regression. Ann Oncol. 2018;29(7):1575–81. https://doi.org/10.1093/annonc/mdy139.
107. Lanitis E, Dangaj D, Irving M, Coukos G. Mechanisms regulating T-cell infiltration and activity in solid tumors. Ann Oncol. 2017;28(suppl_12):xii18–32. https://doi.org/10.1093/annonc/mdx238.
108. Bonavida B, Chouaib S. Resistance to anticancer immunity in cancer patients: potential strategies to reverse resistance. Ann Oncol. 2017;28(3):457–67. https://doi.org/10.1093/annonc/mdw615.
109. Guida M, Tommasi S, Strippoli S, et al. The search for a melanoma-tailored chemotherapy in the new era of personalized therapy: a phase II study of chemo-modulating temozolomide followed by fotemustine and a cooperative study of GOIM (Gruppo Oncologico Italia Meridionale). BMC Cancer. 2018;18(1):552. https://doi.org/10.1186/s12885-018-4479-2.
110. Bradley SD, Chen Z, Melendez B, et al. BRAFV600E co-opts a conserved MHC class I internalization pathway to diminish antigen presentation and CD8+ T-cell recognition of melanoma. Cancer Immunol Res. 2015;3(6):602–9. https://doi.org/10.1158/2326-6066.CIR-15-0030.
111. Kuske M, Westphal D, Wehner R, et al. Immunomodulatory effects of BRAF and MEK inhibitors: implications for melanoma therapy. Pharmacol Res. 2018;136:151–9. https://doi.org/10.1016/j.phrs.2018.08.019.
112. Allegrezza MJ, Rutkowski MR, Stephen TL, et al. Trametinib drives T-cell-dependent control of KRAS-mutated tumors by inhibiting pathological myelopoiesis. Cancer Res. 2016;76(21):6253–65.
113. Heinhuis KM, Ros W, Kok M, Steeghs N, Beijnen JH, Schellens JHM. Enhancing antitumor response by combining immune checkpoint inhibitors with chemotherapy in solid tumors. Ann Oncol. 2019;30(2):219–35. https://doi.org/10.1093/annonc/mdy551.
114. Serrano-del Valle A, Naval J, Anel A, Marzo I. Novel forms of immunomodulation for cancer therapy. Trends Cancer. 2020;6(6):518–32. https://doi.org/10.1016/j.trecan.2020.02.015.
115. Liu R, Hu R, Zeng Y, Zhang W, Zhou H-H. Tumour immune cell infiltration and survival after platinum-based chemotherapy in high-grade serous ovarian cancer subtypes: a gene expression-based computational study. EBioMedicine. 2020;51:102602. https://doi.org/10.1016/j.ebiom.2019.102602.
116. Ugurel S, Paschen A, Becker JC. Dacarbazine in melanoma: from a chemotherapeutic drug to an immunomodulating agent. J Investig Dermatol. 2013;133(2):289–92. https://doi.org/10.1038/jid.2012.341.
117. Di Giacomo AM, Ascierto PA, Pilla L, et al. Ipilimumab and fotemustine in patients with advanced melanoma (NIBIT-M1): an open-label, single-arm phase 2 trial. Lancet Oncol. 2012;13(9):879–86. https://doi.org/10.1016/S1470-2045(12)70324-8.
118. Cheal Cho W, Jour G, Aung PP. Role of angiogenesis in melanoma progression: update on key angiogenic mechanisms and other associated components. Semin Cancer Biol. 2019;59:175–86. https://doi.org/10.1016/j.semcancer.2019.06.015.
119. Albini A, Bruno A, Noonan DM, Mortara L. Contribution to tumor angiogenesis. From innate immune cells within the tumor microenvironment: implications for immunotherapy. Front Immunol. 2018;9:527. https://doi.org/10.3389/fimmu.2018.00527.
120. Mennitto A, Huber V, Ratta R, et al. Angiogenesis and immunity in renal carcinoma: can we turn an unhappy relationship into a happy marriage? J Clin Med. 2020;9(4):930. https://doi.org/10.3390/jcm9040930.
121. Jeyakumar G, Kim S, Bumma N, et al. Neutrophil lymphocyte ratio and duration of prior anti-angiogenic therapy as biomarkers in metastatic RCC receiving immune checkpoint inhibitor therapy. J Immunother Cancer. 2017;5:82. https://doi.org/10.1186/s40425-017-0287-5.
122. Mansfield AS, Nevala WK, Lieser EA, Leontovich AA, Markovic SN. The immunomodulatory effects of bevacizumab on systemic immunity in patients with metastatic melanoma. Onco Targets Ther. 2013;2(5):e24436. https://doi.org/10.4161/onci.24436.

123. Verzoni E, Ferro S, Procopio G, et al. Potent natural killer (NK) and myeloid blood cell rimodelling by cabozantinib (Cabo) in re-treated metastatic renal cell carcinoma (RCC) patients. Ann Oncol. 2018;29(suppl_8):viii303–31. https://doi.org/10.1093/annonc/mdy283.

124. Rinchai D, Verzoni E, Huber V, et al. Pazopanib induces dramatic but transient contraction of myeloid suppression compartment in favor of adaptive immunity. bioRxiv; 2020. doi: https://doi.org/10.1101/2020.05.01.071613.

125. Stehle F, Schulz K, Fahldieck C, et al. Reduced immunosuppressive properties of axitinib in comparison with other tyrosine kinase inhibitors. J Biol Chem. 2013;288(23):16334–47. https://doi.org/10.1074/jbc.M112.437962.

126. Cannarile MA, Weisser M, Jacob W, et al. Colony-stimulating factor 1 receptor (CSF1R) inhibitors in cancer therapy. J Immunother Cancer. 2017;5:53. https://doi.org/10.1186/s40425-017-0257-y.

127. Fleming V, Hu X, Weber R, et al. Targeting myeloid-derived suppressor cells to bypass tumor-induced immunosuppression. Front Immunol. 2018;9:398. https://doi.org/10.3389/fimmu.2018.00398.

128. Jordan S, Tung N, Casanova-Acebes M, et al. Dietary intake regulates the circulating inflammatory monocyte pool. Cell. 2019;178(5):1102–1114.e17. https://doi.org/10.1016/j.cell.2019.07.050.

129. Adawi M, Watad A, Brown S, Aazza K, Aazza H, Zouhir M, Sharif K, Ghanayem K, Farah R, Mahagna H, Fiordoro S, Sukkar SG, Bragazzi NL, Mahroum N. Ramadan fasting exerts immunomodulatory effects: insights from a systematic review. Front Immunol. 2017;8:1144. https://doi.org/10.3389/fimmu.2017.01144.

130. ClinicalTrials.gov identifier: NCT03454282. Impact of dietary intervention on tumor immunity: the DigesT Trial (DIgesT).

131. Vernieri C, Ligorio F, Zattarin E, et al. Fasting-mimicking diet plus chemotherapy in breast cancer treatment. Nat Commun. 2020;11:4274. https://doi.org/10.1038/s41467-020-18194-1.

132. El Sissy C, Kirilovsky A, Van Den Eynde M, et al. The consensus Immunoscore adapted to biopsies in patients with locally advanced rectal cancer: Potential clinical significance for a "Watch and Wait" strategy. J Clin Oncol. 2019;37(15_suppl):2628.

133. Marliot F, Chen X, Kirilovsky A, et al. Analytical validation of the Immunoscore and its associated prognostic value in patients with colon cancer. J Immunother Cancer. 2020;8(1):e000272. https://doi.org/10.1136/jitc-2019-000272.

134. Yang J, Dong M, Shui Y, et al. A pooled analysis of the prognostic value of PD-L1 in melanoma: evidence from 1062 patients. Cancer Cell Int. 2020;20:96. https://doi.org/10.1186/s12935-020-01187-x.

135. Davis AA, Patel VG. The role of PD-L1 expression as a predictive biomarker: an analysis of all US Food and Drug Administration (FDA) approvals of immune checkpoint inhibitors. J Immunother Cancer. 2019;7:278. https://doi.org/10.1186/s40425-019-0768-9.

136. Madore J, Vilain RE, Menzies AM, Kakavand H, Wilmott JS, Hyman J, Yearley JH, Kefford RF, Thompson JF, Long GV, Hersey P, Scolyer RA. PD-L1 expression in melanoma shows marked heterogeneity within and between patients: implications for anti-PD-1/PD-L1 clinical trials. Pigment Cell Melanoma Res. 2015;28:245–53. https://doi.org/10.1111/pcmr.12340.

137. Ugurel S, Schadendorf D, Horny K, et al. Elevated baseline serum PD-1 or PD-L1 predicts poor outcome of PD-1 inhibition therapy in metastatic melanoma. Ann Oncol. 2020;31(1):144–52. https://doi.org/10.1016/j.annonc.2019.09.005.

Part II
Targeted Therapies in Skin Cancers

Chapter 5
Dabrafenib and Trametinib

Katarzyna Kozak, Tomasz Świtaj, and Piotr Rutkowski

Pharmacological Properties and Early Development

Dabrafenib (GSK2118436) is a reversible, ATP-competitive inhibitor of the *BRAF* V600 kinase. Dabrafenib inhibits BRAF kinases with in vitro IC50 values of 0.65, 0.5, and 1.84 nM for BRAF V600E, BRAF V600K, and BRAF V600D enzymes, respectively [1]. In preclinical studies, dabrafenib inhibited tumor growth in models of melanoma (A375P) and colorectal cancer (Colo205). Inhibition of the *BRAF* V600E kinase reduces ERK phosphorylation and proliferation of tumor cells through G1-phase cell cycle arrest [2]. In in vivo studies, mice transplanted with human *BRAF* V600E-mutated melanoma (A375P F11) received dabrafenib at doses of 0.1, 1, 10, and 100 mg/kg once daily for 14 days. The inhibition of tumor growth was dose-dependent, with the highest dose inducing complete remission in 50% of mice [3]. In the phase I study BREAK-1, immunohistochemistry was used to analyze the expression of phosphorylated ERK in tissues collected from patients before and during dabrafenib treatment. Compared with baseline, dabrafenib reduced ERK phosphorylation substantially after 1–2 weeks of treatment (median, 83.9%; range, 38.0–93.3%). Similarly, fluorodeoxyglucose-based positron emission tomography (FDG-PET) showed a reduced FDG uptake in 95% of patients after 2 weeks of dabrafenib treatment, with a median reduction in the standardized uptake value (SUVmax) of 60% compared with baseline (range, 19–100%) [4].

Trametinib (GSK1120212, JTP-74057) is an oral, low-molecular-weight, selective inhibitor of the MEK1 and MEK2 kinases. In contrast to *BRAF* mutations, activating *MEK* mutations are very rare in melanoma cells [5]. However, MEK kinases are crucial for the MAPK signaling pathway, because they may be the only

K. Kozak (✉) · T. Świtaj · P. Rutkowski
Department of Soft Tissue/Bone Sarcoma and Melanoma, Maria Sklodowska-Curie National Research Institute of Oncology, Warsaw, Poland
e-mail: katarzyna.kozak@pib-nio.pl

P. Rutkowski, M. Mandalà (eds.), *New Therapies in Advanced Cutaneous Malignancies*, https://doi.org/10.1007/978-3-030-64009-5_5

substrate for both MEK isoforms [6, 7]. In mouse models of colorectal cancer (HT-29 and COLO205) and melanoma (A-375P), trametinib decreased ERK phosphorylation and inhibited the growth of cancer cells carrying the *BRAF*, *NRAS*, and *KRAS* mutations. The inhibition of cell proliferation and G1-phase cell cycle arrest caused apoptosis of tumor cells. The best response to treatment was seen in tumors with *BRAF* mutations. Trametinib given once daily had a long half-life and caused long-term ERK suppression (>24 h). The IC50 values for MEK1 and MEK2 were 0.7–0.9 nmol/l [8, 9]. In a phase I study, the pharmacodynamic properties of trametinib were assessed based on the effects on tumor tissue during treatment (biopsy samples were taken before and 15 days after treatment). At a dose of 2 mg daily, ERK phosphorylation decreased by 30%, Ki-67 phosphorylation decreased by 54%, and p27 phosphorylation increased by 83%. In patients with *BRAF*- and *NRAS*-mutated melanoma, these changes were more pronounced and dose-dependent [10].

By acting on two different kinases (BRAF and MEK), dabrafenib and trametinib jointly block the MAPK signaling pathway. Studies in xenograft models showed that the dabrafenib–trametinib combination inhibited the growth of cancer cells more efficiently than dabrafenib ($p = 0.01$) or trametinib alone ($p = 0.0001$) [11].

Pharmacokinetic Properties of Dabrafenib and Trametinib

Administration of dabrafenib with a meal decreases its bioavailability and delays absorption, with a 51% reduction in the maximum concentration and a 31% reduction in the area under the curve (AUC) compared with the fasting state. Therefore, dabrafenib should be taken ≥1 h before or ≥2 h after a meal. The maximum blood concentration of dabrafenib is reached 2 h after oral ingestion of a single dose, and the mean half-life is 5.2 h. Repeated dosing decreases dabrafenib exposure, which is probably because dabrafenib induces its own metabolism. Age, weight, sex, and race do not significantly affect the pharmacokinetic properties of dabrafenib. Dabrafenib binds highly to plasma proteins (99.7%), mainly albumin. Dabrafenib is metabolized primarily by CYP3A4 and CYP2C8 to hydroxy-dabrafenib, which is then oxidized by CYP3A4 to carboxy-dabrafenib. Carboxy-dabrafenib can be decarboxylated non-enzymatically to desmethyl dabrafenib. Carboxy-dabrafenib is excreted in the bile and urine. Desmethyl dabrafenib can also be formed in the gut and reabsorbed. Desmethyl dabrafenib is metabolized by CYP3A4 to oxidative metabolites. The terminal half-life for dabrafenib is 8 h, for hydroxy dabrafenib 10 h, and for carboxy dabrafenib and desmethyl dabrafenib 21–22 h. Both hydroxy dabrafenib and desmethyl dabrafenib may contribute to the clinical activity of dabrafenib, but the activity of carboxy dabrafenib is probably insignificant [1, 10]. Dabrafenib is a substrate for and an inducer of CYP3A4, a substrate for CYP2C8, and an inducer of CYP2Cs and CYP2B6. Concomitant use of dabrafenib with drugs that are substrates, inducers, or inhibitors of these metabolic enzymes requires caution because of the risk of serious interactions. Particular caution should be exercised when dabrafenib is used in combination with strong inhibitors of CYP3A4, glucuronidation, and/or transport proteins (e.g., ketoconazole, nefazodone, clarithromycin, ritonavir, itraconazole, voriconazole, posaconazole). Conversely, concomitant use of dabrafenib with strong inducers of CYP3A4 or CYP2C8 (e.g., rifampicin, phenytoin, carbamazepine, phenobarbital, St. John's wort) may result in incomplete exposure to dabrafenib. Dabrafenib is excreted as metabolites in feces (71%) and urine (23%). The clearance of dabrafenib is unchanged in patients with mild to moderate renal or hepatic impairment. In severe renal or hepatic impairment, caution should be exercised because dabrafenib has not been tested in these patients [1].

Trametinib is rapidly absorbed in the gastrointestinal tract following oral ingestion. Taking trametinib with a meal decreases its bioavailability and delays absorption, with a 70% reduction in the maximum concentration and a 10% reduction in the AUC compared with the fasting state. After ingestion of a single dose, the maximum blood concentration of trametinib is reached after 1.5 h, and the mean half-life is 5.3 days. Repeated dosing of trametinib leads to accumulation. The mean accumulation ratio for repeated dosing of 2 mg/day is 5.97. Trametinib binds highly to human plasma proteins (97.4%). Trametinib is metabolized mainly by deacetylation, deacetylation with monooxygenation, or in combination with glucuronidation. Oxidation by the CYP3A4 isoenzymes is considered a minor metabolic pathway. Therefore, trametinib has a low risk of drug interactions. However, because biliary metabolism and excretion are the major routes of elimination, trametinib should be used with caution in patients with moderate or severe hepatic impairment. In patients with mild or moderate renal impairment, trametinib clearance remains unchanged [10, 12, 13].

The use of dabrafenib in combination with trametinib did not significantly affect the pharmacokinetics of either drug [1].

Phase I Trials

The phase I study assessing the safety, tolerability, and recommended phase II dose of dabrafenib included 184 patients with incurable solid tumors (156 with metastatic melanoma) [4]. The maximum tolerated dose (MTD) was not reached, and doses up to 300 mg twice daily were well tolerated. Based on these findings, the recommended dose for phase II studies was 150 mg twice daily. Of 36 patients with *BRAF* V600-mutated advanced melanoma who received dabrafenib at a dose of 150 mg twice daily, 18 (50%) achieved a confirmed partial response (PR) or complete response (CR). The median response duration was 6.2 months [95% confidence interval (CI): 4.2–7.7 months]; the median progression-free survival (PFS) was 5.5 months. Of 10 patients with previously untreated brain melanoma metastases, 9 had tumor regression.

The open-label, first-in-human, dose-escalation, phase I study MEK111054 assessed the safety, pharmacokinetics, and pharmacodynamics of trametinib in patients with solid tumors or lymphomas [12]. The dose of 2.0 mg once daily was selected for further evaluation. Only patients with melanoma were included in this evaluation. Of 36 patients with BRAF-mutated advanced melanoma, 30 had not previously received a BRAF inhibitor. In this subgroup, 2 patients achieved a CR and 10 achieved a PR (confirmed response rate, 33%). The median PFS in this subgroup was 5.7 months (95% CI: 4.0–7.4 months). Of 6 patients with prior BRAF inhibitor treatment, 1 had an unconfirmed PR. Of 39 patients with non-BRAF-mutated melanoma, 4 had a confirmed PR (10%).

Activity and Efficacy

The efficacy of dabrafenib in patients with BRAF-mutated metastatic melanoma was assessed in phase II and phase III studies (BRF113710 [BREAK-2], BRF113683 [BREAK-3], BRF113929 [BREAK-MB]) [14–16]. In the phase II trial, 45 patients (59%) with *BRAF* V600E mutations and 2 patients (13%) with V600K mutations achieved a confirmed response. The median PFS was 6.3 months for patients with V600E mutations and 4.5 months for those with V600K mutations; the median overall survival (OS) was 13.1 months and 12.9 months, respectively [14]. Dabrafenib has been approved for the treatment of patients with BRAF-mutated metastatic melanoma based on the results of the randomized phase III trial BREAK-3 that compared the efficacy of dabrafenib and dacarbazine. The study included 250 previously untreated patients who were randomized in a 3:1 ratio to dabrafenib (150 mg twice daily) or dacarbazine (1000 mg/m^2 intravenously every 3 weeks) [17]. The complete or partial response rate was 50% in the dabrafenib arm and 6% in the dacarbazine arm. The PFS hazard ratio was 0.37 (95% CI: 0.23, 0.57), with the median PFS 6.9 months in the dabrafenib arm and 2.7 months in the dacarbazine arm. The median OS was 18.2 months and 15.6 months, respectively. However, the OS in the dacarbazine arm was confounded because patients with disease progression could cross-over to dabrafenib [15, 18].

In monotherapy, trametinib is less effective than dabrafenib for *BRAF*-mutated metastatic melanoma. The phase II study MEK113583 assessed the objective response rate, safety, and pharmacokinetics of trametinib at a dose of 2.0 mg once daily in patients with advanced BRAF-mutated melanoma after failure of prior BRAF inhibitor therapy (group A, $n = 40$) or without prior BRAF inhibition (group B, $n = 57$). In group A ($n = 40$), the clinical activity of trametinib was low: 11 patients (28%) had stable disease (SD), and the median PFS was 1.8 months. In group B, 1 patient (2%) achieved a CR, 13 (23%) achieved a PR, and 29 (51%) had SD (confirmed response rate, 25%); the median PFS was 4.0 months. Trametinib activity was observed in patients with *BRAF* V600E mutations but also in those with rarer mutations (*BRAF* K601E, *BRAF* V600R) [19]. In the randomized, phase III study METRIC (MEK114267), the efficacy of trametinib was compared with chemotherapy (dacarbazine or paclitaxel) in 322 patients with *BRAF* V600E/K-mutated unresectable or metastatic melanoma [20]. Patients were randomized in a 2:1 ratio to trametinib (2 mg once daily) or first-line or second-line chemotherapy (no prior treatment with BRAF or MEK inhibitors or ipilimumab). A cross-over from the chemotherapy arm to the trametinib arm was allowed after confirmation of disease progression. The median PFS was 4.8 months in the trametinib arm and 1.5 months in the chemotherapy arm (HR for disease progression or death in the trametinib arm at baseline was 0.45; 95% CI: 0.33–0.63, $p < 0.001$). After 6 months, the OS rate was 81% in the trametinib arm and 67% in the chemotherapy arm, despite the cross-over (HR for death was 0.54; 95% CI: 0.32–0.92; $p = 0.01$). The objective response rate was 22% for the trametinib arm and 8% for the chemotherapy arm ($p = 0.001$). These results led to the approval of trametinib monotherapy for *BRAF* V600E- or V600K-mutated unresectable or metastatic melanoma [20].

Combined therapy with dabrafenib and trametinib improved treatment outcomes in patients with *BRAF*-mutated melanoma. A phase I/II study assessed the safety, pharmacokinetics, and efficacy of the dabrafenib–trametinib combination in 247 patients with BRAF-mutated advanced melanoma. Part C of this study compared the efficacy of dabrafenib monotherapy with the dabrafenib–trametinib combination. The objective response rate was higher in patients receiving dabrafenib (300 mg/day) and trametinib (2 mg/day) than in patients receiving dabrafenib monotherapy (76% vs. 54%, $p = 0.03$). The median PFS was 9.4 months for the combined treatment and 5.8 months for dabrafenib monotherapy (HR 0.39; 95% CI: 0.25–0.62; $p < 0.001$) [21]. In that study, OS was 30% at 4 years and 28% at 5 years of follow-up [22].

The efficacy of the dabrafenib–trametinib combination as a first-line treatment was assessed in two phase III studies: COMBI-d ($n = 423$) and COMBI-v ($n = 704$). In the COMBI-d study, patients who received dabrafenib monotherapy served as the control arm. The response rate was 69% for the dabrafenib–trametinib combination and 53% for dabrafenib monotherapy ($p = 0.0014$). The median PFS was 11 months for the dabrafenib–trametinib combination and 8.8 months for dabrafenib monotherapy (HR 0.67; 95% CI: 0.53–0.84, $p = 0.0004$); the median OS was 25.1 months and 18.7 months, respectively (HR 0.71, 95% CI: 0.55–0.92; $p = 0.01$) [23]. In addition, compared with dabrafenib monotherapy, the dabrafenib–trametinib combination improved the health-related quality of life and reduced pain [24]. In the phase III COMBI-v study, patients in the control arm received vemurafenib monotherapy. The objective response rate was 64% in the dabrafenib–trametinib combination arm and 51% in the vemurafenib arm ($p < 0.001$) [25]. The dabrafenib–trametinib combination improved OS significantly compared with vemurafenib monotherapy (26.1 vs. 17.8 months; HR = 0.68; 95% CI: 0.56–0.83). The median PFS in the dabrafenib–trametinib arm was 12.1 months and 7.3 months in the vemurafenib arm (HR = 0.61, 95% CI 0.51–0.73) [26].

The pooled analysis of data from these two studies was published in 2019. In total, 563 patients received dabrafenib with trametinib; the median follow-up was 22 months. The rates of 4-year and 5-year PFS in patients receiving dabrafenib with trametinib were 21% (95% CI: 17–24) and 19% (95% CI: 15–22), respectively. The OS rate was 37% (95% CI: 33–42) after 4 years and 34% (95% CI: 30–38) after 5 years. A CR was observed in 109 patients (19%), which was associated with an improvement in long-term results: the 5-year OS rate in this group was 71% (95%

Table 5.1 Results of phase III studies of dabrafenib and trametinib in monotherapy or in combination for advanced melanoma

Drug	BREAK-3 [15] Dabrafenib	METRIC [20] Trametinib	COMBI-d [28] Dabrafenib	COMBI-d [28] Dabrafenib + trametinib	COMBI-v [25, 26] Vemurafenib	COMBI-v [25, 26] Dabrafenib + trametinib
Objective response rate (ORR), %	50	22	53	69	51	64
Median progression-free survival (PFS), months	6.9.	4.8	8.8	11	7.3	11.1
Median overall survival (OS), months	15	15.6	18.7	25.1	17.8	25.9
3-year overall survival rate, %	24	–	32	44	31	45

– not reported

CI 62–79). Multivariate analyses showed that male sex, ECOG performance status 1, lactate dehydrogenase (LDH) level above the upper limit of normal, and metastases to three or more organs were unfavorable factors for PFS and OS [27].

The phase III trials of dabrafenib and trametinib are summarized in Table 5.1.

The example of dramatic response to dabrafenib–trametinib in a patient with metastatic melanoma treated in Department of Soft Tissue/Bone Sarcoma and Melanoma, Maria Sklodowska-Curie National Research Institute of Oncology, Warsaw, Poland is shown in Fig. 5.1.

Efficacy of Dabrafenib Combined with Trametinib in Patients with Brain Melanoma Metastases

Melanoma patients with brain metastases have a poor prognosis. The efficacy of targeted therapy in these patients has been proven in several prospective clinical trials. The first clinical trials among patients with brain melanoma metastases assessed the efficacy of BRAF inhibitors as monotherapy. The largest study to date, in 172 patients with asymptomatic brain metastases, assessed the efficacy of dabrafenib (phase II BREAK-MB study). The intracranial response rate was 39.2% for patients without prior local treatment and 30.8% for patients with disease progression after local treatment. The median overall survival in both cohorts was approximately 31 weeks [16]. A combined inhibition of BRAF and MEK, with dabrafenib plus trametinib, improved outcomes when compared with dabrafenib monotherapy in advanced melanoma without brain metastases. The only prospective clinical trial evaluating the activity of this combination in patients with brain metastases was the phase II trial COMBI-MB [29]. This study enrolled 125 patients with ECOG

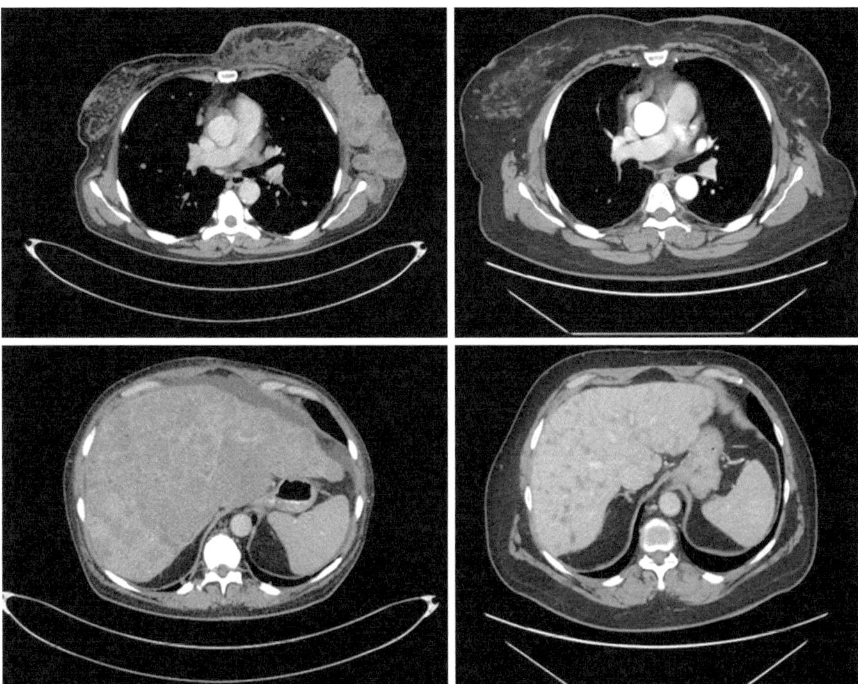

Fig. 5.1 Computed tomography findings before (left) and after 6 months (right) of treatment with dabrafenib and trametinib in a patient with metastatic melanoma

performance status 0–2, with or without prior local treatment for brain metastases. Intracranial response rates of 56–59% were observed regardless of prior local treatment or symptomatic metastases. The responses were most prolonged in patients with asymptomatic brain metastases. However, the median duration of response was significantly shorter than that observed in phase III clinical trials that did not include patients with brain metastases (approximately 6 months vs. 12–14 months) [24, 30, 31]. Symptomatic brain metastases were associated with a particularly poor prognosis (median OS 3–4 months). Nevertheless, the COMBI-MB study showed that the dabrafenib–trametinib combination is effective in patients with melanoma brain metastases. The main advantage of targeted therapy in these patients is a rapid improvement of the general condition.

Stereotactic radiation therapy is often used in patients with melanoma brain metastases. Data on the effects of combining BRAF inhibitors with radiation therapy are contradictory. On one hand, in vitro studies suggest that BRAF inhibitors could sensitize melanoma cells to radiation therapy [32]. On the other hand, this radiosensitizing effect may worsen adverse effects. There is no conclusive evidence that combining targeted therapy with radiation therapy increases the risks for neurotoxicity, brain hemorrhage, or radiation necrosis [33–35]. Molecularly targeted therapy combined with brain radiosurgery has fewer adverse effects than when combined with standard radiation therapy. Skin toxicity is the most common adverse effect of standard radiation therapy (more severe with vemurafenib) [28, 36].

Currently, it is recommended to discontinue BRAF or MEK inhibitors 1 day before and 1 day after stereotactic radiosurgery used to treat brain metastases [33].

The Effects of the Dabrafenib–Trametinib Combination in Patients Previously Treated with BRAF Inhibitors

In a prospective, phase II study in patients with melanoma and documented disease progression on BRAF inhibitors (with or without trametinib) and immunotherapy, a combination of dabrafenib and trametinib was started $\geq$12 weeks after the last targeted therapy. Partial remission was seen in 8 out of 25 patients (32%), and stable disease in 10 (40%); the median PFS was 4.9 months [37]. The efficacy of BRAF/MEK inhibitors rechallenge in clinical practice was confirmed in several retrospective studies: the response rates to BRAF/MEK inhibitors ranged from 27% to 43%, and the median PFS was 5–5.9 months [38–40].

Dabrafenib and Trametinib as Adjuvant Treatment

The efficacy of the dabrafenib–trametinib combination as adjuvant treatment was assessed in the randomized, phase III clinical trial COMBI-AD ($n = 870$). In this study, patients received adjuvant treatment with dabrafenib (300 mg/day) plus trametinib (2 mg/day) for 1 year after surgical treatment of BRAF-mutated, stage III melanoma (stage IIIA with metastases of >1 mm, IIIB, IIIC according to American Joint Committee on Cancer staging system ed. 7); placebo was used in the control arm. The dabrafenib–trametinib combination improved relapse-free survival (RFS) in all patient subgroups (HR [95% CI]: IIIA, 0.61 [0.35–1.07]; IIIB, 0.50 [0.37–0.67; IIIC], 0.48 [0.36–0.64]). The 4-year and 5-year RFS rates were 55% (95% CI, 50–60%) and 52% (95% CI, 48–58%) in the combination arm, and 38% (95% CI, 34–43%) and 36% (95% CI, 32–41%) in the placebo arm. The median distant metastasis-free survival (DMFS) was not reached, but the 5-year DMFS rate was higher in the dabrafenib plus trametinib arm than in the placebo arm (65% vs. 54%; HR, 0.55 [95% CI, 0.44–0.70]) [41, 42].

Toxicity Profile

Skin Toxicity

Dabrafenib causes various cutaneous side effects, which occur due to different mechanisms: inflammatory reactions, proliferation of squamous cells or melanocytes, and hypersensitivity reactions. As they occur frequently during dabrafenib therapy, patients should be under careful dermatologic surveillance [11, 15, 21, 43, 44]. The most common cutaneous side effects of dabrafenib include hyperkeratosis, papillomas, alopecia, and the hand-foot skin syndrome. Phototoxic reactions, common with vemurafenib [45, 46], are rare during dabrafenib treatment. Cutaneous warts, palmar-plantar erythrodysesthesia, and grade 2 or higher cutaneous squamous cell carcinoma (cuSCC)/keratoacanthoma (KA) are found in <20% of patients. Usually, squamous cell carcinoma of the skin is well-differentiated, does not metastasize, and requires surgical removal only. The oncogenesis of cuSCC during dabrafenib treatment is multifactorial, with *RAS* mutations and paradoxical MAPK signaling being implicated [47]. Proliferation of keratinocytes, which leads to skin changes, might be caused by an activation of signaling through *CRAF* dimerization that results from both an inhibition of unmutated *BRAF* and a secondary *BRAF* transactivation [48, 49]. Because dabrafenib has lower specificity toward unmutated *BRAF* and *CRAF*, paradoxical activation of RAF dimers is less likely during dabrafenib treatment, which may explain lower skin toxicity compared with vemurafenib. Anforth et al. showed that dabrafenib-induced cuSCC develops mainly in sites where cuSCC/KA does not usually arise spontaneously (on the arm, thorax, and/or thigh). A *RAS* mutation may occur in as many as half of the cases of cuSCC or papillary hyperkeratotic lesions induced by dabrafenib [50]. Another cutaneous side effect of dabrafenib is panniculitis. Painful, erythematous, subcutaneous nodules are located mainly on the limbs and may be accompanied by fever, pain, and joint swelling [51] (Table 5.2).

Table 5.2 The most common adverse events related to dabrafenib in phase II and III studies

	BREAK-2 [14]		BREAK-3 [15]	
	Grade 3/4	Total	Grade 3/4	Total
Adverse event	*n* (%)	*n* (%)	*n* (%)	*n* (%)
Any event	33 (36)	86 (93)	58 (28)	100 (53)
Arthralgia	1 (1)	30 (33)	2 (1)	36 (19)
Hyperkeratosis	1 (1)	25 (27)	3 (1.5)	67 (36)
Pyrexia	0	22(24)	5 (3)	30 (16)
Asthenia	1 (1)	20 (22)	2 (1)	33 (18)
Headache	2 (2)	19 (21)	0	34 (18)
Nausea	1 (1)	18 (20)	0	26 (14)
Skin papilloma	0	14 (15)	0	42 (22)
Vomiting	1 (1)	14 (15)		
Decreased appetite	1 (1)	12 (13)		
Hair loss	0	11 (12)	1 (<1)	50 (27)
Chills	0	11 (12)		
Diarrhea	1 (1)	10 (11)		
cuSCC/KA	8 (9)	10 (11)	14 (7)	18 (10)
Pruritus	0	9 (10)		
Palmar-plantar hyperkeratosis			4 (2)	36 (19)
Rash			0	56 (30)

cuSCC cutaneous squamous cell carcinoma, *KA keratoacanthoma*

Table 5.3 The most common adverse events related to trametinib in phase III METRIC study [20]

Adverse events	Any grade	Grade 2	Grade 3
($n = 211$)	n (%)	n (%)	n (%)
Rash	121 (57)	40 (19)	16(8)
Diarrhea	91 (43)	13 (6)	0
Fatigue	54 (26)	11 (5)	8 (4)
Peripheral edema	54 (26)	8 (4)	2 (1)
Dermatitis acneiform	40 (19)	20 (9)	2 (1)
Nausea	38 (18)	5 (2)	2 (1)
Alopecia	36 (17)	3 (1)	1 (<1)
Hypertension	32 (15)	6 (3)	26 (12)
Constipation	30 (14)	3 (1)	0
Vomiting	27 (13)	3 (1)	2 (1)

The skin toxicity profile of MEK inhibitors differs from that of dabrafenib. No secondary skin neoplasms were found during treatment with trametinib [20]. The rash that appears during trametinib treatment is maculo-pustular, and it is different from the hyperkeratotic and maculopapular changes observed during dabrafenib treatment. An acne-like eruption, which resembles the lesions caused by epidermal growth factor inhibitors, such as cetuximab, is also associated with trametinib treatment. These eruptions usually occur on the face, chest, and back, possibly due to the greater number of sweat glands in these areas; treatment usually includes topical antibiotics [52] (Table 5.3).

The addition of trametinib to dabrafenib reduced the percentage of typical skin complications seen with dabrafenib, that is, cuSCC/KA, cutaneous warts, and hyperkeratotic lesions [21]. This reduction is related to the inhibition of paradoxical activation of signal transduction in the MAPK pathway via CRAF by the MEK inhibitor [11, 21]. The acne-like lesions characteristic of trametinib monotherapy are also less frequent. Overall, the skin complications of the dabrafenib–trametinib combination are usually mild and manageable, and they do not require dose reduction or treatment discontinuation.

Pyrexia

Fever is a very common complication of the dabrafenib–trametinib combination (51–63%) [23, 25, 41]. It occurs more often than with dabrafenib alone (16–24%) [14, 15] (Table 5.4). The pathophysiological mechanism of fever is unclear, but it is not related to treatment efficacy. Fever usually starts within the first 4 weeks of treatment. In half of the patients, it is recurrent: 1 in 5 patients has ≥4 episodes of fever [53]. Fever may be associated with severe chills, dehydration, and hypotension,

Table 5.4 Incidence of the most common adverse events related to dabrafenib–trametinib therapy in phase III trials (COMBI-v and COMBI-d)

Adverse events	COMBI-v [25]				COMBI-d [23]			
	Dabrafenib + trametinib (n = 350)		Vemurafenib (n = 349)		Dabrafenib + trametinib (n = 209)		Dabrafenib (n = 211)	
	Any grade n (%)	Grade 3 n (%)	Any grade n (%)	Grade 3 n (%)	Any grade n (%)	Grade 3 n (%)	Any grade n (%)	Grade 3 n (%)
Total	343 (98)	167 (48)	345 (99)	198 (57)	199 (95)	66 (32)	203 (96)	72 (34)
Fever	184 (53)	15 (4)	73 (21)	2(<1)	107 (51)	12 (6)	59 (28)	4 (2)
Nausea	121 (35)	1(<1)	125 (36)	2(<1)	63 (30)	0	54 (26)	3 (1)
Diarrhea	112 (32)	4 (1)	131 (38)	1(<1)	51 (24)	1(<1)	30 (14)	2(<1)
Chills	110 (31)	3(<1)	27 (8)	0	62 (30)	0	33 (16)	0
Fatigue	101 (29)	4 (1)	115 (33)	6 (2)	74 (35)	4 (2)	74 (35)	2(<1)
Headache	101 (29)	3(<1)	77 (22)	2(<1)	63 (30)	1(<1)	62 (29)	3 (1)
Vomiting	101 (29)	4 (1)	53 (15)	3(<1)	42 (20)	2(<1)	29 (14)	1(<1)
Hypertension	92 (26)	48 (14)	84 (24)	32 (9)	46 (22)	8 (4)	29 (14)	10 (5)
Arthralgia	84 (24)	3(<1)	178 (51)	15 (4)	51 (24)	1(<1)	8 (27)	0
Rash	76 (22)	4 (1)	149 (43)	30 (9)	48 (23)	0	46 (22)	2(<1)
Pruritus	30 (9)	0	75 (21)	3(<1)				
Alopecia	20 (6)	0	137 (39)	1(<1)	15 (7)	0	55 (26)	0
Hyperkeratosis	15 (4)	0	86 (25)	2(<1)	7 (3)	0	68 (32)	1(<1)
Skin papilloma	6 (2)	0	80 (23)	2(<1)	3 (1)	0	45 (21)	0
cuSCC/KA	5 (1)		63 (18)		5 (2)		20 (9)	

cuSCC cutaneous squamous cell carcinoma, *KA* keratoacanthoma

which in some cases may lead to acute renal failure. An infectious cause of fever should always be ruled out. When fever occurs, treatment should be interrupted. Fever can be treated with paracetamol or nonsteroidal anti-inflammatory drugs [54]. Steroid prophylaxis is sometimes used in patients with frequent relapses [55].

Arthralgia and Myalgia

Arthralgia is associated with dabrafenib. It can be seen in one or more joints. During dabrafenib monotherapy, joint pain occurs in 23–35% of patients, but in dabrafenib–trametinib combination it is less frequent (16–28%) [14, 15]. Joint pain is rarely ≥grade 3 (about 1%). Usually, joint pain is managed with standard analgesics, and it does not warrant treatment discontinuation or dose adjustment.

Myalgia occurs in 19% of patients treated with dabrafenib plus trametinib [25]. Similar to joint pain, myalgia is usually mild and disappears with analgesics.

Gastrointestinal Toxicity

The most common gastrointestinal complications of dabrafenib include nausea (14–26%), diarrhea (11–14%), and vomiting (14–15%) [14, 15, 23]. The incidence of gastrointestinal complications with trametinib monotherapy is similar. In the METRIC study, diarrhea was observed in 43% of patients, nausea in 18%, and vomiting in 13% of patients [20]. Compared with dabrafenib monotherapy, the dabrafenib–trametinib combination causes a two-fold increase in the incidence of diarrhea (18–34% vs. 9–14%); nausea (30–40%) and vomiting (20–28%) are also more common [23] (Table 5.3). Gastrointestinal complications occur most frequently at the beginning of treatment, usually within the first 2 months; they are most often grade 1 or 2. Symptomatic treatment (oral rehydration, loperamide, electrolyte supplementation) is sufficient for good symptom control. Other causes of diarrhea, such as bacterial, viral, or parasitic infections, should be ruled out.

Cardiovascular Events

Overall, the dabrafenib–trametinib combination is associated with a higher risk of cardiac complications than dabrafenib monotherapy. The most common cardiac complications are arterial hypertension and reduced left ventricular ejection fraction (LVEF). Pulmonary embolism and QTc prolongation are less frequent.

In clinical trials, hypertension was observed in 11–26% of patients who received dabrafenib and trametinib, in 14% of patients who received dabrafenib, and in 5% of those who received trametinib [20, 23, 31, 56]. Two pathophysiological mechanisms of hypertension during treatment with BRAF or MEK inhibitors have been described. One mechanism is dysregulation of the renin–angiotensin system due to the inhibition of BRAF and MEK signaling. The other mechanism is a reduced production and bioavailability of nitric oxide (NO). The inhibition of the MAPK pathway disturbs the vascular endothelial growth factor signaling pathway, which regulates NO synthesis. Reduced production or bioavailability of NO causes vasoconstriction, leukocyte adhesion to the endothelium, increased platelet aggregation, thrombus formation, and increased vascular smooth muscle cell proliferation [57, 58]. These effects, in turn, can cause pulmonary embolism and myocardial infarction.

MEK inhibition can reduce LVEF. Reduced LVEF was observed in 4–8% of patients who received dabrafenib and trametinib, 2% of patients who received dabrafenib, and 7% of those who received trametinib [14, 15, 20, 23, 25]. Mincu et al. showed that patients younger than 55 years of age have a higher risk of LVEF reduction [56]. The pathogenesis of LVEF reduction during treatment with BRAF and MEK inhibitors is not fully understood. The MAPK signaling pathway could be cardioprotective. Inhibition of this pathway can lead to hypertrophy, apoptosis, and myocyte remodeling [56, 59]. LVEF reduction of grade 3 or greater is rare: it occurs in 1% of patients who receive dabrafenib plus trametinib. Heart failure or LVEF reduction by >20% from baseline warrants discontinuation of dabrafenib [56]. In most cases, this complication is reversible.

QTc prolongation is rarely seen with dabrafenib treatment. The addition of trametinib to dabrafenib did not affect the incidence of this complication. Dabrafenib should not be used in patients with unregulated electrolyte disturbances (including magnesium concentrations), long QT syndrome, or taking drugs that prolong the QT interval. During treatment with dabrafenib, it is necessary to monitor the electrocardiogram and electrolytes [56, 60].

Eye Complications

Serous neurosensory detachment (SND) is the most common ocular side effect. It has been associated with the use of trametinib. The incidence of SND is difficult to estimate due to the asymptomatic course in some patients. In clinical trials with BRAF and MEK inhibitors (vemurafenib + cobimetinib, encorafenib + binimetinib) in which optical coherence tomography (OCT) was performed routinely, the incidence was 8–13% [61, 62].

Unlike central serous retinopathy, lesions in SND are usually binocular, multifocal, and symmetrical. SND is often asymptomatic. In some patients, it causes reduced visual acuity, color vision disorders, or photophobia. Trametinib treatment should be interrupted in patients with SND. In most patients, SND resolves without permanent sequelae [63].

Uveitis and conjunctivitis are ocular side effects of dabrafenib. Usually, treatment with topical steroids is sufficient. In most patients, it is mild and does not require treatment modification.

Retinal vein occlusion (<1%) is a very rare but serious complication of BRAF and MEK inhibitors. Treatment with dabrafenib and trametinib should be discontinued in patients with retinal vein occlusion [1, 13, 58].

Summary of Approval and Regulatory Indications

Dabrafenib (Tafinlar®) as monotherapy or in combination with trametinib (Mekinist®) is indicated for the treatment of adult patients with unresectable or metastatic melanoma with a *BRAF V600* mutation. Trametinib may be also used in monotherapy in this indication. Dabrafenib in combination with trametinib is also approved for the adjuvant treatment of patients with stage III melanoma with *BRAF V600* mutations following complete resection.

Additionally, beyond melanoma combination of dabrafenib and trametinib is approved for the treatment of adult patients with metastatic non-small cell lung cancer (NSCLC) with BRAF V600 mutation and for therapy of patients with locally advanced or metastatic anaplastic thyroid cancer (ATC) with BRAF V600 mutation and with no satisfactory locoregional treatment options (the latter is FDA label only). The recommended dose of dabrafenib, when used in combination with trametinib, is 150 mg twice daily.

The recommended dose of dabrafenib, either used as monotherapy or in combination with trametinib, is 150 mg (two 75 mg capsules) twice daily (corresponding to a total daily dose of 300 mg). The recommended dose of trametinib, either used as monotherapy or in combination with dabrafenib, is 2 mg once daily. Two dabrafenib capsule strengths, 50 mg and 75 mg, and two trametinib capsule strengths, 2 mg and 0.5 mg, are available for management of dose modification requirements. The management of adverse reactions may require treatment interruption, dose reduction, or treatment discontinuation.

Trametinib may be used as monotherapy for the treatment of adult patients with unresectable or metastatic melanoma with a BRAF V600 mutation. This indication seems justified when BRAF inhibitor is contraindicated and there are no options of immunotherapy. Trametinib monotherapy has not demonstrated clinical activity in patients who have progressed on a prior BRAF inhibitor therapy. Treatment with BRAF and MEK inhibitors should be initiated and supervised by a physician experienced in the administration of anti-cancer medicinal products.

References

1. Tafinlar EPAR Product information. European Medicines Agency. Available from https://www. ema.europa.eu/en/documents/product-information/tafinlar-epar-product-information_en.pdf.
2. Laquerre S. AM, Moss K. i wsp. A selective Raf kinase inhibitor induces cell death, Mol. atrohccleB-REm, B88. CTsa.
3. Rheault TR, Stellwagen JC, Adjabeng GM, et al. Discovery of Dabrafenib: a selective inhibitor of Raf kinases with antitumor activity against B-Raf-driven tumors. ACS Med Chem Lett. 2013;4:358–62.
4. Falchook GS, Long GV, Kurzrock R, et al. Dabrafenib in patients with melanoma, untreated brain metastases, and other solid tumours: a phase 1 dose-escalation trial. Lancet. 2012;379:1893–901.
5. Samatar AA, Poulikakos PI. Targeting RAS-ERK signalling in cancer: promises and challenges. Nat Rev Drug Discov. 2014;13:928–42.
6. Montagut C, Settleman J. Targeting the RAF-MEK-ERK pathway in cancer therapy. Cancer Lett. 2009;283:125–34.
7. Salama AK, Kim KB. MEK inhibition in the treatment of advanced melanoma. Curr Oncol Rep. 2013;15:473–82.
8. Yamaguchi T, Kakefuda R, Tajima N, Sowa Y, Sakai T. Antitumor activities of JTP-74057 (GSK1120212), a novel MEK1/2 inhibitor, on colorectal cancer cell lines in vitro and in vivo. Int J Oncol. 2011;39:23–31.
9. Gilmartin AG, Bleam MR, Groy A, et al. GSK1120212 (JTP-74057) is an inhibitor of MEK activity and activation with favorable pharmacokinetic properties for sustained in vivo pathway inhibition. Clin Cancer Res. 2011;17:989–1000.
10. Falchook GS, Lewis KD, Infante JR, et al. Activity of the oral MEK inhibitor trametinib in patients with advanced melanoma: a phase 1 dose-escalation trial. Lancet Oncol. 2012;13:782–9.

11. King AJ, Arnone MR, Bleam MR, et al. Dabrafenib; preclinical characterization, increased efficacy when combined with trametinib, while BRAF/MEK tool combination reduced skin lesions. PLoS One. 2013;8:e67583.
12. Infante JR, Fecher LA, Falchook GS, et al. Safety, pharmacokinetic, pharmacodynamic, and efficacy data for the oral MEK inhibitor trametinib: a phase 1 dose-escalation trial. Lancet Oncol. 2012;13:773–81.
13. Mekinist EPAR Product Information. European Medicines Agency. Available from https://www.ema.europa.eu/en/documents/product-information/mekinist-epar-product-information_en.pdf.
14. Ascierto PA, Minor D, Ribas A, et al. Phase II trial (BREAK-2) of the BRAF inhibitor dabrafenib (GSK2118436) in patients with metastatic melanoma. J Clin Oncol. 2013;31:3205–11.
15. Hauschild A, Grob JJ, Demidov LV, et al. Dabrafenib in BRAF-mutated metastatic melanoma: a multicentre, open-label, phase 3 randomised controlled trial. Lancet. 2012;380:358–65.
16. Long GV, Trefzer U, Davies MA, et al. Dabrafenib in patients with Val600Glu or Val600Lys BRAF-mutant melanoma metastatic to the brain (BREAK-MB): a multicentre, open-label, phase 2 trial. Lancet Oncol. 2012;13:1087–95.
17. Fleming ID, Cooper JS, Henson DE, editors. Soft tissue sarcoma, in American Joint Committee on Cancer Staging MAnual. 5th ed. Philadelphia, PA: Lippincott-Reven; 1997. p. 149–56.
18. Hauschild A, Grob JJ, Demidov LV, et al. An update on BREAK-3, a phase III, randomized trial: Dabrafenib (DAB) versus dacarbazine (DTIC) in patients with BRAF V600E-positive mutation metastatic melanoma (MM). J Clin Oncol. 2013;31(15_suppl):9013.
19. Kim KB, Kefford R, Pavlick AC, et al. Phase II study of the MEK1/MEK2 inhibitor Trametinib in patients with metastatic BRAF-mutant cutaneous melanoma previously treated with or without a BRAF inhibitor. J Clin Oncol. 2013;31:482–9.
20. Flaherty KT, Robert C, Hersey P, et al. Improved survival with MEK inhibition in BRAF-mutated melanoma. N Engl J Med. 2012;367:107–14.
21. Flaherty KT, Infante JR, Daud A, et al. Combined BRAF and MEK inhibition in melanoma with BRAF V600 mutations. N Engl J Med. 2012;367:1694–703.
22. Long GV, Eroglu Z, Infante JR et al. Five-year overall survival (OS) update from a phase II, open-label trial of dabrafenib (D) and trametinib (T) in patients (pts) with BRAF V600 — mutant unresectable or metastatic melanoma (MM). J Clin Oncol 2017; 35 (supl.; abstr. 9505).
23. Long GV, Stroyakovskiy D, Gogas H, et al. Combined BRAF and MEK inhibition versus BRAF inhibition alone in melanoma. N Engl J Med. 2014;371:1877–88.
24. Long GV, Stroyakovskiy D, Gogas H, et al. Dabrafenib and trametinib versus dabrafenib and placebo for Val600 BRAF-mutant melanoma: a multicentre, double-blind, phase 3 randomised controlled trial. Lancet. 2015;386:444–51.
25. Robert C, Karaszewska B, Schachter J, et al. Improved overall survival in melanoma with combined dabrafenib and trametinib. N Engl J Med. 2015;372:30–9.
26. Robert C, Karaszewska B, Schachter J, et al. Three-year estimate of overall survival in COMBI-v, a randomized phase 3 study evaluating first-line dabrafenib (D) + trametinib (T) in patients (pts) with unresectable or metastatic BRAF V600E / K – mutant cutaneous melanoma [Abstract no. 3696]. Ann Oncol. 2016;27(6):1–36.
27. Robert C, Grob JJ, Stroyakovskiy D, et al. Five-year outcomes with dabrafenib plus trametinib in metastatic melanoma. N Engl J Med. 2019;381:626–36.
28. Long GV, Flaherty KT, Stroyakovskiy D, et al. Dabrafenib plus trametinib versus dabrafenib monotherapy in patients with metastatic BRAF V600E/K-mutant melanoma: long-term survival and safety analysis of a phase 3 study. Ann Oncol. 2017;28:1631–9.
29. Davies MA, Saiag P, Robert C, et al. Dabrafenib plus trametinib in patients with BRAF(V600)-mutant melanoma brain metastases (COMBI-MB): a multicentre, multicohort, open-label, phase 2 trial. Lancet Oncol. 2017;18:863–73.
30. Schadendorf D, Amonkar MM, Stroyakovskiy D, et al. Health-related quality of life impact in a randomised phase III study of the combination of dabrafenib and trametinib versus dabrafenib monotherapy in patients with BRAF V600 metastatic melanoma. Eur J Cancer. 2015;51:833–40.

31. Robert C, Karaszewska B, Schachter J, Rutkowski P. Three-year estimate of overall survival in COMBI-v, a randomized phase 3 study evaluating first-line dabrafenib (D) + trametinib (T) in patients with unresectable or metastatic BRAF V600E/K-mutant cutaneous melanoma. Ann Oncol. 2016;27(6):1–36. LBA40

32. Ugurel S, Thirumaran RK, Bloethner S, et al. B-RAF and N-RAS mutations are preserved during short time in vitro propagation and differentially impact prognosis. PLoS One. 2007;2:e236.

33. Anker CJ, Grossmann KF, Atkins MB, Suneja G, Tarhini AA, Kirkwood JM. Avoiding severe toxicity from combined BRAF inhibitor and radiation treatment: consensus guidelines from the Eastern Cooperative Oncology Group (ECOG). Int J Radiat Oncol Biol Phys. 2016;95:632–46.

34. Ly D, Bagshaw HP, Anker CJ, et al. Local control after stereotactic radiosurgery for brain metastases in patients with melanoma with and without BRAF mutation and treatment. J Neurosurg. 2015;123:395–401.

35. Rompoti N, Schilling B, Livingstone E, et al. Combination of BRAF inhibitors and brain radiotherapy in patients with metastatic melanoma shows minimal acute toxicity. J Clin Oncol. 2013;31:3844–5.

36. Hecht M, Zimmer L, Loquai C, et al. Radiosensitization by BRAF inhibitor therapy-mechanism and frequency of toxicity in melanoma patients. Ann Oncol. 2015;26:1238–44.

37. Schreuer M, Jansen Y, Planken S, et al. Combination of dabrafenib plus trametinib for BRAF and MEK inhibitor pretreated patients with advanced BRAF(V600)-mutant melanoma: an open-label, single arm, dual-centre, phase 2 clinical trial. Lancet Oncol. 2017;18:464–72.

38. Tietze JK, Forschner A, Loquai C, et al. The efficacy of re-challenge with BRAF inhibitors after previous progression to BRAF inhibitors in melanoma: a retrospective multicenter study. Oncotarget. 2018;9:34336–46.

39. Cybulska-Stopa B, Rogala P, Czarnecka AM, et al. BRAF and MEK inhibitors rechallenge as effective treatment for patients with metastatic melanoma. Melanoma Res; 2020.

40. Valpione S, Carlino MS, Mangana J, et al. Rechallenge with BRAF-directed treatment in metastatic melanoma: a multi-institutional retrospective study. Eur J Cancer. 2018;91:116–24.

41. Schadendorf D, Hauschild A, Santinami M, et al. Patient-reported outcomes in patients with resected, high-risk melanoma with BRAF(V600E) or BRAF(V600K) mutations treated with adjuvant dabrafenib plus trametinib (COMBI-AD): a randomised, placebo-controlled, phase 3 trial. Lancet Oncol. 2019;20:701–10.

42. Hauschild A, Dummer R, Santinami M et al. Long-term benefit of adjuvant dabrafenib + trametinib (D + T) in patients (pts) with resected stage III BRAF V600-mutant melanoma: five-year analysis of COMBI-AD. Presented at: 2020 ASCO Virtual Scientific Program; May 29–31. Abstract 10001. J Clin Oncol 38, no. 15_suppl.

43. Vanneste L, Wolter P, Van den Oord JJ, Stas M, Garmyn M. Cutaneous adverse effects of BRAF inhibitors in metastatic malignant melanoma, a prospective study in 20 patients. J Eur Acad Dermatol Venereol. 2015;29:61–8.

44. Rutkowski P, Blank C. Dabrafenib for the treatment of BRAF V600-positive melanoma: a safety evaluation. Expert Opin Drug Saf. 2014;13:1249–58.

45. Chapman PB, Hauschild A, Robert C, et al. Improved survival with vemurafenib in melanoma with BRAF V600E mutation. N Engl J Med. 2011;364:2507–16.

46. Larkin J, Del Vecchio M, Ascierto PA, et al. Vemurafenib in patients with BRAF(V600) mutated metastatic melanoma: an open-label, multicentre, safety study. Lancet Oncol. 2014;15:436–44.

47. Su F, Viros A, Milagre C, et al. RAS mutations in cutaneous squamous-cell carcinomas in patients treated with BRAF inhibitors. N Engl J Med. 2012;366:207–15.

48. Heidorn SJ, Milagre C, Whittaker S, et al. Kinase-dead BRAF and oncogenic RAS cooperate to drive tumor progression through CRAF. Cell. 2010;140:209–21.

49. Hatzivassiliou G, Song K, Yen I, et al. RAF inhibitors prime wild-type RAF to activate the MAPK pathway and enhance growth. Nature. 2010;464:431–5.

50. Anforth R, Tembe V, Blumetti T, Fernandez-Penas P. Mutational analysis of cutaneous squamous cell carcinomas and verrucal keratosis in patients taking BRAF inhibitors. Pigment Cell Melanoma Res. 2012;25:569–72.
51. Mossner R, Zimmer L, Berking C, et al. Erythema nodosum-like lesions during BRAF inhibitor therapy: report on 16 new cases and review of the literature. J Eur Acad Dermatol Venereol. 2015;29:1797–806.
52. Anforth R, Liu M, Nguyen B, et al. Acneiform eruptions: a common cutaneous toxicity of the MEK inhibitor trametinib. Australas J Dermatol. 2014;55:250–4.
53. Menzies AM, Ashworth MT, Swann S, et al. Characteristics of pyrexia in BRAFV600E/K metastatic melanoma patients treated with combined dabrafenib and trametinib in a phase I/II clinical trial. Ann Oncol. 2015;26:415–21.
54. Atkinson V, Long GV, Menzies AM, et al. Optimizing combination dabrafenib and trametinib therapy in BRAF mutation-positive advanced melanoma patients: guidelines from Australian melanoma medical oncologists. Asia Pac J Clin Oncol. 2016;12(Suppl 7):5–12.
55. Menzies AM, Long GV. Dabrafenib and trametinib, alone and in combination for BRAF-mutant metastatic melanoma. Clin Cancer Res. 2014;20:2035–43.
56. Mincu RI, Mahabadi AA, Michel L, et al. Cardiovascular adverse events associated with BRAF and MEK inhibitors: a systematic review and meta-analysis. JAMA Netw Open. 2019;2:e198890.
57. Totzeck M, Hendgen-Cotta UB, Luedike P, et al. Nitrite regulates hypoxic vasodilation via myoglobin-dependent nitric oxide generation. Circulation. 2012;126:325–34.
58. Heinzerling L, Eigentler TK, Fluck M, et al. Tolerability of BRAF/MEK inhibitor combinations: adverse event evaluation and management. ESMO Open. 2019;4:e000491.
59. Banks M, Crowell K, Proctor A, Jensen BC. Cardiovascular effects of the MEK inhibitor, trametinib: a case report, literature review, and consideration of mechanism. Cardiovasc Toxicol. 2017;17:487–93.
60. Welsh SJ, Corrie PG. Management of BRAF and MEK inhibitor toxicities in patients with metastatic melanoma. Ther Adv Med Oncol. 2015;7:122–36.
61. Ascierto PA, McArthur GA, Dreno B, et al. Cobimetinib combined with vemurafenib in advanced BRAF(V600)-mutant melanoma (coBRIM): updated efficacy results from a randomised, double-blind, phase 3 trial. Lancet Oncol. 2016;17:1248–60.
62. Dummer R, Ascierto PA, Gogas HJ, et al. Overall survival in patients with BRAF-mutant melanoma receiving encorafenib plus binimetinib versus vemurafenib or encorafenib (COLUMBUS): a multicentre, open-label, randomised, phase 3 trial. Lancet Oncol. 2018;19:1315–27.
63. Carvajal RD, Schwartz GK, Tezel T, Marr B, Francis JH, Nathan PD. Metastatic disease from uveal melanoma: treatment options and future prospects. Br J Ophthalmol. 2017;101:38–44.

Chapter 6
Vemurafenib and Cobimetinib

Hanna Koseła-Paterczyk and Piotr Rutkowski

Pharmacological Properties and Early Development

Vemurafenib Pharmacodynamics

Vemurafenib is a small molecule oral BRAF serine/threonine kinase inhibitor. In preclinical studies, the safety of the drug was initially tested in animals. Vemurafenib administered to rats and dogs for 28 days at doses increasing to 1000 mg/kg/day did not induce toxicity at any dose level. Further studies on long-term use (26 weeks in rats, 13 weeks in dogs) confirmed the safety of the drug. The doses used in rats were significantly higher than the effective doses in humans. Interestingly, no dermal toxicity was seen in the animals while taking the drug [1].

Vemurafenib dosing studies were conducted, among others, using BRAF V600E colon cancer xenograft models. In this model, tumor growth was inhibited at a dose of 6 mg/kg (AUC0–24 ~ 50 μM h), tumor stabilization was observed at a dose of 20 mg/kg (AUC0–24 ~ 200 μM h), and significant tumor regression was noted at 20 mg/kg twice daily (AUC0–24 ~ 300 μM h). The studied melanoma xenograft models (COLO829, LOX) showed similar sensitivity to the drug [2]. Preclinical studies have shown that vemurafenib can strongly inhibit BRAF kinases with activating mutations in codon 600. In ERK phosphorylation and cellular antiproliferation tests on available melanoma cell lines, it was shown that the concentration inhibiting 50 (IC50) cell proliferation with the V600 mutation found (V600E, V600R, 12 V600D, and V600K) ranged from 0.016 to 1.131 μM (Table 6.1) [3]. In the phase I BRIM-1 study, immunohistochemical analysis of phosphorylated ERK,

H. Koseła-Paterczyk (✉) · P. Rutkowski
Department of Soft Tissue/Bone Sarcoma and Melanoma, Maria Sklodowska-Curie National Research Institute of Oncology, Warsaw, Poland
e-mail: Hanna.Kosela-Paterczyk@pib-nio.pl; Piotr.Rutkowski@pib-nio.pl

P. Rutkowski, M. Mandalà (eds.), *New Therapies in Advanced Cutaneous Malignancies*, https://doi.org/10.1007/978-3-030-64009-5_6

Table 6.1 Vemurafenib inhibitory activity against selected BRAF kinases

Kinase	Inhibitory concentration IC50 (nM)
BRAF V600E	10
BRAF V600K	7
BRAF V600R	9
BRAF V600D	7
BRAF V600G	8
BRAF V600M	7

cyclin D1, and Ki-67 expression in tissues taken from patients before treatment and on day 15 was performed. There was a significant reduction in the level of phosphorylation of ERK, cyclin D1, and Ki-67 in all samples taken on day 15 of treatment. Response to treatment increased with increasing dose, which was reflected in the inhibition of MEK and ERK phosphorylation [4, 5].

Vemurafenib Pharmacokinetics

The absolute bioavailability and the effect of food on the absorption of vemurafenib are unknown. Age, weight, gender, and race had no significant effect on the pharmacokinetic parameters. The highest blood levels of vemurafenib are found 4 h after a single oral dose. Vemurafenib has a long half-life, with a dose of 960 mg twice daily, the serum half-life is approximately 51 h. The drug is highly bound (>99%) to plasma proteins, mainly albumin [3]. It is metabolized by hepatic cytochrome P450 isoforms. Vemurafenib is a substrate and inducer of the CYP3A4 enzyme, a moderate CYP1A2 inhibitor, and a mild CYP2D6 and 2C9 inhibitor. Concomitant use of vemurafenib with drugs that are substrates, inducers, or inhibitors of these metabolic enzymes requires caution as there is a risk of serious interactions [6]. Particular caution should be taken when vemurafenib is used in combination with strong CYP3A4 inhibitors, glucuronidation, and/or transporting proteins (e.g., ritonavir, saquinavir, telithromycin, ketoconazole, itraconazole, voriconazole, posaconazole, nefazodone, atazanavir). Conversely, concomitant use of strong P-glycoprotein inducers, glucuronidation, and/or CYP3A4 may result in incomplete exposure to vemurafenib (e.g., rifampicin, carbamazepine, phenytoin, or St. John's Wort) [3].

Vemurafenib is mainly excreted in feces (>94%). Urinary excretion is below 1%. The estimated apparent clearance of vemurafenib in the population of patients with metastatic melanoma is 29.3 L/day. In patients with mild or moderate renal or hepatic dysfunction, the clearance of this drug was unchanged. Caution should be exercised in patients with severe renal or hepatic impairment as vemurafenib has not been evaluated in this population. Its effects on fertility have not been determined. Due to the lack of data on the passage of vemurafenib and its metabolites into breast milk, it should not be used during breastfeeding [3].

Cobimetinib Pharmacodynamics

Cobimetinib is a selective, reversible, allosteric inhibitor of the second generation of MEK1 and MEK2 proteins, the inhibitory concentration (IC50) in MEK1 is 4.2 nM. In studies on BRAF mutant melanoma cells, IC50 values associated with inhibition of cellular phosphorylation and ERK1/2 proliferation were 1.8 nM and 8 nM, respectively. Inhibition of cellular ERK1/2 activity has also been observed in other tumor cell lines that are dependent on abnormal ERK/MAPK signaling, for example, with the *KRAS* and *BRAF* mutation. Cobimetinib also causes C-RAF protein to move to the cell membrane in cancer cells with the KRAS mutation [7]. In vivo efficacy was observed for cell lines with the BRAF and KRAS mutation both when used alone or in combination with a PI3K inhibitor [8, 9]. In preclinical models, cobimetinib in combination with vemurafenib has been shown to inhibit reactivation of the MAPK pathway through MEK1/2 by concomitant action against mutant BRAFV600 and MEK proteins in melanoma cells. This results in stronger inhibition of intracellular signaling and less proliferation of tumor cells [10]. The 21 days treatment/7 days break schedule was chosen because of the smaller tumor growth during the dosing interval compared to the 14 days treatment/14 days break schedule [11].

Cobimetinib Pharmacokinetics

The drug has high oral bioavailability. Absolute bioavailability was estimated at 46% due to intestinal metabolism. Absorption was not affected by a simultaneous meal or increased gastric pH [12]. The drug's metabolism is mainly through the CYP3A4 enzyme in the intestinal mucosa [13]. The half-life is between 26 and 53 h. Cobimetinib is mainly excreted in feces (75%), to a lesser extent in urine. After intravenous administration of 2 mg cobimetinib, the mean plasma clearance (CL) was 10.7 l/h. The mean apparent clearance in patients with malignancies after oral administration of 60 mg was 13.8 l/h. The drug binds to plasma proteins in over 90% (mainly in unchanged form), is quickly and extensively transported to tissues, where it reaches high concentrations [14].

Animal studies have shown reduced penetration into the brain tissue [8]. The dosing regimen of treatment 21 days/7 days off maximum tolerated dose was determined during phase I dose escalation to 60 mg per day [11]. Cobimetinib Cmax and AUC values are dose-proportional and this drug has an average elimination half-life of approximately 40 h with low systemic clearance (11.7 l/h), that is, complete elimination from the systemic circulation after treatment can take up to 2 weeks. The pharmacokinetics of cobimetinib is linear in the dosage range from ~3.5 mg to 100 mg. Cobimetinib is not affected by the administration of vemurafenib. Based on a population pharmacokinetic analysis, gender, race, ethnicity, baseline ECOG performance level, and mild to moderate renal impairment did not affect the pharmacokinetics of cobimetinib. Its pharmacokinetics in children and adolescents, and carcinogenicity have not been studied. Cobimetinib was not genotoxic in standard studies [12, 15].

The concomitant administration of strong CYP3A inhibitors (e.g., itraconazole or grapefruit juice—increasing the drug concentration) and CYP3A inducers (e.g., carbamazepine, phenytoin, St. John's Wort—reducing the drug concentration) should be avoided during treatment with cobimetinib. Concomitant intake of P-gp inhibitors such as cyclosporin and verapamil has the potential to increase cobimetinib plasma concentrations [10]

Activity and Efficacy in Melanoma

Vemurafenib Monotherapy

Clinical trials on vemurafenib began in 2006. Currently, BRIM (the BRAF inhibitor in melanoma) phase I, II, and III studies are completed. They led to the registration of vemurafenib as a monotherapy in adults with unresectable melanoma or metastatic melanoma that had the *BRAF V600* mutation. The results of these studies are summarized in Table 6.2.

Table 6.2 Summary of phase I–III results of clinical trials assessing the efficacy of vemurafenib in patients with stage IIIc or stage IV melanoma

Clinical trial	Inclusion criteria	Number of patients	The objective response rate (%)	Median PFS (months)	Median OS (months)
Phase I study (*extension phase*) BRIM-1 [4]	BRAF (+) melanoma, stage IIIc/IV ≥ first line of systemic treatment	32	81 (56)[a]	7	Not reached
Phase II study (BRIM-2) [13]	BRAF (+) melanoma, stage IIIc/IV ≥ first line of systemic treatment	132	53	6.8	15.9
Phase III study (BRIM-3) [14]	BRAF (+) stage IIIc/ IV melanoma without prior systemic treatment	675	48	5.3	13.2

PFS progression-free survival, *OS* overall survival
[a]According to an independent assessment

Phase I Study (BRIM-1)

The multicenter phase I study consisted of two phases. The dose-escalation phase was performed in patients with metastatic solid tumors after previous systemic treatment and no other therapeutic options available [4]. In turn, the extension phase only included patients with advanced melanoma with the BRAF V600E mutation. Treatment was initiated at a dose of 160 mg twice daily. Side effects in the form of rashes, joint pain, fatigue, and cutaneous squamous cell cancer (SCC) were observed after exceeding the dose of 720 mg two times a day. The maximum tolerated dose established for phase II studies was 960 mg twice daily. In the follow-up phase, 32 patients with metastatic melanoma *BRAF V600E* mutated received vemurafenib in dose 960 mg twice daily. The objective response rate in this group of patients was 81% (56% according to an independent assessment), two patients achieved complete response (CR) and 24 patients achieved partial response (PR). The estimated median progression-free survival (PFS) was over 7 months, the median overall survival (OS) was not reached. Responses to treatment were observed regardless of the location of the metastatic lesions. It was also noted in patients who received in the escalation phase a lower dose than the currently recommended dose.

Phase II Study (BRIM-2)

The results of the phase II study (BRIM-2) were presented at the American Society of Clinical Oncology (ASCO) conference in 2011. The inclusion criteria included patients with advanced/metastatic melanoma with confirmed *BRAF V600E* mutation after prior systemic treatment. The presence of active metastatic lesions in the central nervous system (CNS) was an exclusion criterion (allowed was inclusion of patients with metastases to the CNS without progression after prior local treatment for at least 3 months). The primary objective of the study was the overall response rate to treatment. 132 patients were included in the study. Response rate to treatment was 53%, including CR in 6% and PR in 47%. The median PFS was 6.8 months [95% CI (confidence interval), 5.6–8.1], the median OS was 15.9 months (95% CI 11.6–18.3). Although 24% of patients received ipilimumab after progression during treatment with vemurafenib, the median OS remained the same also after excluding this group of patients. The overall survival rates in the 6th, 12th, and 18th month (estimated value) were 77%, 58%, and 43% respectively. Toxicity of grade 3 experienced 63% of patients, in most cases it was cutaneous toxicity and joint pain. In contrast, grade 4 toxicity occurred in only 3% of patients. Due to toxicity, 45% of patients required dose reduction [13].

Phase III Study (BRIM-3)

The phase III clinical study (BRIM-3) was a multicenter randomized trial comparing the efficacy of vemurafenib to dacarbazine in the first line of treatment. Included were 675 patients with unresectable stage IIIC or IV melanoma with confirmed *BRAF* mutation who had not received systemic treatment. Patients with stable metastases in the central nervous system could also be included in the study. Patients were randomly assigned to one of two arms in a 1:1 ratio. In one arm, patients received vemurafenib at a dose of 960 mg twice a day, in the other arm dacarbazine was administered intravenously at a dose of 1000 mg/m^2 every 3 weeks. The primary objective of the study was to evaluate overall survival and progression-free survival. The median OS for vemurafenib was 13.2 months (1-year survival was 55% for vemurafenib and 43% for dacarbazine). The median PFS was 5.3 and 1.6 months for vemurafenib and dacarbazine, respectively. The study showed a relative reduction in risk of death by 63% and of tumor progression by 74% after treatment with vemurafenib. The objective response rate in the group of patients treated with vemurafenib was 48% (in the group with dacarbazine it was 5%), although the majority of patients receiving vemurafenib had a positive response to treatment. The incidence of adverse events was similar to that observed in clinical phase I and II. Keratoacanthoma (KA—squamous cell keratoma) or squamous cell carcinoma of the skin was found at least once in 18% of the subjects in the vemurafenib arm; 38% of patients required dose reduction due to toxicity [14].

Figure 6.1 shows an example of partial response to vemurafenib treatment in a patient treated at Maria Sklodowska-Curie National Research Institute of Oncology, Department of Soft Tissue/Bone Sarcoma and Melanoma Warsaw.

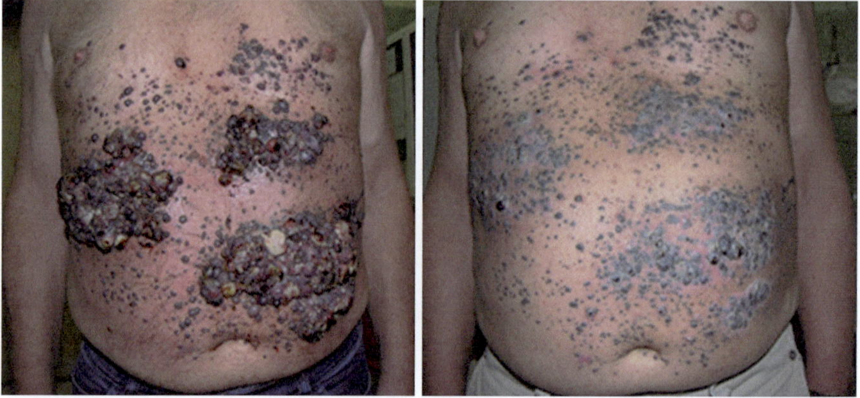

Fig. 6.1 Partial response of metastatic cutaneous melanoma to vemurafenib monotherapy (courtesy of T. Switaj)

Vemurafenib and Cobimetinib

Most patients treated with BRAF inhibitors experience disease progression after some time due to the development of drug resistance mechanisms in melanoma cells. One of these mechanisms is bypassing the blockade of BRAF, resulting in the excessive activity of the MAPK kinase pathway again, due to the stimulation of MEK proteins [15, 16].

In recent years, the results of clinical trials conducted among patients with metastatic melanoma have been published, showing the superiority of the simultaneous blocking of BRAF and MEK proteins over the separate use of BRAF inhibitors. The first study compared the efficacy of the combination of dabrafenib with trametinib with dabrafenib and placebo in first-line treatment in patients diagnosed with metastatic BRAF-mutated melanoma. The primary endpoint of the study was PFS. The use of the drug combination was associated with PFS prolongation. Simultaneous inhibition of BRAF and MEK led to a 25% relative reduction in the risk of disease progression compared to dabrafenib alone, with a significantly higher response rate and longer OS. The incidence of side effects was similar in both groups, but more often dose modifications were made in the dabrafenib- and trametinib-treated group. Squamous cell carcinoma of the skin was less common among patients treated with the combination of drugs than in the group receiving the BRAF inhibitor alone. Fever occurred in a larger number of patients taking two drugs at the same time (51% vs. 28%) and was more severe in this group (toxicity grade 3: 6% for the combination of drugs vs. 2% alone) [17, 18]. Another randomized study had a similar structure, but the drug used as monotherapy instead of dabrafenib was vemurafenib, and the endpoint was OS [19].

The use of MEK inhibitors in monotherapy is also an effective treatment, prolonging both PFS and OS compared to dacarbazine treatment [20]. Although no randomized trial comparing the efficacy of MEK inhibitor monotherapy and BRAF inhibitor therapy has been performed, the results of available studies indicate that MEK blockade alone is less effective, and the use of MEK inhibitors in the treatment of patients with metastatic melanoma should be limited to drug combinations [21]. Table 6.3 shows a summary of clinical trial results for combination therapy with vemurafenib and cobimetinib in patients with advanced BRAF (+) melanoma.

Early-Phase Studies

The first study assessing primarily the safety, but also the efficacy of the MEK inhibitor cobimetinib in the diagnosis of advanced melanoma was the Ib phase NO25395 (BRIM7) study, where the drug was used in combination with vemurafenib [11]. 129 patients with metastatic melanoma with confirmed *BRAF*

Table 6.3 Summary of clinical trial results for combination therapy with vemurafenib and cobimetinib in patients with advanced BRAF (+) melanoma

Authors	Study characteristics	Patients number	Primary endpoint	OS rates and median	PFS median	Overall response rate
Ribas et al. [11]	Ib phase study with V + C dose-escalation cohort	129	Safety of drug combination and identification of the dose-limiting toxicity and the maximum tolerated dose	After a year: patients previously treated with V—32%, previously untreated with BRAF—83%; median OS 28.5 months in the group not previously treated with BRAF inhibitors compared to 8.4 months in the group after progression to V	After previous progression to V: 2.8 months. No previous BRAF inhibitor therapy: 13.7 months	After previous progression to V: 15% Without previous BRAF inhibitor therapy: 88%
Larkin et al. [22]	A phase III randomized trial comparing the combination of V + C and V monotherapy	495	PFS as assessed by the investigator	After 9 months: V 73% (95% CI: 65–80), V + C—81% (95% CI: 75–87), HR: 0.65 (95% CI: 0.42–1.00; $p = 0.046$) Updated data (median observation 18.5 months): median OS 22.3 months (95% CI: 20.3—not reached) in group V + C compared to 17.4 months (95% CI: 15.0–19.8) in the group with V (HR: 0.70; 95% CI: 0.55–0.90; $p = 0.005$) The percentage of 1-year OS was 74.5% in the V + C group compared with 63.8% in the group with V, while the 2-year OS percentage was 48.3% and 38.0%, respectively	V—6.2 months (95% CI: 5.6–7.4) V + C—9.9 months (95% CI: 9.0—not reached) HR: 0.51 (95% CI: 0, 39–0.68; $p < 0.001$) Median PFS after a mean follow-up of 14 months was 12.3 months in the V + C combination group and 7.2 months in the V group alone	V 50% V + C 70% ($p < 0.001$)

C cobimetinib, *OS* overall survival, *PFS* progression-free survival, *V* vemurafenib
Other studies on the drug combination

mutation were enrolled in this large, single-arm study, 63 patients never received a BRAF inhibitor, and 66 had prior disease progression during BRAF inhibitor therapy. The main endpoint of the study was to evaluate the safety of the drug combination and to assess dose-limiting toxicity and to determine the maximum tolerated dose. The secondary endpoint was treatment efficacy. During the escalation phase, patients received vemurafenib 720 mg or 960 mg twice daily continuously and cobimetinib 60 mg, 80 mg, or 100 mg once daily for 14 days in 28-day cycles or 21 days dosing with a 7-day break, or continuously. The maximum tolerated dose of the combination was finally established: vemurafenib 960 mg twice daily in combination with cobimetinib 60 mg once daily for 21 days with a weekly break. Dose-limiting toxicity occurred in four patients. One patient receiving vemurafenib 960 mg twice daily and cobimetinib 80 mg once daily for 2 weeks, followed by a 2-week break had a grade 3 fatigue for more than a week. Another patient treated with vemurafenib 960 mg twice daily and cobimetinib 60 mg daily for 3 weeks followed by a weekly break experienced a grade 3 QTc prolongation. Dose-limiting toxicity was also found in two patients during treatment with vemurafenib 960 mg twice daily and cobimetinib 60 mg taken continuously—one had gingivitis and grade 3 fatigue, the other had joint and muscular pain. In all dosing schedules, the most common side effects were diarrhea (83 patients, 64%), non-acne-like rash (77 patients, 60%), increased liver enzymes (64 patients, 50%), fatigue (62 patients, 48%), nausea (58 patients, 45%), and photosensitivity (52 patients, 40%). Most of them were mild to moderate in severity. The most common grade 3 or 4 adverse reactions were cutaneous squamous cell carcinoma (12 patients, 9%), increased alkaline phosphatase (11 patients, 9%), and anemia (9 patients, 7%).

Objective responses were reported in 55 of 63 patients (87%) who had not received prior BRAF inhibitor therapy, including 6 (10%) with complete response. The median PFS in this group of patients was 13.7 months, with a median follow-up of 12.7 months. The median duration of response was 12.5 months. The percentage of 1-year OS was 83% (95% CI, 73–93%). Among patients previously treated with a BRAF inhibitor, objective responses were reported in 10 of 66 patients (15%), and the median PFS in this group was 2.8 months. The percentage of 1-year OS in this subgroup of patients was 32% (95% CI, 19–45%) [11]. Worse prognosis recorded among patients treated after earlier progression during BRAF inhibitor therapy confirms the results of older studies, which showed that only a small percentage of these patients will benefit from the addition of MEK inhibitor in such a clinical situation. This indicates a more complex mechanism of acquired melanoma cell resistance to BRAF blockade than excessive MEK protein activation alone, and that the combination of a BRAF inhibitor and MEK should be used from the commencement of treatment [23].

Updated data presented at the American Society of Clinical Oncology (ASCO) conference in 2015 showed a median OS of 28.5 months in the group not previously treated with BRAF inhibitors compared to a median of 8.4 months in the group after progression after using vemurafenib [24].

Phase III

Positive results of the cited phase I trial were the basis for conducting a multicenter randomized phase III trial comparing the efficacy of the vemurafenib + cobimetinib to vemurafenib + placebo combination (coBRIM) [22]. Patients were randomized in a 1:1 ratio. 495 patients with locally advanced/metastatic melanoma with *BRAF V600* mutation were included in the study. Only patients with no previous systemic treatment were included. At randomization, the presence of negative prognostic factors was well balanced between both groups of patients. Internal organ metastases were present in 59% of patients in the combination therapy group and in 62% of patients in the control group. 46% and 43% of patients, respectively, had elevated lactate dehydrogenase. The median follow-up time for the originally published results was 7.3 months. The primary endpoint of the study was PFS as assessed by the investigators. The median PFS was 9.9 months in the drug combination group and 6.2 months in the control group (HR 0.51 [95% CI: 0.39–0.68]; $p < 0.001$). Response to treatment was found in the study group in 68% of patients compared with 45% in the group receiving vemurafenib alone ($p < 0.001$). Complete response to treatment was found in 10% of patients in the combination therapy group and 4% in the control group. PFS prolongation among patients treated with the drug combination was observed in all previously defined patient subgroups. Based on the stage analysis, it was found that the 9-month OS in the group treated with the drug combination was 81% compared to 73% in the monotherapy group. Adverse reactions associated with the combination of vemurafenib and cobimetinib and safety of therapy are discussed in the next section. The median PFS reported after an average follow-up of 14 months was 12.3 months in the drug combination group and 7.2 months in the vemurafenib alone group and the response rate was 70% and 50%, respectively [25]. Equally important, the Co-BRIM study showed that, compared to vemurafenib, combination treatment with vemurafenib and cobimetinib is associated with a reduction in disease symptoms, fatigue, improvement of social functioning and quality of life related to health assessed using the quality of life questionnaire (EORTC QLQC30, European Organization for Research and Cancer Quality of Life Questionnaire) [26].

At the end of 2015, at the Congress of Society of Melanoma Research were presented the results of this study updated after a longer observation (median observation of 18.5 months), which formed the basis for the registration of cobimetinib in the United States and the European Union. Median OS was 22.3 months (95% CI: 20.3—not achieved) in the vemurafenib/cobimetinib combination group compared to 17.4 months (95% CI: 15.0–19.8)) in the group in which vemurafenib was used as monotherapy (HR: 0.70; 95% CI: 0.55–0.90; $p = 0.005$). The percentages of annual OS were 74.5% in the combined treatment group compared to 63.8% in the monotherapy group, while the percentages of 2-year OS were 48.3% and 38.0%, respectively [27].

Figure 6.2 shows an example of response to vemurafenib and cobimetinib used in second line of therapy in a patient treated at Maria Sklodowska-Curie National

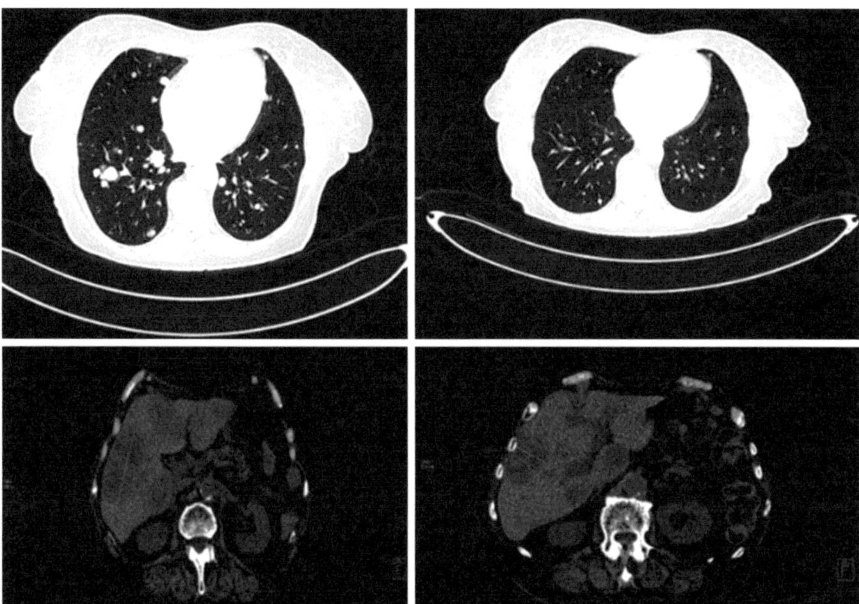

Fig. 6.2 Partial response in lung and liver metastases of *BRAF*-mutated melanoma during vemurafenib and cobimetinib (own material)

Research Institute of Oncology, Department of Soft Tissue/Bone Sarcoma and Melanoma Warsaw.

In 2018, there were published results of a negative clinical study on the efficacy and safety of vemurafenib in adjuvant therapy in patients with high risk of recurrence after surgery (study BRIM-8). It was an international, double-blind, placebo-controlled trial. The study enrolled 498 patients, after radical surgical treatment, with *BRAF*-positive cutaneous melanoma diagnosed in stage IIC–IIIA–IIIB (cohort 1) or stage IIIC (cohort 2). Patients were randomized to the arm where they received vemurafenib at a dose of 960 mg 2× daily or to the arm with appropriately selected placebo. The treatment lasted 52 weeks. The primary endpoint of the study was disease-free survival (DFS) evaluated separately in each cohort. Cohort 2 enrolled 184 patients (93 received vemurafenib and 91 placebo), and cohort 1 enrolled 314 patients (157 to the vemurafenib group and 157 to placebo). At the time of analysis, the median follow-up was 33.5 months in cohort 2 and 30.8 months in cohort 1. In cohort 2 (stage IIIC), the median DFS was 23.1 months (95% PU 18.6–26.5) in the vemurafenib group versus 15.4 months (95% PU 11.1–35.9) in the placebo group (HR 0.8; 95% PU 0.54–1.18; log-rank $p = 0.26$). In cohort 1 (stage IIC–IIIA–IIIB), median DFS was not reached in the vemurafenib group versus 36.9 months (95% PU 21.4-not reached) in the placebo group (HR 0.54; 95% PU 0, 37–0.78; log-rank $p = 0.001$). However, this result was not significant due to the predetermined hierarchical condition of the primary disease-free survival analysis in cohort 2 to demonstrate a significant benefit of disease-free survival [28].

The efficacy of melanoma treatment has increased in the last decade with the introduction of checkpoint inhibitors (anti-PD-1, anti PDL-1, or anti-CTA-4 antibodies) as well as BRAF and/or MEK inhibitors for the subgroup of patients with the *BRAF V600* mutation. From basic research, it is known that BRAF/MEK-targeted therapies have an impact on the tumor microenvironment that justify their combination in treatment with PD-1/PD-L1 inhibitors. The results of the phase Ib clinical trial (ClinicalTrials.gov, number NCT01656642) were published in which was assessed the safety and antitumor activity of the combination of atezolizumab (anti-PD-L1) and vemurafenib or cobimetinib + vemurafenib in patients with disseminated BRAF (+) melanoma. The confirmed objective response rate was 71.8% (95% confidence interval 55.1–85.0). The estimated average duration of response was 17.4 months (95% confidence interval 10.6–25.3), and the response was maintained in 39.3% of patients after 29.9 months of follow-up. This is a highly toxic treatment—Grade 3 or 4 side effects occurred in more than 60% of patients. Adverse reactions leading to permanent discontinuation of any study medication were reported in 28 patients. The most common such toxicity was increased transaminase levels [29].

A randomized, double-blind, placebo-controlled phase III study was conducted (IMspire150). Included were patients with unresectable stage IIIc–IV, *BRAF V600*-positive melanoma. Subjects were randomly assigned 1:1 to 28-day cycles of atezolizumab, vemurafenib, and cobimetinib (study group) or atezolizumab placebo, vemurafenib, and cobimetinib (control group). In cycle 1, all patients received vemurafenib and cobimetinib only. Atezolizumab placebo was added from cycle 2. The primary outcome was investigator-assessed PFS. 514 were enrolled and randomly assigned to the study group ($n = 256$) or control group ($n = 258$). At a median follow-up of 18.9 months PFS was significantly prolonged with atezolizumab versus control (15.1 vs 10.6 months; hazard ratio [HR] 0.78; 95% CI 0.63–0.97; $p = 0.025$). Investigator-assessed confirmed objective response rates were similar between the study (66.3%; 95% CI 60.1–72.1) and control groups (65%; 58.7–71). Rates of complete response (15.7% vs 17.1%), partial response (50.6% vs 48%), and stable disease (22.7% vs 22.8%) were also similar between the study and control groups. However, median duration of response was longer in the atezolizumab group (21 months; 95% CI 15·1 to not estimable) compared with the control group (12.6 months; 10.5–16.6). Most common adverse events (>30%) in the atezolizumab and control groups were blood creatinine phosphokinase increased (51.3% vs 44.8%), diarrhea (42.2% vs 46.6%), rash (40.9%, both groups), arthralgia (39.1% vs 28.1%), pyrexia (38.7% vs 26%), alanine aminotransferase increased (33.9% vs 22.8%), and lipase increased (32.2% vs 27.4%). In 13% of patients in the atezolizumab group and 16% in the control group, all treatment was stopped due to side effects [30].

At the ESMO 2019 congress were presented the results of a negative clinical study on the efficacy and safety of a combination of cobimetinib and atezolizumab compared to pembrolizumab in patients with metastatic melanoma without the *BRAF* mutation. In patients diagnosed with melanoma without the presence of the BRAF mutation, the MAPK pathway is also activated, and emerging data suggest that inhibition of MAPK may enhance the antitumor immune response to checkpoint inhibitors. In a phase I study, the combination of MEK inhibitor (cobimetinib) and anti-PD-L1 antibody (atezolizumab) showed promising antitumor activity. Therefore, a phase III randomized trial was conducted to assess whether this combination would improve treatment efficacy compared to pembrolizumab monotherapy in patients with previously untreated advanced melanoma without the *BRAF V600* mutation. Patients were stratified by PD-L1 expression, LDH level, and geographical location, and were randomly assigned 1: 1 to the arm with the combination of cobimetinib (60 mg, days 1–21) and atezolizumab (840 mg, every 2 weeks) in 28-day cycles or pembrolizumab (200 mg, every 3 weeks). Treatment continued until the loss of clinical benefit, of unacceptable toxicity or withdrawal of consent. The primary endpoint was PFS. Secondary endpoints are objective response rate (ORR), disease control index (DCR), OS, and safety. 446 patients were included in the study; 68% of patients had PD-L1 positive tumors and 25% had elevated LDH levels. The median follow-up was 7 months (range 0–15). The use of the drug combination did not significantly improve PFS compared to pembrolizumab (median 5.5 vs. 5.7 months; HR 1.15; 95% CI 0.88–1.50; $P = 0.295$). The results were consistent across all patient subgroups. ORR was 26% for combinations vs 32% for monotherapy; DCR was 46% vs 44%. Median OS was not reached in any arm (HR 1.06; 95% CI 0.69–1.61). Adverse reactions were consistent with the known safety profiles of individual drugs. Grade ≥3 adverse reactions occurred in 67% of patients receiving the combination vs 33% of patients alone. Adverse reactions leading to treatment discontinuation occurred in 12% vs 6% [31].

Toxicity Profile

The combination of vemurafenib and cobimetinib in the phase III study was associated with a statistically insignificantly higher incidence of some side effects than with vemurafenib alone [10, 22]. Side effects associated with the combination include: central serous retinopathy, toxic effect on the gastrointestinal system (diarrhea, nausea, or vomiting), sensitivity to sunlight, increased aminotransferase levels or elevated levels of creatine kinase (Tables 6.4 and 6.5). Most (>50%) of them occurred in grade 1 or 2 according to Common Terminology Criteria for Adverse Events (CTCAE). Grade 3 adverse reactions occurred with similar frequencies in both groups (49%). Slightly more common among patients receiving two drugs were CTCAE grade 4 adverse reactions (9% in the control group vs. 13% in the combined treatment group). Almost half of them in the study group were caused by asymptomatic laboratory abnormalities (increased transaminase or creatine kinase activity). The most common adverse reaction (4%) in grade 4 was elevated creatine kinase (this is a known adverse reaction associated with MEK blockade) [32]), although most of the side effects seen with increases in creatine kinase (66%) were grade 1 or 2. Another adverse effect characteristic of the use of MEK inhibitors is ocular toxicity reminiscent of central serous retinopathy, referred to in the literature

Table 6.4 Summary of the safety of vemurafenib in combination with cobimetinib versus vemurafenib + placebo [22]

	Vemurafenib + placebo (n = 239)	Vemurafenib + cobimetinib (n = 254)
Patients with at least one adverse event n (%)	233 (98)	250 (98)
Patients with at least one adverse event of the following:		
Grade ≥3, n (%)	142 (59)	165 (65)
Grade 5, n (%)	3 (1.3)	6 (2.3)
Serious adverse events, n (%)	60 (25)	75 (30)
Adverse events leading to vemurafenib discontinuation, n (%)	32 (13)	35 (14)
Adverse events leading to cobimetinib/placebo discontinuation, n (%)	33 (14)	42 (17)
Adverse events leading to both vemurafenib and cobimetinib discontinuation, n (%)	28 (12)	32 (13)

Table 6.5 Summary of selected adverse events [22]

Adverse events, n (%)	Vemurafenib + placebo (n = 239)					Vemurafenib + cobimetinib (n = 254)				
	Grade 1	Grade 2	Grade 3	Grade 4	All	Grade 1	Grade 2	Grade 3	Grade 4	All
Cutaneous squamous cell carcinomas	0	0	27 (11)	0	27(11)	0	1(<1)	6(2)	0	7(3)
Keratoacanthoma	1 (<1)	1(<1)	18(8)	0	20(8)	0	0	2(1)	0	2(1)
Central serous retinopathy	1(<1)	0	0	0	1(<1)	26(10)	18(7)	6(2)	1(<1)	51 (20)
Reduced left ventricular ejection fraction	0	4(2)	3(1)	0	7(3)	2(1)	14(6)	3(1)	0	19 (7)
QT prolongation	8(3)	2(1)	3(1)	0	13(5)	6(2)	2(1)	1(<1)	0	9(4)

as transient drug-induced retinopathy [33, 34]. 86% of patients in the above study experienced grade 1 (clinically asymptomatic) or type 2 (moderate reduction in visual acuity) ocular toxicity. In most cases, it resolved without any additional treatment, as a result of cobimetinib dose reduction or temporary discontinuation of treatment. Side effects such as squamous cell carcinomas or basal cell carcinomas (skin toxicity associated with the development of secondary skin tumors and keratoproliferative changes through paradoxical activation of the MAPK signaling pathway), alopecia or joint pain have been less commonly observed in the combination group. Clinically significant cardiologic adverse reactions (QT prolongation or reduced left ventricular ejection fraction) were rare but with similar frequency in both groups. Six deaths in the study group and three deaths in the control group were associated with the occurrence of treatment adverse effects. Despite differences in the type and frequency of adverse reactions between the two groups, the incidence of toxicity leading to treatment discontinuation was similar (12% in the control group and 13% in the group receiving the drug combination). Women of childbearing potential should use effective contraception during and for 3 months after treatment. Patients during combination therapy require regular skin monitoring, preferably dermatoscopic. Figures 6.3 and 6.4 show cutaneous toxicity of vemurafenib therapy.

An interesting analysis was published assessing the effect of adverse effects of vemurafenib and cobimetinib treatment on treatment efficacy. This study aimed to assess the effect of early adverse events on OS, PFS, and objective response to treatment in a pooled secondary analysis of patients treated in the first line with vemurafenib or vemurafenib and cobimetinib in clinical trials in BRIM3 and coBRIM. The analysis included 583 participants who received vemurafenib as monotherapy and 247 who received vemurafenib with cobimetinib. Adverse events requiring dose adjustment of vemurafenib/cobimetinib during the first 28 days of treatment were significantly associated with OS (risk ratio (HR) [95% CI]: dose reduction/discontinuation = 0.79 [0.65–0.96]; withdrawal drug = 1.18 [0.71–1.96]; $p = 0.032$), PFS

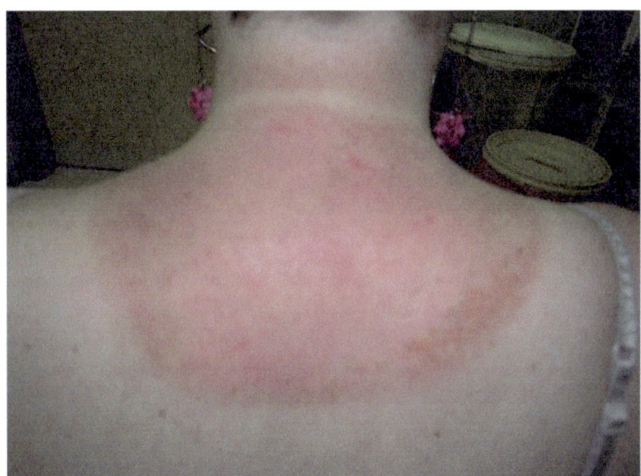

Fig. 6.3 Hypersensitivity to sunlight during vemurafenib treatment (courtesy of K. Kozak)

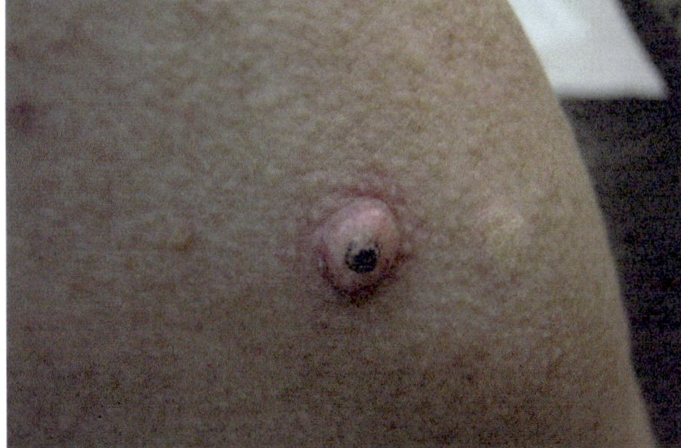

Fig. 6.4 Squamous cell carcinoma in a patient during vemurafenib treatment (courtesy of K. Kozak)

(HR [95% CI]: reduced/interrupted dose = 0.82 [0.67–0.99]; discontinued drug = 1.58 [0.97–2.58]; p = 0.017), and objective response to treatment (odds ratio (OR) [95% CI]: reduced/interrupted dose = 1.35 [0.99–1, 85]; discontinued drug = 0.17 [0.06–0.43]; p = <0.001). Joint pain occurring during the first 28 days of treatment with vemurafenib or vemurafenib and cobimetinib was also significantly associated with favorable OS (p = 0.026), PFS (p = 0.042), and objective response (p = 0.047) [35].

Summary of Approval and Regulatory Indications

In August 2011, the American Food and Drug Administration (FDA) registered vemurafenib (trade name Zelboraf) for the treatment of patients with unresectable/metastatic melanoma with a confirmed *BRAF V600* mutation. The European Medicines Agency (EMA) approved vemurafenib in February 2012. Cobimetinib (trade name Cotellic) was approved in November 2015 by the FDA to be used in combination with vemurafenib to treat unresectable/metastatic melanoma with a confirmed *BRAF V600* mutation. The EMA approved cobimetinib in the above indication in September 2015.

References

1. Bollag G, et al. Clinical efficacy of a RAF inhibitor needs broad target blockade in BRAF-mutant melanoma. Nature. 2010;467(7315):596–9.
2. Yang H, et al. RG7204 (PLX4032), a selective BRAFV600E inhibitor, displays potent antitumor activity in preclinical melanoma models. Cancer Res. 2010;70(13):5518–27.
3. Zelboraf. Summary of product characteristics.
4. Flaherty KT, et al. Inhibition of mutated, activated BRAF in metastatic melanoma. N Engl J Med. 2010;363(9):809–19.
5. Flaherty KT, Yasothan U, Kirkpatrick P. Vemurafenib. Nat Rev Drug Discov. 2011;10(11):811–2.
6. Ravnan MC, Matalka MS. Vemurafenib in patients with BRAF V600E mutation-positive advanced melanoma. Clin Ther. 2012;34(7):1474–86.
7. Hatzivassiliou G, et al. Mechanism of MEK inhibition determines efficacy in mutant KRAS-versus BRAF-driven cancers. Nature. 2013;501(7466):232–6.
8. Choo EF, et al. Preclinical disposition of GDC-0973 and prospective and retrospective analysis of human dose and efficacy predictions. Drug Metab Dispos. 2012;40(5):919–27.
9. Hoeflich KP, et al. In vivo antitumor activity of MEK and phosphatidylinositol 3-kinase inhibitors in basal-like breast cancer models. Clin Cancer Res. 2009;15(14):4649–64.
10. Kobimetynib. Cotellic. Summary of product characteristics.
11. Ribas A, et al. Combination of vemurafenib and cobimetinib in patients with advanced BRAF(V600)-mutated melanoma: a phase 1b study. Lancet Oncol. 2014;15(9):954–65.
12. Musib L, et al. Absolute bioavailability and effect of formulation change, food, or elevated pH with rabeprazole on cobimetinib absorption in healthy subjects. Mol Pharm. 2013;10(11):4046–54.
13. Sosman JA, et al. Survival in BRAF V600-mutant advanced melanoma treated with vemurafenib. N Engl J Med. 2012;366(8):707–14.

14. Chapman PB, et al. Improved survival with vemurafenib in melanoma with BRAF V600E mutation. N Engl J Med. 2011;364(26):2507–16.
15. Van Allen EM, et al. The genetic landscape of clinical resistance to RAF inhibition in metastatic melanoma. Cancer Discov. 2014;4(1):94–109.
16. Rizos H, et al. BRAF inhibitor resistance mechanisms in metastatic melanoma: spectrum and clinical impact. Clin Cancer Res. 2014;20(7):1965–77.
17. Long GV, et al. Combined BRAF and MEK inhibition versus BRAF inhibition alone in melanoma. N Engl J Med. 2014;371(20):1877–88.
18. Long GV, et al. Dabrafenib and trametinib versus dabrafenib and placebo for Val600 BRAF-mutant melanoma: a multicentre, double-blind, phase 3 randomised controlled trial. Lancet. 2015;386(9992):444–51.
19. Robert C, et al. Improved overall survival in melanoma with combined dabrafenib and trametinib. N Engl J Med. 2015;372(1):30–9.
20. Flaherty KT, et al. Improved survival with MEK inhibition in BRAF-mutated melanoma. N Engl J Med. 2012;367(2):107–14.
21. Ascierto PA, Marincola FM, Atkins MB. What's new in melanoma? Combination! J Transl Med. 2015;13:213.
22. Larkin J, et al. Combined vemurafenib and cobimetinib in BRAF-mutated melanoma. N Engl J Med. 2014;371(20):1867–76.
23. Johnson DB, et al. Combined BRAF (Dabrafenib) and MEK inhibition (Trametinib) in patients with BRAFV600-mutant melanoma experiencing progression with single-agent BRAF inhibitor. J Clin Oncol. 2014;32(33):3697–704.
24. http://meetinglibrary.asco.org/content/143297-156.
25. http://www.esmo.org/Conferences/PastConferences/European-Cancer-Con-gress-2015/News/Greater-Clinical-BenefitObtained-in-Advanced-BRAFV600-mutated-Melanoma-with-CobimetinibVemurafenib-Over-Vemurafenib-Is-Consistent-Across-Mutation-Subtypes
26. Dreno B, et al. Health-related quality of life impact of cobimetinib in combination with vemurafenib in patients with advanced or metastatic BRAF(V600) mutation-positive melanoma. Br J Cancer. 2018;118(6):777–84.
27. Atkinson V., Larkin J., McArthur G. i wsp. Improved overall survival (OS) with cobimetinib (COBI) + vemurafenib (V) in advanced BRAF-mutated melanoma and biomarker correlates of efficacy. Society for Melanoma Research 2015. LBA 1.
28. Maio M, et al. Adjuvant vemurafenib in resected, BRAF(V600) mutation-positive melanoma (BRIM8): a randomised, double-blind, placebo-controlled, multicentre, phase 3 trial. Lancet Oncol. 2018;19(4):510–20.
29. Sullivan RJ, et al. Atezolizumab plus cobimetinib and vemurafenib in BRAF-mutated melanoma patients. Nat Med. 2019;25(6):929–35.
30. Gutzmer R, et al. Atezolizumab, vemurafenib, and cobimetinib as first-line treatment for unresectable advanced BRAF(V600) mutation-positive melanoma (IMspire150): primary analysis of the randomised, double-blind, placebo-controlled, phase 3 trial. Lancet. 2020;395(10240):1835–44.
31. Arance AM, Gogas H, Dreno B, et al. Combination treatment with cobimetinib (C) and atezolizumab (A) vs pembrolizumab (P) in previously untreated patients (pts) with BRAFV600 wild type (wt) advanced melanoma: primary analysis from the phase 3 IMspire170 trial. Ann Oncol. 2019;30(suppl_5):v851–934. https://doi.org/10.1093/annonc/mdz394.
32. Leijen S, et al. Phase I dose-escalation study of the safety, pharmacokinetics, and pharmacodynamics of the MEK inhibitor RO4987655 (CH4987655) in patients with advanced solid tumors. Clin Cancer Res. 2012;18(17):4794–805.
33. McCannel TA, et al. Bilateral subfoveal neurosensory retinal detachment associated with MEK inhibitor use for metastatic cancer. JAMA Ophthalmol. 2014;132(8):1005–9.
34. Urner-Bloch U, et al. Transient MEK inhibitor-associated retinopathy in metastatic melanoma. Ann Oncol. 2014;25(7):1437–41.
35. Hopkins AM, et al. Effect of early adverse events on response and survival outcomes of advanced melanoma patients treated with vemurafenib or vemurafenib plus cobimetinib: a pooled analysis of clinical trial data. Pigment Cell Melanoma Res. 2019;32(4):576–83.

Chapter 7
Encorafenib and Binimetinib

Iwona Lugowska and Paweł Rogala

Introduction

BRAF/MEK inhibitor combinations are established treatments for *BRAF V600*-mutant melanoma based on demonstrated benefits on progression-free survival (PFS) and overall survival (OS) [1–3].

Binimetinib in combination with encorafenib demonstrated safety and early efficacy in metastatic melanomas. FDA approved binimetinib in 2018 in combination with encorafenib for the treatment of metastatic melanomas. In the COLUMBUS Phase III trial, it was demonstrated to double the progression-free survival (14.9 months) compared to vemurafenib alone (7.3 months) in patients with BRAF-mutated metastatic melanoma. Nowadays encorafenib and binimetinib have currently been evaluated in over 70 clinical trials in a variety of cancers. However, high costs and limited durable responses must be taken into account compared to immunotherapy regimens in the decision-making process in melanoma [4, 5].

I. Lugowska
Early Phase Clinical Trials Unit, Maria Sklodowska Curie National Research Institute of Oncology, Warsaw, Poland
e-mail: iwona.lugowska@pib-nio.pl

P. Rogala (✉)
Department of Soft Tissue/Bone Sarcoma and Melanoma, Maria Sklodowska Curie National Research Institute of Oncology, Warsaw, Poland
e-mail: progala@coi.pl

P. Rutkowski, M. Mandalà (eds.), *New Therapies in Advanced Cutaneous Malignancies*, https://doi.org/10.1007/978-3-030-64009-5_7

Pharmacological Properties

Encorafenib

Encorafenib is a potent and highly selective ATP-competitive small-molecule RAF kinase inhibitor and suppresses the RAF/MEK/ERK pathway in tumor cells expressing several mutated forms of BRAF kinase. Encorafenib inhibits in vitro and in vivo BRAF V600E/D/K-mutant melanoma cell growth and BRAF V600E-mutant colorectal cancer cell growth. The pharmacokinetics of encorafenib is dose linear after single and multiples doses. After repeat once-daily dosing, steady-state conditions were reached within 15 days. After oral administration, encorafenib is rapidly absorbed with a median Tmax of 1.5 to 2 h with at least 86% absorption. The AUC is not changed with a high-fat, high-calorie meal. The accumulation ratio of approximately 0.5 is likely due to the auto-induction of CYP3A4; however, encorafenib exposure is not altered in the presence of gastric pH-altering agents.

Encorafenib is moderately bound to human plasma proteins (the mean (SD) blood-to-plasma concentration ratio is 0.58 (0.02) and the mean (CV%) apparent volume of distribution (Vz/F) is 226 L (32.7%)). Approximately 20 different metabolites of encorafenib have been identified and are excreted to equal parts in urine and feces. Approximately only 2 and 5% of the absorbed encorafenib are excreted unchanged in urine and feces, respectively. The median (range) encorafenib terminal half-life (T1/2) was 6 h. The half-maximal inhibitory concentration (IC50) of encorafenib against BRAF V600E, BRAF, and CRAF enzymes is 0.35, 0.47, and 0.30 nM, respectively.

Elimination of encorafenib occurs mainly through metabolism via cytochrome P450 (CYP) enzymes (CYP3A4, CYP2C19, and CYP2D6), and the drug is a relatively potent reversible inhibitor of UGT1A1, CYP2B6, CYP2C9, and CYP3A4/5, and induces CYP1A2, CYP2B6, CYP2C9, and CYP3A4. Encorafenib was found to be a substrate of the P-glycoprotein (P-gp) transporters. Food intake delays the absorption of encorafenib but does not alter overall drug exposure. Hence, encorafenib capsules are allowed to be ingested regardless of food consumption. In vitro, encorafenib inhibited the hepatic transporter OCT1, but is unlikely to be an effective inhibitor clinically. Based on a population pharmacokinetic analysis, age was found to be a significant covariate on encorafenib volume of distribution; however, due to high variability, these findings are unlikely to be clinically meaningful. No clinically significant changes in encorafenib exposure are expected based upon gender, body weight, race, or ethnicity. The higher total encorafenib exposure was observed in patients with mild hepatic impairment (Child-Pugh Class A), so patients with moderate to severe hepatic impairment may have a higher risk of toxicity than patients with mild hepatic impairment due to prolonged exposure. Therefore, in patients with moderate or severe hepatic impairment, encorafenib is not recommended. No formal clinical study has been conducted to evaluate the effect of renal impairment on the pharmacokinetics of encorafenib [6].

Binimetinib

Binimetinib is an ATP-uncompetitive, reversible inhibitor of the kinase activity of mitogen-activated extracellular signal-regulated kinase 1/2 (MEK1/2). Binimetinib is involved in upstream regulation of the extracellular signal-related kinase (ERK) pathway, and effectively inhibits the growth of BRAF- and NRAS-mutant melanoma. Pharmacokinetic (PK) data demonstrate a maximal-tolerated dose of 60 mg BID and a maximal-proposed clinical dose of 45 mg BID. After repeat twice-daily dosing concomitantly with encorafenib, steady-state conditions for binimetinib were reached within 15 days with no major accumulation. Binimetinib pharmacokinetics is dose linear and is rapidly absorbed with a median Tmax of 1.5 h. Binimetinib maximal concentration in the serum (Cmax) is 458 ng/mL with an area under the curve (AUC) of 1648 h ng/mL. A high-fat, high-calorie meal decreased Cmax, but AUC remains unchanged. PK is also not altered by a gastric pH-altering agent. Binimetinib is 97.2% bound to human plasma proteins in vitro. Following a single oral dose with C-14-labeled binimetinib, 60% of the circulating radioactivity was from the parent drug and not metabolites. Metabolites of the drug detected in human hepatocyte incubations showed products of direct glucuronidation of binimetinib as well as an N-desmethylated metabolite. In vitro, CYP1A2 and CYP2C19 catalyze the formation of the active metabolite representing <20% of the clinical binimetinib exposure. Due to no formal clinical study, UGT1A1 inducers or inhibitors should be administered with caution. Binimetinib is a weak reversible inhibitor of CYP1A2 and CYP2C9. Although in vitro experiments indicate that binimetinib is a substrate of P-glycoprotein (P-gp) and breast cancer resistance protein (BCRP), inhibition of P-gp or BCRP is unlikely to result in clinically important differences in concentrations. Elimination of the drug is approximately two-third in the feces and one-third in the urine. Based on a population pharmacokinetic analysis, age, sex, or body-weight do not have a clinically important effect on the systemic exposure of binimetinib [7].

Combination of Encorafenib and Binimetinib

Encorafenib and binimetinib both inhibit the MAPK pathway, resulting in higher antitumor activity. Additionally, the combination of encorafenib and binimetinib prevented the emergence of resistance in *BRAF V600E*-mutant human melanoma xenografts in vivo. In terms of availability, no differences in exposure have been observed clinically when binimetinib is co-administered with encorafenib, and the effects of organ impairment on the pharmacokinetics of combination have not been evaluated clinically.

Early Development

Encorafenib

The preclinical results have shown that *BRAF V600E*-mutated mouse xenograft (A375 and HMEX1906 models) showed that encorafenib effectively inhibits tumor growth at dose 5mg/kg twice daily (BID), but increased dose up to 20mg/kg is necessary to prevent the development of resistance. This finding suggested the dose-dependency of encorafenib efficacy [8].

The phase I study with 89 patients enrolled (half of the patients had already undergone pretreatment with BRAF inhibitors) proved the safety profile of encorafenib. The maximum tolerated dose (MTD) 450 mg once daily was defined; however, due to frequent occurrence of dose-limiting toxicities in the expansion cohort, 300 mg once daily was evolved as the recommended phase II dose for encorafenib monotherapy. The response rate in BRAFi-pretreated patients was 10% in the dose-escalation cohort and 22% in the extension one. The most common drug-related adverse events included nausea, myalgia, palmoplantar erythrodysesthesia, arthralgia, and hyperkeratosis. In contrast to the BRAFi, cSCC was rare (3–4% of patients) [8].

Binimetinib

In preclinical studies in vivo, binimetinib was efficient in numerous tumor xenograft models that harbor *b-Raf* or *Ras* mutations. The highest greatest preclinical efficacy was observed in melanoma. Pancreatic carcinoma, colon carcinoma, fibrosarcoma, and NSCLC (EGFR T790M) resulted in varying degrees of antitumor activity. MEK inhibitors might affect angiogenesis, and tumor cell apoptosis, by increasing the pro-apoptotic protein BIM [9, 10].

Based on the first in human study, the maximum tolerable dose (MTD) of binimetinib was assessed in a multicenter, open-label phase I study in subjects with advanced solid tumors. The study design was based on a 3 + 3 dose-escalation schema where binimetinib was administered twice daily (BID) in 21-day treatment cycles. The dose-limiting toxicity was observed in two of three evaluable subjects at 80 mg BID and the MTD was determined to be 60 mg BID in the first portion of the study. In the second expansion phase, an unexpected number of ocular toxicities was observed which prompted a dose reduction to 45 mg BID as a recommended phase II dose [11]. In a phase Ib/II, an open-label study of ribociclib + binimetinib in NRAS-mutant melanoma enrolled 14 patients. The most common treatment-related toxicities included CPK elevation, rash, edema, anemia, nausea, diarrhea, and fatigue. Six patients achieved a partial response and six had stable disease. Combined LEE011 + binimetinib showed promising preliminary antitumor activity in *NRAS*-mutant melanoma and led to further clinical trials [12].

Combination of Encorafenib and Binimetinib

Preclinical and clinical data suggested that the combination of BRAF/MEK inhibitors increased the efficacy over monotherapy, and thus may overcome/delay resistance in *BRAF*-mutant metastatic melanoma. Therefore, in phase Ib/II study was evaluated the combination of encorafenib (LGX818) and binimetinib (MEK162) to determine the maximum tolerated dose (MTD) and recommended phase II dose (RP2D). Thirty patients with solid tumours were enrolled, and there were 23 patients with melanoma [9 BRAFi-naïve, 14 BRAFi-pretreated]. The most common adverse events were nausea, diarrhea, fatigue, visual impairment, and headache. No events of fever, hyperkeratosis, or squamous cell carcinoma were observed. There was 1/9 complete response in BRAFi-naïve melanoma patients, and partial responses were observed in 7/9 (78%) BRAFi-naïve melanoma patients, 3/14 (21%) BRAFi-pretreated melanoma patients. These preliminary data indicated the need for further exploration of this combination in the phase II study (LGX818 600 mg QD + MEK162 45 mg BID).[13].

Clinical Phase II/III Studies

Activity, Efficacy, and Toxicity Profile

The LOGIC trial was an open-label, two-stage, multicenter study to evaluate the efficacy, safety profile, and MTD of encorafinib in combination with binimetinib or buparlisib, or infigratinib, or capmatinib, or ribociclib, after progression on treatment with encorafenib monotherapy. Patients diagnosed with unresectable/metastatic melanoma with confirmed *BRAF* mutation, without previous treatment with BRAFi, were recruited for the study. In Part I of the study, patients were enrolled in encorafenib monotherapy until disease progression. In Part II, after progression, the patients received encorafenib and other drugs depending on the molecular evaluation of the resistance mechanisms. Due to the small number of recruited patients (only 15), the obtained data were impossible to interpret, which did not allow for the development of reliable results [14].

The LOGIC-2 trial is similar to the LOGIC trial – patients received encorafenib and binimetinib in the first line, instead of encorafenib alone as in the LOGIC trial. After disease progression, depending on the genetic profile of the tumor, patients were assigned to one of the four arms to receive encorafenib and binimetinib and buparlisib, or infigratinib, or capmatinib, or ribociclib. The estimated completion date of this trial is June 2022 [15, 16].

In a phase III study (NEMO), the use of binimetinib at a dose of 45 mg orally twice daily was evaluated in a group of patients with unresectable stage IIIC or IV melanoma with the presence of the *NRAS* mutation (treatment-naïve patients or after prior immunotherapy) compared with dacarbazine administered 1000 mg/m^2

intravenously q3w. Patients were randomized in a 2: 1 ratio. PFS was the primary endpoint. The study included 402 patients (269 in the binimetinib group and 133 in the dacarbazine group). The median follow-up time was 1.7 months; median PFS was 2.8 months (95% CI: 2.8–3.6) in the binimetinib treatment group and 1.5 months (95% CI: 1.5–1.7) in the dacarbazine group. The median follow-up for OS was 9.2 months. At the time of analysis, the median OS for the binimetinib group was 11.0 months and for the dacarbazine group was 10.1 months. Treatment with binimetinib was associated with a higher percentage of complete responses (15% vs. 7%) and disease control (58% vs. 25%) compared to dacarbazine. In the group receiving binimetinib, adverse events in degree 3 or 4 were found in at least 5% of patients with increased CPK activity (19%) and hypertension (7%). Serious adverse events were reported in 34% of patients in the binimetinib group and 22% in the dacarbazine group. Adverse events led to dose reductions in 61% of patients receiving binimetinib. The most common adverse events are presented in Table 7.1. Despite some confirmed activity of binimetinib in the group of patients with advanced melanomas with the presence of the *NRAS* mutation and improvement of

Table 7.1 The most common adverse events in the NEMO trial [17]

Adverse event n	Binimetinib (*n* = 269)			Dacarbazine (*n* = 114)		
	Grades 1–2	Grade 3	Grade 4	Grades 1–2	Grade 3	Grade 4
Rash	87 (32%)	11 (4%)	0	1 (1%)	0	0
Dermatitis acneiform	88 (33%)	7 (3%)	0	1 (1%)	0	0
Diarrhea	104 (39%)	4 (1%)	0	12 (11%)	1 (1%)	0
Nausea	75 (28%)	4 (1%)	0	36 (32%)	1 (1%)	0
Vomiting	51 (19%)	6 (2%)	0	14 (12%)	0	0
Blood creatine phosphokinase increased	61 (23%)	33 (12%)	19 (7%)	3 (3%)	0	0
Peripheral edema	93 (36%)	1 (<1%)	0	3 (3%)	0	0
Fatigue	54 (20%)	6 (2%)	0	33 (29%)	3 (3%)	0
Asthenia	40 (15%)	8 (3%)	0	14 (12%)	5 (4%)	0
Hypertension	17 (6%)	20 (7%)	0	2 (2%)	2 (2%)	0
Aspartate aminotransferase increased	29 (11%)	6 (2%)	0	4 (4%)	0	0
Decreased appetite	29 (11%)	2 (1%)	0	17 (15%)	1 (1%)	0
Ejection fraction decreased	20 (7%)	10 (4%)	0	1 (1%)	1 (1%)	0
Alanine aminotransferase increased	15 (6%)	7 (3%)	0	5 (4%)	2 (2%)	0
General physical health deterioration	7 (3%)	9 (3%)	2 (1%)	2 (2%)	0	0
Anemia	14 (5%)	4 (1%)	1 (<1%)	5 (4%)	6 (5%)	0
Lymphopenia	3 (1%)	3 (1%)	1 (<1%)	3 (3%)	3 (3%)	0
Neutropenia	1 (<1%)	2 (1%)	0	11 (10%)	5 (4%)	5 (4%)
Thrombocytopenia	2 (1%)	0	1 (<1%)	13 (11%)	2 (2%)	2 (2%)

PFS in relation to the comparator, the results of this study did not lead to the approval of binimetinib monotherapy in this patient population [17].

In Part I of the COLUMBUS trial, 577 patients with advanced/metastatic *BRAF* V600-mutant melanoma were assigned to one of three groups in a 1:1:1 ratio: encorafenib treatment 450 mg once daily in combination with binimetinib 45 mg twice daily, encorafenib 300 mg once daily, and vemurafenib at a dose of 960 mg twice daily. They were not previously treated systemically or received first-line immunotherapy. The primary endpoint was PFS. Median PFS was independently assessed 14.9 months for encorafenib plus binimetinib combination treatment (95% CI: 11.0–18.5) compared to 7.3 months for vemurafenib monotherapy (95% CI: 5.6–8.2) and 9.6 months (95% CI: 7.5–14.8) for encorafenib monotherapy. Median PFS by local assessment was similar. The hazard ratio (HR) for the combination versus vemurafenib was 0.54 ($p = 0.001$) and 0.75 for the combination versus encorafenib ($p = 0.051$). Interestingly, this is the first study to show differences in treatment outcomes between different BRAF inhibitors (encorafenib vs. vemurafenib); this indicates the high specificity of encorafenib for inhibition of BRAF signaling.

The combination treatment with encorafenib at a dose of 450 mg daily with binimetinib at a dose of 45 mg twice daily (combo 450 mg) reduced the risk of death compared to vemurafenib at a dose of 960 mg twice daily (HR 0.61 [95% CI: 0.47–0.79], $p < 0.001$). The median OS was 33.6 months (95% CI: 24.4–39.2) for patients treated with combo 450 mg compared with 16.9 months (95% CI: 14.0–24.5) for patients treated with monotherapy with vemurafenib. The 3-year OS rate for the combination of encorafenib and binimetinib was 47%. Combination therapy was well tolerated and slightly different from other anti-BRAF/MEK combination therapies. Adverse events reported more frequently in the encorafenib–binimetinib combination group included gastrointestinal side effects (diarrhea, constipation, vomiting, and abdominal pain), increased CPK activity (mainly asymptomatic), and blurred vision. Adverse events reported at a lower frequency in the group with combination therapy than in cohorts treated with BRAF inhibitors monotherapy were skin-related adverse events (such as pruritus, hyperkeratosis, rash, palmar-plantar erythrodysesthesia syndrome, dry skin, sunburn, skin warts), alopecia, photosensitivity reactions, joint, and muscle pain, decreased appetite, and weight gain. Grade 3–4 adverse events were reported in fewer patients in the encorafenib plus binimetinib group (58%) than in either the encorafenib (66%) or vemurafenib (63%) groups. The most common adverse events reported in the combination therapy group were: increased level of gamma-glutamyl transpeptidase (9%) and hypertension (6%). Adverse events requiring dose reduction or dose interruption were reported in 48% of patients with combination therapy, 70% with encorafenib monotherapy, and 61% with vemurafenib monotherapy. Fever occurred less frequently with the combination of encorafenib with binimetinib (18%) and with encorafenib monotherapy (16%) than with vemurafenib (30%). Discontinuation of treatment related to adverse events occurred in a similar percentage of patients with combination therapy and with encorafenib monotherapy (13%). Adverse events specific to MEK inhibition, such as exudative serous retinopathy (20%) and left ventricular

Table 7.2 The most common adverse events in the COLUMBUS trial (arms with encorafenib) [18–21]

Adverse event %	Encorafenib 300 mg + binimetinib (*n* = 257)		Encorafenib 300 mg (*n* = 276)		Encorafenib 450 mg + binimetinib (*n* = 192)	
	All grades	Grades 3–4	All grades	Grades 3–4	All grades	Grades 3–4
Rash	15	1	43	5	23	1
Diarrhea	28	2	12	1	36	3
Nausea	27	2	36	3	41	2
Vomiting	15	<1	25	4	30	2
Blood creatine phosphokinase increased	20	5	1	0	23	7
Pyrexia	17	0	16	0	18	4
Fatigue	22	1	26	1	29	2
Dry skin	8	0	28	0	14	0
γ-glutamyltransferase increased	14	5	11	4	15	9
Hyperkeratosis	10	0	39	3	14	1
Ejection fraction decreased	6	1	3	1	8	2
Alanine aminotransferase increased	11	5	4	1	13	6
Palmoplantar erythrodysesthesia syndrome	4	<1	47	11	7	0
Joint pain	22	1	43	8	26	1
Alopecia	13	0	49	<1	14	0

dysfunction (2%), occurred more frequently with combination therapy (details are provided in Table 7.2). Based on the presented results, the combination treatment with encorafenib and binimetinib was registered by the Food and Drug Administration (FDA) in the United States in June 2018 [18–20].

Part II of the COLUMBUS study was designed to assess the contribution of binimetinib to the encorafenib and binimetinib combination. Patients were treated with encorafenib at a dose of 300 mg once a day and with binimetinib 45 mg twice daily (*n* = 258) with encorafenib monotherapy at a dose of 300 mg once a day (*n* = 86; in total, 280 patients were treated with encorafenib monotherapy in Parts I and II). The median PFS for the combination with encorafenib 300 mg was 12.9 months (95% CI: 10.1–14.0)—which suggests a dose-dependency of the BRAF inhibitor in combination therapy in favor of the dose used in Part I of the study—and was significantly longer than with encorafenib monotherapy 9.2 months (95% CI: 7.4, 11.0) (HR 0.77; *p* = 0.029). The confirmed ORR was 65.9% (95% CI: 59.8, 71.7) for combination therapy and 50.4% (95% CI: 44.3, 56.4) for encorafenib 300 mg (Parts I and II) [21] (See Table 7.3).

Table 7.3 The summary of the COLUMBUS trial results [18–21]

	Encorafenib 450 mg + binimetinib ($n = 192$)		Encorafenib 300 mg + binimetinib ($n = 258$)		Encorafenib 300 mg (Part I and II) ($n = 280$)		Vemurafenib ($n = 191$)	
	Central assessment	Local assessment	Central assessment	Local assessment	Central assessment	Local assessment	Central assessment	Local assessment
Median PFS (95% CI) (months)	14.9 (11.0–18.5)	14.8 (10.4–18.4)	12.9 (10.1–14.0)	12.9 (10.9–14.8)	9.2 (7.4–11.0)	9.2 (7.4–11.1)	7.3 (5.6–8.2)	7.3 (5.7–8.5)
ORR (95% CI) (%)	63 (56–70)	75 (68–81)	66 (60–72)	73 (67–78)	50 (44–56)	56 (50–62)	40 (33–48)	49 (42–57)
CR (%)	8	16	8	11	5	8	6	7
PR (%)	55	59	58	62	45	49	35	42
Median DOR (95% CI) (months)	16.6 (12.2–20.4)	16.2 (11.1–20.4)	12.7 (9.3–15.1)	13.1 (10.8–16.6)	12.9 (8.9–15.5)	13.0 (9.5–15.0)	12.3 (6.9–16.9)	8.4 (5.8–11.0)

CR complete response, *PFS* progression-free survival, *PR* partial response, *ORR* overall response rate, *DOR* duration of response

Approval and Regulatory Indications

Encorafenib (450 mg once daily) in combination with binimetinib is indicated for the treatment of adult patients with unresectable or metastatic melanoma with a *BRAF V600* mutation.

Encorafenib (300 mg once daily) in combination with cetuximab is indicated for the treatment of adult patients with metastatic colorectal cancer (CRC) with a *BRAF V600E* mutation, who have received prior unsuccessful systemic therapy.

Summary

The BRAF/MEK inhibitors, encorafenib and binimetinib, is the third FDA/EMA-approved combination used in *BRAF*-positive melanoma. The phase III study showed a very good safety profile and improvement in PFS and OS. A direct comparison of monotherapy showed better results in the arm with encorafenib over vemurafenib. It could be associated with the longest half-life of encorafenib dissociation among BRAF inhibitors.

Nowadays, in the *BRAF*-mutated melanoma patients receiving a combination of BRAF/MEK inhibitors, the median overall survival is more than 2 years and the median progression-free survival is 11–14 months. The rapid responses are observed on the therapy with BRAF/MEK inhibitors in melanomas; however, due to activation of the mechanism of resistance, duration of response is limited. Therefore, BRAF/MEK inhibitors should be considered as the first choice in patients with symptomatic disease and/or a high tumor burden, as well as the results from the randomized phase III trials assessing the sequence of target therapy over immunotherapy are urgently needed. The therapy with BRAF/MEK inhibitors is recommended by the European Society for Medical Oncology (ESMO), National Comprehensive Cancer Network (NCCN), and national guidelines as an option in selected clinical situations in melanoma patients with *BRAF*-positive mutation [1, 3, 5].

References

1. Rutkowski P, Wysocki PJ, Nasierowska-Guttmejer A, et al. Cutaneous melanomas. Oncol Clin Pract. 2019:15. https://doi.org/10.5603/OCP.2018.0055.
2. Rutkowski P. (red.). Nowe terapie w czerniakach. Wyd. 2. Via Medica, Gdańsk; 2017.
3. NCCN Clinical Practice Guidelines in Oncology. Melanoma v. 2. 2019.
4. Dummer R, Ascierto PA, Gogas HJ, et al. Encorafenib plus binimetinib versus vemurafenib or encorafenib in patients with BRAF-mutant melanoma (COLUMBUS): a multicentre, open-label, randomized phase 3 trial. Lancet Oncol. 2018;19(5):603–15.
5. Grob JJ. Is there any interest in a new BRAF–MEK inhibitor combination in melanoma? Lancet Oncol. 2018;19(5):P580–1.

6. https://www.ema.europa.eu/en/medicines/human/EPAR/braftovi#product-information-section
7. https://www.ema.europa.eu/en/medicines/human/EPAR/mektovi#product-information-section
8. Delord JP, Robert C, Nyakas M, et al. Phase I dose-escalation and -expansion study of the BRAF inhibitor encorafenib (LGX818) in metastatic *BRAF*-mutant melanoma. Clin Cancer Res. 2017;23(18):5339–48.
9. Winski S, Anderson D, Bouhana K, et al. MEK162 (ARRY-162), a novel MEK ½ inhibitor, inhibits tumor growth regardless of KRas/Raf pathway mutations. http://www.arraybiopharma.com
10. Lee P, Wallace E, Marlow A, et al. Preclinical development of ARRY-162, a potent and selective MEK 1/2 inhibitor. http://www.arraybiopharma.com
11. Bendell J, Papadopoulos K, Jones S, et al. A phase 1 dose-escalation study of MEK inhibitor MEK162 (ARRY-438162) in patients with advanced solid tumors. AACR-NCI-EORTC 2011.
12. Sosman JA, Kittaneh M, Lolkema MP, et al. A phase 1b/2 study of LEE011 in combination with Binimetinib (MEK162) in patients with advanced *NRAS*-mutant melanoma: early encouraging clinical activity. Chicago: ASCO; 2014.
13. Kefford R, Sullivan RJ, Miller WH Jr, et al. Phase Ib/II, open-label, dose-escalation study of LGX818, an oral selective BRAF inhibitor, in combination with MEK162, an oral MEK1/2 inhibitor, in patients with BRAF V600-dependent advanced solid tumors: preliminary results. J Transl Med. 2014;12(Suppl 1):6.
14. Biopharma A. LGX818 in combination with agents (MEK162; BKM120; LEE011; BGJ398; INC280) in advanced BRAF melanoma (LOGIC). https://clinicaltrials.gov/ct2/show/NCT01820364
15. Dummer R, Sandhu S, Hassel JC et al. LOGIC2: Phase 2, multi-center, open-la-bel study of sequential encorafenib/binimetinib combination followed by a rational combination with targeted agents after progression, to overcome resistance in adult patients with locally advanced or metastatic. ESMO 2015, Denver Post P187.
16. Biopharma A. LGX818 and MEK162 in combination with a third agent (BKM120, LEE011, BGJ398 or INC280) in advanced BRAF melanoma (LOGIC-2). https://clinical-trials.gov/ct2/show/NCT02159066
17. Dummer R, Schadendorf D, Ascierto PA, et al. Binimetinib versus dacarbazine in patients with advanced NRAS-mutant melanoma (NEMO): a multicentre, open-label, randomised, phase 3 trial. Lancet Oncol. 2017;18(4):435–45.
18. Dummer R, Ascierto PA, Gogas HJ, et al. Encorafenib plus binimetinib versus vemurafenib or encorafenib in patients with BRAF-mutant melanoma (COLUMBUS): a multicentre, open-label, randomised phase 3 trial. Lancet Oncol. 2018;19(5):603–15.
19. Dummer R, Ascierto PA, Gogas H, et al. Overall survival in COLUMBUS: a phase 3 trial of encorafenib (ENCO) plus binimetinib (BINI) vs vemurafenib (VEM) or enco in BRAF-mutant melanoma. J Clin Oncol. 2018;36(suppl):9504.
20. Dummer R, Ascierto PA, Gogas H i w. Overall survival in patients with BRAF-mutant melanoma receiving encorafenib plus binimetinib versus vemurafenib or encorafenib (COLUMBUS): a multicentre, open-label, randomised, phase 3 trial. Lancet Oncol. 2018;19(10):1315–27.
21. Dummer R, Ascierto PA, Gogas HJ. i wsp. Results of COLUMBUS Part 2: a phase 3 trial of encorafenib plus binimetinib versus encorafenib in BRAFmutant melanoma. ESMO Congress 2017, Madrid.

Chapter 8
Vismodegib

Monika Dudzisz-Śledź and Piotr Rutkowski

Pharmacological Properties and Early Development

Vismodegib (GDC-0449) is a small molecule inhibitor of smoothened, a key component of the hedgehog (Hh) signaling pathway [1]. Hh signaling pathway is a key regulator of cell growth and differentiation. Hh pathway is inactive in most normal adult tissues, and this pathway reactivation is involved in the pathogenesis of several malignancies [2]. The transmembrane receptor patched (PTCH) is a negative regulator of the transmembrane receptor smoothened (SMO). PTCH is the receptor for the Hh ligand and inhibits SMO until the Hh ligand binds, allowing SMO to signal. Signaling by SMO results in activation of GLI (glioma-associated oncogene) transcription factors and induction of Hh target genes, including *GLI1* and *PTCH1* [3, 4]. Vismodegib is an SMO inhibitor (GDC-0449; 2-chloro-N-[4-chloro-3-pyridin-2-yl-phenyl]-4-methanesulfonyl benzamide, molecular weight 421.30 g/mol) that blocks Hh signaling by binding to SMO and inhibiting activation of downstream Hh target genes. It was developed by high throughput screening of a small molecule compound library and subsequently optimization through medicinal chemistry [1, 3]. Vismodegib is about 10 times more potent than the natural product SMO antagonist, cyclopamine, at inhibiting Hh pathway activity [5].

The antitumor activity of vismodegib has been shown in a mouse model of medulloblastoma and in primary human tumor cell xenograft models, including colorectal and pancreatic cancer [1, 3, 6].

The safety of vismodegib was assessed in the open-label, multicenter, two-stage phase 1 study in patients with solid tumors refractory to current therapies or for

M. Dudzisz-Śledź (✉) · P. Rutkowski
Department of Soft Tissue/Bone Sarcoma and Melanoma, Maria Sklodowska-Curie National Research Institute of Oncology, Warsaw, Poland
e-mail: monika.dudzisz-sledz@pib-nio.pl

P. Rutkowski, M. Mandalà (eds.), *New Therapies in Advanced Cutaneous Malignancies*, https://doi.org/10.1007/978-3-030-64009-5_8

which no standard therapy existed ($n = 68$) [1, 7–9]. The patients received vismodegib at 150 mg/d ($n = 41$), 270 mg/d ($n = 23$), or 540 mg/d ($n = 4$). The purpose of this study was to assess the safety, tumor responses, pharmacokinetics, and pharmacodynamic down-modulation of *GLI1* expression in noninvolved skin. Thirty-three patients had metastatic (mBCC) or locally advanced basal cell carcinoma (laBCC), and 35 had other solid tumors (8 pancreatic cancer, 3 colorectal cancer, 3 mesothelioma, 3 small cell lung cancer, 1 medulloblastoma and others); 95.5% were ECOG 0–1 and 4.5% were ECOG 2. The majority of patients were previously treated with surgery (98.5%), radiotherapy (52.9%), and/or systemic therapy (70.6%). Median age was 54 (range 26–84). Stage 1 of this study was a dose escalation phase, designed to estimate the maximum tolerated dose (MTD) of vismodegib. Patients received a single oral dose of vismodegib on day 1, followed by daily administration at the same dose beginning on day 8. Seven patients received vismodegib in dose 150 mg/d, 9 received 270 mg/d, and 4 received 540 mg/d. The treatment was discontinued in case of dose-limiting toxicities, other intolerable side effects, disease progression (PD), and lack of benefit from treatment, based on the investigator's decision. Part 2 of this study included an expansion cohort of 12 patients with solid tumors (none with BCC) who started continuous daily dosing at 150 mg/d on day 1, to assess the safety profile, pharmacokinetics, and pharmacodynamics of vismodegib. Based on the study protocol amendment, additional 2 cohorts were added. One cohort ($n = 16$, including 10 with advanced BCC), to investigate pharmacokinetic properties of a new vismodegib formulation at 150 mg/d; and second cohort ($n = 20$) with advanced BCC who received vismodegib at the dose 150 or 270 mg/d, to evaluate safety and efficacy, based on encouraging response of 2 patients in stage 1 with advanced BCC. Patients were treated until PD, unacceptable toxicity, or study withdrawal. The safety assessment was done based on the National Cancer Institute's Common Terminology Criteria for Adverse Events, version 3.0 (NCI-CTCAE v. 3.0). The efficacy was assessed according to the Response Evaluation Criteria in Solid Tumors version 1.0 (RECIST v. 1.0) in patients with measurable disease. The radiology assessment was done at baseline and then every 8 weeks. For patients with laBCC with radiographically nonmeasurable lesions, tumors were assessed by physical examination. A complete response (CR) was defined as complete disappearance of a palpable or visible lesions and a partial response (PR) was defined as a reduction of more than 50% in the diameter of a palpable or visible lesions. For pharmacokinetics assessment, baseline and weekly plasma samples were collected from patients in stages 1 and 2 of this study for the first 4 weeks, and then at monthly intervals. Total and unbound plasma levels of vismodegib were determined using liquid chromatography-tandem mass spectrometry. The steady-state levels of GDC-0449 (Css) were calculated by averaging all available concentrations after 21 days of daily dosing. For pharmacodynamic assessment of *GLI1* expression, RNA was extracted from biopsy specimens of noninvolved skin or hair follicles at baseline and at 7 and 21 days after the start of daily dosing. Expression of *GLI1* was assessed using quantitative real-time polymerase chain reaction (qRT-PCR) assay. The role of vismodegib binding to plasma protein alpha-1-acid glycoprotein (AAG) was also studied.

Vismodegib was generally well-tolerated. No dose-limiting toxicities were observed. The most frequently reported adverse events (AEs), observed in $\geq$30% of patients, were muscle spasms, dysgeusia, fatigue, alopecia, and nausea. Grade (G) 5 (fatal) AEs related to PD were reported in 5 patients. No other G5 AEs were reported. G4 AEs were reported in 6 patients (8.8%): hyponatremia, fatigue, pyelonephritis, presyncope, paranoia, and hyperglycemia. In one patient with mBCC with prior history of testicular cancer, papillary thyroid carcinoma, and mucoepidermoid carcinoma, G4 resectable pancreatic adenocarcinoma was newly diagnosed during treatment with vismodegib, but this AE was assessed as unrelated to study treatment by the treating physician. 29.4% of patients experienced G3 AEs, and the most common G3 AEs were hyponatremia (7 patients), abdominal pain (5), and fatigue (4). Hyponatremia and fatigue were generally reversible with temporary discontinuation of the study drug.

In this study, responses were only observed in patients with advanced BCC or medulloblastoma. The overall response rate (ORR = CR + PR) in advanced BCC was 58% (19 of 33). One patient with medulloblastoma had response to treatment. Four patients with other solid tumors achieved stable disease (SD) as the best response: 2 with adenocystic carcinoma, 1 with pancreatic carcinoma, and 1 with metastatic carcinoid.

Pharmacokinetics studies showed that with multiple daily dosing, all doses showed similar steady-state concentrations. An unusual pharmacokinetic profile with an unexplained elimination half-life of more than 7 days and accumulation that unexpectedly reached a pleteau within the first 14 days was found and further studied [9]. The recommended phase II dose was established at 150 mg/d [1]. Analysis of tissue (normal skin punch biopsies and hair follicles) on day 7 or 21 after the initiation of therapy showed down-modulation of *GLI1* mRNA expression compared with *GLI1* expression in pretreatment tissue specimens [1].

Activity and Efficacy

The efficacy of vismodegib in BCC was assessed in pivotal phase IIb study ERIVANCE and in two other phase II studies, STEVIE and MIKIE [10–13].

ERIVANCE was a nonrandomized, single-arm, multicenter, international, pivotal, phase IIb clinical trial assessing the efficacy and safety of vismodegib 150 mg in patients with laBCC and mBCC (NCT00833417) [10, 14]. ORR by central review was the primary endpoint. The response was assessed by central and investigator review based on RECIST v. 1.0. The secondary endpoints were objective response rate (ORR) by investigator review, duration of response (DOR), progression-free survival (PFS), overall survival (OS), safety and quality of life (QoL). The safety assessment was done based on NCI-CTCAE v. 3.0 and included treatment-emergent adverse events (TEAEs), defined as AEs occurring between the first administration of vismodegib and 30 days after the last dose. In the primary analysis of the ERIVANCE BCC study, the ORR based on independent review was 30% in mBCC and 43% in laBCC. ORR by investigator review was 45% in mBCC and 60% in laBCC patients. Finally a total of 104 patients, 33 with mBCC, and 71 with laBCC were enrolled into this study. At the data cut off (39 months after completion of accrual), 8 patients (8%) were treated with vismodegib and continued study procedures, and 69 patients (66%) remained in survival follow-up. Ninety-six patients discontinued treatment, mostly due to PD (27.9%), patient decision (26.0%), and AEs (21.2%). In this updated analysis including final efficacy data and long-term safety data investigator-assessed ORR was 48.5% in the mBCC group (all PR) and 60.3% in the laBCC group. At the data cut off, 97.7% of mBCC and 90.1% of laBCC patients discontinued the study. Median duration of treatment with vismodegib was 12.9 months in the mBCC group and 12.7 months in the laBCC group. Median time to overall response was 57.0 days in the mBCC cohort and 140.0 days in the laBCC cohort. The median PFS was 9.3 months for patients with mBCC and 12.9 months for those with laBCC. All patients experienced ≥ 1 TEAE. G $\geq$ 3 AEs were reported in more than half of the patients ($n = 58$, 55.8%). The most frequent AE with G at least 3 were weight decrease (8.7%), and muscle spasms (5.8%) followed by fatigue, decreased appetite, diarrhea, and squamous cell cancer (SCC). Patients who received vismodegib for more than 12 months experienced more TEAEs ($n = 56$) (muscle spasms, alopecia, dysgeusia, weight decreased, fatigue, and nausea) compared to patients with <12 months treatment duration.

The efficacy of vismodegib in BCC has been confirmed in the post-approval single-arm, multicenter, open label phase II study (NCT01367665) [12, 15, 16]. Patients with laBCC and mBCC not eligible for surgery or radiotherapy, without other satisfactory treatment options, were enrolled into this study. The patients received vismodegib at the daily dose 150 mg, in 28-days cycles, until PD or unacceptable toxicity, withdrawal of consent, death, or other reasons based on the investigator's decision. The primary objective was safety assessed by the investigators on day 1 of each cycle based on NCI-CTCAE v. 4.0. Secondary endpoints included investigator-assessed objective response based on clinical assessments according to RECIST v. 1.1, DOR, time to response, PFS, OS, and QoL assessed by Skindex-16. Measurable tumors accessible by physical examination were assessed every 4–8 weeks and CT or MRI scans were done every 8–16 weeks if necessary. Eligible patients were aged 18 years or older with histologically confirmed (per local guidelines) laBBC or mBCC, ECOG 0–2 with adequate organ function. Patients with Gorlin-Goltz syndrome (GGS) could be enrolled if all other criteria were met. Median duration of treatment was 8.6 (0–44) months. Response rates based on investigator's assessment in patients with histologically confirmed measurable disease at baseline were 68.5% (95% CI: 65.7–71.3) in patients with laBCC and 36.9% (95% CI: 26.6–48.1) in patients with mBCC. The safety profile was comparable to that in the ERIVANCE study. Most patients (98%) had at least 1 TEAE. Serious TEAEs occurred in 289 patients (23.8%). TEAE were the main reason for treatment discontinuation. TEAE leading to treatment discontinuation were mostly G1 and G2. The most common (>20% incidence) TEAEs were muscle spasms (807), alopecia (747), dysgeusia (663), decreased weight (493), decreased appetite (303) and asthenia (291). Longer exposure (>12 months) was not correlated with increased incidence or severity of new TEAEs. No association between increased creatine phosphokinase (CPK) activity and muscle spasm was observed. The majority of the most common TEAEs ongoing at time of treatment discontinuation resolved by 12 next months. The safety was similar in patients with and without GGS.

A review of the QoL outcomes was published in 2018. The QoL was assessed based on the Skindex-16 scale [16]. Skindex-16 is a 16-item questionnaire covering 3 domains: emotion, symptom and function. Median change from baseline (each domain) was assessed at Cycle 2 Day 1, Cycle 7 Day 1, and the end of study in all patients and subgroups (by sex, age, lesion location). Negative changes $\geq$10 points indicated a clinically meaningful improvement. Treatment with vismodegib was associated with clinically meaningful improvement in the emotional domain in all subgroups at all time points in laBCC. Emotion scores were consistent with clinical response. Symptom scores in the overall population were maintained through end of study, clinically meaningful improvements were observed at Cycle 7 Day 1 in patients aged 65 years and females and at Cycle 2 Day 1 and end of study in patients with lesion locations other than head/neck. No clinically meaningful improvements were seen for function scores in patients with laBCC, or for any domain scores at any time point in patients with mBCC.

The analysis done based on Italian subgroup of patients enrolled into this study showed a safety profile consistent with the whole population [17]. Among 182 Italian patients, adverse events occurred with similar incidence to the overall population. Overall response rate was 67.1% in laBCC, 20% in metastatic BCC; CR rate was 33.1% overall and 37.4% in laBCC. Median time to response was 2 months in patients with CR versus 3.6 months overall. Quality of life improved from baseline.

The efficacy of vismodegib based on studies ERIVANCE and STEVIE is summarized in Table 8.1.

The MIKIE study (NCT01815840) was designed to assess different dosing schedules of vismodegib. In this study, patients with BCC and BCC were randomized 1:1 to vismodegib 150 mg once daily in an intermittent schedule of 12 weeks vismodegib followed by 8 weeks placebo (group A, $n = 116$) or 24 weeks induction followed by an intermittent schedule of 8 weeks placebo followed by 8 weeks vismodegib (group B, $n = 113$) [13]. The eligible patients were at least 18 years old, with multiple BCC, including participants with GGS, with at least 6 clinically evident BCC lesions, ECOG 0–2, with adequate organ function. The primary endpoint was percentage reduction from baseline in the number of clinically evident basal cell carcinomas at week 73. The secondary endpoints were safety, discontinuation of treatment, reduction in the total size of the three target lesions (based on the sum of the longest diameters), at least 50% reduction in the number of BCC lesions, number of new BCC lesions at week 73, and disease recurrence. The tumor responses were assessed by the investigator by physical examination and counts of basal cell carcinomas every 8 weeks. The laboratory tests were done every 8 weeks. Adverse events were assessed at visits every 4 weeks. The median duration of treatment was 71.4 weeks in treatment group A and 68.4 weeks in treatment group B. The mean number of BCC lesions at week 73 was reduced from baseline by 62.7% (95% CI 53.0–72.3) in group A and 54.0% (43.6–64.4) in group B. Treatment

Table 8.1 Efficacy of vismodegib based on ERIVANCE and STEVIE studies results [12, 14]

	ERIVANCE mBCC (long-term analysis)	ERIVANCE laBCC (long-term analysis)	STEVIE mBCC	STEVIE laBCC
n	33	63	84	1077
ORR, n (%) [95% CI]	16 (48.5) [30.8–66.2]	38 (60.3) [47.2–71.7]	31 (36.9) [26.6–48.1]	738 (68.5) [65.7–71.3]
CR	0	20	4	360
PR	16	18	27	378
SD	14	15	39	270
PD	2	6	9	21
DOR, median, months [95% CI]	14.8 [5.6–17.0]	26.2 [9.0–37.6]	13.9 [9.2–NE]	23.0 [20.4–26.7]
PFS, median, months	9.3 [7.4–16.6]	12.9 [10.2–28.0]	13.1 [12.0–17.7]	23.2 [21.4–26.0]
OS, median, [95% CI]	33.4 [18.1–NE]	NE [NE]	NA	NA
1-year survival rate, %	78.7	93.2	NA	NA
2-year survival rate,5	62.3%	85.5%	NA	NA

CI confidence interval, *NE* not estimable, *CR* complete response, *PR* partial response, *SD* stable disease, *PD* progressive disease, *OS* overall survival, *PFS* progression free survival, *laBCC* locally advanced basal cell carcinoma, *mBCC* metastatic basal cell carcinoma, *ND* no data available, *DOR* duration of response

tolerability was similar in both groups. Treatment was discontinued in 50 patients in group A (44%) and 57 patients in group B (50%). The main reason for the discontinuation of study treatment in both groups were TEAEs. Overall, 53 (23%) of 229 patients discontinued study treatment due to AEs. More patients in treatment group B (30) discontinued the study due to AEs than patients in treatment group A (23). The most common treatment-related AEs G at least 3 were muscle spasms in 4 patients in treatment group A and in 12 patients in treatment group B, increased blood CPK (1 vs. 4) and hypophosphatemia (0 vs. 3). Serious TEAEs were noted in 22 patients in treatment group A and in 19 patients in treatment group B. This study results indicate that intermittent treatment of patients with multiple BCC with vismodegib could be a useful therapeutic option.

The efficacy and safety results of BCC treatment with vismodegib from clinical trials have been confirmed with data from clinical practice.

In 2014, the results of open-label, multicenter expanded access study (EAS) in patients with advanced BCC not eligible for radiotherapy or surgery ($n = 119$) were published (NCT01160250) [18]. Patients were treated with vismodegib in a dose 150 mg daily until PD or intolerable toxicity. The median age of patients was 62 years (24–100), 61.0 (26–92) in the laBCC group ($n = 62$) and 63.0 (24–100) in the mBCC group ($n = 57$). The median duration of treatment was 5.5 months. Objective responses were observed in 46.4% of evaluable patients with laBCC

(n = 56) and 30.8% of patients with mBCC (n = 39). Median (range) time to objective response was 2.6 months (1.0–11.0) for laBCC patients and 2.6 (1.4–12.6) for patients with mBCC. Response was negatively associated with prior systemic therapy in patients with laBCC (p = 0.002). Mean follow-up for safety was 6.5 months. The most common AEs reported in this study were muscle spasms (70.6%), dysgeusia (70.6%), alopecia (58.0%), and diarrhea (25.2%).

In 2015, the preliminary effectiveness and safety in the first 66 newly diagnosed locally advanced basal cell carcinoma (BCC) patients treated with vismodegib from the RegiSONIC disease registry were published [19]. RegiSONIC (NCT01604252) is a multicenter prospective observational cohort study designed to collect real-world data on the diagnosis and treatment of patients with advanced BCC (aBCC) and/or Gorlin-Goltz syndrome (GGS). Patients were enrolled into 3 cohorts: newly diagnosed (vismodegib-naive) aBCC patients, aBCC patients who previously received vismodegib in a Genentech-sponsored study, or patients with GGS who have aBCC or multiple BCCs of any stage. The efficacy was assessed based on investigator assessment. The patients were followed up every 3 months. By September 12, 2014, a total of 285 non-GGS newly diagnosed laBCC patients were enrolled. The median age of the patients was 68 years. Sixty-six (23%) patients were treated with vismodegib. The median (follow-up was 13.2 months (0.16–26.8). The ORR was 68% (95% CI: 56–79), CR was achieved in 29 patients (44%), PR in 16 (24%). The DOR was 5.95 months (0.03–22.08). AEs were reported in 53 patients (80%) and were consistent with known safety profile of vismodegib and included ageusia/dysgeusia, muscle spasms, alopecia, and weight loss. Eight serious adverse events (SAEs) were reported, and 9 AEs were leading to treatment discontinuation. All AEs leading to treatment discontinuation and 1 SAE (acute renal failure) were considered related to vismodegib.

Many patients with unresectable BCC are aged ≥65 years. To assess the safety and efficacy of vismodegib in the patients at least 65 years old, Chang et al. analyzed and published the data from 2 clinical trials: ERIVANCE and EAS [20]. In the ERIVANCE study, 33 (46%) patients with laBCC and 14 (42%) patients with mBCC were aged ≥65 years. In the EAS, 27 (43%) patients with laBCC and 26 (46%) patients with mBCC were aged ≥65 years. Comorbidities were more frequent in older patients. Median duration of treatment in patients with aBCC aged ≥65 years and <65 years were 9.2 and 10.2 months in ERIVANCE BCC, respectively, and 5.5 and 5.4 months in the EAS, respectively. The efficacy of vismodegib was similar across analyzed cohorts. In the ERIVANCE study, the investigator-assessed best ORR was 46.7% and 72.7% in patients with laBCC aged ≥65 and <65 years, respectively. In the EAS, the best ORR was 45.8% and 46.9% in patients with laBCC aged ≥65 and <65 years, respectively. Among patients with mBCC, the best ORR was 35.7% and 52.6% in patients aged ≥65 and <65 years, respectively, in the ERIVANCE BCC study, and 33.3% and 28.6% in patients aged ≥65 and <65 years, respectively in the EAS. In both studies, the treatment tolerability was similar in patients aged ≥65 and <65 years. No new safety signals were found. This analysis confirmed similar efficacy and safety regardless of age [20].

As BCC is characteristic feature of the Gorlin-Goltz syndrome (GGS) (the nevoid basal cell carcinoma syndrome, NBCCS), vismodegib has been also tested in patients with BCC in the course of GGS. Vismodegib has been tested in patients with GGS as BCC treatment and prophylaxis in the phase II study (NCT00957229). This was a randomized, double-blind, placebo-controlled trial. The primary endpoint of this study was reduction in the incidence of new BCCs that were eligible for surgical resection with vismodegib versus placebo after 3 months. The secondary endpoints included a reduction in the rate of appearance of smaller basal-cell carcinomas on the upper back with vismodegib versus placebo, reduction in the size of existing BCCs, reduction in size of existing surgically eligible BCCs, duration of the effect against BCC after drug discontinuation, change in Hh target-gene expression in BCCs, and safety. This study has shown that vismodegib reduces the BCC tumor burden and blocks the growth of new BCCs in patients with the basal cell nevus syndrome. Forty-one patients were followed with the mean of 8 months (1–15). The rate and size of new surgically eligible BCCs were lower with vismodegib than with placebo, as was the size of existing clinically significant BCCs. In some patients, the regression of BCCs was observed. No PD was observed during treatment with vismodegib. More than half of patients receiving vismodegib (54%) had discontinued the medication due to AEs. Only 1 of 5 eligible patients was able to continue vismodegib for 18 months. Patients receiving vismodegib had more G3 or G4 AEs as compared with patients receiving placebo. After vismodegib discontinuation, dysgeusia and muscle cramps ceased within 1 month. Scalp and body hair started to regrow within 3 months [21].

In 2016, Chang et al. published the results of treatment of patients with GGS based on data from 2 clinical trials: ERIVANCE and EAS [22]. The authors assessed the best ORR and AEs in patients with advanced BCC with GGS and without GGS. In the ERIVANCE study, all patients diagnosed with GGS were in the laBCC group (22). In the EAS study, 12 patients in the laBCC group and 7 patients in the mBCC group were diagnosed with GGS. Based on the analysis of the results, the authors concluded that vismodegib demonstrated comparable efficacy and safety against BCC in patients with and without GGS. In the ERIVANCE BCC study, the investigator-assessed best ORR in patients with GGS with laBCC was 81% (95% CI: 58–95%) and in patients without GGS, it was 50% (95% CI: 34–66%). In the EAS, the best ORR was 33% (95% CI: 10–65%) in patients with GGS and 50% (95% CI: 35–65%) in patients without GGS. In the EAS, the best ORR among patients with GGS with mBCC was 50% (95% CI: 12–88%) and those without GGS had 27% (95% CI: 13–46%). No specific trends in the incidence of AEs were observed across studies. The most frequent AEs in patients with GGS were alopecia (86 and 58% in ERIVANCE BCC and in EAS, respectively), muscle spasms (77 and 63%), weight decrease (68 and 5%), and dysgeusia (59 and 74%), The most frequent AEs in patients without GGS were alopecia (57 and 58% in ERIVANCE BCC and in EAS, respectively), muscle spasms (66 and 72%), weight decrease (40 and 18%), and dysgeusia (49 and 70%).

The data about use of vismodegib in BCC in clinical practice including drug rechallenge after disease recurrence have been published based on reports from different countries [23–25].

Herms et al. (2019) published the results of an observational retrospective study conducted in nine oncodermatology sites in France. They included 119 patients with laBCC treated with vismodegib in a standard dose who discontinued treatment after reaching CR. Eighteen patients (15.5%) had GGS. Ninety-one patients (76.5%) were included in the STEVIE study, 7 (5.9%) in the MIKIE study, and 21 (17.6%) after marketed authorization in France. The primary objective was to evaluate median relapse-free survival (RFS) and secondary objectives were risk factors associated with RFS, relapse, and death and treatment modalities after relapse and their efficacy. The median RFS was 18.4 months (95% CI: 13.5–24.8 months). The RFS rate at 36 months was 35.4% (95% CI: 22.5–47.9%) for the total population and 40.0% (95% CI: 25.7–53.7%) for patients without GGS. The only variable independently associated with a higher risk of relapse was location on the limbs and trunk (hazard ratio, 2.77; 95% CI: 1.23–6.22; $p = 0.019$). 27 patients (50%) who's disease relapsed during follow-up after vismodegib discontinuation were retreated with vismodegib, with an objective response in 23 (ORR 85%; CR 37%; PR 48%) and eligibility for surgery in 24 (42%). Based on the results of this study, the authors concluded that long-term response after vismodegib discontinuation is frequently observed and most patients with disease recurrence respond to vismodegib rechallenge [25].

Bernia et al. (2018) published the results of the use of vismodegib in the treatment of advanced and/or multiple BCC at a cancer center over 5 years [24]. Twenty-two patients were treated in this site, 20 with laBCC and 2 with mBCC with lymph node involvement. The patients received oral vismodegib 150 mg/d until disease progression or unacceptable toxicity. Some patients discontinued treatment due to CR. Median follow-up was 21 months (3–59 months). The mean treatment duration was 11.8 months. Nine patients (41%) achieved CR, 10 had (45%) PR, and 3 patients had SD (14%). The ORR was 86%. Two patients relapsed after a median of 21 months. All of the patients had AEs. The main AEs were mild dysgeusia, alopecia, and muscle cramps.

The efficacy of vismodegib in clinical practice was also described in a population of 42 patients with BCC treated in Poland in three centers. This group of patients accounts for over 50% of all patients treated with vismodegib in Poland. Five of those patients were diagnosed with GGS [23]. This report was to assess the efficacy of vismodegib based on RECIST 1.1 criteria and safety with AEs reported according to CTCAE. The median of the treatment duration was 8.25 months (0.75–68); the median of the observation of patients treated for less than 12 months was 8 months (6–11), and for those treated for more than 12 months, it was 14 months (12–68). The treatment results were assessed after 6 and 12 months. This assessment was done based on data from 29 patients after 6 months and 17 patients after 12 months. CR was achieved in 3/29 (10.3%) and 3/16 (17.6%) patients after 6 and 12 months of treatment, respectively. PR was reported in 13/29 (44.8%) and 5/16 (29.4%) patients, respectively, and stable disease in 13/29 (44.8%) and 8/16 (50.0%) patients, respectively. 7/42 (16.6%) patients within the period of 3–28 months of treatment experienced PD. One patient with brain metastases died due to PD. All patients with GGS achieved a response (CR or PR). AEs were reported in 31/42 (73.8%) patients, more than one AE in a single patient was reported in 22/42 (52.3%)

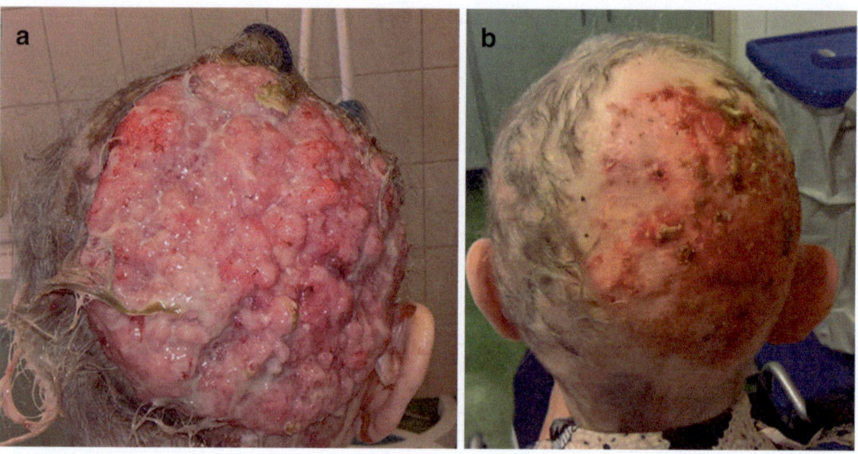

Fig. 8.1 Response to treatment with vismodegib in laBCC: (**a**) before treatment, (**b**) after few months of treatment

patients. The most frequently reported AEs were muscle cramps (in 20 patients; 47.6%), hair loss (12; 28.5%), loss of appetite (12; 28.5%), dysgeusia (10; 23.8%), asthenia/fatigue (5; 11.9%), body weight loss (4; 9.5%), increased creatine kinase level (3; 7.1%), and nausea (2; 4.7%). No serious adverse events were reported [23]. The example of substantial response to vismodegib treatment in patients with laBCC treated in Department of Soft Tissue/Bone Sarcoma and Melanoma, Maria Sklodowska-Curie National Research Institute of Oncology, Warsaw, Poland is shown in Fig. 8.1.

Due to tolerability issues, the patients often require treatment interruption and appropriate management of AEs. The most common AEs seen with vismodegib in the ERIVANCE and STEVIE trials were muscle spasms, alopecia, taste disturbance (dysgeusia and ageusia), fatigue, nausea, and weight loss. In the US RegiSONIC study, the most common AEs (any grade) reported by patients who were treated with vismodegib were muscle spasms, taste disturbances, and alopecia. AEs associated with vismodegib are generally seen early in the treatment course. These common AEs are class-specific. They are assigned to the role of the Hh signaling pathway in muscle metabolism and in the renewal of progenitor cells as part of natural cell turnover. Muscle spasms were reported by 71.2% of patients in the ERIVANCE study, 64% in the STEVIE study, and 47% in the RegiSONIC study. Median time to onset of muscle spasms was 1.9, 2.8, and 1.3 months in the ERIVANCE (12-month update), STEVIE and RegiSONIC studies, respectively. Taste disturbance was reported by more than 50% of patients in clinical trials. Taste disturbances were typically seen within 1–2 months, and alopecia was often reported about 3 months after vismodegib treatment was started. Most AEs related to treatment with vismodegib are mild or moderate, but they can substantially impact patient's QoL. They also impact the treatment tolerability and continuation. Most of them resolve after stopping of vismodegib treatment. Treatment breaks can be needed to improve the tolerance [26]. In the STEVIE study, 368 of 499 assessed patients (74%) had not treatment break due to AEs, 76 patients (15%) had one break, 41 (8%) had two treatment breaks, and 14 (3%) had three or more breaks due to AEs.

Hanke et al. summarized and published the results of treatment of 321 patients with BCC treated with vismodegib in clinical practice in the United States. It was longitudinal, retrospective cohort study to investigate the treatment patterns and characteristics of patients treated with vismodegib in clinical practice. The data were taken from a US commercial insurance claims database. Eligible patients were adult patients with at least 1 claim for vismodegib from January 2012 to December 2015. 47% of patients underwent surgery and 36% of patients were treated with radiotherapy within the 6 months before and after vismodegib initiation. About 20% of the patients required one or more treatment breaks of ≥30 days each before treatment discontinuation. Median duration of vismodegib treatment before the first treatment break was 4.0 months and before discontinuation was 5.5 months. Older age (>65 years) and absence of GGS were associated with increased risk for treatment interruption or discontinuation [27].

The important question is whether the patient can discontinue treatment after CR on vismodegib with the option to rechallenge in case of PD. Interesting results of retrospective analysis of treatment of 27 patients with BCC with vismodegib were published in 2020 by Eecke et al. [28]. The authors analyzed the efficacy and safety data after long-term follow-up of patients treated with vismodegib for aBCC in one center. They focused on underlying genetic mechanisms of primary and secondary resistance to vismodegib. The targeted sequencing of Hh pathway genes in seven tumor samples from 4 patients with primary or secondary resistance to vismodegib was conducted. The patients were followed for 29.9 months (mean, range: 1–77.7 months). The treatment duration was 13.3 months (mean, 1–64.5 months). The ORR was 93% (25/27 patients), 18 patients achieved PR, 7 patients had CR and 1 patient maintained CR up to >3 years after vismodegib discontinuation. Six patients (24%) developed secondary resistance during treatment. Tissue samples from 7 patients were used for sequencing of the Hh pathway genes *PTCH1*, *SMO*, *SUFU*, *GLI1*, and *GLI2*. Mutations in Hh pathway genes *PTCH1* and *SMO* were found. In 3 patients with secondary resistance to vismodegib, acquired pathogenic *SMO* mutations in resistant tumor tissue were detected. The primary resistance to vismodegib was observed in 1 patient with Bazex–Dupré–Christol syndrome and 1 patient with sporadic BCC. Patients who achieved CR during treatment seemed to maintain the long treatment responses after vismodegib discontinuation. The duration of response after vismodegib discontinuation was assessed in 19 patients in whom the response maintained until vismodegib discontinuation (excluding the 6 patients who developed secondary resistance). The mean duration of response was 11.4 months after vismodegib discontinuation (1.1–40.1) in 12 evaluable patients. One patient maintained CR until data cut off, up to 40.1 months after vismodegib discontinuation. The rate of secondary resistance was 24%. No new safety signals were observed, but progression of multiple sclerosis was reported in one patient.

The maintenance therapy with vismodegib was assessed in the observational retrospective study conducted in one site. Forty-two patients with BCC who achieved

CR after treatment with vismodegib were enrolled (35 males, 7 females). The median age of the patients was 75.2 years. The patients included in the study were treated with vismodegib in a standard dose 150 mg/day until CR was achieved. The median duration of treatment was 7.1 (range 1–22) months. After CR of BCC the patients continued vismodegib therapy with the "drug holiday" regimen receiving a once-weekly maintenance dosage of 150 mg vismodegib for 1 year ($n = 27$, 64%) or discontinued vismodegib treatment ($n = 15$, 36%) due to severe AEs, such as severe alopecia and muscle pain. All patients were followed up for 1 year on monthly basis [29]. Patients who received maintenance treatment had no recurrence of BCC during the 1-year follow-up period. Mild dysgeusia in 48% (13/27) of patients and mild muscle pain in 29.6% (8/27) were reported. The BCC recurrence during the 1-year follow-up rate among patients who discontinued vismodegib treatment was 26.6% (4/15). In this group, all AEs previously reported resolved. The maintenance dose of vismodegib effectively eliminated BCC recurrence and reduced the severity of AEs.

A key limitation to vismodegib treatment is development of resistance by BCC, which limits the duration of response. The secondary resistance is observed in about 20% of responders [30].

Chang et al. described the case series of BCC tumor regrowth within or immediately adjacent to (within 1 cm) the prior tumor bed of a vismodegib-responsive tumor in patients continuing treatment with vismodegib. The authors analyzed the records of 28 consequent patients with laBCC or mBCC treated with continuous administration of vismodegib; 21% of patients treated with vismodegib developed at least 1 tumor regrowth during this treatment. The mean time to regrowth detection by clinical examination was 56.4 weeks. The authors attributed this tumor regrowth to secondary resistance [30].

Atwood et al. analyzed the molecular abnormalities potentially leading to primary and secondary resistance to vismodegib. They found that 50% of resistant BCCs operate under two distinct modes of resistance: disruption of ligand responsiveness and release of autoinhibition. They identified *SMO* mutations in 50% (22 of 44) of resistant BCCs and showed that these mutations maintain Hh signaling in the presence of SMO inhibitors [31].

Pricl et al. described the molecular mechanisms of resistance to vismodegib in two BCC cases. In the first case, with PD after 2 months of treatment with vismodegib (primary resistance), the new SMO G497W mutation was found. In the second case, with CR after 5 months of treatment and a subsequent PD after 11 months of treatment with vismodegib (secondary resistance), a *PTCH1* nonsense mutation in both the pre- and the posttreatment specimens was found, and the SMO D473Y mutation in the posttreatment specimens only [32].

Sharpe et al. described the genetic alterations responsible for resistance to Hh inhibitors. This resistance is associated with Hh pathway reactivation, predominantly through mutation of the drug target *SMO* and to a lesser extent through concurrent copy number changes in *SUFU* (suppressor of fused) and *GLI2*. They also found and further studied the intra-tumor heterogeneity observed in the case of resistance [33].

There are currently running studies to find the predictive factors for response to vismodegib therapy in BCC.

Sternfeld et al. analyzed the response of laBCC to systemic treatment with vismodegib by changes in the expression levels of Hh pathway genes. The most important indicator of the Hh pathway activity is expression of *GLI1*. They analyzed tissue samples taken before and after treatment with vismodegib in 12 patients with laBCC. Sixteen Hh pathway genes changed significantly from before to after treatment, and the only gene with a significantly different expression at baseline between patients with CR and PR to vismodegib was *GAS1* ($p = 0.014$). The baseline expression level of GAS1 seems to be predictive of the response of locally advanced BCC to vismodegib [34].

The increased risk of SCC (squamous cell cancer) has been reported in correlation with treatment with vismodegib based on case reports in the literature [35, 36].

The analysis of data from the STEVIE study has shown that SCC has been diagnosed in 51 patients (4%) with advanced BCC in this study. Most patients were aged >75 years. Diagnosed SCCs were mostly located in sun-exposed skin areas. Among such 51 patients with SCC, 18 patients had a history of cutaneous SCC, 3 patients had a history of Bowen disease, and 2 patients had a history of actinic keratosis [12].

Bhutani et al. analyzed the data from 1675 patients and found that the use of vismodegib was not associated with an increased risk of subsequent development of SCC (adjusted hazard ratio, 0.57; 95% CI: 0.28–1.16) [37].

Vismodegib is approved for mBCC and laBCC not eligible for surgery and radiotherapy. As per current NCCN guidelines (v.1, 2020), vismodegib can be considered in case of laBCC in which curative RT and curative surgery are not feasible and in case of mBCC [38].

Vismodegib, although not approved, has been also assessed in neoadjuvant treatment of BCC. Several authors reported their experience using vismodegib in neoadjuvant setting in the treatment of laBCC, including periocular laBCC, to maximally decrease the tumor size and allow for downstaging of surgical resection, including ocular preservation. Neoadjuvant treatment of patients with laBCC has been also assessed in clinical trials [39–50].

The first results of VISMONEO study (NCT02667574), published in 2018, showed that preoperative treatment with vismodegib can allow downstaging of surgical procedure in patients with laBCC localized in functionally sensitive locations [47]. VISMONEO is an open-label, noncomparative, multicenter, phase II study. Patients with at least one histologically confirmed BCC of the face, inoperable or operable with functional or major aesthetic sequelae risk were included. The patients were treated before surgery with vismodegib in a dose 150 mg. The treatment duration was 4–10 months. The patients were operated on after obtaining the best response. Primary endpoint was the percentage of BCC patients with tumor downstaging following surgical resection. Fifty-five patients with laBCC were enrolled into this study, with median age 73.1 years. At the time of study entry, 4 patients were inoperable, 15 were operable with a major functional risk, and 36 were operable with a minor functional risk or a major aesthetic risk; 44 patients from 55 enrolled, achieved response, and had a surgery after vismodegib treatment (80.0%).

In 27 patients, CR was achieved and confirmed by pathology results after surgery. Main AEs were dysgeusia, muscle spasms, alopecia, fatigue, and weight loss (20% of patients with grade ≥3).

In 2019, Gonzales et al. published the results of treatment of 8 patients with periocular laBCC [48]. In case of laBCC located on face, especially periocular laBCC, decreasing tumor size before definitive surgery may be extremely important. Mohs micrographic surgery is the best option in periocular laBCC because of high cure rate and sparing of normal tissue. The patients were treated with vismodegib in a dose 150 mg daily. Treatment was continued until maximal clinical response, PD, unacceptable toxicity, or withdrawal. Mean age of enrolled patients was 76 years. Seven patients (87.5%) had CR and 1 had (12.5%) PD. Maximal CR was achieved at 4.8 months. Patients were operated at the mean time of 7.3 months. Mohs micrographic surgery allowed to confirm a complete histologic response in 5 of 6 (83.3%) cases. One patient refused surgery. One patient progressed. All 7 patients who achieved CR were disease-free after a mean follow-up of 12.4 months. All patients experienced AEs. The most common AEs included dysgeusia (100%), muscle spasms (100%), weight loss (75%), and hair loss (50%). One (12.5%) patient discontinued treatment due to intolerable muscle spasms.

Sagiv et al. published in 2019 the results of retrospective interventional study which included 8 patients with a T4 periocular BCC treated with neoadjuvant vismodegib prior to definitive surgery [49]. Six patients had recurrent disease. One patient had an unresectable tumor, 6 were treated with intention to avoid an orbital exenteration, 1 patient was treated to avoid face disfigurement with surgery. Median duration of treatment was 14 months (4–36 months). All patients underwent an eye-sparing surgery following neoadjuvant treatment with vismodegib and all final surgical margins were negative for tumor. Five patients achieved CR to vismodegib with no microscopic residual BCC found in pathology. Three patients had a significant PR with residual tumor found on pathology. At last follow-up, a mean of 18 (6–43) months after surgery, all patients were off-vismodegib and disease-free.

Toxicity Profile

The detailed description of safety assessment in specific clinical trials can be found in the sections of this chapter dedicated to early development and efficacy assessment.

In this section, the summary of safety profile has been presented based on the last updated version of summary of product characteristics (10.2020). The most common adverse drug reactions (ADR) occurring in ≥30% of patients treated with vismodegib were muscle spasms (74.6%), alopecia (65.9%), dysgeusia (58.7%), weight decreased (50.0%), fatigue (47.1%), nausea (34.8%), and diarrhea (33.3%) [51, 52].

Tabulated list of adverse reactions (ADRs) are presented in Table 8.2 by system organ class and absolute frequency. Frequencies are defined as: very common (≥1/10), common (≥1/100 to <1/10), uncommon (≥1/1000 to <1/100), rare

Table 8.2 ADRs occurring in patients treated with vismodegib [51, 52]

System organ class	Very common	Common	Frequency not known
Metabolism and nutrition disorders	Decreased appetite	Dehydration	
Nervous system disorder	Dysgeusia Ageusia	Hypogeusia	
Gastrointestinal disorders	Nausea Diarrhea Constipation Vomiting Dyspepsia	Abdominal pain upper Abdominal pain	
Hepatobiliary disorders		Hepatic enzymes increased[a]	Drug-induced liver injury[b]
Skin and subcutaneous tissue disorders	Alopecia Pruritus Rash	Madarosis Abnormal hair growth	Stevens-Johnson Syndrome (SJS)/ Toxic Epidermal Necrolysis (TEN), Drug Reaction with Eosinophilia and Systemic Symptoms (DRESS) and Acute Generalized Exanthematous Pustulosis (AGEP)[c]
Musculoskeletal and connective tissue disorders	Muscle spasms Arthralgia Pain in extremity	Back pain Musculoskeletal chest pain Myalgia Flank pain Musculoskeletal pain Blood creatine phosphokinase increased[f]	Epiphyses premature fusion[d]
Endocrine disorders			Precocious puberty[d]
Reproductive system and breast disorders			Amenorrhea[e]
General disorders and administration site conditions	Weight decreased Fatigue Pain	Asthenia	

All reporting is based on ADRs of all grades using NCI-CTCAE v. 3.0 except where noted

[a]Includes preferred terms: liver function test abnormal, blood bilirubin increased, gamma-glutamyl transferase increased, aspartate aminotransferase increased, alkaline phosphatase increased, liver hepatic enzyme increased

[b]Cases of drug-induced liver injury have been reported in patients during post-marketing use

[c]Cases of SCAR (including SJS/TEN, DRESS and AGEP) have been reported in patients during post-marketing use

[d]Individual cases have been reported in patients with medulloblastoma during post-marketing use

[e]Of the 138 patients with advanced BCC, 10 were women of childbearing potential. Among these women, amenorrhea was observed in 3 patients (30%)

[f]Observed in patients during a post-approval study with 1215 safety evaluable patients

($\geq$1/10,000 to <1/1000), very rare (<1/10,000), not known (cannot be estimated from the available data).

Within each frequency grouping, ADRs are presented in the order of decreasing seriousness.

The safety of vismodegib has been evaluated in four open label phase 1 and 2 clinical trials with 138 patients treated for BCC (mBCC and laBCC) with at least one dose of vismodegib at doses $\geq$150 mg. Safety was assessed also in a post-approval study that included 1215 advanced BCC patients treated with vismodegib 150 mg daily and evaluable for safety. The safety profile observed was consistent across studies and in both mBCC and laBCC patients.

Summary of Approval and Regulatory Indications

Vismodegib has been approved in the EU in July 2013 for the treatment of adult patients with: symptomatic metastatic basal cell carcinoma, locally advanced basal cell carcinoma inappropriate for surgery or radiotherapy. In the United States, it has been approved in Jan 2012 for the treatment of adults with metastatic basal cell carcinoma, or with locally advanced basal cell carcinoma that has recurred following surgery or who are not candidates for surgery, and who are not candidates for radiation [51, 52].

In clinical trials, treatment with vismodegib was continued until disease progression or until unacceptable toxicity. Treatment interruptions of up to 4 weeks were allowed based on individual tolerability. Benefit of continued treatment should be regularly assessed, with the optimal duration of therapy varying for each individual patient. The recommended dose is one 150 mg capsule taken once daily. No dose adjustment is required in patients $\geq$65 years of age. Mild and moderate renal impairment is not expected to impact the elimination of vismodegib and no dose adjustment is needed. Very limited data are available in patients with severe renal impairment. Patients with severe renal impairment should be carefully monitored for adverse reactions. No dose adjustment is required in patients with mild, moderate, or severe hepatic impairment. The safety and efficacy of vismodegib in children and adolescents aged below 18 years have not been established. Vismodegib can result in severe birth defects or embryo-fetal death. Vismodegib is embryotoxic and teratogenic in animals. Due to the risk of embryo-fetal death or severe birth defects caused by vismodegib, women taking vismodegib must not be pregnant or become pregnant during treatment and for 24 months after the final dose. Vismodegib is present in semen, and due to this, men should use condom when having sex in female partner while taking vismodegib and for 2 months after the final dose. Patients should be advised to notify their healthcare provider immediately if they suspect that they or their female partner may be pregnant. Concomitant treatment with strong CYP inducers (e.g., rifampicin, carbamazepine, or phenytoin) should be avoided, as a risk for decreased plasma concentrations and decreased efficacy of vismodegib cannot be excluded [51, 52].

References

1. LoRusso PM, Rudin CM, Reddy JC, et al. Phase I trial of hedgehog pathway inhibitor vismodegib (GDC-0449) in patients with refractory, locally advanced or metastatic solid tumors. Clin Cancer Res. 2011;17:2502.
2. Scales SJ, de Sauvage FJ. Mechanisms of hedgehog pathway activation in cancer and implications for therapy. Trends Pharmacol Sci. 2009;30:303–12.
3. Robarge KD, Brunton SA, Castanedo GM, et al. GDC-0449-a potent inhibitor of the hedgehog pathway. Bioorg Med Chem Lett. 2009;19:5576–81.
4. Rubin LL, de Sauvage FJ. Targeting the hedgehog pathway in cancer. Nat Rev Drug Discov. 2006;5:1026–33.
5. Romer JT, Kimura H, Magdaleno S, et al. Suppression of the Shh pathway using a small molecule inhibitor eliminates medulloblastoma in Ptc11/2p532/2 mice. Cancer Cell. 2004;6:229–40.
6. Yauch RL, Gould SE, Scales SJ, et al. A paracrine requirement for hedgehog signalling in cancer. Nature. 2008;455:406–10.
7. Von Hoff DD, LoRusso PM, Rudin CM, et al. Inhibition of the hedgehog pathway in advanced basal-cell carcinoma. N Engl J Med. 2009;361:1164–72.
8. Rudin CM, Hann CL, Laterra J, et al. Treatment of medulloblastoma with hedgehog pathway inhibitor GDC-0449. N Engl J Med. 2009;361:1173–8.
9. Graham RA, Lum BL, Cheet S, et al. Pharmacokinetics of hedgehog pathway Inhibitor vismodegib (GDC- 0449) in patients with locally advanced or metastatic solid tumors: the role of alpha-1-acid glycoprotein binding. Clin Can Res. 2011;17:2512–20.
10. Sekulic A, Migden MR, Oro AE, et al. Efficacy and safety of vismodegib in advanced basal-cell carcinoma. N Engl J Med. 2012;366:2171–9.
11. Sekulic A, Migden MR, Lewis K, et al. Pivotal ERIVANCE basal cell carcinoma (BCC) study: 12-month update of efficacy and safety of vismodegib in advanced BCC. J Am Acad Dermatol. 2015;72:1021.
12. Basset-Seguin N, Hauschild A, Kunstfeld R, et al. Vismodegib in patients with advanced basal cell carcinoma: primary analysis of STEVIE, an international, open-label trial. Eur J Cancer. 2017;86:334–48.
13. Dréno B, Kunstfeld R, Hauschild A, et al. Two intermittent vismodegib dosing regimens in patients with multiple basal-cell carcinomas (MIKIE): a randomised, regimen-controlled, double-blind, phase 2 trial. Lancet Oncol. 2017;18:404–12.
14. Sekulic A, Migden MR, Basset-Seguin N, Garbe C, Gesierich A, Lao CD, et al. Long-term safety and efficacy of vismodegib in patients with advanced basal cell carcinoma (BCC): 24-month update of the pivotal ERIVANCE BCC study. BMC Cancer. 2017;17(1):332.
15. Basset-Seguin N, Hauschild A, Grob JJ, et al. Vismodegib in patients with advanced basal cell carcinoma (STEVIE): a pre-planned interim analysis of an international, open-label trial. Lancet Oncol. 2015;16(6):729–36.
16. Hansson J, Bartley K, Grob JJ, et al. Assessment of quality of life using Skindex-16 in patients with advanced basal cell carcinoma (BCC) treated with vismodegib in the STEVIE study. Eur J Dermatol. 2018;28:775–83.
17. Bossi P, Peris K, Calzavara-Pinton P, et al. Cohort analysis of safety and efficacy of vismodegib in Italian patients from the Phase II, multicenter STEVIE study. Future Oncol. 2020;16(16):1091–100.
18. Chang AL, Solomon JA, Hainsworth JD, et al. Expanded access study of patients with advanced basal cell carcinoma treated with the Hedgehog pathway inhibitor, vismodegib. J Am Acad Dermatol. 2014;70(1):60–9.
19. Lacouture ME, Tang JY, Rogers GS, et al. The RegiSONIC disease registry: Preliminary effectiveness and safety in the first 66 newly diagnosed locally advanced basal cell carcinoma (BCC) patients treated with vismodegib. J Clin Oncol. 2015;33(15_suppl):9023.
20. Chang ALS, Lewis KD, Arron TS, et al. Safety and efficacy of vismodegib in patients aged ≥65 years with advanced basal cell carcinoma. Oncotarget. 2016;7(46):76118–24.

21. Tang JY, Mackay-Wiggan JM, Aszterbaum M, et al. Inhibiting the hedgehog pathway in patients with the basal-cell nevus syndrome. N Engl J Med. 2012;366(23):2180–8.
22. Chang AL, Arron ST, Migden MR, et al. Safety and efficacy of vismodegib in patients with basal cell carcinoma nevus syndrome: pooled analysis of two trials. Orphanet J Rare Dis. 2016;11(1):120.
23. Słowińska M, Maciąg A, Dudzisz-Śledź M, et al. Vismodegib in the treatment of basal cell carcinoma – polish clinical experience in the frame of therapeutic program. Oncol Clin Pract. 2019;15(3):139–49.
24. Bernia E, Llombart B, Serra-Guillén C, et al. Experience with vismodegib in the treatment of advanced basal cell carcinoma at a cancer center. Actas Dermosifiliogr. 2018;109(9):813–20.
25. Herms F, Lambert J, Grob JJ, et al. Follow-up of patients with complete remission of locally advanced basal cell carcinoma after vismodegib discontinuation: a multicenter french study of 116 patients. J Clin Oncol. 2019;37:3275.
26. Fife K, Herd R, Lalondrelle S, et al. Managing adverse events associated with vismodegib in the treatment of basal cell carcinoma. Future Oncol. 2017;13(2):175–84.
27. Hanke CW, Mhatre SK, Oliveri D, et al. Vismodegib use in clinical practice: analysis of a united states medical claims database. J Drugs Dermatol. 2018;17(2):143–8.
28. Van Eecke L, Vander Borght S, Vanden Bempt I, et al. Vismodegib treatment in patients with advanced basal cell carcinoma: long term efficacy and safety data with focus on secondary resistance and underlying resistance mechanism. Int J Clin Expl Dermatol. 2020;5(1):7–12.
29. Scalvenzi M, Cappello M, Costa C, et al. Low-dose vismodegib as maintenance therapy after locally advanced basal cell carcinoma complete remission: high efficacy with minimal toxicity. Dermatol Ther (Heidelb). 2020;10(3):465–8.
30. Chang ALS, Oro AE. Initial assessment of tumor regrowth after vismodegib in advanced Basal cell carcinoma. Arch Dermatol. 2012;148(11):1324–5.
31. Atwood SX, Sarin KY, Whitson RJ, et al. Smoothened variants explain the majority of drug resistance in basal cell carcinoma. Cancer Cell. 2015;27:342.
32. Pricl S, Cortelazzi B, Dal Col V, et al. Smoothened (SMO) receptor mutations dictate resistance to vismodegib in basal cell carcinoma. Mol Oncol. 2015;9(2):389–97.
33. Sharpe HJ, Pau G, Dijkgraaf GJ, et al. Genomic analysis of smoothened inhibitor resistance in basal cell carcinoma. Cancer Cell. 2015;27(3):327–41.
34. Sternfeld A, Rosenwasser-Weiss S, Ben-Yehuda G. Gene-related response of basal cell carcinoma to biologic treatment with vismodegib. Sci Rep. 2020;10(1):1244.
35. Mohan SV, Chang J, Li S, et al. Increased risk of cutaneous squamous cell carcinoma after vismodegib therapy for basal cell carcinoma. JAMA Dermatol. 2016;152:527.
36. Saintes C, Saint-Jean M, Brocard A, et al. Development of squamous cell carcinoma into basal cell carcinoma under treatment with vismodegib. J Eur Acad Dermatol Venereol. 2015;29(5):1006–9.
37. Bhutani T, Abrouk M, Sima CS, et al. Risk of cutaneous squamous cell carcinoma after treatment of basal cell carcinoma with vismodegib. J Am Acad Dermatol. 2017;77:713.
38. NCCN Guidelines. Basal cell skin cancer. Version 1. 2020.
39. Kahana A, Worden FP, Elner VM. Vismodegib as eye-sparing adjuvant treatment for orbital basal cell carcinoma. JAMA Ophthalmol. 2013;131:1364–6.
40. Yin VT, Pfeiffer ML, Esmaeli B. Targeted therapy for orbital and periocular basal cell carcinoma and squamous cell carcinoma. Ophthalmic Plast Reconstr Surg. 2013;29:87–92.
41. Ally MS, Aasi S, Wysong A, et al. An investigator-initiated open-label clinical trial of vismodegib as a neoadjuvant to surgery for high risk basal cell carcinoma. J Am Acad Dermatol. 2014;71:904–11.e1.
42. Demirci H, Worden F, Nelson CC, et al. Efficacy of vismodegib (erivedge) for basal cell carcinoma involving the orbit and periocular area. Ophthalmic Plast Reconstr Surg. 2015;31:463–6.
43. Sofen H, Gross KG, Goldberg LH, et al. A phase II, multicenter, open-label, 3-cohort trial evaluating the efficacy and safety of vismodegib in operable basal cell carcinoma. J Am Acad Dermatol. 2015;73:99–105.e1.

44. Ching JA, Curtis HL, Braue JA, et al. The impact of neoadjuvant hedgehog inhibitor therapy on the surgical treatment of extensive basal cell carcinoma. Ann Plast Surg. 2015;74(suppl 4):S193–7.
45. Kwon GP, Ally MS, Bailey-Healy I, et al. Update to an open-label clinical trial of vismodegib as neoadjuvant before surgery for high-risk basal cell carcinoma (BCC). J Am Acad Dermatol. 2016;75:213–5.
46. Alcalay J, Tauber G, Fenig E, et al. Vismodegib as a neoadjuvant treatment to Mohs surgery for aggressive basal cell carcinoma. J Drugs Dermatol. 2015;14:219–23.
47. Mortier L, Bertrand N, Basset-Seguin N et al. Vismodegib in neoadjuvant treatment of locally advanced basal cell carcinoma: First results of a multicenter, open-label, phase 2 trial (VISMONEO study). J Clin Oncol. 2018; 36(suppl; abstr 9509).
48. González AR, Etchichury D, Gil ME, Del Aguila R. Neoadjuvant vismodegib and Mohs micrographic surgery for locally advanced periocular basal cell carcinoma. Ophthalmic Plast Reconstr Surg. 2019;35(1):56–61.
49. Sagiv O, Nagarajan P, Ferrarotto R, et al. Ocular preservation with neoadjuvant vismodegib in patients with locally advanced periocular basal cell carcinoma. Br J Ophthalmol. 2019;103(6):775–80.
50. Su MG, Potts LB, Tsai JH. Treatment of periocular basal cell carcinoma with neoadjuvant vismodegib. Am J Ophthalmol Case Rep. 2020;19:100755.
51. Erivedge (vismodegib), Summary of product characteristics. Last update 10.2020. https://www.ema.europa.eu/en/documents/product-information/erivedge-epar-product-information_en.pdf
52. Erivedge (vismodegib) capsules, for oral use, prescribing information.

Chapter 9
Sonidegib

Monika Dudzisz-Śledź

Pharmacological Properties and Early Development

Sonidegib (LDE225), N-(6-((2S,6R)-2,6-dimethylmorpholino)pyridin-3-yl)-2-methyl-40-(trifluoromethoxy)biphenyl- 3-carboxamide is a selective inhibitor of smoothened (SMO), which was identified in a cell-based high-throughput screening. It is an orally available, potent and selective, small molecular inhibitor of the hedgehog (Hh) pathway. Hh signaling pathway is a key regulator of cell growth and differentiation and plays a key role during embryogenesis, maintenance of adult tissue, and maintenance of stem cells [1, 2]. This pathway is inactive in most normal adult tissues with only limited activity in some processes, including hair growth and maintenance of taste [3]. Hh pathway reactivation is involved in the pathogenesis of several malignancies. Aberrant activation of the Hh pathway results in tumorigenesis and is associated with basal cell carcinoma (BCC) and medulloblastoma [4–7]. The transmembrane receptor patched (PTCH) is a negative regulator of the transmembrane receptor smoothened (SMO). PTCH is the receptor for the Hh ligand and inhibits SMO until the Hh ligand binds, allowing SMO to signal. Signaling by SMO results in the activation of glioma-associated oncogene (GLI) transcription factors and induction of Hh target genes, including *GLI1* and *PTCH1* [8]. LDE225 acts by binding to and inhibiting the activity of the SMO transmembrane protein. This results in complete suppression of GLI and tumor regression. The IC50 of sonidegib in humans is 11 nM [9]. Sonidegib has a high affinity for SMO. LDE225 has high tissue penetration and the ability to cross the blood-brain barrier. Sonidegib has high oral bioavailability based on the preclinical studies. This drug is not a derivative of cyclopamine and is structurally distinct from vismodegib [10]. The capsules for oral

M. Dudzisz-Śledź (✉)
Department of Soft Tissue/Bone Sarcoma and Melanoma, Maria Sklodowska-Curie National Research Institute of Oncology, Warsaw, Poland
e-mail: monika.dudzisz-sledz@pib-nio.pl

P. Rutkowski, M. Mandalà (eds.), *New Therapies in Advanced Cutaneous Malignancies*, https://doi.org/10.1007/978-3-030-64009-5_9

administration contain sonidegib in diphosphate form, although the 200 mg relates only to the free base content, as this increases its bioavailability. An in vitro study has shown that cells with SMO mutations display resistance to sonidegib [11–13].

Sonidegib was assessed in the first-in-human phase I study (NCT00880308). The purpose of this study is to determine the maximum tolerated dose (MTD), dose-limiting toxicities (DLT), safety, tolerability, pharmacokinetics (PK), pharmacodynamics, biomarkers in skin and tumor biopsies, and preliminary antitumor activity of sonidegib in patients with advanced solid tumors [12]. A total of 103 patients whose disease progressed despite standard therapy or for whom no standard therapy was available were enrolled in this study. Among 103 patients, 16 patients with BCC and 9 patients with medulloblastoma were enrolled. The patients in Eastern Cooperative Oncology Group (ECOG) 0–2 and with adequate bone marrow, renal, and liver function were eligible for the study. The patients were treated with oral sonidegib at doses ranging from 100 mg to 3000 mg once daily and 250 to 750 mg twice daily, every day. The safety was assessed according to Common Terminology Criteria for Adverse Events (CTCAE) v. 3.0 and included laboratory tests, physical examination, vital signs, weight, and periodic electrocardiogram recordings. The safety assessments were done from the first dose of sonidegib until 28 days after the last dose. Additional assessments of creatine phosphokinase (CPK) were included. Tumor samples, fresh or archival, as well biopsies from normal skin were collected from all patients before treatment, at the end of cycles 1 and 2, and within 14 days after the last dose. The *GLI1* expression and Hh pathway activation status were evaluated. The tumor assessment was done at baseline and then every 8 weeks. The efficacy was done according to RECIST v. 1.0 (response evaluation criteria in solid tumors) and the Neuro-Oncology Criteria of Tumor Response (for medulloblastoma only). For PK tests blood samples were collected during the study.

Sonidegib was generally well tolerated. The adverse events (AEs) were similar to those reported for other medications in the same class of drugs. The AEs reported by the patients were mostly mild (G- grade, G1, and G2). The treatment-emergent AEs (TEAEs) were manageable and reversible after treatment discontinuation. Most common treatment-related G1 and G2 AEs reported by >10% of patients included nausea, dysgeusia, anorexia, vomiting, muscle spasms, myalgia, increased serum creatine kinase, fatigue/asthenia, and alopecia. G3 and G4 AEs experienced by <5% of all treated patients included weight loss, myalgia, hyperbilirubinemia, dizziness, and asthenia. No deaths due to drug-related AEs were reported. A total of 17 patients required dose reduction and 20 patients permanently discontinued treatment due to AEs, mostly CPK elevation. Elevated CPK was assessed as dose-limiting toxicity in 19 patients treated with doses ≥800 mg once daily and ≥250 mg twice daily. Reversible dose-limiting CPK elevation was observed in 18% of patients across all doses. CPK elevation was of skeletal muscle origin and without evidence of cardiac muscle injury. There was no clear relationship between the incidence of muscle cramps/spasms and elevated CPK.

Sonidegib was rapidly absorbed following oral administration and had a long elimination half-life. The median Tmax was 2 h for all dosing regimens and doses administered. The maximum tolerated dose in a phase I study in patients with advanced solid tumors was determined to bc 800 mg daily and 250 mg twice daily. Twice-daily dosing of sonidegib provided a higher systemic exposure than equivalent once-daily doses. However, no clinical advantage was observed for twice-daily dosing. Therefore, the once-daily dosing regimen was recommended for further studies and is currently recommended in clinical practice [12].

A total of 99 patients were evaluable for tumor response. Partial response (PR) was observed over the dose range of 100 to 1500 mg. Sonidegib showed clinically relevant antitumor activity in patients with locally advanced (laBCC) or metastatic basal cell carcinoma (mBCC) and relapsed medulloblastoma. 6 of 16 patients with BCC and 3 of 9 patients with medulloblastoma achieved objective tumor responses (PR or CR; CR, complete response). There was a strong association between tumor response and Hh pathway activation. Stable disease (SD) as best response was observed in 24 patients, with a duration of SD > 6 months in three patients with lung adenocarcinoma, spindle cell sarcoma, and BCC. Sonidegib exhibited a dose- and exposure-dependent inhibition of *GLI1* mRNA expression (a marker for Hh pathway activation) in tumor tissue and normal skin biopsies from patients with advanced solid tumors [12].

In 2014 the data from the single-center open-label study to assess the absorption, distribution, metabolism, and excretion of sonidegib were published. Six healthy nonsmoking male volunteers (mean age of 33 years) were enrolled in this study. The subjects received a single oral dose of 800 mg ^{14}C-sonidegib under fasting conditions. Blood, plasma, urine, and fecal samples were collected predose, postdose in-house (days 1–22), and during 24-h visits (weekly, days 29–43; biweekly, days 57–99). Safety and tolerability were also evaluated and included vital signs, laboratory tests, ECGs, and AEs. The CTCAE v. 4.03 was used. The mean estimated total absorption of the radiolabeled sonidegib was 6–7%. Absorbed sonidegib was distributed extensively into the tissues and was metabolized slowly. The half-life of sonidegib reported in this study was similar to that in the phase I study. The elimination of absorbed sonidegib occurred predominantly or exclusively by oxidative and hydrolytic metabolism. No unchanged sonidegib was detected in urine, and only small amounts were found in the feces. Unabsorbed sonidegib was excreted through the feces and metabolites were also mostly excreted through the feces. The data from this study suggest a strong positive food effect on sonidegib absorption. The single 800-mg dose of sonidegib was well tolerated in healthy male subjects in this study. Two subjects experienced G1 AEs suspected to be related to sonidegib, including myalgia and pain in an extremity [14].

Sonidegib is mostly metabolized by the liver. The effect of mild or moderate hepatic impairment on the PK of sonidegib was assessed in phase I, multicenter, open-label parallel-group study [15]. The investigators assessed the PK and safety of sonidegib in subjects with different degrees of hepatic impairment and compared with results from healthy subjects. A total of 33 subjects were enrolled in this study and received sonidegib in a single dose of 800 mg. The results, published in 2018, indicated that dose adjustment is not necessary in patients with mild, moderate, or severe hepatic impairment. Sonidegib exposures were similar or decreased in subjects with hepatic impairment compared with the subjects with normal hepatic function. Sonidegib was generally well tolerated.

The PK of sonidegib was additionally assessed in a population study published in 2016. This study was conducted in healthy subjects and patients with advanced solid tumors to characterize PK, determine variability, and estimate covariate effects. Based on this study results, the authors concluded that no sonidegib dose adjustment was needed for mild hepatic impairment, mild and moderate renal impairment, age, weight, gender, or ethnicity. Proton pump inhibitors (PPI) co-administration reduced sonidegib bioavailability by 30% [16].

The effect of esomeprazole, a proton pump inhibitor (PPI) on the oral absorption and PK of sonidegib in healthy volunteers was assessed in a phase I study. Forty-two healthy subjects received either sonidegib alone (in a single dose 200 mg) or sonidegib in combination with esomeprazole (40 mg for 5 days before and on day of sonidegib administration), under fasting condition. The results, published in 2016, indicated that there was a modest reduction in the extent of sonidegib absorption by esomeprazole. No obvious metabolic drug-drug interaction between sonidegib and esomeprazole was reported. Both drugs were well tolerated [17].

Activity and Efficacy

Sonidegib was approved for the treatment of laBCC based on the results of the BOLT study (NCT01327053). The BOLT study was a multicenter, randomized, double-blind, phase II trial [13, 18–21]. Patients with histologically confirmed, laBCC not amenable to radiotherapy or curative surgery, or mBCC were randomized in a 1:2 ratio to receive 200 mg or 800 mg oral sonidegib daily. Two doses were selected based on phase I clinical study results. The dose 200 mg was the lowest active dose and dose 800 mg was the highest active well-tolerated dose. As sonidegib 200 mg/d was expected to be less active than dose 800 mg/d, the patients were randomly assigned to these doses in a 1:2 ratio. The eligible patients were adult patients with ECOG 0–2, and with adequate bone marrow, liver, and renal function. The randomization was stratified by disease stage (laBCC v. mBCC), histological subtype (aggressive v. nonaggressive), and geographical region. The aggressive subtypes were micronodular, infiltrative, multifocal, basosquamous, or sclerosing BCCs and nonaggressive subtypes included nodular and superficial BCCs. The aggressive tumors were diagnosed in 40 patients (51%) treated with sonidegib 200 mg and 76 patients (50%) in the group receiving sonidegib 800 mg/d. The patients were treated with sonidegib capsules taken orally once-daily up to 42 months or until progressive disease (PD), unacceptable toxicity, withdrawal of consent, discontinuation at the discretion of the investigator, death, or study termination. The primary endpoint was objective response rate [ORR = CR + PR] based on central review. Secondary endpoints included ORR based on investigator review, CR rate, duration of response (DOR), and progression-free survival (PFS) based on central and investigator review, overall survival (OS), and safety. Tumor assessments were done at baseline, during treatment and post-treatment follow-up, and at discontinuation of the study, using BCC-modified RECIST for laBCC and RECIST v. 1.1 for mBCC. Tumor response was assessed based on central and investigator review. CRs and PRs required further confirmation on repeated assessments done after at least 4 weeks. Safety was assessed based on CTCAE v. 4.03, from the first dose of study drug administration until 30 days after the last dose. Fresh tumor biopsy samples were collected at screening, week 9, week 17, and at the end of treatment to measure *GLI1* expression. The quantitative RT-PCR was done in all valid samples to detect *GLI1* expression. Fresh tumor biopsies were also done to confirm the response or to assess the response in case of any confounding lesions. Changes in disease-related symptoms, functioning, and quality of life (QoL) were assessed by investigators at baseline and weeks 9 and 17 during treatment then every 8 weeks during year 1 and every 12 weeks thereafter. The European Organisation for Research and Treatment of Cancer Quality of Life Questionnaire-Core 30 (QLQ-C30) and the module-specific for head and neck cancers (H&N35) were used. All enrolled patients were required to use highly effective methods of contraception during the study and for 6 months after the last dose of sonidegib.

A total of 230 patients were enrolled in this study, 79 in the 200 mg/d sonidegib group, and 151 in the 800 mg/d sonidegib group; 194 patients had laBCC and 36 had mBCC. Baseline characteristics were generally similar in the two groups. The median age of patients in the sonidegib 200 mg/d group was 67 (25–92) and in the sonidegib 800 mg group was 65 (24–93). More than 50% of patients were ≥65 years. More than 60% of patients were male.

At the 6-month analysis, with the median follow-up of 13.9 months, tumor assessments after baseline were done for 227 (99%) patients. A total of 144 (63%) patients discontinued treatment, primarily because of AEs, the patient's decision, or PD [13]; 20 (36%, 95% CI 24–50) of 55 patients in the 200 mg dose group and 39 (34%, 25–43) of 116 patients in the 800 mg group achieved an objective response. The ORR by central review in laBCC patients treated with sonidegib 200 mg daily was 43% and in patients with mBCC was 15%. Disease control was observed in more than 90% of patients treated with 200 mg sonidegib and in approximately 80% of patients treated with 800 mg sonidegib. Responses >6 months in patients with laBCC were observed in 12 (39%) of 31 responders taking 200 mg sonidegib and 17 (38%) of 45 responders taking 800 mg sonidegib. The median duration of exposure to sonidegib for patients was 8.9 months in the 200 mg dose group and 6.5 months in the 800 mg dose group. Most patients treated with sonidegib had stable or improved disease-related symptoms, functioning, and health status based on QoL assessments. Decreases in *GLI1* expression from baseline at weeks 9 and 17 were similar in the two treatment groups. At week 17, substantial decreases from baseline in *GLI1* expression were seen in patients with disease control. There was the only patient with PD who had tumors available for *GLI1* assessment. In this patient, *GLI1* expression increase by 10% was observed.

These results were confirmed in subsequent analyses done with 12, 18, 30, and 42 months follow-up. Sonidegib demonstrated sustained tumor responses in patients with both laBCC and mBCC. The ORR, PFS, and DOR are presented in Tables 9.1 and 9.2.

Table 9.1 Summary of efficacy data from the BOLT study for laBCC treated with sonidegib 200 mg/d, based on central review (approved dose and indication, n = 66) in subsequent analyses [18–21]

	6 months follow-up (primary analysis)	12 months follow-up [19]	18 months follow-up [20]	30 months follow-up [20]	42 months follow-up [21]
ORR (%); 95% CI	47.0% (34.6–59.7)	57.6% (44.8-69.7)	56.1% (43.3–68.3)	56.1% (43.3–68.3)	56% (43–68)
DOR	NR	NR	NR	26.1 months	26.1 months
PFS	NR	22.1 months	22.1 months	22.1 months	22.1 months

ORR objective response rate, *DOR* duration of response, *PFS* progression-free survival, *NE* not estimable, *CI* confidence interval, *NR* not reached

Table 9.2 Summary of efficacy data from the BOLT study for laBCC and mBCC based on central review, follow-up at 42 months [21]

	laBCC 200 mg (n = 66)	laBCC 800 mg (n = 128)	mBCC 200 mg (n = 13)	mBCC 800 mg (n = 23)
ORR (%), 95%CI	56 (43–68)	46.1 (37.2–55.1)	8 (0.2–36)	17 (5–39)
DOR, median, months, 95%CI	26.1 (NE)	23.3 (12.2–29.6)	24.0 (NE)	NE (NE)
PFS, median, months	22.1 (NE)	24.9 (19.2–33.4)	13.1 (5.6–33.1)	11.1 (7.3–16.6)

ORR objective response rate, *DOR* duration of response, *PFS* progression-free survival, *NE* not estimable, *CI* confidence interval

In the analysis done with 12 months follow-up, efficacy in laBCC was generally similar to or improved and in mBCC was similar to that observed in the primary analysis. Response rates in laBCC based on central review were 57.6% and 43.8% in the 200 mg/d and 800 mg/d groups, respectively and in mBCC were 7.7% and 17.4% in the 200 mg/d and 800 mg/d, respectively.

The results were similar for aggressive and nonaggressive histology. The disease response rates in patients with aggressive and nonaggressive subtypes per central review were 59.5% v. 55.2% in the 200 mg/d group and 44.0% v. 43.4% in the 800 mg/d group, respectively. The median duration of response was not reached in either arm. In patients with mBCC, median time to tumor response was 1.8 and 1.0 months in the 200 mg/d and 800 mg/d arms and in patients with laBCC, 4.0 and 3.8 months, respectively [19].

After 30 months of follow-up, ORR was 56.1% for patients treated with sonidegib in dose 200 mg/d based on central review and 71.2% based on investigators review in laBCC. ORR in mBCC was 7.5% in central and 23.1% in investigator review, respectively. The median duration of response was 26.1 months (based on central review) and 15.7 months (based on investigators review) in laBCC and 24.0 months (central) and 18.1 months (investigator) in mBCC. Five patients with laBCC and three with mBCC in the arm receiving sonidegib in dose 200 mg/d died. Median overall survival (OS) was not reached in either population. Two-year OS rates were 93.2% in patients with laBCC and 69.3% in patients with mBCC. In laBCC, efficacy was similar regardless of tumor aggressiveness based on pathology [20].

In 2019 the last update with 42 months follow-up was published. The median duration of exposure to sonidegib was 11.0 months in the group treated with dose 200 mg/d and 6.6 months in the group treated with dose 800 mg/d; 8% in sonidegib 200mg/d group and 3.3% in sonidegib 800 mg/d group remained on treatment by the 42-month cut-off. The ORR was higher in patients with laBCC than for patients with mBCC. ORR for laBCC patients was 56% (43–68) in the 200 mg/d group and 46.1% (37.2–55.1) in the 800 mg/d group. For patients with mBCC, ORR were 8% (0.2–36) and 17% (5–39) for the 200 mg/d and 800-mg groups, respectively. Disease control rate (DCR) exceeded 90% both in patients with laBCC and in those with mBCC treated with sonidegib 200 mg/d. The median DOR for responders receiving sonidegib 200 mg/d was 26.1 months, responses ≥6 months were seen in 23 of 37 responders with laBCC receiving sonidegib 200 mg/d [21].

The activity of sonidegib was evaluated as a topical treatment in patients with BCC associated with Gorlin Goltz syndrome (GGS), also known as nevoid basal cell carcinoma syndrome (NBCCS). The characteristic feature of GGS is the high penetrance of inactivating mutations of the *PTCH1* gene leading to the development of multiple BCCs. The preclinical data suggest that sonidegib has a high potential to interfere with the Hh pathway in BCCs after topical treatment. It was a double-blind, randomized, vehicle-controlled study to assess the local tolerability, safety, PK, and pharmacodynamics of sonidegib used topically in patients with GGS and BCCs [22]. A total of 8 GGS patients with 27 BCCs were treated twice daily with 0.75% LDE225 cream or vehicle for 4 weeks. The application of 0.75% LDE225 cream was well tolerated. No skin irritation was observed. Of 13 BCCs treated with sonidegib, 3 showed CR, 9 showed PR, and 1 no clinical response. One PR was observed in BCCs treated with vehicle, no other clinical responses were observed in BCCs treated with vehicle.

Another study to determine the safety, local tolerability, PK and PD of LDE225 on sporadic superficial, and nodular skin BCC was started in 2009 (NCT01033019). This study was terminated as the data from the study showed insufficient efficacy [23].

The primary resistance to other Hh pathway inhibitor vismodegib occurs in about 50% of patients and the secondary resistance was reported in about 20% of patients [24–26].

In 2016 the results of an investigator-initiated open-label study with sonidegib used for the treatment of patients with BCC resistant to vismodegib were published (NCT01529450) [26]. The purpose of this study was to determine the efficacy of sonidegib in BCCs refractory to vismodegib. Nine patients were enrolled in this study. SMO mutations were identified using biopsy samples from the target BCC lesions. 5 patients experienced PD, and 3 patients achieved SD and discontinued sonidegib either due to adverse events ($n = 1$) or due to further surgery ($n = 2$). The response in 1 patient was not evaluable. The median duration of treatment with sonidegib was 6 weeks (3–58 weeks). The entire coding regions for SMO were sequenced. SMO mutations were identified in 5 of 8 available baseline tumor samples. There were mutations related to those previously reported functional resistance in vitro to either sonidegib or vismodegib. None of these patients experienced a response to treatment, 4 patients experienced PD, and 1 patient achieved SD. In conclusion, patients with advanced BCCs who were previously resistant to treatment with vismodegib were also resistant to sonidegib. The results of this study indicate that patients who have developed treatment resistance to an SMO inhibitor may continue to experience tumor progression in response to other SMO inhibitors.

Currently, there is a postauthorization study recruiting patients with locally advanced BCC who are not amenable to curative surgery or radiation therapy (NCT04066504). This is a noninterventional, multinational, and multicenter study to assess the safety of sonidegib administered in routine clinical practice [27].

Toxicity Profile

In the preclinical studies, sonidegib was tested in dogs and rats. The majority of the adverse effects of sonidegib can be attributed to its pharmacological mechanism of action. The effects in rats and dogs were similar. Most effects occurred close to the intended human exposures. These effects observed at clinically relevant exposures include the closure of bone growth plates, effects on growing teeth, effects on the male and female reproductive tract, atrophy of the hair follicles with alopecia, gastrointestinal toxicity with bodyweight loss, and effects on lymph nodes. At exposures above the clinical exposure, an additional target organ was the kidney [28].

Carcinogenicity studies have not been performed with sonidegib, but sonidegib was not genotoxic in studies conducted in vitro and in vivo [28].

Sonidegib was shown to be fetotoxic in rabbits, as evidenced by abortion and/or complete resorption of fetuses and teratogenic resulting in severe malformations at very low exposure. Teratogenic effects included vertebral, distal limb and digit malformations, severe craniofacial malformations, and other severe midline defects. Fetotoxicity in rabbits was also seen at very low maternal exposure. There was reduced fertility at low exposure in female rats. For sonidegib-treated male rats, exposure at approximately two-fold the clinical exposure did not impact male fertility [28].

In phase II study the safety of sonidegib was assessed in 229 patients with BCC treated with sonidegib in dose 200 mg ($n = 79$) or 800 mg ($n = 150$) [28]. The most common adverse drug reactions (ADRs) occurring in $\geq 10\%$ of patients treated with sonidegib 200 mg were muscle spasms, alopecia, dysgeusia, fatigue, nausea, musculoskeletal pain, diarrhea, weight loss, decreased appetite, myalgia, abdominal pain, headache, pain, vomiting, and pruritus. The most common grade G3 and G4 ADRs occurring in $\geq 2\%$ of patients treated with sonidegib in dose 200 mg were fatigue, weight decrease, and muscle spasms. The frequency of ADRs was greater in patients treated with sonidegib in dose 800 mg than in patients treated with sonidegib in dose 200 mg, except for musculoskeletal pain, diarrhea, abdominal pain, headache, and pruritus. The most commonly reported G3 and G4 laboratory abnormalities with an incidence of ≥5% occurring in patients treated with sonidegib 200 mg were lipase increase and blood CPK increase. Based on a summary of product characteristics, ADRs reported in patients treated with sonidegib in dose 200 mg/d are listed in Table 9.3 and the most frequent laboratory abnormalities are listed in Table 9.4.

ADRs are listed by Medical Dictionary for Regulatory Activities (MedDRA) version 18 system organ class. Within each system organ class, the ADRs are ranked by frequency, with the most frequent reactions first. Within each frequency

Table 9.3 ADRs (all grades) observed in the phase II pivotal study in patients treated with sonidegib in a dose 200 mg/day (n = 79) [28]

Primary system organ class (the preferred term)	Frequency
Metabolism and nutrition disorders:	
Decreased appetite	Very common
Dehydration	Common
Nervous system disorders:	
Dysgeusia	Very common
Headache	Very common
Gastrointestinal disorders:	
Nausea	Very common
Diarrhea	Very common
Abdominal pain	Very common
Vomiting	Very common
Dyspepsia	Common
Constipation	Common
Gastroesophageal reflux disorder	Common
Skin and subcutaneous tissue disorders:	
Alopecia	Very common
Pruritus	Very common
Rash	Common
Abnormal hair growth	Common
Musculoskeletal and connective tissue disorders:	
Muscle spasms	Very common
Musculoskeletal pain	Very common
Myalgia	Very common
Myopathy	Common
[muscular fatigue and muscular weakness]	
Reproductive system and breast disorders:	
Amenorrhea[a]	Very common
General disorders and administration site conditions:	
Fatigue	Very common
Pain	Very common
Investigations:	
Weight decrease	Very common

[a]Of the 79 patients receiving sonidegib in dose 200 mg/day, 5 were women of childbearing age. Among these women, amenorrhea was observed in 1 patient (20%)

Table 9.4 The laboratory abnormalities reported based on CTCAE version 4.03 [28]

Laboratory test	Frequency, all G
Hematological parameters:	
Hemoglobin decreased	Very common
Lymphocyte count decreased	Very common
Biochemistry parameters:	
Serum creatinine increased	Very common
Serum creatine phosphokinase (CPK) increased	Very common
Blood glucose increased	Very common
Lipase increased	Very common
Alanine aminotransaminase (ALT) increased	Very common
Aspartate aminotransaminase (AST) increased	Very common
Amylase increased	Very common

grouping, adverse drug reactions are presented in order of decreasing seriousness. Besides, the corresponding frequency category for each adverse drug reaction is based on the following convention: very common ($\geq 1/10$); common ($\geq 1/100$ to $< 1/10$); uncommon ($\geq 1/1000$ to $< 1/100$); rare ($\geq 1/10,000$ to $< 1/1000$); very rare ($< 1/10,000$); not known (cannot be estimated from the available data).

ADRs can limit the utility of sonidegib by leading to treatment discontinuation in many patients. The awareness and appropriate management of most frequent ADRs reported by patients during treatment with sonidegib are crucial. Most ADRs can be attributed to the mechanism of action of this drug and it is believed that such ADRs belong to the class effect of inhibitors of the Hedgehog (Hh) signaling pathway [28].

Management of severe or intolerable adverse reactions may require temporary dose interruption, with or without a subsequent dose reduction, or in some cases discontinuation. When dose interruption is required, it is advised to consider resuming sonidegib at the same dose after resolution of the adverse reaction to $\leq$ G1. If dose reduction is required, then the dose should be reduced to 200 mg every other day. If the same adverse drug reaction occurs following the change to alternate daily dosing and does not improve, it is advised to consider treatment discontinuation. Due to the long half-life of sonidegib, the full effect of a dose interruption or dose reduction of sonidegib is expected to occur after a few weeks. Detailed information about recommended dose modifications and management for symptomatic CPK elevations and muscle-related adverse reactions is included in the summary of product characteristics [28].

Sonidegib 800 mg once daily does not prolong the corrected QT interval and the approved 200 mg dose is not expected to cause clinically significant QTc prolongation [28, 29].

Sonidegib may cause embryo-fetal death or severe birth defects when administered to pregnant women. In animal studies, sonidegib has been shown to be teratogenic and fetotoxic. Women taking sonidegib must not be pregnant or become pregnant during treatment and for 20 months after the end of treatment [28].

Concomitant treatment with strong CYP inducers (e.g., rifampicin, carbamazepine, or phenytoin) should be avoided, as a risk for decreased plasma concentrations and decreased efficacy of sonidegib cannot be excluded. Sonidegib is primarily metabolized by CYP3A4, and concomitant administration of strong inhibitors or inducers of CYP3A4 can increase or decrease sonidegib concentrations significantly. Special care should be taken when using concomitantly other drugs that may cause muscle-related toxicity. Patients should be carefully followed. If muscle symptoms develop the dose adjustments should be considered [28].

In the BOLT study based on the primary analysis published in 2015, fewer patients in the group treated with dose 200 mg/d experienced AEs than in the group receiving dose 800 mg/d. The most common adverse events were muscle spasms, dysgeusia, alopecia, nausea, increased CPK, weight decrease, and fatigue. Less patients in the group treated with dose 200 mg/d experienced AEs leading to dose interruptions or reductions (25 [32%] of 79 patients vs 90 [60%] of 150) or treatment discontinuation (17 [22%] v. 54 [36%]) than in the group receiving dose 800 mg/d. The most frequent adverse events leading to discontinuation of treatment were muscle spasms, dysgeusia, weight decrease, and nausea. The most commonly reported AEs G3 and G4 were increased CPK (5 [6%] in the 200 mg group v.19 [13%] in the 800 mg group) and increased lipase (4 [5%] v. 8 [5%]). Serious adverse events (SAEs) were reported in 11 (14%) of 79 patients in the 200 mg group and 45 (30%) of 150 patients in the 800 mg group. Secondary malignancies were noted in 5 patients in the 200 mg group and 11 patients in the 800 mg group. No deaths related to study drug were reported [13].

In the 12-month follow-up, there were no new safety signals reported in this study. G3 and G4 AEs and AEs leading to treatment discontinuation were less frequent with sonidegib 200 mg/d than with sonidegib 800 mg/d (38.0% v. 59.3% and 27.8% v. 37.3%, respectively). Dose modification or interruption due to AEs was required in 38.0% and 64.0% of patients, and treatment discontinuation because of AEs occurred in 27.8% (200 mg) and 37.3% (800 mg) of patients. AEs were observed less commonly in the group receiving sonidegib 200 mg/d than in the group receiving sonidegib 800 mg/d; 97.0% of patients in the sonidegib 200 mg/d group and 100% in the group receiving sonidegib 800 mg/d experienced at least 1 AE. SAEs regardless of causality were reported in 16.5% of patients treated with sonidegib 200 mg/d and 32.7% in patients receiving the dose 800 mg/d. The most common SAEs reported in this analysis were rhabdomyolysis (1.3% v. 3.3%) and elevated CPK (1.3% v. 2.7%). None of the cases of rhabdomyolysis were confirmed by an independent review [19]. In the analyses done after 18 and 30 months follow-up, the safety profile of the dose 200 mg was continuously better than 800 mg [20].

The last published analysis of safety data from the BOLT study collected after 42 months of follow-up showed, that reported AEs were consistent with the known safety profile of sonidegib, with no new or late-onset safety concerns emerging at 42 months. Most AEs in the 200 mg/d group were G1 and G2 and most AEs were manageable and reversible with dose interruptions or reductions, with no overall impact on efficacy. In the 200 mg/d arm, the AEs that most frequently led to treatment discontinuation were muscle spasms, asthenia, dysgeusia, nausea, fatigue, weight loss, and decreased appetite. The AEs most frequently leading to treatment discontinuation in the 800 mg arm included muscle spasms, alopecia, weight loss, decreased appetite, dysgeusia, nausea, fatigue, dehydration, and elevated CPK. The detailed frequency of AEs G1–G2 v. G3–G4 reported in ≥20% of patients treated with sonidegib 200 mg and 800 mg/d are shown in Table 9.5 [21].

The summary of AEs reported in patients treated with sonidegib 200 mg/d in BOLT study based on analyses with 12, 30, and 42-months follow-up is presented in Table 9.6

Table 9.5 Adverse events in ≥20% of patients treated with sonidegib 200 mg and 800 mg daily, based on the safety data collected after 42-month follow-up. Based on Dummer et al. [21]

AE	200 mg G1–G2 (%)	200 mg G3–G4 (%)	800 mg G1–G2 (%)	800 mg G3–G4 (%)
Muscle spasms	51.9	2.5	64.0	5.3
Alopecia	49.4	NA	58.0	NA
Dysgeusia	44.3	NA	60.0	NA
Nausea	38.0	1.3	44.7	2.7
Diarrhea	30.4	1.3	24.0	0.0
CPK increase	24.1	6.3	24.0	13.3
Weight decrease	25.3	5.1	36.7	6.7
Fatigue	31.6	1.3	34.7	2.0
Appetite decrease	21.5	1.3	31.3	4.0

CPK creatine kinase, *NA* not applicable

Table 9.6 AEs reported in patients treated with sonidegib 200 mg/d in BOLT study based on analyses with 12, 30, and 42-months follow-up ($n = 79$). Based on Dummer et al. [21]

	12 months FU	30 months FU	42 months FU
All AEs, *n* (%)	77 (98)	77 (98)	77 (98)
AEs G3 and G4, *n* (%)	30 (38)	34 (43)	34 (43)
All TRAEs, *n* (%)	70 (89)	70 (89)	70 (89)
TRAEs G3 and G4, *n* (%)	22 (28)	24 (30)	25 (32)
SAEs, *n* (%)	13 (17)	16 (20)	16 (20)
Treatment-related SAEs, *n* (%)	2 (3)	3 (4)	4 (5)
AEs leading to discontinuation, *n* (%)	22 (28)	24 (30)	24 (30)
AEs leading to dose interruption and/or reduction, *n* (%)	30 (38)	34 (43)	34 (43)

FU follow-up, *AE* adverse event, *SAE* serious adverse event, *TRAE* treatment-related adverse event, *G* grade

Summary of Approval and Regulatory Indications

Sonidegib is approved in the EU for the treatment of adult patients with locally advanced basal cell carcinoma (BCC), who are not amenable to curative surgery or radiation therapy. In the US it is approved for the treatment of adult patients with locally advanced basal cell carcinoma (BCC) that has recurred following surgery or radiation therapy, or those who are not candidates for surgery or radiation therapy. It was approved by the FDA (the US Food and Drug Administration) in July 2015 and by the EMA (the European Medicines Agency) in August 2015.

The recommended dose is 200 mg sonidegib taken orally, once daily. Sonidegib must be taken at least 2 hours after a meal and at least 1 hour before the following meal to prevent an increased risk of adverse reactions due to higher exposure of sonidegib when taken with a meal. Treatment should be continued as long as clinical benefit is observed or until unacceptable toxicity [28].

PK studies showed that there are no clinically relevant effects of age, body weight, gender, and creatinine clearance on the systemic exposure of sonidegib [16, 28]. The dose adjustment is not required in older patients ($\geq$65 years), patients with mild-or-moderate renal impairment, and patients with hepatic impairment. No efficacy and safety data are available in patients with severe renal impairment.

No data are available about the safety and efficacy of sonidegib in children and adolescents aged below 18 years with BCC.

References

1. McMahon AP, Ingham PW, Tabin CJ. Developmental roles and clinical significance of hedgehog signaling. Curr Top Dev Biol. 2003;53:1–114. https://doi.org/10.1016/s0070-2153(03)53002-2.
2. Blanpain C, Fuchs E. Epidermal homeostasis: a balancing act of stem cells in the skin. Nat Rev Mol Cell Biol. 2009;10(3):207–17. https://doi.org/10.1038/nrm2636.
3. Leavitt E, Lask G, Martin S. Sonic Hedgehog pathway inhibition in the treatment of advanced basal cell carcinoma. Curr Treat Options in Oncol. 2019;20(11):84. https://doi.org/10.1007/s11864-019-0683-9.
4. Scales SJ, de Sauvage FJ. Mechanisms of Hedgehog pathway activation in cancer and implications for therapy. Trends Pharmacol Sci. 2009;30(6):303–12. https://doi.org/10.1016/j.tips.2009.03.007.
5. Amakye D, Jagani Z, Dorsch M. Unraveling the therapeutic potential of the Hedgehog pathway in cancer. Nat Med. 2013;19(11):1410–22. https://doi.org/10.1038/nm.3389.
6. Teglund S, Toftgård R. Hedgehog beyond medulloblastoma and basal cell carcinoma. Biochim Biophys Acta. 2010;1805(2):181–208. https://doi.org/10.1016/j.bbcan.2010.01.003.
7. Pasca di Magliano M, Hebrok M. Hedgehog signalling in cancer formation and maintenance. Nat Rev Cancer. 2003;3(12):903–11. https://doi.org/10.1038/nrc1229.
8. Rubin LL, de Sauvage FJ. Targeting the Hedgehog pathway in cancer. Nat Rev Drug Discov. 2006;5(12):1026–33. https://doi.org/10.1038/nrd2086.
9. Pan S, Wu X, Jiang J, Gao W, Wan Y, Cheng D, Han D, Liu J, Englund NP, Wang Y, Peukert S, Miller-Moslin K, Yuan J, Guo R, Matsumoto M, Vattay A, Jiang Y, Tsao J, Sun F, Pferdekamper AC, Dodd S, Tuntland T, Maniara W, Kelleher JF III, Yao YM, Warmuth M, Williams J, Dorsch

M. Discovery of NVP-LDE225, a potent and selective smoothened antagonist. ACS Med Chem Lett. 2010;1(3):130–4. https://doi.org/10.1021/ml1000307.

10. Wang C, Wu H, Katritch V, Han GW, Huang XP, Liu W, Siu FY, Roth BL, Cherezov V, Stevens RC. Structure of the human smoothened receptor bound to an antitumour agent. Nature. 2013;497(7449):338–43. https://doi.org/10.1038/nature12167.

11. Sharpe HJ, Pau G, Dijkgraaf GJ, Basset-Seguin N, Modrusan Z, Januario T, Tsui V, Durham AB, Dlugosz AA, Haverty PM, Bourgon R, Tang JY, Sarin KY, Dirix L, Fisher DC, Rudin CM, Sofen H, Migden MR, Yauch RL, de Sauvage FJ. Genomic analysis of smoothened inhibitor resistance in basal cell carcinoma. Cancer Cell. 2015;27(3):327–41. https://doi.org/10.1016/j.ccell.2015.02.001.

12. Rodon J, Tawbi HA, Thomas AL, Stoller RG, Turtschi CP, Baselga J, Sarantopoulos J, Mahalingam D, Shou Y, Moles MA, Yang L, Granvil C, Hurh E, Rose KL, Amakye DD, Dummer R, Mita AC. A phase I, multicenter, open-label, first-in-human, dose-escalation study of the oral smoothened inhibitor Sonidegib (LDE225) in patients with advanced solid tumors. Clin Cancer Res. 2014;20(7):1900–9. https://doi.org/10.1158/1078-0432.Ccr-13-1710.

13. Migden MR, Guminski A, Gutzmer R, Dirix L, Lewis KD, Combemale P, Herd RM, Kudchadkar R, Trefzer U, Gogov S, Pallaud C, Yi T, Mone M, Kaatz M, Loquai C, Stratigos AJ, Schulze HJ, Plummer R, Chang AL, Cornélis F, Lear JT, Sellami D, Dummer R. Treatment with two different doses of sonidegib in patients with locally advanced or metastatic basal cell carcinoma (BOLT): a multicentre, randomised, double-blind phase 2 trial. Lancet Oncol. 2015;16(6):716–28. https://doi.org/10.1016/s1470-2045(15)70100-2.

14. Zollinger M, Lozac'h F, Hurh E, Emotte C, Bauly H, Swart P. Absorption, distribution, metabolism, and excretion (ADME) of ^{14}C-sonidegib (LDE225) in healthy volunteers. Cancer Chemother Pharmacol. 2014;74(1):63–75. https://doi.org/10.1007/s00280-014-2468-y.

15. Horsmans Y, Zhou J, Liudmila M, Golor G, Shibolet O, Quinlan M, Emotte C, Boss H, Castro H, Sellami D, Preston RA. Effects of mild to severe hepatic impairment on the pharmacokinetics of sonidegib: a multicenter, open-label, parallel-group study. Clin Pharmacokinet. 2018;57(3):345–54. https://doi.org/10.1007/s40262-017-0560-2.

16. Goel V, Hurh E, Stein A, Nedelman J, Zhou J, Chiparus O, Huang PH, Gogov S, Sellami D. Population pharmacokinetics of sonidegib (LDE225), an oral inhibitor of hedgehog pathway signaling, in healthy subjects and in patients with advanced solid tumors. Cancer Chemother Pharmacol. 2016;77(4):745–55. https://doi.org/10.1007/s00280-016-2982-1.

17. Zhou J, Quinlan M, Glenn K, Boss H, Picard F, Castro H, Sellami D. Effect of esomeprazole, a proton pump inhibitor on the pharmacokinetics of sonidegib in healthy volunteers. Br J Clin Pharmacol. 2016;82(4):1022–9. https://doi.org/10.1111/bcp.13038.

18. Chen L, Silapunt S, Migden MR. Sonidegib for the treatment of advanced basal cell carcinoma: a comprehensive review of sonidegib and the BOLT trial with 12-month update. Future Oncol (London, England). 2016;12(18):2095–105. https://doi.org/10.2217/fon-2016-0118.

19. Dummer R, Guminski A, Gutzmer R, Dirix L, Lewis KD, Combemale P, Herd RM, Kaatz M, Loquai C, Stratigos AJ, Schulze HJ, Plummer R, Gogov S, Pallaud C, Yi T, Mone M, Chang AL, Cornélis F, Kudchadkar R, Trefzer U, Lear JT, Sellami D, Migden MR. The 12-month analysis from Basal Cell Carcinoma Outcomes with LDE225 Treatment (BOLT): A phase II, randomized, double-blind study of sonidegib in patients with advanced basal cell carcinoma. J Am Acad Dermatol. 2016;75(1):113–125.e115. https://doi.org/10.1016/j.jaad.2016.02.1226.

20. Lear JT, Migden MR, Lewis KD, Chang ALS, Guminski A, Gutzmer R, Dirix L, Combemale P, Stratigos A, Plummer R, Castro H, Yi T, Mone M, Zhou J, Trefzer U, Kaatz M, Loquai C, Kudchadkar R, Sellami D, Dummer R. Long-term efficacy and safety of sonidegib in patients with locally advanced and metastatic basal cell carcinoma: 30-month analysis of the randomized phase 2 BOLT study. J Eur Acad Dermatol Venereol. 2018;32(3):372–81. https://doi.org/10.1111/jdv.14542.

21. Dummer R, Guminksi A, Gutzmer R, Lear JT, Lewis KD, Chang ALS, Combemale P, Dirix L, Kaatz M, Kudchadkar R, Loquai C, Plummer R, Schulze HJ, Stratigos AJ, Trefzer U, Squittieri N, Migden MR. Long-term efficacy and safety of sonidegib in patients with advanced basal

cell carcinoma: 42-month analysis of the phase II randomized, double-blind BOLT study. Br J Dermatol. 2020;182(6):1369–78. https://doi.org/10.1111/bjd.18552.

22. Skvara H, Kalthoff F, Meingassner JG, Wolff-Winiski B, Aschauer H, Kelleher JF, Wu X, Pan S, Mickel L, Schuster C, Stary G, Jalili A, David OJ, Emotte C, Antunes AM, Rose K, Decker J, Carlson I, Gardner H, Stuetz A, Bertolino AP, Stingl G, De Rie MA. Topical treatment of Basal cell carcinomas in nevoid Basal cell carcinoma syndrome with a smoothened inhibitor. J Invest Dermatol. 2011;131(8):1735–44. https://doi.org/10.1038/jid.2011.48.

23. To Evaluate the Safety, Local Tolerability, PK and PD of LDE225 on Sporadic Superficial and Nodular Skin Basal Cell Carcinomas (sBCC). https://clinicaltrials.gov/ct2/show/NCT01033019.

24. Chang AL, Solomon JA, Hainsworth JD, Goldberg L, McKenna E, Day BM, Chen DM, Weiss GJ. Expanded access study of patients with advanced basal cell carcinoma treated with the Hedgehog pathway inhibitor, vismodegib. J Am Acad Dermatol. 2014;70(1):60–9. https://doi.org/10.1016/j.jaad.2013.09.012.

25. Chang AL, Oro AE. Initial assessment of tumor regrowth after vismodegib in advanced Basal cell carcinoma. Arch Dermatol. 2012;148(11):1324–5. https://doi.org/10.1001/archdermatol.2012.2354.

26. Danial C, Sarin KY, Oro AE, Chang AL. An investigator-initiated open-label trial of sonidegib in advanced basal cell carcinoma patients resistant to vismodegib. Clin Cancer Res. 2016;22(6):1325–9. https://doi.org/10.1158/1078-0432.Ccr-15-1588.

27. Post-authorization safety study on the long term safety of sonidegib in patients with locally advanced cell carcinoma. https://ClinicalTrials.gov/show/NCT04066504.

28. Odomzo® (sonidegib) summary of product characteristics. October 2020. https://www.ema.europa.eu/en/documents/product-information/odomzo-epar-product-information_en.pdf

29. Odomzo® (sonidegib) capsules, for oral use: US prescribing infomation. 2015.

Part III
Immunological Strategies in Advanced Melanoma

Chapter 10
Ipilimumab in Melanoma: An Evergreen Drug

Francesco Spagnolo, Enrica Tanda, and Mario Mandalà

Introduction

Ipilimumab is a fully human monoclonal antibody (IgG1κ) that activates the immune system by targeting the cytotoxic T-lymphocyte antigen 4 (CTLA-4), a co-receptor with inhibitory properties expressed by T lymphocytes. CTLA-4 is physiologically involved in maintaining self-tolerance. When T lymphocytes are activated through recognition of an antigen exposed on the surface of the antigen-presenting cells (signal 1) and the interaction between the CD28 co-stimulatory receptor and the CD80 and CD86 molecules (signal 2), they start expressing CTLA-4 on their surface. CTLA-4 has greater affinity for the CD80 and CD86 molecules than CD28 and displace their interaction, eliciting an inhibitory signal to the T cell rather than an activating one (see Fig. 10.1) [1]. CTLA-4 is also a target gene of the Forkhead box P3 transcription factor (FOXP3), which is a crucial factor in the genesis of regulatory T-cell lineage [2]. The role of CTLA-4 and the function of regulatory T cells are closely related. In fact, subjects harboring the homozygous mutation in FOXP3 suffer from an autoimmune X-linked hereditary syndrome, known as IPEX, with clinical manifestations of polyendocrinopathy and enteropathy [3]. These signs and symptoms are similar to some of the most frequent immune-related adverse events observed in patients treated with anti-CTLA-4 antibodies [4]. Therefore, the inhibition of CTLA-4 is a therapeutic strategy based both on the enhancement of the T

F. Spagnolo (✉) · E. Tanda
Oncologia Medica 2, IRCCS Ospedale Policlinico San Martino, Genoa, Italy
e-mail: francesco.spagnolo@hsanamrtino.it

M. Mandalà
University of Perugia, Unit of Medical Oncology, Ospedale Santa Maria Misericordia, Perugia, Italy
e-mail: mario.mandala@unipg.it

P. Rutkowski, M. Mandalà (eds.), *New Therapies in Advanced Cutaneous Malignancies*, https://doi.org/10.1007/978-3-030-64009-5_10

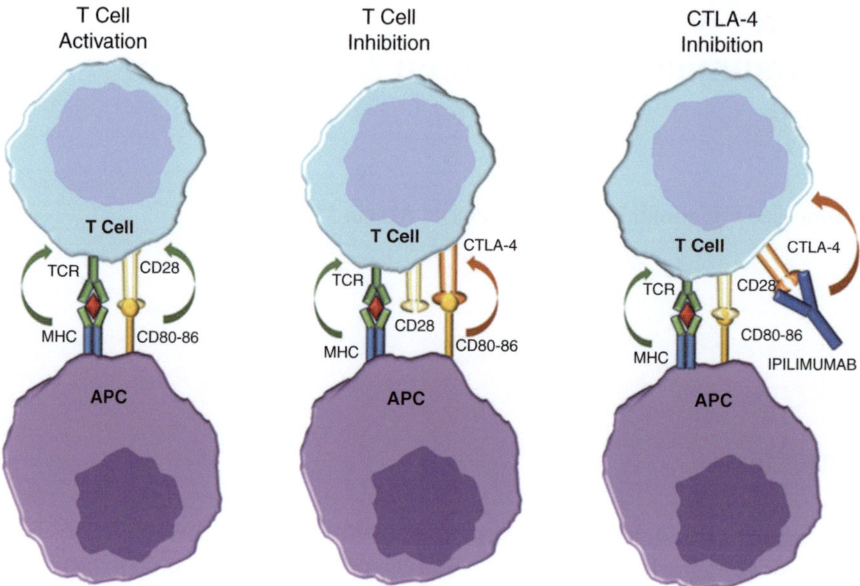

Fig. 10.1 Mechanism of action of ipilimumab. CTLA-4 is an inhibitory molecule present on T cells: during the interaction between antigen-presenting cells and lymphocytes, CTLA4 competes with co-stimulatory signals and interrupts T-cell priming. By blocking CTLA-4, the inhibitory effect on the priming phase is released leading to unrestricted T-cell activation

effector lymphocytes and the inhibition of regulatory T-cell lymphocytes. The anti-CTLA-4 tremelimumab and ipilimumab were the first fully humanized anti-CTLA-4 antibodies that underwent clinical testing, and, in 2011, ipilimumab 3 mg per kilogram (IPI3) every 3 weeks for 4 administrations was the first immune-checkpoint inhibitor which received the FDA approval for the treatment of a solid tumor, after the results of the MDX010–20 phase 3 trial in patients with advanced melanoma [5].

The purpose of this chapter is to report the most relevant results of ipilimumab from selected clinical trials and real world studies, to discuss how the introduction of ipilimumab into clinical practice challenged the evaluation of tumor response and management of toxicity, and to discuss the role of ipilimumab in the era of anti-PD-1 agents.

Ipilimumab as Single Agent for the Treatment of Advanced Melanoma

In the MDX010–20 phase 3 trial, patients with pretreated advanced melanoma were randomized in a 3:1:1 ratio to receive either ipilimumab plus gp100 (403 patients), ipilimumab alone (137 patients), or gp100 alone (136 patients). Ipilimumab was administered with or without gp100 at a dose of 3 mg per kilogram of body weight for up to four treatments (induction); patients who derived a benefit but ultimately had progressive disease (PD) could receive reinduction therapy, consisting of other 4 ipilimumab infusions. The primary endpoint was overall survival (OS). The median OS was 10.0 and 10.1 months among patients receiving ipilimumab plus gp100 or ipilimumab alone, respectively, as compared with 6.4 months among patients receiving gp100 alone. Severe (grade 3–4) immune-related adverse events (irAEs) occurred in 10–15% of patients receiving ipilimumab, and 7 patients died due to an immune-related toxicity [5]. The most common autoimmune side effects included skin rash, endocrine deficiencies, and colitis. In the ipilimumab-alone group, the overall response rate (ORR) was 10.9%, with a disease control rate (DCR) of 28.5%. Despite the small absolute benefit in terms of median OS and the low response rate, analyses of survival showed that 2-year OS was 21.6–23.5% in patients who received ipilimumab as compared with 13.7% for gp100 alone, which is clinically significant [5] (Table 10.1). Based on the results of this study, ipilimumab 3 mg/kg every 3 weeks for a total of 4 administrations received the approval by the regulatory agencies for the treatment of metastatic melanoma.

Ipilimumab was found to stimulate a dose-dependent effect on both clinical activity and toxicity [6, 15], leading to the investigation of higher doses in further studies (Tables 10.1 and 10.2). In the randomized, phase 2 CA184–022 clinical trial, 217 patients with previously treated advanced melanoma were randomly assigned to receive ipilimumab at either a dose of 10 mg/kg, 3 mg/kg, or 0.3 mg/kg every 3 weeks for four administrations followed by maintenance therapy every 3 months. The primary endpoint was best ORR, which was 11.1% for 10 mg/kg and 4.2% for 3 mg/kg, while no objective responses were achieved with 0.3 mg/kg. The dose-dependent effect on clinical activity was also noted in terms of toxicity, with irAEs of any grade being observed in 70%, 65%, and 26% of patients who received the doses of 10 mg/kg, 3 mg/kg, and 0.3 mg/kg, respectively. No grade 3–4 gastrointestinal irAEs were observed at the lowest dose, as compared as 16% and 3% for ipilimumab 10 mg/kg and 3 mg/kg, respectively [6]. In the phase 3 study of ipilimumab 10 mg per kilogram plus dacarbazine as a first-line treatment for patients with advanced melanoma, 502 subjects were randomized in a 1:1 ratio to receive either ipilimumab 10 mg per kilogram (IPI10) plus dacarbazine or dacarbazine plus placebo. Patients with stable disease (SD) or an objective response and no toxic effects were eligible to receive maintenance therapy with ipilimumab or placebo every 12 weeks. The primary endpoint was OS, which was significantly longer in the group receiving ipilimumab (11.2 months vs. 9.1 months). Similar to that observed in the MDX010–20 phase 3 trial, despite the difference in terms of median OS was only 2.1 months, the landmark analysis of survival revealed a clinically meaningful long-term benefit, with 20.8% of patients who received ipilimumab being alive at 3 years versus 12.2% in the dacarbazine group. Grade 3–4 adverse events occurred in 56.3% of patients treated with ipilimumab plus dacarbazine, with no drug-related deaths [7].

The efficacy and safety of IPI3 and IPI10 was then directly compared in a randomized phase 3 trial. Median OS was 15.7 months (95% CI 11.6–17.8) for IPI10 compared with 11.5 months (95% CI 9.9–13.3) for IPI3 (hazard ratio 0.84, 95%

Table 10.1 Summary of results of selected clinical trials with ipilimumab as single agent or in combination with other drugs for the treatment of patients with advanced melanoma. Only data for treatment regimens including ipilimumab are reported

Name of study, first author and date of publication	Study design	Treatment regimen	Median OS (months)	Median PFS (months)	Overall response rate (%)	2-year OS (%)	3-year OS (%)	Grade 3–4 irAEs (%)
MDX010–20, Hodi 2010 [5]	Phase 3	IPI3 every 3 weeks for 4 cycles	10.0–10.1	2.76–2.86	6–11	22–24	NA	10–15
CA184–022, Wolchok 2010 [6]	Phase 2	IPI10 every 3 weeks for 4 cycles, followed by IPI10 every 3 months	11.4	NA	11	30	NA	18
		IPI3 every 3 weeks for 4 cycles, followed by IPI3 every 3 months	8.7	NA	4	24	NA	5
		IPI0.3 every 3 weeks for 4 cycles, followed by IPI0.3 every 3 months	8.6	NA	0	18	NA	0
CA184–024, Robert 2011 [7]	Phase 3	IPI10 plus DTIC every 3 weeks for 4 cycles, followed by DTIC	11.2	NA	15	29	21	38
CA184–169, Ascierto 2017 [8]	Phase 3	IPI10 every 3 weeks for 4 cycles	15.7	2.8	15	39	31	34
		IPI3 every 3 weeks for 4 cycles	11.5	2.8	12	31	23	18
CheckMate-064, Weber 2016 [9]	Phase 2	NIVO→IPI	Not reached	NA	56	NA	NA	63
		IPI → NIVO	16.9	NA	31	NA	NA	50
CheckMate-069, Hodi 2016 [10]	Phase 2	IPI3 + NIVO1	Not reached	Not reached	59	64	NA	54
		IPI3 every 3 weeks for 4 cycles	Not reached	3.0	11	54	NA	20
CheckMate-067, Wolchok 2017 [11] Larkin 2019 [12]	Phase 3	IPI3 + NIVO1	Not reached (>60.0)	11.5	58	64	58	59
		IPI3 every 3 weeks for 4 cycles	19.9	2.9	19	45	34	28
CheckMate-511, Lebbé 2019 [13]	Phase 3b/4	IPI3 + NIVO1	Not reached	8.94	51	NA	NA	48
		IPI1 + NIVO3	Not reached	9.92	46	NA	NA	34
Keynote-029, Long 2017 [14]	Phase 1b	Pembrolizumab 2 mg/kg plus IPI1 every 3 weeks for four cycles, followed by pembrolizumab 2 mg/kg every 3 weeks	Not reached	Not reached	61	NA	NA	27

IPI1 + NIVO3 nivolumab 3 mg/kg plus ipilimumab 1 mg/kg every 3 weeks for four cycles, followed by nivolumab 3 mg/kg every 2 weeks; *IPI3 + NIVO1* nivolumab 1 mg/kg plus ipilimumab 3 mg/kg every 3 weeks for four cycles, followed by nivolumab 3 mg/kg every 2 weeks; *IPI → NIVO* IPI3 every 3 weeks for 4 cycles, followed by NIVO3 every 2 weeks for 6 doses, followed by NIVO3 maintenance therapy every 2 weeks; *NIVO→IPI* NIVO3 every 2 weeks for 6 doses, followed by IPI3 every 3 weeks for 4 cycles, followed by NIVO3 maintenance therapy every 2 weeks

Table 10.2 Summary of safety with different doses of ipilimumab as single agent or in combination with anti-PD-1

Treatment regimen	Grade 3–4 irAEs (%)	Discontinuation rate due to any grade irAEs (%)	Studies
Iplimumab 0.3 mg/kg	0	2	CA184–022 [6]
Iplimumab 3 mg/kg	5–28	5–19	MDX010–20 [5], CA184–022 [6], CA184–169 [8], CheckMate-069 [10], CheckMate-067 [12] [11]
Iplimumab 10 mg/kg	18–34	11–31	CA184–022 [6], CA184–169 [8]
Iplimumab 10 mg/kg + dacarbazine	38	36	CA184–024 [7]
Iplimumab 3 mg/kg + nivolumab 1 mg/kg	48–59	33–39	CheckMate-069 [10], CheckMate-067 [11], CheckMate-511 [13]
Iplimumab 1 mg/kg + nivolumab 3 mg/kg	34	24	CheckMate-511 [13]
Pembrolizumab 2 mg/kg + Iplimumab 1 mg/kg	27	26	Keynote-029 [14]

CI 0.70–0.99), but more treatment-related serious adverse events occurred in patients who received the higher dose (37% versus 18%) [8]. Despite the impact on OS, which is particularly appreciated in terms of chance of long-term survival (3-year OS was 31% for IPI10 versus 23% for IPI3), the higher dosage of ipilimumab did not receive the FDA approval for the treatment of advanced melanoma, partly due to the upcoming results of anti-PD-1 agents, which took the place of ipilimumab as the first-line immunotherapy for metastatic melanoma patients [16, 17].

Long-Term Efficacy and Effectiveness

Despite the impact of ipilimumab on clinical activity outcomes such as ORR and progression-free survival (PFS) was not meaningful (Table 10.1), long-term follow-up demonstrated its great efficacy and effectiveness in at least a subset of patients. In a pooled analysis of long-term survival data from phase 2 and phase 3 trials of ipilimumab in advanced melanoma, among 1.861 patients, median OS was 11.4 months (95% CI, 10.7 to 12.1 months), but the survival curve began to plateau around year 3, with follow-up of up to 10 years. Three-year survival rates were 22%, 26%, and 20% for all patients, treatment-naive patients, and previously treated patients, respectively. Including data from the expanded access program, median OS was 9.5 months (95% CI, 9.0 to 10.0 months), with a plateau at 21% in the survival curve beginning around year 3, demonstrating the effectiveness of ipilimumab in an unselected population [18]. In the 5-year analysis of the phase 3 study with IPI10 plus dacarbazine versus dacarbazine plus placebo, 5-year OS was 18.2% for the experimental arm and 8.8% for the control [19]. The long-term chance for survival in the chemotherapy group was higher as compared with historical data [20], probably due to a subset of patients who received ipilimumab after PD with chemotherapy.

Efficacy, Clinical Activity, and Safety of Re-induction

Some data suggested that re-induction upon disease progression in patients who derived a clinical benefit from the induction treatment with ipilimumab may be a valid approach to overcome immune tolerance in selected patients. Disease-control was regained in 48–75% of patients receiving re-induction in clinical trials and expanded access programs, and ORR ranged from 12% to 38%, with no toxicity concerns, as the incidence of treatment-related AEs observed during retreatment was similar to that observed during induction [5, 21, 22]. However, the sample size was too small for retreatment to be worth regulatory agencies approval, and further evaluation of this strategy in randomized clinical trials was not necessary due to the anti-PD-1 agent's breakthrough.

Clinical Activity of Ipilimumab in Patients with Brain Metastases

The incidence of brain metastases in melanoma patients is common and associated with poor prognosis [23]. Evidence of intracranial tumor responses after ipilimumab treatment was reported in both clinical trials and real world experiences (Table 10.3) [24–28]. Despite that, survival outcomes remained poor, especially in patients receiving corticosteroids due to brain metastases symptoms [23, 27].

The Evaluation of Antitumor Response to Ipilimumab

Conventional response criteria, such as Response Evaluation Criteria in Solid Tumors (RECIST), were developed based on data from cytotoxic chemotherapy trials and are not always appropriate to assess the activity of immunotherapy. Indeed, ipilimumab may achieve tumor regression and obtain long-lasting disease control even after an initial increase in tumor burden or appearance of new lesions, which would be defined as PD by conventional criteria. Therefore, immune-related response criteria were developed to assess the specific antitumor effects of immune-checkpoint inhibitors: by such criteria, the appearance of new lesions or initial increase in tumor burden is not assessed as PD and must be confirmed through a subsequent tumor assessment [29]. Responses and SD assessed by immune-related criteria were observed in an additional 10% of metastatic melanoma patients treated

Table 10.3 Summary of results of phase 2 clinical trials and selected real world studies

Author and date of publication	Study design and number of patients with brain metastases	Treatment regimen	Median OS (months)	Median PFS (months)	Overall response rate	Overall intracranial response rate	Symptoms due to brain metastases
Heller 2011 [24]	Retrospective analysis of IPI10 EAP (N = 165)	IPI10	NA	1-year OS: 20%	NA	NA	0%
Weber 2011 [25]	Retrospective analysis of a phase 2 study (N = 12)	IPI10	14.0	NA	NA	NA	NA
Di Giacomo 2012 [26]	Phase 2 (N = 20)	IPI10 plus fotemustine	12.7	3.4	40%	NA	0%
Margolin 2012 [27]	Phase 2 (N = 72)	IPI10	3.7–7.0[a]	1.3–2.7[a]	5–10%[a]	5–16%[a]	100–0%[a]
Queirolo 2014 [28]	Retrospective analysis of the Italian IPI3 EAP (N = 146)	IPI3	4.3	3.1	12%	NA	0%

EAP expanded access program, *IPI3* ipilimumab 3 mg/kg, *IPI10* ipilimumab 10 mg/kg, *NA* not available, *OS* overall survival, *PFS* progression-free survival
[a]Symptomatic and asymptomatic patients, respectively

with ipilimumab and were associated with improved survival [29]. Immune-related criteria have been improved and updated over time. In 2017, a consensus guideline was developed and published by the RECIST working group for the use of RECIST version 1.1 criteria in cancer immunotherapy trials [30]. This guideline, named iRE-CIST, describes a standard approach to tumor assessment in patients with advanced solid tumors treated with immunotherapy, to warrant consistent design and to facilitate the collection of data. The most relevant difference between conventional RECIST 1.1 and iRECIST is the definition of immune-related unconfirmed progressive disease (iUPD), which is defined on the basis of RECIST 1.1 principles, but requires confirmation at a subsequent tumor assessment: if PD is not confirmed, the sum of diameters of target lesions is reset so that iUPD needs to occur again and then be confirmed by further tumor growth for immune-related confirmed progressive disease to be defined. This allows atypical responses, such as delayed responses that occur after pseudoprogression, to be identified [30].

The Management of Immune-Related Adverse Events

The introduction of immune-checkpoint inhibitors in clinical practice was a new challenge not only for the evaluation of antitumor response, but also because a new class of treatment-related adverse events emerged. Indeed, unlike chemotherapy, immune-checkpoint inhibitors can induce a spectrum of toxicities of autoimmune pathogenesis, namely irAEs. Due to the autoimmune pathogenesis, the milestone for the management of irAEs is corticosteroids therapy. Despite the immunosuppressive properties of corticosteroids, especially at higher doses, their use for the management of toxicities did not seem to affect the effectiveness of ipilimumab [31]. The corticosteroid dosages, routes of administration, and duration of tapering depend on the type and severity of the irAEs. In corticosteroid-refractory cases, other immunomodulatory agents such as infliximab (an anti-TNFα agent) and vedolizumab ($\alpha_4\beta_7$ integrin inhibitor) must be used in case of colitis, mycophenolate in case of hepatitis, myositis, bullous dermopathies, lupus, nephritis, interstitial lung disease, while plasmapheresis and immunoglobulin infusions are more commonly employed in case of neurotoxicity (in particular Guillain–Barré-like syndromes) [31]. The majority of severe toxicities, with the exception of dermatologic and endocrine irAEs, require permanent ipilimumab discontinuation [31–33]. Temporary treatment suspensions are generally required for grade 2 irAEs, with the exception of skin rash and asymptomatic endocrine events [31–33]. Toxicities involving the endocrine glands are treated with substitute hormones rather than corticosteroids [31–33]. Guidelines for the management of immune-mediated toxicities have been developed and improved over time. The most recent guidelines are those provided by The National Comprehensive Cancer Network (NCCN) [31], the European Society for Medical Oncology (ESMO) [32], and the American Society of Clinical Oncology (ASCO) [33].

Besides the use of immunomodulatory agents, other key factors are early recognition of irAEs and a proper baseline assessment. The history of autoimmune diseases must be collected to anticipate possible flares, and laboratory tests and physical examination should be performed before each ipilimumab infusion [34].

The clinical activity as well as toxicity of anti-CTLA-4 immunotherapy was proven to be dose-dependent [6, 8] (Table 10.2), unlike immunotherapy with anti-PD-1 [31, 35]. Moreover, immunotherapy with anti-CTLA-4 is associated with a higher rate of grade 3–4 irAEs (24% in a recent meta-analysis) [36], as compared with patients who received anti-PD-I drugs (5–8%) [37]. In patients receiving the combination of IPI3 and nivolumab 1 mg/kg (NIVO1) the rate of severe toxicities was as high as nearly 50% [17], while the reverse dosage was associated with grade 3–4 irAEs in 33.9% of patients [13].

Ipilimumab in Combination with Targeted Therapy

Strong evidence supports the notion that MAPK kinase-targeted therapy has immunomodulatory properties and enhances immune activation [38], hence clinical trials investigating the combination of ipilimumab with targeted therapy were initiated. However, the first attempt combining BRAF inhibitor vemurafenib with ipilimumab failed due to severe toxicities [39]. In the first cohort, vemurafenib 960 mg bid was administered as a single agent for 1 month, followed by the combination with ipilimumab; dose-limiting toxicities (DLTs) of grade 3 elevations in aminotransferase levels developed in four patients 2–5 weeks after the first infusion of ipilimumab in combination with vemurafenib. In the second cohort, vemurafenib 720 mg bid was given upfront in combination with ipilimumab: among the first four patients who received such regimen, elevations in aminotransferase levels (grade 3 in two patients and grade 2 in one patient) developed within 3 weeks after starting ipilimumab [39].

The safety of combination therapy of ipilimumab with BRAF inhibitor dabrafenib with or without MEK inhibitor trametinib was also halted due to severe treatment-related AEs. In the group of patients receiving ipilimumab plus dabrafenib and trametinib, among seven patients, two developed colitis followed by intestinal perforation [40].

The pursue of a combination regiment with BRAF and MEK inhibitors was abandoned, as new combination approaches were made possible with the more manageable anti-PD-1 agents, which were proven to be safe even in combination with BRAF plus MEK inhibitors [41].

Ipilimumab in Combination with Anti-PD-1 Drugs

In 2015, the results of the CheckMate-069 phase 2 trial [10] led to accelerated FDA approval of a combination of ipilimumab plus nivolumab for patients with BRAF wild-type, advanced melanoma (Table 10.1). After the results of the CheckMate-067 phase 3 trial, ipilimumab plus nivolumab was granted accelerated approval in January 2016 to include patients with BRAF-mutant melanoma [17]. In this phase

3 clinical study, a total of 945 treatment-naive patients with advanced melanoma were randomly assigned 1:1:1 to receive either nivolumab 1 mg/kg + ipilimumab 3 mg/kg every 3 weeks for 4 doses then nivolumab 3 mg/kg every 2 weeks (IPI3 + NIVO1), or nivolumab 3 mg/kg every 2 weeks + ipilimumab-matched placebo, or ipilimumab 3 mg/kg every 3 weeks for 4 doses + nivolumab-matched placebo. The primary endpoints were PFS and OS. Notably, the study was not designed for a formal statistical comparison between the combination group and the nivolumab monotherapy group. The 5-year update showed a PFS of 36%, 29%, and 8%, in the nivolumab + ipilimumab, nivolumab alone, and ipilimumab arms, respectively, with a 5-year OS of 52%, 44%, and 26% [12]. However, these results were obtained at the cost of higher toxicity. In fact, 59% of patients who received nivolumab + ipilimumab had grade 3–4 AEs, versus 23% and 28% in the nivolumab and ipilimumab arms, respectively. The most frequent grade 3–4 AEs leading to treatment discontinuation were diarrhea and colitis for all groups [11, 12, 17].

In order to overcome the difficulty of the higher rate of severe toxicity of the IPI3 + NIVO1, the KEYNOTE-029 phase 1b trial was conducted to evaluate the anti-PD-1 pembrolizumab + low-dose ipilimumab (1 mg/kg) for four cycles every 3 weeks, followed by pembrolizumab alone. An incidence of grade 3–4 irAEs of 27% was observed with this combination, numerically lower than that observed in CheckMate-067 trial with IPI3 + NIVO1. Treatment was permanently discontinued due to a treatment-related AE in 14% of patients. The ORR was 61%, and 1-year estimates for PFS and OS were 69% and 89%, respectively [14]. A similar approach was also investigated in the CheckMate-511 study, which was a phase 3b/4 trial conducted to assess if NIVO3 + IPI1 had a lower incidence of grade 3–5 AEs than the approved NIVO1 + IPI3 regimen. The incidence of treatment-related G3-G5 AEs in the two arms, primary endpoint of the study, was significantly lower in the NIVO3 + IPI1 arm compared with NIVO1 + IPI3 (34% vs. 48%; $p = 0.006$) [13]. Despite the study was not designed to demonstrate the non-inferiority of NIVO3 + IPI1 to NIVO1 + IPI3 in terms of clinical activity, in descriptive analyses ORR was 45.6% for NIVO3 + IPI1 *versus* 50.6% for NIVO1 + IPI3, with a median PFS of 9.9 and 8.9 months in the NIVO3 + IPI1 and NIVO1 + IPI3 arms, respectively [13].

Ipilimumab in Sequence with Anti-PD-1 Drugs

Concurrent administration of the immune-checkpoint inhibitors nivolumab and ipilimumab has shown greater efficacy than either agent alone, albeit with a higher rate of severe treatment-related adverse events [17]. The randomized phase 2 trial CheckMate-064 was designed to assess whether sequential administration of nivolumab followed by ipilimumab with a planned switch, or the reverse sequence, could maximize efficacy while maintaining an acceptable toxicity profile [9]. One hundred and forty patients were randomized 1:1 to receive, in the induction period, nivolumab 3 mg/kg every 2 weeks for 6 doses, followed by ipilimumab 3 mg/kg every 3 weeks for 4 cycles (NIVO→IPI cohort), or the reverse sequence (IPI → NIVO cohort). In the continuation phase, all patients were treated with nivolumab 3 mg/kg every 2 weeks until PD or unacceptable toxicity. Primary endpoint was the incidence of G3–5 AEs until the end of the induction period [9]. At week 25, the incidence of grade 3–5 AEs in the two groups was similar: 50% for NIVO→IPI and 43% for IPI → NIVO. No treatment-related deaths occurred. The most common grade 3–4 irAEs was colitis (15% in patients receiving NIVO→IPI and 20% in those treated with the IPI → NIVO sequence). Types and frequencies of AEs leading to discontinuation during the whole study were similar between groups (37% for the NIVO→IPI sequence versus 33% for IPI → NIVO); the most frequent irAEs leading to treatment permanent discontinuation were colitis, increased AST/ALT, and diarrhea. In terms of clinical activity and efficacy, the overall response rate at week 25 was higher for patients who received NIVO→IPI as compared with the reverse IPI → NIVO sequence (41% versus 20%), and more patients in the NIVO→IPI cohort were alive at 1 year than in the IPI → NIVO cohort (76% versus 54%) [9].

Biomarkers

Ipilimumab achieves a great clinical benefit in a small proportion of melanoma patients, highlighting the strong need to investigate predictive biomarkers. Despite that, no validated predictive biomarker has been identified yet to select patients who derive a benefit from such treatment.

Several blood biomarkers have shown their prognostic role, including baseline and post-treatment changes in leukocyte counts [42–46], lactate dehydrogenase [43–45, 47, 48], C-reactive protein [45, 47], and soluble CTLA-4 [49], but the retrospective and non-randomized nature of most studies, the small sample sizes, short follow-up time, and variability in the investigated biomarkers did not allow to properly assess their predictive potential [50]. In the largest study assessing the relevance of leucocyte counts in patients receiving ipilimumab for advanced melanoma, the derived neutrophil-to-lymphocyte ratio [absolute neutrophil counts/(white cell counts—absolute neutrophil counts)] and baseline absolute neutrophil counts were found to be associated with risk of death and progression, with higher values being associated with increased risk [42]. However, the role of such indexes as predictive biomarkers was not further investigated in clinical studies.

The investigation of CTLA-4 gene polymorphisms has also shown a promising biomarker to select patients with a higher chance of response to ipilimumab and long-term survival. In a multicenter study on 173 patients who received ipilimumab for advanced melanoma within the Italian Expanded Access, an association of CTLA-4 gene variants with response to therapy and long-term survival was found in subjects carrying the −1577G/G or CT60G/G genotypes [51]. Moreover, the CTLA-4 gene variant −1661A > G was found to be associated with a higher risk of endocrine irAEs [52].

Despite various biomarkers being correlated with improved response rate and long-term survival upon treatment with ipilimumab, their predictive value remains unclear so far, as most of these biomarkers are also well known as prognostic markers [50].

Adjuvant Setting

In 2015, after a significant impact on recurrence-free survival (RFS) was observed in the EORTC 18071 phase 3 trial for patients with completely resected high-risk stage III melanoma, IPI10 was approved for this indication by the FDA only. CA 184–029 (EORTC 18071) is a randomized phase 3 clinical trial which compared the anti-CTLA-4 agent ipilimumab 10 mg/kg every 3 weeks for four cycles, followed by maintenance doses every 3 months for up to 3 years versus placebo, in patients with resected stage III melanoma (excluding lymph node metastasis ≤ 1 mm in patients with stage IIIA melanoma, and excluding subjects with in-transit metastases for stage IIIB/IIIC). The 5-year RFS was 41% vs. 30% in the ipilimumab and placebo arms, respectively (HR for recurrence or death: 0.76; 95% CI 0.64 to 0.89). Ipilimumab also gave an advantage in terms of DMFS: 48% of patients were alive and metastasis-free at 5 years in the experimental arm versus 39% for placebo (HR for distant metastasis or death: 0.76; 95% CI 0.64 to 0.92) [53, 54]. Moreover, OS was significantly longer in the ipilimumab group (HR for death: 0.72; 95% CI 0.58 to 0.88), with 65% of patients treated with ipilimumab being alive at 5 years vs. 54% in the placebo arm. The subgroup analysis emphasized the superiority of ipilimumab in the ulcerated primary population and in patients with ≥ 3 involved lymph nodes [53, 54]. Despite these encouraging efficacy results, ipilimumab was associated with severe toxicities. Grade 3–4 irAEs were observed in more than 50% of patients, and 5 patients died (1.1%) in the intervention arm due to immune-related toxicities (3 colitis, 1 myocarditis, 1 Guillain–Barré syndrome) [53]. Of 471 patients who started ipilimumab, 240 patients (51%) discontinued treatment due to treatment-related adverse events. Due to the unacceptable toxicity profile, adjuvant ipilimumab at 10 mg/kg has not been approved in Europe, but received FDA approval only.

The EORTC 18071 had no active comparator in the control arm. In the E1609 study, the safety and efficacy of ipilimumab 10 mg/kg or 3 mg/kg was compared with high dose interferon in patients with resected stage IIIB, IIIC, and IV M1a/ M1b melanoma. Treatment with ipilimumab 3 mg/kg improved OS compared with high-dose interferon (HR: 0.78; 95% CI 0.61 to 1.00), while ipilimumab 10 mg/kg showed only a trend toward improvement in OS (HR 0.88; 95% CI 0.69 to 1.12) that was not statistically significant. The study was not powered for the comparison between the two doses of ipilimumab; however, exploratory analyses of OS and RFS with ipilimumab 3 mg/kg and 10 mg/kg suggested that low-dose ipilimumab was at least as effective as high-dose ipilimumab. Additionally, more patients in the ipilimumab 10 mg/kg group experienced a grade 3 or higher treatment-related AE than those who received ipilimumab 3 mg (58% and 37%, respectively), and more patients discontinued treatment due to an AE of any grade (54% with ipilimumab 10 mg/kg and 35% with ipilimumab 3 mg/kg). Eight patients treated with high-dose ipilimumab died to an AE considered at least possibly related to study treatment compared with 3 patients treated with low-dose ipilimumab [55, 56]. Based on the results of the E1609 study, in cases where adjuvant treatment with ipilimumab still represents an option, ipilimumab 3 mg/kg seems to have an advantage over the approved dosage of ipilimumab 10 mg/kg.

In advanced disease, ipilimumab was outperformed in terms of both efficacy and safety by the anti-PD-1 agents nivolumab and pembrolizumab [16, 17], and their efficacy was then investigated in the adjuvant setting. In the CheckMate-238 randomized phase 3 clinical trial, patients with resected stage IIIB, IIIC, and IV melanoma were randomized to receive either nivolumab 3 mg/kg every 2 weeks for a year or ipilimumab 10 mg/kg every 3 weeks for four cycles and then every 12 weeks for up to a year. At a median follow-up of 36 months, patients receiving nivolumab had superior RFS compared with patients on ipilimumab for an HR of 0.68 (95% CI, 0.56–0.82). At 3 years, 58% of patients were free of relapse in the nivolumab group as compared with 45% for ipilimumab [57]. Nivolumab was superior to ipilimumab regardless of PD-L1 expression, disease stage, and BRAF mutation status [58, 59]. Most importantly, severe treatment-related AEs were significantly lower in patients treated with nivolumab compared with ipilimumab (14% vs. 46%, respectively); treatment was discontinued because of any AE in less than 10% of patients who received the anti-PD-1 agent compared with 43% of patients receiving ipilimumab [59]. Similar to that observed in patients with advanced melanoma, nivolumab was shown to be both more effective and better tolerated than ipilimumab also in the adjuvant setting. Exploratory biomarkers, such as tumor interferon-gamma gene expression signature, tumor mutational burden, tumor CD8+ T-cell infiltration, and myeloid-derived suppressor cell levels, correlated with RFS with both nivolumab and ipilimumab, highlighting their role as prognostic but not predictive biomarkers [57].

In the ongoing CheckMate-915 trial, a randomized phase 3 study evaluating nivolumab plus ipilimumab at a very low dose (1 mg/kg every 6 weeks) versus nivolumab alone for the adjuvant treatment of patients with resected stage IIIB/C/D or stage IV melanoma, the combination treatment failed to provide a statistically significant benefit for the co-primary endpoint of RFS in patients whose tumors expressed PD-L1 < 1% (Bristol-Myers Squibb Press Release, Wednesday, November 20, 2019; https://news.bms.com/press-release/corporatefinancial-news/bristol-myers-squibb-announces-update-checkmate-915-opdivo-niv). The study will continue to assess the other co-primary endpoint of RFS in the intent-to-treat population.

The combination of ipilimumab with nivolumab was also assessed in another adjuvant trial for patients with resected stage IV melanoma. In the randomized, placebo-controlled, phase 2 trial IMMUNED, patients with stage IV melanoma with no evidence of disease after surgery or radiotherapy were randomized 1:1:1 to receive either nivolumab plus ipilimumab (1 mg/kg of nivolumab every 3 weeks plus 3 mg/kg of ipilimumab every 3 weeks for four doses, followed by 3 mg/kg of nivolumab every 2 weeks), nivolumab monotherapy (3 mg/kg every 2 weeks), or placebo. The HR for recurrence for nivolumab plus ipilimumab versus placebo was 0.23 (97.5% CI, 0.12–0.45), and for nivolumab versus placebo was 0.56 (0.33–0.94). In the nivolumab plus ipilimumab group, RFS was 75% and 70% at 1 and 2 years, respectively, versus 52% and 42% for nivolumab monotherapy, and 32% and 14% for placebo. However, severe irAEs were reported at a rate as high as 71% in the combination group, as compared to 27% with nivolumab as a single agent [60]. The results of this study highlight the possible role of combination treatment in patients with melanoma at a very high risk of recurrence, such as resected stage IV, but regimens with lower dosages of ipilimumab could be preferred to decrease the risk of severe and potentially fatal toxicities.

Neoadjuvant Setting

Patients with high-risk resectable stage III/IV melanoma have poor outcomes even after adjuvant treatments [61]. A strong rationale supports the use of immune-checkpoint inhibitors in the neoadjuvant rather than the adjuvant setting, as the presence of the tumor and associated tumor-infiltrating lymphocytes might result in a stronger antitumor immune response. In fact, in the OpACIN trial, the use of neoadjuvant immunotherapy was associated with a greater increase of tumor-resident T-cell clones in peripheral blood compared with adjuvant immunotherapy [62]. Despite that, anti-PD-1 as a single agent did not achieve a sufficient rate of pathological complete responses to be worth further investigation in the neoadjuvant setting [63, 64]. The combination of IPI3 with NIVO1, which is the regimen currently approved in the advanced setting, had a high clinical activity at the cost of a very high rate of severe toxicities [62, 64, 65]. Thus, based on the results of the studies conducted so far, the best immunotherapy regimen to be further investigated in the neoadjuvant setting seemed to be IPI1 plus NIVO3, which achieved similar results than those obtained with IPI3 plus NIVO1 in terms of clinical activity, but with a lower rate of toxicities [65].

The Role of Ipilimumab in the Era of Anti-PD-1 Drugs

Ipilimumab is currently employed in combination with nivolumab as an upfront treatment in patients with advanced melanoma, regardless of the presence of a BRAF mutation. In patients who received previous treatment with a single-agent anti-PD-1 drug, ipilimumab still has a role as a subsequent treatment, with similar safety and clinical activity as that observed in clinical trials with anti-PD-1 naïve patients. However, no prospective clinical trials exist in this setting, and data are still scarce and mostly of retrospective nature [66–68]. The results of two studies recently presented at ASCO 2020 suggest that in single-agent anti-PD-1 resistant patients, the addition of ipilimumab to the anti-PD-1 treatment may be more effective than ipilimumab alone [69, 70]. Despite that, the use of ipilimumab is not indicated by the regulatory agencies in this setting. Ipilimumab should not be administered neither before nor after anti-PD-1 agents with a planned switch (without evidence of PD), as investigated in CheckMate-064 trial, due to a similar rate of severe toxicities as observed with concurrent administration but with lower activity [9].

In patients with high-risk, resected melanoma, IPI10 should not be considered an option anymore, due to the higher toxicity and lower efficacy than anti-PD-1 agents, as highlighted in CheckMate-238 study [59], and BRAF plus MEK inhibitors in BRAF-mutant patients [71]. In fact, even if a direct comparison between ipilimumab and BRAF and MEK inhibitors does not exist, the overlapping results in terms of RFS of the placebo arms in both studies facilitate cross-trial comparison [53, 71]. The preliminary results of CheckMate-915 clinical trial showed that very low doses of ipilimumab (1 mg/kg every 6 weeks) in combination with nivolumab may not be superior to anti-PD-1 alone in patients with PD-L1 expression <1% [press release], while the IMMUNED study suggested that IPI3 + NIVO1 may have a role for the adjuvant treatment of resected stage IV melanoma, despite toxicity concerns [60].

Finally, even if it has not received an indication by the regulatory agencies yet, low-dose ipilimumab in combination with nivolumab (IPI1 + NIVO3) may have an important role as a neoadjuvant treatment for clinically positive stage III melanoma, as single-agent nivolumab did not provide sufficient pathological responses to be a valuable option in this setting [62, 64, 65, 72].

References

1. Pardoll DM. The blockade of immune checkpoints in cancer immunotherapy. Nat Rev Cancer. 2012;12(4):252–64.
2. Hori S, Nomura T, Sakaguchi S. Control of regulatory T cell development by the transcription factor Foxp3. Science. 2003;299(5609):1057.
3. Barzaghi F, Passerini L, Bacchetta R. Immune dysregulation, polyendocrinopathy, enteropathy, x-linked syndrome: a paradigm of immunodeficiency with autoimmunity. Front Immunol. 2012;3:211.
4. Queirolo P, Boutros A, Tanda E, et al. Immune-checkpoint inhibitors for the treatment of metastatic melanoma: a model of cancer immunotherapy. Semin Cancer Biol. 2019;59:290–7. https://doi.org/10.1016/j.semcancer.2019.08.001.
5. Hodi FS, O'Day SJ, McDermott DF, et al. Improved survival with ipilimumab in patients with metastatic melanoma. N Engl J Med. 2010;363(8):711–23.
6. Wolchok JD, Neyns B, Linette G, et al. Ipilimumab monotherapy in patients with pretreated advanced melanoma: a randomised, double-blind, multicentre, phase 2, dose-ranging study. Lancet Oncol. 2010;11(2):155–64.
7. Robert C, Thomas L, Bondarenko I, et al. Ipilimumab plus dacarbazine for previously untreated metastatic melanoma. N Engl J Med. 2011;364(26):2517–26.
8. Ascierto PA, Del Vecchio M, Robert C, et al. Ipilimumab 10 mg/kg versus ipilimumab 3 mg/kg in patients with unresectable or metastatic melanoma: a randomised, double-blind, multicentre, phase 3 trial. Lancet Oncol. 2017;18(5):611–22.

9. Weber JS, Gibney G, Sullivan RJ, et al. Sequential administration of nivolumab and ipilimumab with a planned switch in patients with advanced melanoma (CheckMate 064): an open-label, randomised, phase 2 trial. Lancet Oncol. 2016;17(7):943–55.

10. Hodi FS, Chesney J, Pavlick AC, et al. Combined nivolumab and ipilimumab versus ipilimumab alone in patients with advanced melanoma: 2-year overall survival outcomes in a multicentre, randomised, controlled, phase 2 trial. Lancet Oncol. 2016;17(11):1558–68.

11. Wolchok JD, Chiarion-Sileni V, Gonzalez R, et al. Overall survival with combined nivolumab and ipilimumab in advanced melanoma. N Engl J Med. 2017;377(14):1345–56.

12. Larkin J, Chiarion-Sileni V, Gonzalez R, et al. Five-year survival with combined nivolumab and ipilimumab in advanced melanoma. N Engl J Med. 2019;381(16):1535–46.

13. Lebbé C, Meyer N, Mortier L, et al. Evaluation of two dosing regimens for nivolumab in combination with ipilimumab in patients with advanced melanoma: results from the phase IIIb/IV checkmate 511 trial. J Clin Oncol Off J Am Soc Clin Oncol. 2019;37(11):867–75.

14. Long GV, Atkinson V, Cebon JS, et al. Standard-dose pembrolizumab in combination with reduced-dose ipilimumab for patients with advanced melanoma (KEYNOTE-029): an open-label, phase 1b trial. Lancet Oncol. 2017;18(9):1202–10.

15. Altomonte M, Di Giacomo A, Queirolo P, et al. Clinical experience with ipilimumab 10 mg/kg in patients with melanoma treated at Italian centres as part of a European expanded access programme. J Exp Clin Cancer Res CR. 2013;32(1):82.

16. Robert C, Ribas A, Schachter J, et al. Pembrolizumab versus ipilimumab in advanced melanoma (KEYNOTE-006): post-hoc 5-year results from an open-label, multicentre, randomised, controlled, phase 3 study. Lancet Oncol. 2019;20(9):1239–51. https://doi.org/10.1016/S1470-2045(19)30388-2.

17. Hodi FS, Chiarion-Sileni V, Gonzalez R, et al. Nivolumab plus ipilimumab or nivolumab alone versus ipilimumab alone in advanced melanoma (CheckMate 067): 4-year outcomes of a multicentre, randomised, phase 3 trial. Lancet Oncol. 2018;19(11):1480–92.

18. Schadendorf D, Hodi FS, Robert C, et al. Pooled analysis of long-term survival data from phase II and phase III trials of ipilimumab in unresectable or metastatic melanoma. J Clin Oncol Off J Am Soc Clin Oncol. 2015;33(17):1889–94.

19. Maio M, Grob J-J, Aamdal S, et al. Five-year survival rates for treatment-naive patients with advanced melanoma who received ipilimumab plus dacarbazine in a phase III trial. J Clin Oncol Off J Am Soc Clin Oncol. 2015;33(10):1191–6.

20. Korn EL, Liu P-Y, Lee SJ, et al. Meta-analysis of phase II cooperative group trials in metastatic stage IV melanoma to determine progression-free and overall survival benchmarks for future phase II trials. J Clin Oncol. 2008;26(4):527–34.

21. Chiarion-Sileni V, Pigozzo J, Ascierto PA, et al. Ipilimumab retreatment in patients with pretreated advanced melanoma: the expanded access programme in Italy. Br J Cancer. 2014;110(7):1721–6.

22. Neyns B, Weber JS, Lebbé C, Maio M, Harmankaya K, Hamid O, O'Day S, Chin KM, Opatt McDowell D, Cykowski L, McHenry B, Wolchok JD. Ipilimumab (Ipi) retreatment at 10 mg/kg in patients with metastatic melanoma previously treated in phase II trials. J Clin Oncol. 2013;31:abstract 9059.

23. Spagnolo F, Picasso V, Lambertini M, et al. Survival of patients with metastatic melanoma and brain metastases in the era of MAP-kinase inhibitors and immunologic checkpoint blockade antibodies: a systematic review. Cancer Treat Rev. 2016;45:38–45.

24. Heller KN, Pavlick AC, Hodi FS, et al. Safety and survival analysis of ipilimumab therapy in patients with stable asymptomatic brain metastases. J Clin Oncol. 2011;29(15_suppl):8581.

25. Weber JS, Amin A, Minor D, et al. Safety and clinical activity of ipilimumab in melanoma patients with brain metastases: retrospective analysis of data from a phase 2 trial. Melanoma Res. 2011;21(6):530–4.

26. Di Giacomo AM, Ascierto PA, Pilla L, et al. Ipilimumab and fotemustine in patients with advanced melanoma (NIBIT-M1): an open-label, single-arm phase 2 trial. Lancet Oncol. 2012;13(9):879–86.

27. Margolin K, Ernstoff MS, Hamid O, et al. Ipilimumab in patients with melanoma and brain metastases: an open-label, phase 2 trial. Lancet Oncol. 2012;13(5):459–65.
28. Queirolo P, Spagnolo F, Ascierto PA, et al. Efficacy and safety of ipilimumab in patients with advanced melanoma and brain metastases. J Neuro-Oncol. 2014;118(1):109–16.
29. Wolchok JD, Hoos A, O'Day S, et al. Guidelines for the evaluation of immune therapy activity in solid tumors: immune-related response criteria. Clin Cancer Res. 2009;15(23):7412.
30. Seymour L, Bogaerts J, Perrone A, et al. iRECIST: guidelines for response criteria for use in trials testing immunotherapeutics. Lancet Oncol. 2017;18(3):e143–52.
31. Thompson JA, Schneider BJ, Brahmer J, et al. Management of immunotherapy-related toxicities, version 1.2019, NCCN clinical practice guidelines in oncology. J Natl Compr Cancer Netw. 2019;17(3):255–89.
32. Haanen JBAG, Carbonnel F, Robert C, et al. Management of toxicities from immunotherapy: ESMO Clinical Practice Guidelines for diagnosis, treatment and follow-up. Ann Oncol Off J Eur Soc Med Oncol. 2017;28(suppl_4):iv119–42.
33. Brahmer JR, Lacchetti C, Schneider BJ, et al. Management of immune-related adverse events in patients treated with immune checkpoint inhibitor therapy: American Society of clinical oncology clinical practice guideline. J Clin Oncol Off J Am Soc Clin Oncol. 2018;36(17):1714–68.
34. Champiat S, Lambotte O, Barreau E, et al. Management of immune checkpoint blockade dysimmune toxicities: a collaborative position paper. Ann Oncol. 2016;27(4):559–74.
35. Kumar V, Chaudhary N, Garg M, et al. Current diagnosis and management of immune related adverse events (irAEs) induced by immune checkpoint inhibitor therapy. Front Pharmacol. 2017;8:49.
36. Bertrand A, Kostine M, Barnetche T, et al. Immune related adverse events associated with anti-CTLA-4 antibodies: systematic review and meta-analysis. BMC Med. 2015;13:211.
37. Wang P-F, Chen Y, Song S-Y, et al. Immune-related adverse events associated with anti-PD-1/PD-L1 treatment for malignancies: a meta-analysis. Front Pharmacol. 2017;8:730.
38. Cooper ZA, Juneja VR, Sage PT, et al. Response to BRAF inhibition in melanoma is enhanced when combined with immune checkpoint blockade. Cancer Immunol Res. 2014;2(7):643–54.
39. Ribas A, Hodi FS, Callahan M, et al. Hepatotoxicity with combination of vemurafenib and ipilimumab. N Engl J Med. 2013;368(14):1365–6.
40. Minor DR, Puzanov I, Callahan MK, et al. Severe gastrointestinal toxicity with administration of trametinib in combination with dabrafenib and ipilimumab. Pigment Cell Melanoma Res. 2015;28(5):611–2.
41. Ascierto PA, Ferrucci PF, Fisher R, et al. Dabrafenib, trametinib and pembrolizumab or placebo in BRAF-mutant melanoma. Nat Med. 2019;25(6):941–6.
42. Ferrucci PF, Ascierto PA, Pigozzo J, et al. Baseline neutrophils and derived neutrophil-to-lymphocyte ratio: prognostic relevance in metastatic melanoma patients receiving ipilimumab. Ann Oncol. 2016;27(4):732–8.
43. Zaragoza J, Caille A, Beneton N, et al. High neutrophil to lymphocyte ratio measured before starting ipilimumab treatment is associated with reduced overall survival in patients with melanoma. Br J Dermatol. 2016;174(1):146–51.
44. Martens A, Wistuba-Hamprecht K, Geukes Foppen M, et al. Baseline peripheral blood biomarkers associated with clinical outcome of advanced melanoma patients treated with ipilimumab. Clin Cancer Res Off J Am Assoc Cancer Res. 2016;22(12):2908–18.
45. Valpione S, Martinoli C, Fava P, et al. Personalised medicine: development and external validation of a prognostic model for metastatic melanoma patients treated with ipilimumab. Eur J Cancer. 2015;51(14):2086–94.
46. Sacdalan DB, Lucero JA, Sacdalan DL. Prognostic utility of baseline neutrophil-to-lymphocyte ratio in patients receiving immune checkpoint inhibitors: a review and meta-analysis. OncoTargets Ther. 2018;11:955–65.
47. Simeone E, Gentilcore G, Giannarelli D, et al. Immunological and biological changes during ipilimumab treatment and their potential correlation with clinical response and survival in patients with advanced melanoma. Cancer Immunol Immunother. 2014;63(7):675–83.

48. Kelderman S, Heemskerk B, van Tinteren H, et al. Lactate dehydrogenase as a selection criterion for ipilimumab treatment in metastatic melanoma. Cancer Immunol Immunother. 2014;63(5):449–58.
49. Pistillo MP, Fontana V, Morabito A, et al. Soluble CTLA-4 as a favorable predictive biomarker in metastatic melanoma patients treated with ipilimumab: an Italian melanoma intergroup study. Cancer Immunol Immunother. 2019;68(1):97–107.
50. Hopkins AM, Rowland A, Kichenadasse G, et al. Predicting response and toxicity to immune checkpoint inhibitors using routinely available blood and clinical markers. Br J Cancer. 2017;117(7):913–20.
51. Queirolo P, Dozin B, Morabito A, et al. Association of CTLA-4 gene variants with response to therapy and long-term survival in metastatic melanoma patients treated with ipilimumab: an Italian melanoma intergroup study. Front Immunol. 2017;8:386.
52. Queirolo P, Dozin B, Morabito A, et al. CTLA-4 gene variant -1661A>G may predict the onset of endocrine adverse events in metastatic melanoma patients treated with ipilimumab. Eur J Cancer. 2018;97:59–61.
53. Eggermont AMM, Chiarion-Sileni V, Grob J-J, et al. Adjuvant ipilimumab versus placebo after complete resection of high-risk stage III melanoma (EORTC 18071): a randomised, double-blind, phase 3 trial. Lancet Oncol. 2015;16(5):522–30.
54. Eggermont AMM, Chiarion-Sileni V, Grob J-J, et al. Prolonged survival in stage III melanoma with ipilimumab adjuvant therapy. N Engl J Med. 2016;375(19):1845–55.
55. Tarhini AA, Lee SJ, Hodi FS, et al. A phase III randomized study of adjuvant ipilimumab (3 or 10 mg/kg) versus high-dose interferon alfa-2b for resected high-risk melanoma (U.S. Intergroup E1609): Preliminary safety and efficacy of the ipilimumab arms. J Clin Oncol. 2017;35(15_suppl):9500.
56. Tarhini AA, Lee SJ, Hodi FS, et al. United States Intergroup E1609: a phase III randomized study of adjuvant ipilimumab (3 or 10 mg/kg) versus high-dose interferon-α2b for resected high-risk melanoma. J Clin Oncol. 2019;37(15_suppl):9504.
57. Weber JS, Del Vecchio M, Mandala M, et al. Adjuvant nivolumab (NIVO) versus ipilimumab (IPI) in resected stage III/IV melanoma: 3-year efficacy and biomarker results from the phase 3 CheckMate 238 trial. Annals of Oncology. 2019;30(suppl_5):v533–63. https://doi.org/10.1093/annonc/mdz255.
58. Weber JS, Mandalà M, Del Vecchio M, et al. Adjuvant therapy with nivolumab (NIVO) versus ipilimumab (IPI) after complete resection of stage III/IV melanoma: Updated results from a phase III trial (CheckMate 238). J Clin Oncol. 2018;36(15_suppl):9502.
59. Weber J, Mandala M, Del Vecchio M, et al. Adjuvant nivolumab versus Ipilimumab in resected stage III or IV melanoma. N Engl J Med. 2017;377(19):1824–35.
60. Zimmer L, Livingstone E, Hassel JC, et al. Adjuvant nivolumab plus ipilimumab or nivolumab monotherapy versus placebo in patients with resected stage IV melanoma with no evidence of disease (IMMUNED): a randomised, double-blind, placebo-controlled, phase 2 trial. Lancet. 2020;395(10236):1558–68.
61. Spagnolo F, Boutros A, Tanda E, Queirolo P. The adjuvant treatment revolution for high-risk melanoma patients. Semin Cancer Biol. 2019;59:283–9.
62. Blank CU, Rozeman EA, Fanchi LF, et al. Neoadjuvant versus adjuvant ipilimumab plus nivolumab in macroscopic stage III melanoma. Nat Med. 2018;24(11):1655–61.
63. Huang AC, Orlowski RJ, Xu X, et al. A single dose of neoadjuvant PD-1 blockade predicts clinical outcomes in resectable melanoma. Nat Med. 2019;25(3):454–61.
64. Amaria RN, Reddy SM, Tawbi HA, et al. Neoadjuvant immune checkpoint blockade in high-risk resectable melanoma. Nat Med. 2018;24(11):1649–54.
65. Rozeman EA, Menzies AM, van Akkooi ACJ, et al. Identification of the optimal combination dosing schedule of neoadjuvant ipilimumab plus nivolumab in macroscopic stage III melanoma (OpACIN-neo): a multicentre, phase 2, randomised, controlled trial. Lancet Oncol. 2019;20(7):948–60.

66. Bowyer S, Prithviraj P, Lorigan P, et al. Efficacy and toxicity of treatment with the anti-CTLA-4 antibody ipilimumab in patients with metastatic melanoma after prior anti-PD-1 therapy. Br J Cancer. 2016;114(10):1084–9.
67. Aya F, Gaba L, Victoria I, et al. Ipilimumab after progression on anti-PD-1 treatment in advanced melanoma. Future Oncol. 2016;12(23):2683–8.
68. Zimmer L, Apuri S, Eroglu Z, et al. Ipilimumab alone or in combination with nivolumab after progression on anti-PD-1 therapy in advanced melanoma. Eur J Cancer. 2017;75:47–55.
69. Olson D, Luke JJ, Poklepovic AS, et al. Significant antitumor activity for low-dose ipilimumab (IPI) with pembrolizumab (PEMBRO) immediately following progression on PD1 Ab in melanoma (MEL) in a phase II trial. J Clin Oncol. 2020;38(15_suppl):10004.
70. Pires Da Silva I, Ahmed T, Lo S, et al. Ipilimumab (IPI) alone or in combination with anti-PD-1 (IPI+PD1) in patients (pts) with metastatic melanoma (MM) resistant to PD1 monotherapy. J Clin Oncol. 2020;38(15_suppl):10005.
71. Hauschild A, Dummer R, Schadendorf D, et al. Longer follow-up confirms relapse-free survival benefit with adjuvant dabrafenib plus trametinib in patients with resected BRAF V600-mutant stage III melanoma. J Clin Oncol Off J Am Soc Clin Oncol. 2018;36(35):JCO1801219.
72. Spagnolo F, Croce E, Boutros A, et al. Neoadjuvant treatments in patients with high-risk resectable stage III/IV melanoma. Expert Rev Anticancer Ther. 2020;20(5):403–13.

Chapter 11
Nivolumab in Melanoma: An Overview of Medical Literature and Future Perspectives

Luigia Stefania Stucci, Annalisa Todisco, Mario Mandalà, and Marco Tucci

Introduction

The first approval of Nivolumab for the treatment of advanced melanoma occurred in December 2014 on the basis of results of either phase I CA209-003 or phase III CA209-037 trials [1, 2]. Thus, the Food and Drug Administration (FDA) approved Opdivo® for pretreated locally advanced or metastatic melanoma patients. From the early indication of Ipilimumab® and Vemurafenib® in 2011, Dabrafenib and Trametinib in 2013, and Pembrolizumab in 2014, Opdivo was the seventh innovative drug approved for the treatment of metastatic melanoma. In 2015, FDA approved the combination of Nivolumab and Ipilimumab in BRAF V600 wild-type unresectable or metastatic melanoma and in the early 2016 for advanced melanoma, independently of the BRAF mutational status. Finally, in December 2017 and July 2018, the FDA and the European Medicine Agency (EMA) extended the Nivolumab indication to the adjuvant setting in melanoma patients with stage III as well as resected with "No Evidence of Disease" (NED).

L. S. Stucci · A. Todisco
Dipartimento di Scienze Biomediche ed Oncologia Umana, UO Oncologia Medica Universitaria, Università di Bari "Aldo Moro", Bari, Italy

M. Mandalà
University of Perugia, Unit of Medical Oncology, Ospedale Santa Maria Misericordia, Perugia, Italy
e-mail: mario.mandala@unipg.it

M. Tucci (✉)
Dipartimento di Scienze Biomediche ed Oncologia Umana, UO Oncologia Medica Universitaria, Università di Bari "Aldo Moro", Bari, Italy

IRCCS, Tumori Institute Giovanni Paolo II, Bari, Italy
e-mail: marco.tucci@uniba.it

© The Author(s), under exclusive license to Springer Nature Switzerland AG 2021
P. Rutkowski, M. Mandalà (eds.), *New Therapies in Advanced Cutaneous Malignancies*, https://doi.org/10.1007/978-3-030-64009-5_11

Based on the results shown by these agents, great efforts in discovering new immune checkpoint inhibitors (ICIs) to ameliorate the overall clinical results for the treatment of melanoma are ongoing in several prospective clinical trials.

Of note, in the wake of enthusiasm generated by the anti-PD1 combination with anti-CTLA4, the association of Nivolumab with other ICIs has been explored in clinical trials, and both LAG3 inhibitors and anti-NTKR agents showed promising results. In particular, the combination with anti-CTLA4 MoAbs produced relevant results in terms of duration and depth of response, although a high incidence of serious adverse events (AEs) has been reported. In this chapter, we review the activity, efficacy, and toxicity of nivolumab in metastatic and adjuvant setting and summarize new potential therapeutic strategies, which could potentially expand its spectrum of activity in melanoma.

Nivolumab in Advanced Disease

The CA209-003 was the first phase I trial testing the tolerability and activity of Nivolumab in advanced solid cancer, followed by phase II Checkmate 172 and 037 and phase III Checkmate 037 and 066, which explored the efficacy of Nivolumab in advanced melanoma [1–5].

Checkmate 003, a phase I open-label, multicenter, multidose, dose-escalation trial, investigated the safety, clinical activity, pharmacodynamic, and immunologic effect of nivolumab (MDX-1106) in patients with advanced refractory solid tumors [1]. Patients with metastatic melanoma, advanced colorectal cancer (CRC), castrate-resistant prostate cancer, non-small-cell lung cancer (NSCLC), or renal cell carcinoma (RCC) received a single intravenous infusion (i.v.) of MDX-1106 in a dose-escalating program at 0.1–10 mg/kg every 2 weeks up to 96 weeks or until progressive disease, unacceptable toxic effects as well as withdrawal of consent. The primary endpoint of the study was safety and tolerability. An emendation of the study allowed the collection of data concerning the overall survival (OS). The last 5 years' update [1] included a cohort of 270 patients bearing advanced melanoma (n. 107, 39,6%), NSCLC (n. 129, 47,8%), or RCC (n. 34, 12,6%). In melanoma cohort, 57% and 6.5% of patients experienced any grade or grade 3–4 AEs, respectively. The majority of AEs involved the skin (40.2%), the gastroenteric tract (18.7%), the endocrine system (13.1%), and the liver (8.4%). An objective overall response (ORR) according to the RECISTs criteria was achieved in 31.8% of patients, while a stable (SD) and a progressive disease was reported in 21.5% (23/107) in 38.3% (41/107) of patients, respectively. The 5-year OS was 34.2%, with a median OS of 17.3 months. Poor prognostic factors included liver and bone metastases, whereas good performance status (PS) and development of treatment-related AEs positively impacted on OS. At the median follow-up of 30 months, the progression-free survival (PFS) was 26% in patients receiving Nivolumab at 3 mg/kg. It is noteworthy that many responders ($n = 21$) who discontinued the drug for any reason, apart from the progression, maintained a response longer than 16 weeks.

The efficacy of Nivolumab in melanoma patients who progressed after Ipilimumab and/or a BRAF inhibitor was tested in Checkmate 037, a phase III randomized trial comparing Nivolumab vs. chemotherapy [2]. Four hundred and five patients were randomly assigned 2:1 to receive Nivolumab (3 mg/kg i.v. every 2 weeks) or investigator's choice chemotherapy (Dacarbazine, DTIC or Carboplatin and Paclitaxel) and were stratified on the basis of PD-L1 expression, BRAF status, and best response to Ipilimumab. Treatment beyond progression was only allowed in the Nivolumab arm. Primary endpoints were the ORR and OS. The study did not meet its co-primary survival endpoint, Nivolumab showed higher and durable response without any benefit in terms of survival compared to chemotherapy [2]. Median OS was of 15.7 months in the Nivolumab arm and 14.4 months in patients receiving chemotherapy (HR: 0.95; CI: 0.73–1.24), the median PFS was 3.1 months vs. 3.7 months (HR:1.0; CI: 0.78 to 1.436). The ORR was 27% and 10% with nivolumab and chemotherapy, respectively; the median duration of response favored the nivolumab arm (32 months vs 13 months). In addition, a lower rate of grade 3–4 AEs (14% in Nivolumab vs. 34% in the chemotherapy arm) was demonstrated. The ECOG PS, brain metastases, and high LDH levels were associated with poor survival. The reported AEs in the Nivolumab arm involved skin (38%), GI (18%), liver (11%), and endocrine glands (7.8%). The reasons for failing to meet the primary endpoint can be only hypothesized: (1) the high percentage of patients with brain metastases or elevated LDH levels; (2) the crossover to anti-PD1 or anti-PDL1 antibody for patients progressing upon chemotherapy; (3) the higher proportion of patients dropped out after assignment to the chemotherapy arm and before starting chemotherapy.

The efficacy of *Nivolumab* vs Dacarbazine in the first-line treatment of BRAF wt advanced melanoma patients was investigated in Checkmate 066 trial [3]. This was a randomized phase III, double-blind clinical study that enrolled 418 BRAF wt melanoma patients to receive 1:1 Nivolumab (3 mg/kg every 2 weeks) or Dacarbazine (1000 mg/mq every 3 weeks). Patients with clinical benefit from Nivolumab or without significant AEs could be treated beyond progression. Crossover to Nivolumab was allowed for patients who progressed during Dacarbazine, in an open-label extension phase of the trial. The primary endpoint was the OS while the secondary endpoints were PFS and ORR. The median OS with Nivolumab vs Dacarbazine was 37.5 months vs. 11.2 months, whereas the 3-year OS rate was of 51.2% vs. 21.6%. Median PFS was 5.1 and 2.2 months, respectively, whereas the 3-year PFS rate was 32.2% and 2.9% for Nivolumab and Dacarbazine groups, respectively. The benefit of Nivolumab in terms of mOS was reached regardless of the PD-L1 expression. The secondary endpoint of the study was ORR. Complete and partial responses, respectively, were reported for 19.0% (40 of 210) and 23.8% (50 of 210) of patients in the nivolumab group compared with 1.4% (3 of 208) and 13.0% (27 of 208) of patients in the dacarbazine group.

The benefit was obtained even for patients with brain metastases or elevated LDH. Indeed, a clinical response was observed up to 160 weeks after starting treatment, regardless of therapy discontinuation. In addition, the long-term survival at 3 years was seen independently of the radiological response. Post hoc analysis of OS in patients who discontinued treatment due to disease progression showed that mOS from randomization was 21.5 months in patients treated with Ipilimumab following Nivolumab, 35.4 and 17.4 months for those treated with Nivolumab or Ipilimumab after Dacarbazine, respectively. Among 68 patients who discontinued Nivolumab and received Ipilimumab, 10.3% obtained an OR. Grade 3–4 AEs occurred in 15% of patients treated with Nivolumab and 17.6% of patients in the Dacarbazine arm, whereas no deaths due to AEs were registered.

Based on results of phase III CheckMate 037, the efficacy of Nivolumab has been investigated in *Checkmate 172, which enrolled a* challenging subgroup of patients excluded from clinical trials: Briefly, CheckMate 172 was a phase II single-arm study that explored the use of Nivolumab in previously treated, unresectable, stage III or IV melanoma (regardless of BRAF mutation status) patients who progressed upon Ipilimumab. Furthermore, patients with different melanoma subtypes, brain metastases, autoimmune diseases, ECOG 2 and previous grade 3–4 immune-related AEs (irAEs) were included [4, 5]. Patients received 3 mg/kg of Nivolumab every 2 weeks up to 2 years. Primary endpoint of the study was the safety; secondary endpoints included (1) incidence of all grade ≥ 3 not conventional AEs, (2) median time to onset and resolution of grade 3/4 select AEs, and (3) OS. Exploratory endpoints were safety, tolerability, and OS. Among challenging subgroups, patients who experienced an Ipilimumab-related grade 3/4 irAE and those with autoimmune disease showed the longest median OS (21.5 months and 18. months, respectively) without difference with overall population (median OS, 21.4 months). Patients with brain metastases and ECOG PS 2 had a lower median OS (11.6 months and 2.4 months, respectively). The 18-month OS rate was 53.8% in the general population and 42.3%, 18.8%, 59.3%, and 58.2% in patients with brain metastases, ECOG 2, Ipilimumab-related grade 3/4 irAE, and autoimmune disease, respectively. These data confirmed the worse outcome of patients with a poor ECOG PS, although the majority of them harbored additional adverse clinical prognostic factors including brain metastases (27.3%), rare histotypes such as mucosal melanoma (13.6%) and high LDH levels (78.8%).

The 18-month median OS was 25.3 months in non-acral cutaneous melanoma, 25.8 months in acral cutaneous melanoma, 12.6 months in uveal melanoma and 11.5 months in mucosal melanoma patients, while the OS rate was 57.5%, 59%, 34.8%, and 31.5%, respectively, thus confirming the known worse prognosis of mucosal and uveal melanomas. Similar to Checkmate 003, the most common toxicities were cutaneous (26.4% any grade, 1.2% grade 3 or 4), endocrine (16.9% any grade, 1.8% grade 3 or 4), gastrointestinal (13.5% any grade, 1.4% grade 3 or 4), hepatic (8.2% any grade, 2.8% grade 3 or 4), pulmonary (2.2% any grade, 0.5% grade 3 or 4), and renal (1.7% any grade, 0.1% grade 3 or 4). Patients with ECOG 2 and autoimmune disease experienced toxicities at gastrointestinal tract and endocrine system. Interestingly, this analysis produced relevant insights for the management of patients who experienced immune-related AEs following the treatment with ipilimumab, but also of those with a concomitant autoimmune disease. The first subgroup had a lower incidence of grade 3/4 AEs as compared to the general population (11.9% versus 18.2%), the latter showed limited grade 3–4 AEs and, interestingly, the OS that resulted similar to the overall population, thus suggesting that these patients can be safely treated with anti-PD1.

Although subgroup analyses of CheckMate 066 and CheckMate 172 provided a proof of principle of Nivolumab activity as monotherapy in patients with brain metastasis, the most robust data on the activity as a single agent or in combination derive from the phase 2 CheckMate 204 study and the anti-PD-1 Brain Collaboration (ABC) Trial, a phase II trial of Nivolumab Plus Ipilimumab or Nivolumab alone in patients with melanoma brain metastases [6, 7] .

In the ABC study, 60 were asymptomatic, and, of these, 35 received a combination of nivolumab and ipilimumab (cohort A) and 25 received nivolumab monotherapy (cohort B). Sixteen patients who had failed local therapy or were neurologically symptomatic and/or had leptomeningeal disease (LMD) received nivolumab monotherapy (cohort C). Intracranial responses were achieved in 51%, 20%, and 6%, and 12-month OS was 63%, 60%, and 31% in cohorts A, B, and C, respectively. The intracranial OR in cohort A was 59% for treatment-naive patients and 25% in patients previously treated with BRAF inhibitors. However, ABC was not designed/powered to be comparative between treatment arms [6].

The safety and efficacy of nivolumab and ipilimumab was also evaluated in CheckMate 204. In the most recent update, 119 patients had been treated: 101 patients with asymptomatic MBMs and 18 patients with either symptomatic MBMs or who were receiving up to 4 mg of oral dexamethasone. The intracranial RR was 54% in patients with asymptomatic MBMs, including CRs in 29%. The 6-month intracranial PFS was 63% and the median PFS was not reached. In patients who were either symptomatic or requiring steroids at the time of treatment initiation, the RR was 22%, although only 1/11 patients (9%) receiving steroids experienced a response [7, 8].

Efficacy of Ipilimumab Plus Nivolumab Regimen

CheckMate 067 is one of the most relevant trials evaluating the combination of ICIs. The trial was designed to compare the combo regimen vs Ipilimumab but was underpowered to compare the combo regimen with Nivolumab. Patients were randomized to receive one of the following strategies: (1) Nivolumab plus Ipilimumab for four doses followed by Nivolumab alone, (2) Nivolumab alone or (3) Ipilimumab alone [9]. The median OS at 60 months was longer than 60 months (median not reached), 36.9 months, and 19.9 months, in the Nivolumab/Ipilimumab, Nivolumab alone, and Ipilimumab alone cohorts, respectively. With regard to the landmark analysis, the 5-year OS was 52%, 44%, and 26%, in the Nivolumab/Ipilimumab, Nivolumab alone and in the Ipilimumab cohorts, respectively. The ORR was 58% in the Nivolumab/Ipilimumab group, 45% in the Nivolumab group, and 19% in the Ipilimumab group with 22%, 19%, and 6% of CR, respectively. This advantage was observed in all subgroups, independently of BRAF mutation status, PD-L1 expression as well as extension of disease. In addition, patients who discontinued treatment early for an AE had a survival benefit almost similar to the overall population [10]

Ongoing Promising Clinical Trials

Results of CA224-020, a phase 1/2 study evaluating Relatlimab (LAG3 inhibitor) with and without Nivolumab for the treatment of solid tumors were presented at ESMO 2017 [11]. The lymphocyte activation gene 3 (LAG3) is an additional target of ICI that negatively regulates the activity of effector T cells. Based on the dual inhibition of the LAG3 and PD1 activity exerted by Relatlimab and Nivolumab, a signal of potential clinical benefit in previously treated metastatic or unresectable melanoma patients resistant to an anti-PD(L)1 MoAb has been demonstrated. The ORR was 11.5%, the disease Control Rate (DCR) 49%, with a safety profile similar to Nivolumab alone, while the response rate was higher in patients with LAG-3 expression $\geq 1\%$. Based on these results, a randomized, double-blind, phase II/III study of Relatlimab in combination with Nivolumab versus Nivolumab alone in previously untreated metastatic or unresectable (CA224-047) melanoma is actually ongoing

Bempegaldesleukin (NKTR-214) is a CD122-preferential IL-2 pathway agonist able to increase tumor-infiltrating lymphocytes, T-cell clonality, and PD-1 expression. Safety and tolerability of NKTR-214 was proven in PIVOT-02 phase 1/2 trial. After over 18 months of follow-up, in untreated advanced melanoma, NKTR-214 plus Nivolumab showed clinical activity, with an ORR of 53%, and a remarkable 34% of CR, independently of PD-L1 expression [12].

The PIVOT IO 001, a phase III, randomized, open-label study of NKTR-214 plus Nivolumab vs Nivolumab monotherapy in patients with untreated advanced melanoma is still ongoing (NCT03635983).

Nivolumab in Adjuvant Setting

Adjuvant therapy is actually considered the best option for stage III melanoma patients in order to reduce the risk of recurrence. Recently, ipilimumab at 10 mg/kg showed a significant improvement in terms of RFS and OS in stage III melanoma compared to placebo but with a high incidence of severe irAEs [13]. Moreover, new options have emerged and the results from the CheckMate 238 and the IMMUNED trials have been reported [14, 15].

The CheckMate 238 trial investigated the efficacy of Nivolumab vs Ipilimumab in stage IIIB/C and radically resected stage IV melanoma patients. Patients were randomly assigned 1:1 to receive Nivolumab 3 mg/kg every 2 weeks or Ipilimumab 10 mg/kg every 4 weeks for 4 doses and every 12 weeks thereafter for 1 year or less or until disease recurrence or unacceptable toxicity. The primary endpoint was recurrence-free survival (RFS), and exploratory endpoints included distant metastasis-free survival (DMFS) and OS. Furthermore, exploratory analyses included predictive biomarkers of outcome. At a median follow-up of 36 months, the Nivolumab arm had better RFS compared with the Ipilimumab arm (hazard ratio

[HR] = 0.68; 95% confidence interval [CI] = 0.56–0.82, $p < 0.0001$). The 3-year RFS rate was 58% vs 45% with Nivolumab and Ipilimumab, respectively. Distant metastasis-free survival was improved in the Nivolumab arm as well (HR = 0.78; 95% CI = 0.62–0.99). Surrogate analyses suggested that a high tumor mutational burden, the interferon-gamma gene expression signature, as well as a high infiltration of $CD8^+$ T cells and low density of myeloid-derived suppressor cell correlate with improved RFS in both arms. The majority of first-occurrence treatment-related adverse events (TRAEs) with adjuvant Nivolumab occurred early during treatment (0–3 months) while rarely (<2.5%) after the last dose. Almost all TRAEs were solved within 6 months. No association was observed between early TRAEs and RFS [16].

With regard to the radically resected stage IV disease, the IMMUNED study has been recently reported [15]. The IMMUNED was a phase II randomized clinical trial evaluating Nivolumab/Ipilimumab vs single-agent Nivolumab vs placebo, in patients with radically resected or irradiated stage IV disease and considered to be at high risk for recurrence. This was the first prospective randomized placebo-controlled clinical study in patients with stage IV melanoma without evidence of disease. Overall, 167 patients with high-risk stage IV disease were randomly assigned to Nivolumab at 3 mg/kg (with maintenance Nivolumab), Nivolumab at 1 mg/kg plus Ipilimumab at 3 mg/kg (with maintenance Nivolumab) or placebo. Notwithstanding the limited median time of treatment with the combination therapy (6.4 weeks), it yielded a 2-year recurrence-free survival rate of 70%, which compared favorably with Nivolumab (42%) or placebo (14%). Relapses occurred in 81% of the placebo arm, 56% of the Nivolumab arm, and 27% of the combination arm. Distant relapses were reported in 44%, 39%, and 14%, respectively. Nivolumab alone was better tolerated than the combo regimen, with lower incidence of grade 3 or 4 AEs and less toxicity leading to treatment discontinuation. The combination of ICIs has been further evaluated in the phase III CheckMate-915 study. This trial included 1943 patients with IIIB/C and radically resected stage IV melanoma patients.

Participants were treated with 240 mg of intravenous Nivolumab every 2 weeks and 1 mg/kg Ipilimumab every 6 weeks or 480 mg of Nivolumab every 4 weeks for 12 months. Results are not still available, preliminary data suggest modest RFS benefit with the combination in patients with PD-L1 levels lower than 1% [17].

Nivolumab in the Neoadjuvant Setting

The outcome of patients with palpable node, locally advanced stage III melanoma still remains poor. The neoadjuvant approach is well suited for melanoma: prototype tumor for drug development, there is accessible tissue, and provides rapid results. Nevertheless, some caveat should be considered including patients not responding might deteriorate losing the opportunity of curative surgery, irAEs might hamper surgery, neoadjuvant therapies require more patient management, timing scans, day clinic appointments, and surgery planning. Nivolumab alone or in combination with ipilimumab has been investigated in four major clinical trials [18–21]. Amaria et al. reported results from a randomized phase 2 study of neoadjuvant nivolumab versus combined ipilimumab with nivolumab in 23 patients with high-risk resectable melanoma. Treatment with combined ipilimumab and nivolumab yielded high response rates (RECIST ORR 73%, pCR 45%) but substantial toxicity (73% grade 3 trAEs), whereas treatment with nivolumab monotherapy yielded modest responses (ORR 25%, pCR 25%) and low toxicity (8% grade 3 trAEs). Immune correlates of response were identified, demonstrating higher lymphoid infiltrates in responders to both therapies and a more clonal and diverse T-cell infiltrate in responders to nivolumab monotherapy. Blank et al. reported the results of the OpACIN trial, a randomized phase Ib trial [22]. A total of 20 patients with palpable stage III melanoma were randomized to four cycles of adjuvant or neoadjuvant Ipilimumab 3 mg/kg plus Nivolumab 1 mg/kg treatment (two cycles before and after surgery). In the neoadjuvant arm, all patients underwent complete lymph node dissection after at least one course of neoadjuvant therapy. One patient in the adjuvant arm discontinued therapy due to disease progression. The other patients discontinued the therapy due to development of grade 3/4 AEs. Nine of ten patients in the neoadjuvant arm were evaluated for a pathologic response, and seven of them achieved a response: three patients obtained a pCR, three patients achieved "near" pCR, defined as $\leq$10% of viable tumor cells; one patient experienced a partial pathologic response (pPR), defined as $\leq$50% viable tumor cells. Two patients without PR relapsed. At a median follow-up of 21.6 months in this group, none of the seven patients with a PR relapsed. In terms of AEs, 90% patients stopped therapy due to grade 3/4 AEs. In relation to the severe toxicity of the standard Ipilimumab plus Nivolumab dosing schedule, the OpACIN-neo-trial was designed to identify a less toxic dosing schedule of Ipilimumab plus Nivolumab. Patients had resectable stage III melanoma only involving lymph nodes, and measurable disease according to the Response Evaluation Criteria in Solid Tumors (RECIST) version 1.1. Patients were randomly assigned (1:1:1) to one of three neoadjuvant dosing schedules: group A, two cycles of Ipilimumab 3 mg/kg plus Nivolumab 1 mg/kg once every 3 weeks intravenously; group B, two cycles of Ipilimumab 1 mg/kg plus Nivolumab 3 mg/kg once every 3 weeks intravenously; or group C, two cycles of Ipilimumab 3 mg/kg once every 3 weeks directly followed by two cycles of Nivolumab 3 mg/kg once every 2 weeks intravenously. The primary endpoints were the proportion of patients with grade 3–4 irAEs within the first 12 weeks and the proportion of patients achieving a radiological objective response and PR at 6 weeks. Patients were enrolled and randomly assigned to one of the three groups: 30 patients in group A, 30 in group B, and 26 in group C. During the first 12 weeks, grade 3–4 irAEs were observed in 12 (40%) of 30 patients in group A, six (20%) of 30 in group B, and 13 (50%) of 26 in group C. The difference in grade 3–4 toxicity between groups B and A was 20% (95% CI −46 to 6; p = 0·158) and between groups C and A was 10% (−20 to 40; p = 0·591). The most common grade 3–4 AE was the increase in liver enzymes in group A and colitis in group C. A patient in group A died 9.5 months after starting the treatment because of late-onset immune-related encephalitis. Nineteen (63%) of 30 patients in group A, 17 (57%) of 30 in group B, and nine (35%) of 26 in group C achieved a radiological objective response, while PR occurred in 24 (80%) patients in group A, 23 (77%) in group B, and 17 (65%) in group C. With regard to immune biomarkers, subgroup analyses revealed IFN-gamma signature and TMB correlated with response while PDL-1 expression did not. Moreover, low bacterial alpha diversity was associated with severe irAEs and poor anti-melanoma responses. In addition, similarly to the Opacin trial, the neoadjuvant immunotherapy led to a greater expansion of tumor-resident T-cell clones in the peripheral blood as compared with adjuvant treatment [23]. Immune signature analysis demonstrated that patients with a high IFN/T-cell/BATF3 signature had a better clinical outcome [24–26] as well as high/intermediate IFN signatures identified patients showing long-term responses.

Based on these evidences, OpACIN-neo identified a tolerable neoadjuvant dosing schedule (group B: two cycles of Ipilimumab 1 mg/kg plus Nivolumab 3 mg/kg) that gains a PR in a high proportion of patients. However, the optimal duration of neoadjuvant therapy is not yet standardized (Identification of the Optimal Combination Dosing Schedule of Neoadjuvant Ipilimumab Plus Nivolumab in macroscopic stage III melanoma [20]. Very recently, the PRADO trial has been designed in an attempt to reduce the extension of surgery and tailor the adjuvant strategy according to the response to the neoadjuvant approach [21].

Several neoadjuvant studies in melanoma are ongoing or planned to be started in the near future. A randomized phase II trial will investigate the activity of Nivolumab with or without Ipilimumab or Relatlimab (anti-LAG-3 monoclonal antibody) before surgery in patients with resectable stage IIIB–IV melanoma (NCT02519322). Immunotherapy with Nivolumab, Ipilimumab or Relatlimab may restrain the ability of the immune system to counterattack tumor cell growing and spreading. Upfront treatment with Nivolumab alone or in combination with Ipilimumab or Relatlimab might reduce the tumor size and limit the removal of normal nearby tissue. Moreover, a pilot phase I trial study is exploring VX15/2503 (Pepinemab) with or without Ipilimumab and/or Nivolumab for treatment of inoperable stage IIIB–D melanoma patients (NCT03769155). Another ongoing study is a phase II neoadjuvant trial of Nivolumab in combination with HF10 oncolytic viral therapy in resectable stage IIIB, IIIC, and IVM1a melanoma (Neo-NivoHF10) (NCT03259425).

References

1. Topalian SL, Hodi FS, Brahmer JR, et al. Five-year survival and correlates among patients with advanced melanoma, renal cell carcinoma, or non–small cell lung cancer treated with nivolumab. JAMA Oncol. 2019;5:1411–20.
2. Larkin J, Minor D, D'Angelo S, et al. Overall survival in patients with advanced melanoma who received nivolumab versus investigator's choice chemotherapy in CheckMate 037: a randomized, controlled, open-label phase III trial. J Clin Oncol. 2018;36:383–90.
3. Ascierto P, Long GV, Robert C, et al. Survival outcomes in patients with previously untreated BRAF wild-type advanced melanoma treated with nivolumab therapy: three-year follow-up of a randomized phase 3 trial. JAMA Oncol. 2019;5(2):187–94.

4. Schadendorf D, Ascierto PA, Haanen J, et al. Safety and efficacy of nivolumab in challenging subgroups with advanced melanoma who progressed on or after ipilimumab treatment: a single-arm, open-label, phase II study (CheckMate 172). Eur J Cancer. 2019;121:144–53.

5. Nathan P, Ascierto PA, Haanen J, et al. Safety and efficacy of nivolumab in patients with rare melanoma subtypes who progressed on or after ipilimumab treatment: a single-arm, open-label, phase II study (CheckMate 172). Eur J Cancer. 2019;119:168–78.

6. Long GV, Atkinson V, Lo S, et al. Combination nivolumab and ipilimumab or nivolumab alone in melanoma brain metastases: a multicentre randomised phase 2 study. Lancet Oncol. 2018;19(5):672–81.

7. Tawbi HA, Forsyth PA, Algazi A, et al. Combined nivolumab and Ipilimumab in melanoma metastatic to the brain. NEJM. 2018;379(8):722–30.

8. Tawbi HA, Forsyth PA, Hodi S, et al. Efficacy and safety of the combination of nivolumab (NIVO) plus ipilimumab (IPI) in patients with symptomatic melanoma brain metastases (CheckMate204). J Clin Oncol. 2019;37(15_suppl):9501.

9. Larkin J, Chiarion-Sileni V, Gonzalez R, et al. Five-year survival with combined nivolumab and ipilimumab in advanced melanoma. N Engl J Med. 2019;381:1535–46.

10. Schadendorf D, Wolchok JD, Hodi S, et al. Efficacy and safety outcome in patients with advanced melanoma who discontinued treatment with nivolumab and ipilimumab because of adverse events: a pooled analysis of randomized phase II and III trials. J Clin Oncol. 2017;35(34):3807–14.

11. Ascierto P, Bono P, Bhatia S, et al. Efficacy of BMS-986016, a monoclonal antibody that targets LAG-3, in combination with Nivolumab in pts with melanoma who progressed during prior anti–PD-1/PD-L1 therapy (MEL PRIOR IO) in all-comer and biomarker-enriched populations. Ann Oncol. 2017;28:605–49.

12. Adi D, Tannir NM, al BSE. Bempegaldesleukin (NKTR-214) plus nivolumab in patients with advanced solid tumors: phase I dose-escalation study of safety, efficacy, and immune activation (PIVOT-02). Cancer Discov. 2020;10:1–16.

13. Eggermont AMM, Chiarion-Sileni V, Grob JJ, et al. Prolonged survival in stage III melanoma with ipilimumab adjuvant therapy. NEJM. 2016;375:1845–55.

14. Weber J, del Vecchio M, Mandala M, et al. Adjuvant nivolumab versus ipilimumab in resected stage III/IV melanoma: 3-year efficacy and biomarker results from the phase 3 CheckMate 238 trial. Ann Oncol. 2019;30(S5):v533–63.

15. Zimmer L, Livingstone E, Hasse JC, et al. Adjuvant nivolumab plus ipilimumab or nivolumab monotherapy versus placebo in patients with resected stage IV melanoma with no evidence of disease (IMMUNED): a randomised, double-blind, placebo-controlled, phase 2 trial. Lancet. 2020;395(10236):1558–68.

16. Mandalà M, Larkin J, Ascierto PA, et al. An analysis of nivolumab-mediated adverse events and association with clinical efficacy in resected stage III or IV melanoma (CheckMate 238). J Clin Oncol. 2019;37(15_suppl):9584.

17. Bristol-Myers Squibb Announces Update on CheckMate -915 for Opdivo (Nivolumab) Plus Yervoy (Ipilimumab) Versus Opdivo Alone in Patients with Resected High-Risk Melanoma and PD-L1 <1% [press release] 2019. Princeton, New Jersey, November 20.

18. Amaria RN, Reddy SM, Tawbi HA, et al. Neoadjuvant immune checkpoint blockade in high-risk resectable melanoma. Nat Med. 2018;24(11):1649–54.

19. Rozeman EA, Fanchi L, van Akkooi ACJ, et al. (Neo-)Adjuvant Ipilimumab + Nivolumab (Ipi + Nivo) in palpable stage 3 melanoma - updated relapse free survival (RFS) data from the Opacin trial and first biomarker analyses. Ann Oncol. 2017;28:428–48.

20. Rozeman EA, Menzies AM, van Akkooi ACJ, et al. Identification of the optimal combination dosing schedule of neoadjuvant ipilimumab plus nivolumab in macroscopic stage III melanoma (OpACIN-neo): a multicentre, phase 2, randomised, controlled trial. Lancet Oncol. 2019;20(7):948–60.

21. Blank CU, Pennington T, Versluis JM, et al. First safety and efficacy results of PRADO: a phase II study of personalized response-driven surgery and adjuvant therapy after neoadju-

vant ipilimumab (IPI) and nivolumab (NIVO) in resectable stage III melanoma. J Clin Oncol. 2020;38(15_suppl):10002.

22. Blank CU, Rozeman EA, Fanchi LF, et al. Neoadjuvant versus adjuvant ipilimumab plus nivolumab in macroscopic stage III melanoma. Nat Med. 2018;24(11):1655–61.

23. Batten M, Shanahan ER, Silva IP et al (2019) Low intestinal microbial diversity is associated with severe immune-related adverse events and lack of response to neoadjuvant combination antiPD1, antiCTLA4 immunotherapy [abstract]. In: Proceedings of the American Association for Cancer Research Annual Meeting 2019; Atlanta (GA), Mar 29–Apr 3 AACR, Cancer Res 2019;79:abstract 2822.

24. Spranger S, Dai D, Horton B, et al. Tumor-residing Batf3 dendritic cells are required for effector T cell trafficking and adoptive T cell therapy. Cancer Cell. 2017;31(5):711–23.

25. Spranger S, Bao R, Gajewski TF. Melanoma-intrinsic β-catenin signalling prevents anti-tumour immunity. Nature. 2015;523(7559):231–5.

26. Ayers M, Lunceford J, Nebozhyn M, et al. IFN-γ-related mRNA profile predicts clinical response to PD-1 blokade. J Clin Investig. 2017;127(8):2930–40.

Chapter 12
Pembrolizumab in Melanoma: From Care to Cure

Indini Alice and Mario Mandalà

Introductions

Pembrolizumab (MK-3475) is a humanized monoclonal antibody (mAb) targeting the programmed cell death 1 (PD-1) [1]. Through its binding to human PD-1, pembrolizumab blocks the interaction between PD-1 and its ligands (the programmed cell death ligand 1 [PD-L1], and PD-L2). The result of this interaction is the induction of cytokine production (interferon [IFN]γ, interleukin [IL]-10, IL-12p70, IL-1β, IL-2, IL-6, IL-8, and tumor necrosis factor [TNF]α), thereby promoting the T lymphocytes' activity against tumor cells [2].

Pembrolizumab is administered intravenously and has an immediate and complete bioavailability. As other human mAbs, the pharmacokinetic profile of pembrolizumab is characterized by low clearance and limited volume of distribution [3]. It is catabolized through nonspecific pathways, and its metabolism does not influence the clearance. Also, the following factors had no clinically meaningful effect on the clearance of pembrolizumab: age (range: 15–94 years), sex, race, tumor burden, mild (GFR <90 and ≥60 mL/min/1.73 m^2) or moderate (GFR <60 and ≥30 mL/min/1.73 m^2) renal impairment, or mild hepatic impairment (TB ≤ ULN and AST > ULN or TB between 1 and 1.5 × ULN and any AST). There is insufficient information on whether there are clinically relevant differences in the clearance of pembrolizumab in subjects with severe renal impairment (estimated GFR <30 and

I. Alice
Unit of Medical Oncology, Department of Internal Medicine, Fondazione IRCCS Ca' Granda Ospedale Maggiore Policlinico, Milan, Italy

M. Mandalà (✉)
University of Perugia, Unit of Medical Oncology, Ospedale Santa Maria Misericordia, Perugia, Italy
e-mail: mario.mandala@unipg.it

P. Rutkowski, M. Mandalà (eds.), *New Therapies in Advanced Cutaneous Malignancies*, https://doi.org/10.1007/978-3-030-64009-5_12

$\geq$15 mL/min/1.73 m^2), or moderate (TB >1.5-3 $\times$ ULN and any AST) or severe (TB >3 $\times$ ULN and any AST) hepatic impairment [1].Therefore, there are no recommendations regarding specific dosing modifications based on such intrinsic factors. Given its parental administration and catabolic clearance, food intake and/or drug–drug interactions do not affect its exposure. Indeed, studies on the potential drug–drug interaction with the co-administration of systemic corticosteroids, chemotherapy, epacadostat and axitinib, failed to demonstrate a significant effect on the pharmacokinetics of pembrolizumab.

The formerly approved dose of pembrolizumab for the treatment of melanoma (i.e., 2 mg/kg every 3 weeks [q3w]) has been replaced by a flat dose of 200 mg q3w across different tumor types. In fact, a flat exposure response relationship was demonstrated between pembrolizumab exposure/dose and efficacy or safety, with an exposure at 2 mg/kg q3w being similar to the exposure at 200 mg q3w [4]. The similarity in efficacy between the dose regimens is further supported by the comparisons of response rates and survival outcomes for the tested dose regimens in the melanoma and non-small cell lung cancer (NSCLC) patients' population. Similarly, the alternative dosing regimen of pembrolizumab at 400 mg q6w has recently been approved across different treatment indications, on the basis of modeling and simulation analyses, primarily based on pharmacokinetic exposure matching with approved q3w dosing regimens [4].

Pembrolizumab in Advanced/Metastatic Melanoma

Pembrolizumab was first approved as single agent for the treatment of advanced unresectable/metastatic melanoma based on the results of three major prospective clinical trials, the KEYNOTE-001, the KEYNOTE-002, and the KEYNOTE-006.

KEYNOTE-001 (NCT01295827) was an open-label, phase Ib trial that included multiple cohorts of patients with advanced solid tumors, including melanoma [5, 6]. Patients were randomized to receive pembrolizumab 2 mg/kg q3w, 10 mg/kg q3w, or 10 mg/kg q2w until disease progression, intolerable toxicity, or patient's or investigator's decision to withdraw from treatment. After a protocol amendment, patients with complete response, who were treated with pembrolizumab for >6 months, could discontinue treatment after receiving 2 pembrolizumab doses beyond the first determination of complete response. Patients were eligible to receive a second course of pembrolizumab if they stopped treatment after achieving disease response (either complete, or partial response, or stable disease) after 2 years of treatment with pembrolizumab.

The primary efficacy outcome measure was overall response rate (ORR); secondary efficacy outcome measures were disease control rate (DCR), duration of response (DOR), progression-free survival (PFS), and overall survival (OS). A total of 655 participants with melanoma were enrolled in the three cohorts: 2 mg/kg q3w ($n = 162$), 10 mg/kg q3w ($n = 313$), or 10 mg/kg q2w ($n = 180$). Among these patients, 151 were treatment-naive and 496 had received previous systemic treatment(s). After a median follow-up of 55 months (range, 48–69), the estimated 5-year OS rate was 34% in all patients, and 41% in treatment-naive patients. Median OS was 23.8 months (95% CI, 20.2–30.4) and 38.6 months (95% CI, 27.2–not reached) in the whole study population and in treatment-naive patients, respectively. The 5-year estimated PFS rate was 21% and 29%, respectively. Median PFS was 8.3 months (95% CI, 5.8–11.1) in all patients and 16.9 months (95% CI, 9.3–35.5) in treatment-naive patients. Survival results were similar among the three dose levels of pembrolizumab. DCR was 65% in all patients, and 72% in treatment-naïve patients. Median time to response was 2.8 months in both groups, and median DOR was not reached in the whole population and in the treatment-naïve population, respectively. The ORR was slightly higher in ipilimumab-naive patients (46%) than in ipilimumab-pretreated patients (36%), while DCR was similar between groups (66% and 64%, respectively). Overall, results from this trial confirmed the antitumor activity of pembrolizumab both in treatment-naïve and pretreated patients. Among the 72 patients meeting eligibility criteria for stopping pembrolizumab, 7 (10%) had subsequent progressive disease after stopping therapy, while most (90%) patients had maintained response. The 2-year disease-free survival (DFS) among the 67 patients who stopped therapy after achieving a complete response was ~90%. Four patients, all with complete response after the first treatment course received second course pembrolizumab: best overall response on second course was complete response ($n = 1$), stable disease ($n = 1$), and progressive disease ($n = 2$). Notwithstanding the small number of patients, the authors concluded that survival outcomes upon pembrolizumab re-treatment can provide additional benefit.

The KEYNOTE-002 trial (NCT01704287) was a randomized phase II study for patients with advanced melanoma who had progressed on ipilimumab, previous targeted therapy, or both (if BRAFV600 mutated patients) [7]. Participants were randomized (1:1:1) to receive pembrolizumab 2 mg/kg q3w ($n = 180$), or 10 mg/kg q3w ($n = 181$), or investigator's choice chemotherapy ($n = 179$). The primary endpoints of the study were PFS (as assessed by independent central review) and OS; secondary endpoints were PFS (as assessed by investigators), ORR and DOR. Results of this trial confirmed that pembrolizumab provided a significant improvement of survival in heavily pretreated patients with durable responses [8]. OS improved with pembrolizumab 2 mg/kg (HR 0.86, 95% confidence interval [CI] 0.67–1.10; $p = 0.117$) and 10 mg/kg (HR 0.74, 95% CI 0.57–0.96; $p = 0.011$) versus chemotherapy. Two-year OS rates were 36% (95% CI 28.9–43.0), 38% (95% CI 31.1–45.2) and 30% (95% CI 23.0–36.7) with pembrolizumab 2 mg/kg, 10 mg/kg and chemotherapy, respectively. There was no difference in OS between the two pembrolizumab treatment arms (HR 0.87, 95% CI 0.67–1.12; $p = 0.290$), and OS results were consistent across all protocol-specified subgroups. Adjusting for crossover had limited effect on OS in patients treated with pembrolizumab (both regimens): among participants randomized to chemotherapy, 55% crossed over and subsequently received treatment with pembrolizumab. Also PFS improved with pembrolizumab 2 mg/kg (HR 0.58, 95% CI 0.46–0.73; p < 0.0001) and 10 mg/kg (HR 0.47, 95% CI 0.37–0.60; p < 0.0001) versus chemotherapy. The estimated 2-year PFS was 16% (95% CI 10.9–22.1) with pembrolizumab 2 mg/kg, 22% (95% CI 16.1–28.3) with pembrolizumab 10 mg/kg, versus 0.6% (95% CI 0.1–3.2) with chemotherapy [8]. The ORR was five- to six-fold increased for patients receiving pembrolizumab compared to those receiving chemotherapy (p < 0.0001 for both pembrolizumab doses versus chemotherapy), with no differences between the pembrolizumab doses (p = 0.214). Median DOR was 22.8 months (range 1.4 + to 25.3+) with pembrolizumab 2 mg/kg and was not reached (range 1.1 + to 28.3+) with pembrolizumab 10 mg/kg, compared to 6.8 months (range 2.8–11.3) for chemotherapy.

The third major clinical trial of pembrolizumab in patients with advanced melanoma was the KEYNOTE-006 (NCT01866319), in which patients with ipilimumab-naïve and ≤1 prior therapy for BRAF-mutant disease, were randomized (1:1:1) to receive pembrolizumab 10 mg/kg q2w (n = 279) or q3w (n = 277), or ipilimumab 3 mg/kg q3w (n = 278) [9–11]. A second course of pembrolizumab 200 mg q3w (lasting ≤1 year, that is, 17 cycles of therapy) was offered to patients who achieved DCR with the first course. The primary endpoints of this trial were OS and PFS; secondary endpoints were ORR and DOR. Survival results (both PFS and OS) were similar between the pembrolizumab treatment arms, therefore, the results of the two dosing groups were combined. Overall, 368 (66%) patients in the pembrolizumab groups and 181 (65%) patients in the ipilimumab group received pembrolizumab as first-line systemic treatment. Median OS was 32.7 months (95% CI 24.5–41.6) in the combined pembrolizumab groups and 15.9 months (95% CI 13.3–22.0) in the ipilimumab group (HR 0.73, 95% CI 0.61–0.88, p = 0.00049). 5-year OS was 38.7% (95% CI 34.2–43.1) and 31% (95% CI 25.3–36.9) in the combined pembrolizumab groups and in the ipilimumab group, respectively. Median PFS was 8.4 months (95% CI 6.6–11.3) in the combined pembrolizumab groups versus 3.4 months (95% CI 2.9–4.2) in the ipilimumab group (HR 0.57, 95% CI 0.48–0.67, p < 0.0001). 2-year PFS was 23% (95% CI 19.1–27.1) in the combined pembrolizumab groups and 7.3% (95% CI 3.3–13.3) in the ipilimumab group. DCR was 63% in the combined pembrolizumab groups, and 42% in the ipilimumab group, with a median DOR of 53.5 months (95% CI 50.99-not available) and not reached (95% CI 20.96-not available) in the ipilimumab group.

Two relevant issues raised by the analysis of KEYNOTE-006 results deserve to be addressed. The first regards the optimal treatment duration [11, 12]. Among the 103 (19%) patients who completed 2 years of first-course pembrolizumab, responses were ongoing in 16 (76%) of 21 patients with a complete response, 53 (77%) of 69 patients with a partial response, and 7 (54%) of 13 patients with stable disease. After a median follow-up of 42.9 months (95% CI 39.9–46.3) from treatment completion, 3-year OS from treatment completion was 100% (95% CI 100.0–100.0) for patients achieving complete response, 94.8% (95% CI 84.7–98.3) for patients with partial response, and 66.7% (95% CI 28.2–87.8) for patients with stable disease. The estimated 2-year PFS from completion of pembrolizumab for all 103 patients was 78.4% (95% CI 68.3–85.6), and significantly differed according to disease response, being 85.4% (95% CI 61.3–95.1) for patients achieving complete response, 82.3% (95% CI 70.3–89.8) for patients with partial response, and 39.9% (95% CI 8.1–71.4) for patients with stable disease. Interestingly, patients with complete response who interrupted treatment early per protocol (i.e., those showing complete response after at least 6 months of pembrolizumab, who received two additional doses after the first evidence of complete response and thus did not complete 2 years of treatment), had 2-year PFS of 86.4% (95% CI 63.4–95.4). This PFS rate is superimposable to that observed in patients achieving complete response after completion of 2 years of pembrolizumab, suggesting that the implementation of predictors of long-term benefit could help the optimization of treatment duration [13]. Moreover, real-life experience confirmed a low relapse rate for patients with a complete response, however, relapse was more likely with treatment duration <6 months [14]. This evidence will lead to consider therapy interruption in patients with a complete response that persists at the following radiological evaluation (to be performed at least 4 weeks after), and who have received at least 6 months of anti-PD1 treatment. Table 12.1 displays data from the major clinical trials and real-life experiences of pembrolizumab, supporting the maintenance of response after treatment discontinuation.

The second important issue regards re-treatment with a second course of pembrolizumab in patients achieving disease control with acceptable treatment-related adverse events (AEs). Updated results from KEYNOTE-006 on pembrolizumab re-treatment have recently been presented at the American Society of Clinical Oncology (ASCO) annual meeting 2020 [12]. Overall, 15 patients received second course pembrolizumab with the following distribution of best overall response during first course: complete response ($n = 6$), partial response ($n = 6$), and stable disease ($n = 3$). The median time from the end of first course treatment to the start of second course was 24.5 months (range, 4.9–41.4). Median follow-up in patients who received re-treatment was 25.3 months (range, 3.5–39.4) with a median second course treatment duration of 8.3 months (range, 1.4–12.6). Best overall response upon pembrolizumab re-treatment among patients evaluable for response ($n = 10$) was complete response ($n = 3$), partial response ($n = 5$), stable disease ($n = 3$), and progressive disease ($n = 2$). These data suggest that re-treatment with pembrolizumab in patients who progress after achieving disease control and stopping treatment can still provide additional clinical benefit in the majority of patients.

Data on treatment duration and re-treatment with anti-PD1 derived from real-world experiences partially differ from those of clinical trials. In a recent retrospective report by Betof et al. [15], data of 396 melanoma patients treated with anti-PD1

Table 12.1 Data from clinical trials and real-life experiences of pembrolizumab, supporting maintenance of response after treatment discontinuation

	Number of pts. who stopped anti-PD1/total patients	OR in pts. who stopped anti-PD1	Median off-treatment follow-up, mo	Maintenance of response, %
Ladwa/ Atkinson[a]	29/ ND	100% CR	8	89.6
KEYNOTE-001[b,c]	72/655	67% CR 5% PR	22	90
KEYNOTE-006[d,e]	104/556	30% CR 63% PR 10% SD	42.9	79.6
Real-life series[f]	81/509	43% CR 38% PR 19% SD	11.2	97.5
Real-life series[g]	185[i]/803	63% CR 24% PR 9% SD	18	78.4
Betof et al.[h]	396[j]/ND	25.8% CR 23.5% PR 11.6 SD	21[k]	72.1%[k]

CR complete response, *mo* months, *ND* not determined, *OR* objective response, *PR* partial response, *pts* patients, *SD* stable disease

[a]Ladwa R, Atkinson V. The cessation of anti-PD-1 antibodies of complete responders in metastatic melanoma. Melanoma Res. 2017; 27(2):168–170

[b]Robert C, Ribas A, Hamid O, et al. Three-year overall survival for patients with advanced melanoma treated with pembrolizumab in KEYNOTE-001. J Clin Oncol. 2016; 34:15_suppl, 9503–9503

[c]Hamid O, Robert C, Daud A, et al. Five-year survival outcomes for patients with advanced melanoma treated with pembrolizumab in KEYNOTE-001. Ann Oncol. 2019;30(4):582–588

[d]Robert C, Ribas A, Schachter J, et al. Pembrolizumab versus ipilimumab in advanced melanoma (KEYNOTE-006): post hoc 5-year results from an open-label, multicenter, randomized, controlled, phase 3 study. Lancet Oncol. 2019;20(9):1239–1251

[e]Long GV, Schachter J, Arance A, et al. Long-term survival from pembrolizumab (pembro) completion and pembro retreatment: Phase III KEYNOTE-006 in advanced melanoma. J Clin Oncol 38: 2020 (suppl; abstr 10013). doi: https://doi.org/10.1200/JCO.2020.38.15_suppl.10013

[f]Jansen Y, Rozeman EA, Geukes Foppen M, et al. Real life outcome of advanced melanoma patients who discontinue pembrolizumab (PEMBRO) in the absence of disease progression. J Clin Oncol. 017; 35(suppl): 9539

[g]Jansen YJL, Rozeman AE, Mason R, et al. Discontinuation of anti-PD-1 antibody therapy in the absence of disease progression or treatment limiting toxicity: clinical outcomes in advanced melanoma. Ann Oncol. 2019;30(7):1154–1161

[h]Betof Warner A, Palmer JS, Shoushtari AN, et al.: Long-term outcomes and responses to retreatment in patients with melanoma treated with PD-1 blockade. J Clin Oncol. 2020; 38:1655–1663

[i]Includes patients receiving pembrolizumab ($n = 167$) and nivolumab ($n = 18$)

[j]Includes patients receiving pembrolizumab ($n = 340$) and nivolumab ($n = 56$). Treatment was given outside of a clinical trial in 69.2% of patients

[k]Data on patients with CR only

(either single-agent pembrolizumab, 85.9% of patients; or nivolumab, 14.1% of patients) were presented. Treatment was given outside of a clinical trial in 69.2% of patients. Overall, 102 (25.8%) patients were classified as having complete response as best response before treatment cessation. The authors defined complete response as: (1) being free of radiographic evidence of disease; (2) having evidence of disease after radiographic response, with a biopsy that showed no evidence of viable tumor; or (3) absence of radiographically measurable tumor. With a median follow-up from time of complete response of 21.1 months for patients who were treatment failure-free (range, 1.6–65.6 months), neither the median time to treatment failure (TTF) nor the median OS from time of complete response was reached. The probability of being alive and not requiring additional systemic therapy at 3 years was 72.1% (95% CI, 59.9% to 81.1%) with an estimated 3-year OS from time of complete response of 82.7% (95% CI, 67.9% to 91.1%). Seventy-eight (19.7%) patients who experienced disease progression after discontinuing anti-PD1 therapy received a second-course of immune checkpoint inhibitor therapy (either single-agent anti-PD1, 34 patients; or combined ipilimumab and nivolumab, 44 patients). The BOR to the first anti-PD1 course was complete response in 10 patients, partial response in 18 patients, stable disease in 13 patients; 37 patients had progressive disease. The median time between first-course anti–PD-1 discontinuation and the start of retreatment was 6.3 months (range, 0.3–28.6 months). Five patients (14.7%) responded to retreatment with single-agent anti-PD-1 (2 patients achieved complete response). There was no correlation between BOR to the initial course of anti–PD-1 and response to re-treatment. The median duration of retreatment was 1.6 months (range, <1.0–28.3 months). The estimated median OS for all 78 retreated patients from the start of retreatment was 9.9 months (95% CI, 6.8 to 17.9 months); the 2-year OS was 37.6% (95% CI, 25.5% to 49.7%). According to this report, which is the largest report to date on patients receiving re-treatment with anti-PD1, the rate of progression after treatment discontinuation for complete response appears higher than that observed in KEYNOTE-001 and KEYNOTE-006. Notably, the median treatment duration of patients with complete response was shorter than that in the KEYNOTE-001/-006 cohorts, and the median duration of treatment after achieving a CR was 0 months. Reports from smaller case series of patients who electively discontinued anti-PD1 treatment in patients achieving complete response identified a significantly increased risk of disease relapse in patients treated with anti-PD-1 treatment for <6 months versus >6 months. The available data therefore suggest that the possibility to interrupt anti-PD1 treatment should be proposed and properly discussed with patients experiencing complete response, however, after 6–12 months of treatment which should be continued until the complete response is confirmed. The optimization of treatment management and duration is an interesting field of research, and data on this topic are growing.

Adjuvant Pembrolizumab in Resected High-Risk Melanoma

Pembrolizumab has recently been approved as adjuvant treatment for resected stage III melanoma on the basis of the results of the European Organization for Research and Treatment of Cancer (EORTC) 1325 (KEYNOTE-054) clinical trial (NCT02362594) [16]. Eligible patients had to have either resected stage IIIA (at least one micrometastasis measuring >1 mm in greatest diameter), IIIB, or IIIC melanoma, as defined by the American Joint Committee on Cancer (AJCC) 2009 classification, seventh edition. This randomized, double-blind, phase 3 trial randomized participants (1:1) were to receive pembrolizumab 200 mg q3w ($n = 514$) for a total of 18 doses (approximately 1 year) or until disease recurrence, unacceptable toxicity, or withdrawal of consent, or to receive placebo ($n = 505$). If recurrent disease was documented, patients were eligible for cross-over or repeat treatment with pembrolizumab if recurrence happened after >6 months from stopping therapy. The primary efficacy outcome measures were investigator-assessed relapse-free survival (RFS) in the overall population, and in participants with PD-L1 positive tumors. Secondary endpoints included distant metastasis-free survival and OS. Safety measures and health-related quality of life (QoL) were additional secondary endpoints, and will be discussed further (Toxicity Profile section). After a median follow-up of 36 months, the RFS was 64% in the pembrolizumab group and 44% in the placebo group (HR 0.56, 95% CI 0.47–0.68) [17]. This survival improvement was consistent across subgroups, regardless of PD-L1 expression, BRAF mutation, and the stage of disease. This consistency across subgroups is maintained when using the AJCC Cancer Staging Manual, eighth edition (AJCC-8) [18], compared with the AJCC-7 staging system [19]. Notably, the RFS improvement observed in BRAF-mutated patients was similar to the one observed with adjuvant dabrafenib and trametinib in the COMBI-AD trial (HR 0.47, 3-year RFS: 58% vs. 39%; 19% rate difference) [20]. In the overall population, the 3-year cumulative distant metastases free survival (DMFS) was 22.3% and 37.3% in the pembrolizumab arm and in the placebo arm, respectively (HR 0.55, 95% CI 0.44–0.69) [16]. Future data will provide not only information on OS, but also relevant data on whether to start adjuvant pembrolizumab in all resected stage III patients or start treatment only for those at time of recurrence.

Given the proven benefit in survival outcomes in patients with stage III melanoma, adjuvant pembrolizumab is currently under evaluation in patients with surgically resected high-risk stage II melanoma. In fact, patients with stage IIB, IIC, or stage IIIB melanoma have similar survival rates [18].

KEYNOTE-716 (NCT03553836) is a two-part (adjuvant and rechallenge/crossover) randomized, double-blind, and placebo-controlled phase III study of adjuvant pembrolizumab in adult patients (aged ≥18 years) and pediatric patients (aged 12 to <18 years) with resected stage IIB or IIC cutaneous melanoma. Stage IIB and IIC (according to the AJCC eighth edition) include patients with T category T3b, T4a, and T4b, respectively, with negative sentinel lymph node biopsy, and no evidence of regional or distant metastases. In Part 1, patients are randomized (1:1) to receive adjuvant pembrolizumab/placebo (200 mg q3w for adult patients; 2 mg/kg q3w for pediatric patients) for up to 17 cycles. In Part 2 (unblinded crossover/rechallenge phase), eligible patients with disease recurrence can receive further treatment with pembrolizumab if they meet eligibility criteria [21].

The primary endpoint of the study is RFS (assessed by the site investigator); secondary endpoints include DMFS (assessed by the site investigator), OS, and to assess the safety and tolerability of pembrolizumab. This trial is currently ongoing and recruiting patients. Results from this study will potentially help to define the role of adjuvant pembrolizumab in the management of high-risk stage II melanoma and hopefully improve survival outcomes in this patient population.

Pembrolizumab in Neoadjuvant Setting

Neaodjuvant pembrolizumab has been studied in a phase Ib clinical trial which enrolled patients with measurable resectable clinical stage III or resectable stage IV melanoma (NCT02434354) [22]. After a baseline pretreatment tumor biopsy, 29 patients received a single dose of pembrolizumab 200 mg followed by surgical resection 3 weeks later. After resection and on surgical recovery, patients continued to receive adjuvant pembrolizumab q3w for up to 1 year, or until the time of recurrence or any unacceptable treatment-related toxicity. There were no major toxicities or unexpected delays in surgery or negative surgical outcomes. Six (20.6%) patients had confirmed radiological response, and half of these patients had $\geq 20\%$ reduction per RECIST v 1.1. Twenty-seven patients were evaluable for pathologic response: 5 achieved a complete pathologic response, while 3 achieved a major pathologic response (defined as <10% viable tumor). After a median follow-up of 25 months, all patients achieving complete or major pathologic response remained disease-free, median DFS was not reached, and the 1-year DFS rate was 63%. Twenty paired pretreatment and posttreatment tissue samples were investigated, showing an increase in brisk tumor infiltrating lymphocytes (TILs) upon treatment with pembrolizumab, which also correlated with pathologic response and DFS.

Neoadjuvant pembrolizumab was also studied in combination with high-dose interferon (HDI) in a phase I trial in high-risk patients with locoregionally advanced melanoma (i.e., stage IIIB, IIIC, or IV according to the AJCC seventh edition) (NCT02339324). The primary endpoint of the study was to assess the safety of the combination of pembrolizumab and HDI. Eligible patients received two cycles of pembrolizumab, followed by definitive surgery, and subsequent adjuvant pembrolizumab until the completion of 1-year treatment. HDI was given concurrently in both the preoperative and postoperative treatment periods [23]. Overall, results from this study suggest that combining HDI does increase toxicity without providing substantial benefit to single-agent pembrolizumab.

Toxicity Profile

Treatment with pembrolizumab may be associated with a peculiar spectrum of immune-related adverse events (irAEs) [24]. In most cases, irAEs are mild and transient, but occasionally they can evolve to severe and potentially fatal disease. The most common irAEs during anti-PD1 therapy are dermatologic, followed by endocrinopathies, diarrhea/colitis, hepatotoxicity, although virtually every organ site can be affected [24].

Dermatologic toxicity affects approximately 30–40% of patients receiving pembrolizumab. Most patients develop dermatologic complications as first treatment-related adverse events, with onset an average of 3.6 weeks after treatment initiation. The most common findings are pruritus, cutaneous rash, however, also vitiligo, oral mucositis with dry mouth, and alopecia can be seen. Severe rashes such as Stevens-Johnson syndrome/toxic epidermal necrolysis have been reported in rare cases.

Endocrinopathies are the second most common type of irAEs [25]. The estimated incidence of clinically significant endocrinopathies during immune checkpoint inhibitors is ~10%. However, data from clinical trials vary depending on methods of assessment, diagnosis, and monitoring. The most common endocrinopathies during anti-PD1 treatment affect the thyroid, while hypophysitis is less commonly observed. Type 1 diabetes mellitus and adrenal insufficiency are rare findings.

Diarrhea/colitis is less frequent with anti-PD1 therapy compared with anti-CTLA4, and is usually observed later on during treatment, approximately after 6 weeks from the beginning of pembrolizumab. However, grade 3/4 immune-mediated colitis is seen in approximately 1–2% of patients treated with pembrolizumab [1].

Hepatotoxicity (i.e., elevations in serum levels of aspartate aminotransferase [AST], and alanine aminotransferase [ALT] can be observed most commonly as asymptomatic laboratory abnormalities. The most common time of onset of liver toxicity is 8–12 weeks after treatment initiation. In observational studies of PD-1-blocking antibodies, the rates of inflammatory hepatitis are <5%, and severe (i.e., grade 3–4) hepatotoxicity is even rarer [26].

Pulmonary toxicity is an uncommon but potentially severe toxicity during anti-PD1 treatment [27]. Its clinical manifestation may vary and diagnosis is commonly made after excluding other causative agents (e.g., infections, progressive disease).

Several uncommon irAEs have been described during treatment with pembrolizumab, including acute kidney injury [28], cardiovascular toxicity [1], neurologic syndromes [29], and hematologic disease [30]. Due to their rarity and potentially atypical presentation, irAEs can be particularly challenging for diagnosis and treatment, and often evolve in severe and eventually fatal syndromes.

General recommendations to optimize the outcomes in case of irAEs include rapid identification of symptoms and prompt initiation of local or systemic immunosuppression [31]. Treatment of moderate and severe irAEs usually requires the interruption of anti-PD1 and subsequent initiation of high doses of corticosteroids (i.e., prednisone 1–2 mg/kg/day or equivalent). If corticosteroids are not effective in treating irAEs in the first days, stronger immunosuppressive drugs are needed (e.g., infliximab, mycophenolate mofetil) [31]. With the increasing use of pembrolizumab and other anti-PD1 antibodies for the treatment of several solid tumors, the knowledge on the toxicity profile is growing accordingly. Adequate patient's information and frequent communication between patients, caregivers, and the clinical team is relevant for the successful management of irAEs.

Available data suggest that patients who experienced irAEs during immune checkpoint inhibitors (either anti-CTLA4, or anti-PD1/PD-L1) can be safely retreated with another course of immunotherapy, after careful risk-to-benefit assessment [32, 33]. Elements to be considered include the type of irAE(s), its severity and responsiveness to systemic corticosteroids, and the clinical response to the initial immunotherapy regimen. Moreover, data are limited on the effectiveness of this retreatment approach.

Novel Treatment Strategies and Combination Therapies

Several clinical trials are currently underway in order to improve the outcomes of single-agent anti-PD1 therapy. Most efforts focus on developing combination strategies to increase the therapeutic activity of anti-PD1 and delay the onset of treatment resistance. Another field of current investigation is to potentiate the outcomes of melanoma patients with brain metastases receiving pembrolizumab with the aid of combination strategies.

The following categories of drugs are under investigation as combined therapies with pembrolizumab: immunotherapy agents, including other immune checkpoint inhibitors, and vaccines; cytotoxic chemotherapy; targeted therapy (i.e., BRAF and MEK inhibitors); antiangiogenic drugs. Several other agents have been proposed to be used in combination with pembrolizumab. Table 12.2. shows the major clinical trials of pembrolizumab-based combination therapy currently ongoing for the treatment of advanced/metastatic melanoma.

Conclusions

See Table 12.2. Pembrolizumab changed the way we treat melanoma patients both in advanced and early stage disease. Several clinical trials are currently underway, in order to improve the outcomes of patients receiving single-agent Pembrolizumab. Most efforts focus on developing combination strategies to increase therapeutic activity of Pembrolizumab, delay the onset of treatment resistance, or reverse primary or secondary resistance. Another field of current investigation is to potentiate the outcomes of melanoma patients with brain metastases receiving pembrolizumab, with the aid of combination strategies.

Table 12.2. Summary of the main ongoing clinical trials of pembrolizumab combination therapy in advanced unresectable/metastatic setting for melanoma (source: www.clinicaltrials.gov, accessed July 2020)

Trial name, NCT number	Study design	Disease characteristics, setting	Investigational drug(s)	Combination strategy	Sample size	Primary endpoint(s)
Immunotherapy combinations						
NCT02706353	Phase I/II	Metastatic (any line)	APX500M, pembro	Intralesional CD40 + systemic anti-PD1	41	MTD, RP2D ORR
NCT03132675	Phase II	Metastatic, progressed on anti-PD1	Tavokinogene telseplasmid, pembro	Intralesional pIL-2 and electroporation + systemic anti-PD1	100	ORR
NCT02743819	Phase II	Metastatic, progressed on anti-PD1	Ipilimumab, pembro	Anti-CTLA4 + antiPD1	70	ORR
MASTERKEY-115, NCT04068181	Phase II	IIIB/IV, progressed on anti-PD1	Talimogene laherparepvec, pembro	Intralesional T-VEC + systemic anti-PD1	100	ORR
MK-3475-02B, NCT04305054	Phase II, randomized	Metastatic, first line	MK-7684, pembro	Anti-TIGIT + anti-PD1	135	AE(s)[a] ORR
IMCODE001, NCT03815058	Phase II, randomized	Advanced/metastatic, first line	RO7198457, pembro	Cancer vaccine + anti-PD1	132	PFS
SCIB1-002, NCT04079166	Phase II	Metastatic, first line	SCIB1, pembro	Cancer vaccine and electroporation + anti-PD1	25	AEs ORR
NCT02621021	Phase II, randomized	Metastatic, refractory to first line therapy	Cyclophosphamide, fludarabine, aldesleukin, pembro	TILs + anti-PD1	170	RR
Targeted therapy and TKIs combinations						
IMMU-TARGET, NCT02902042	Phase II, randomized	IIIB-D/IV BRAF+, first line	Encorafenib, binimetinib, pembro	BRAF/MEKi + anti-PD1	145	Incidence of TE-AEs PFS

NCT03149029	Phase II	Advanced/metastatic BRAF+, first line	Dabrafenib, trametinib, pembro	BRAF/MEKi + anti-PD1	50	DCR
NCT03957551	Phase Ib/II	Metastatic, first line (previous BRAF/MEKi allowed)	Cabozantinib, pembro	Multiple target inhibitor + anti-PD1	39	AE(s) ORR
NCT02872259	Phase Ib/II, randomized	Advanced/metastatic BRAF+, first line	BGB324, dabrafenib, trametinib, pembro	AXLi + BRAF/MEKi + anti-PD1	92	ORR AEs
NCT03131908	Phase I/II	Metastatic, PTEN loss, progressed on anti-PD1	GSK263677, pembro	PI3Ki + anti-PD1	41	MTD ORR
NCT03021460	Phase II	Metastatic, first line	Ibrutinib, pembro	BTKi + anti-PD1	51	ORR
Cytotoxic chemotherapy combinations						
NCT02617849	Phase II	Metastatic, first line (previous BRAF/MEKi allowed)	CBDCA, paclitaxel, pembro	Chemotherapy + anti-PD1	30	ORR
NCT02816021	Phase II	Metastatic (any line)	CC-846 (azacytidine), pembro	Chemotherapy + anti-PD1	70	ORR AEs
Antiangiogenic drugs combinations						
LEAP-003, NCT03820986	Phase III, randomized	Metastatic, first line (previous BRAF/MEKi allowed)	Lenvatinib, pembro	VEGFi + anti-PD1	660	PFS OS
LEAP-004, NCT03776136	Phase II	Metastatic, progressed on anti-PD1	Lenvatinib, pembro	VEGFi + anti-PD1	100	ORR
NCT02681549	Phase II	Brain metastases (any line, except previous antiPD1/PD-L1)	Bevacizumab, pembro	VEGFi + anti-PD1	53	BMRR

(continued)

Table 12.2. (continued)

Trial name, NCT number	Study design	Disease characteristics, setting	Investigational drug(s)	Combination strategy	Sample size	Primary endpoint(s)
Other combinations						
NCT03278665	Phase Ib/II	Metastatic, progressed on anti-PD1	4SC-202, pembro	HDACi + anti-PD1	40	AEs
NCT02557321	Phase I/II, randomized	Metastatic, first line	PV-10, pembro	Intralesional Rose Bengal + anti-PD1	192	AEs PFS
NCT03620019	Phase II	Metastatic, first line	Denosumab, pembro, nivo	mAb anti-RANKL + anti-PD1	28	Antitumor effect (circulating biomarkers)

AEs adverse events, *AXLi* inhibitors of AXL, *BMRR* brain metastases response rate, *BRAF/MEKi* BRAF/MEK inhibitors, *BTKi* bruton kinase inhibitor, *CBDCA* carboplatin, *CD-40* cluster of differentiation 40, *CTLA-4* cytotoxic T lymphocyte antigen 4, *DCR* disease control rate, *HDACi* Histone deacetylases inhibitor, *IL-2* interleukin 2, *MTD* maximum tolerated dose, *ORR* objective response rate, *OS* overall survival, *PD-1* programmed cell death 1, *PD-L1* programmed cell death ligand 1, *PFS* progression-free survival, *PI3Ki* Phosphoinositide 3-kinases inhibitor, *PTEN* Phosphatase and tensin homolog, *RANKL* receptor activator of nuclear factor kappa-B ligand, *RP2D* recommended phase 2 dose, *RR* response rate, *T-VEC* talimogene laherparepvec, *TEAE* treatment-emergent adverse events, *TIGIT* T cell immunoreceptor with Ig and ITIM domains, *TILs* tumor infiltrating lymphocytes, *VEGF* vascular endothelial growth factor inhibitor

[a]Includes rate of participants who discontinue study treatment due to an AE

References

1. Merck Sharp & Dohme Corp. KEYTRUDA® (Pembrolizumab) for injection, for intravenous use. Whitehouse Station, NJ: Merck & Co., Inc.; 2020.
2. Brown JA, Dorfman DM, Ma F-R, Sullivan EL, Munoz O, Wood CR, et al. Blockade of programmed death-1 ligands on dendritic cells enhances T cell activation and cytokine production. J Immunol. 2003;170(3):1257–66.
3. Dostalek M, Gardner I, Gurbaxani BM, et al. Pharmacokinetics, pharmacodynamics and physiologically-based pharmacokinetic modelling of monoclonal antibodies. Clin Pharmacokinet. 2013;52:83–124.
4. Freshwater T, Kondic A, Ahamadi M, et al. Evaluation of dosing strategy for pembrolizumab for oncology indications. J Immunother Cancer. 2017;5:43.
5. Robert C, Ribas A, Hamid O, et al. Three-year overall survival for patients with advanced melanoma treated with pembrolizumab in KEYNOTE-001. J Clin Oncol. 2016;34(15_suppl):9503.
6. Hamid O, Robert C, Daud A, et al. Five-year survival outcomes for patients with advanced melanoma treated with pembrolizumab in KEYNOTE-001. Ann Oncol. 2019;30(4):582–8. https://doi.org/10.1093/annonc/mdz011.
7. Ribas A, Puzanov I, Dummer R, et al. Pembrolizumab versus investigator-choice chemotherapy for ipilimumab-refractory melanoma (KEYNOTE-002): a randomised, controlled, phase 2 trial. Lancet Oncol. 2015;16(8):908–18. https://doi.org/10.1016/S1470-2045(15)00083-2.
8. Hamid O, Puzanov I, Dummer R, et al. Final analysis of a randomised trial comparing pembrolizumab versus investigator-choice chemotherapy for ipilimumab-refractory advanced melanoma. Eur J Cancer. 2017;86:37–45. https://doi.org/10.1016/j.ejca.2017.07.022.
9. Robert C, Schachter J, Long GV, et al. Pembrolizumab versus ipilimumab in advanced melanoma. N Engl J Med. 2015;372(26):2521–32. https://doi.org/10.1056/NEJMoa1503093.
10. Schachter J, Ribas A, Long GV, et al. Pembrolizumab versus ipilimumab for advanced melanoma: final overall survival results of a multicentre, randomised, open-label phase 3 study (KEYNOTE-006). Lancet. 2017;390(10105):1853–62. https://doi.org/10.1016/S0140-6736(17)31601-X.
11. Robert C, Ribas A, Schachter J, et al. Pembrolizumab versus ipilimumab in advanced melanoma (KEYNOTE-006): post-hoc 5-year results from an open-label, multicentre, randomised, controlled, phase 3 study. Lancet Oncol. 2019;20(9):1239–51. https://doi.org/10.1016/S1470-2045(19)30388-2.
12. Long GV, Schachter J, Arance A, et al. Long-term survival from pembrolizumab (pembro) completion and pembro retreatment: phase III KEYNOTE-006 in advanced melanoma. J Clin Oncol. 2020;38(15_suppl):10013. https://doi.org/10.1200/JCO.2020.38.15_suppl.10013.
13. Tan AC, Emmett L, Lo S, et al. FDG-PET response and outcome from anti-PD-1 therapy in metastatic melanoma. Ann Oncol. 2018;29(10):2115–20. https://doi.org/10.1093/annonc/mdy330.
14. Jansen YJL, Rozeman EA, Mason R, et al. Discontinuation of anti-PD-1 antibody therapy in the absence of disease progression or treatment limiting toxicity: clinical outcomes in advanced melanoma. Ann Oncol. 2019;30(7):1154–61.
15. Betof Warner A, Palmer JS, Shoushtari AN, et al. Long-term outcomes and responses to retreatment in patients with melanoma treated with PD-1 blockade. J Clin Oncol. 2020;38:1655–63.
16. Eggermont AMM, Blanck CU, Mandalà M, et al. Adjuvant pembrolizumab versus placebo in resected stage III melanoma. N Engl J Med. 2018;378:1789–801.
17. Eggermont AM, Blank CU, Mandalà M, et al. Pembrolizumab versus placebo after complete resection of high-risk stage III melanoma. New recurrence-free survival results from the EORTC 1325-MG/Keynote 054 double-blinded phase III trial at three-year median follow-up. J Clin Oncol. 2020;38(suppl):abstr 10000. doi:https://doi.org/10.1200/JCO.2020.38.15_suppl.10000.
18. Gershenwald JE, Scolyer RA, Hess KR, et al. Melanoma staging: evidence-based changes in the American Joint Committee on Cancer eighth edition cancer staging manual. CA Cancer J Clin. 2017;67(6):472–92.

19. Eggermont AMM, Blank CU, Mandala M, et al. Prognostic and predictive value of AJCC-8 staging in the Phase III EORTC1325/KEYNOTE-054 trial of pembrolizumab vs placebo in resected high-risk stage III melanoma. Eur J Cancer. 2019;116:148–57.
20. Hauschild A, Dummer R, Schadendorf D, et al. Longer follow-up confirms relapse-free survival benefit with adjuvant dabrafenib plus trametinib in patients with resected BRAF V600-mutant stage III melanoma. J Clin Oncol. 2018;36(35):3441–9. https://doi.org/10.1200/JCO.18.01219.
21. Luke JJ, Ascierto PA, Carlino MS, et al. KEYNOTE-716: phase III study of adjuvant pembrolizumab versus placebo in resected high-risk stage II melanoma. Future Oncol. 2020;16(3):4429–38. https://doi.org/10.2217/fon-2019-0666.
22. Huang AC, Orlowski RJ, Xu X, et al. A single dose of neoadjuvant PD-1 blockade predicts clinical outcomes in resectable melanoma. Nat Med. 2019;25(3):454–61.
23. Najjar Y, McCurry D, Lin H, et al. A phase I study of neoadjuvant combination immunotherapy in locally/regionally advanced melanoma. J Clin Oncol. 2019;37(15_suppl):9586.
24. Naidoo J, Page DB, Li BT, et al. Toxicities of the anti-PD-1 and anti-PD-L1 immune checkpoint antibodies. Ann Oncol. 2015;26(12):2375.
25. Barroso-Sousa R, Barry WT, Garrido-Castro AC, et al. Incidence of endocrine dysfunction following the use of different immune checkpoint inhibitor regimens: a systematic review and meta-analysis. JAMA Oncol. 2018;4(2):173.
26. Tsung I, Dolan R, Lao CD, et al. Liver injury is most commonly due to hepatic metastases rather than drug hepatotoxicity during pembrolizumab immunotherapy. Aliment Pharmacol Ther. 2019;50(7):800.
27. Naidoo J, Wang X, Woo KM, et al. Pneumonitis in patients treated with anti-programmed death-1/programmed death ligand 1 therapy. J Clin Oncol. 2017;35(7):709.
28. Mamlouk O, Selamet U, Machado S, et al. Nephrotoxicity of immune checkpoint inhibitors beyond tubulointerstitial nephritis: single-center experience. J Immunother Cancer. 2019;7(1):2.
29. Reynolds KL, Guidon AC. Diagnosis and management of immune checkpoint inhibitor-associated neurologic toxicity: illustrative case and review of the literature. Oncologist. 2019;24(4):435.
30. Noseda R, Bertoli R, Müller L, Ceschi A. Haemophagocytic lymphohistiocytosis in patients treated with immune checkpoint inhibitors: analysis of WHO global database of individual case safety reports. J Immunother Cancer. 2019;7(1):117.
31. Brahmer JR, Lacchetti C, Schneider BJ, et al. Management of immune-related adverse events in patients treated with immune checkpoint inhibitor therapy: American Society of Clinical Oncology Clinical Practice Guideline. J Clin Oncol. 2018;36(17):1714.
32. Pollack MH, Betof A, Dearden H, et al. Safety of resuming anti-PD-1 in patients with immune-related adverse events (irAEs) during combined anti-CTLA-4 and anti-PD1 in metastatic melanoma. Ann Oncol. 2018;29(1):250.
33. Simonaggio A, Michot JM, Voisin AL, et al. Evaluation of readministration of immune checkpoint inhibitors after immune-related adverse events in patients with cancer. JAMA Oncol. 2019;5(9):1310–7. https://doi.org/10.1001/jamaoncol.2019.1022.

Chapter 13
Talimogene Laherparepvec (T-VEC)

Marcin Zdzienicki, Piotr Rutkowski, Evalyn Mulder, and Dirk J. Grunhagen

Introduction

In recent years, significant progress has been made in the treatment of advanced (i.e., stage III and metastatic stage IV) melanoma patients. The emergence of effective systemic therapies (molecular-targeted therapy or systemic checkpoint inhibitors—CPIs) has changed the fate of advanced melanoma patients. The effectiveness of these therapies has also been proven in adjuvant treatment, after surgery in patients at a high risk of recurrence. However, there are still subpopulations of melanoma patients for whom optimal treatment has not been identified. One such unresolved problem is the locoregional recurrences of melanoma, which includes local recurrences, in transit, and satellite metastases.

There are many therapeutic options for patients with locoregional recurrence of melanoma. These are very diverse methods, ranging from simple surgical excision of individual lesions to advanced techniques of local chemotherapy, using isolated limb perfusion. Systemic treatment was used in very advanced cases, as was the case with disseminated disease. Until recently, however, none of the options listed in national and international recommendations could be considered as a standard treatment in this group of patients. Therefore, methods were sought that would allow for effective treatment of locoregional relapse in these patients. The new recently approved option for therapy of unresectable in-transit recurrences

M. Zdzienicki (✉) · P. Rutkowski
Department of Soft Tissue/Bone Sarcoma and Melanoma, Maria Sklodowska-Curie National Research Institute of Oncology, Warsaw, Poland
e-mail: marcin.zdzienicki@pib-nio.pl; piotr.rutkowski@pib-nio.pl

E. Mulder · D. J. Grunhagen
Department of Surgical Oncology, Erasmus Medical Centre Cancer Institute, Rotterdam, The Netherlands
e-mail: e.e.a.p.mulder@erasmusmc.nl; d.grunhagen@erasmusmc.nl

P. Rutkowski, M. Mandalà (eds.), *New Therapies in Advanced Cutaneous Malignancies*, https://doi.org/10.1007/978-3-030-64009-5_13

265

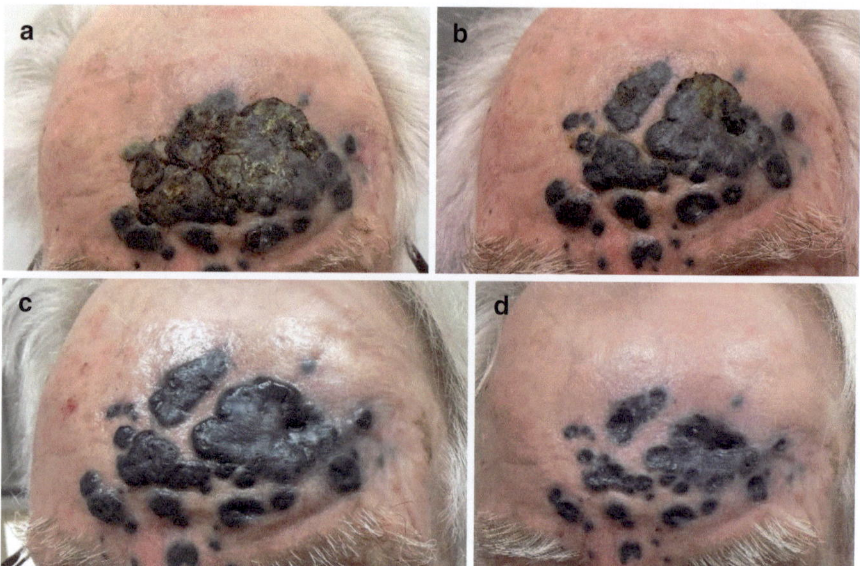

Fig. 13.1 Case–T-VEC treatment of unresectable locoregional recurrence after immunotherapy

(Fig. 13.1) subcutaneous metastases, or lymph nodal involvement (stages IIIB–IVA) with category 1 recommendations in US National Comprehensive Cancer Network (NCCN) guidelines is talimogene laherparepvec (T-VEC, IMLYGIC®)—the first in its class oncolytic virus for intralesional injections.

Phase III Registration Trial

In 2015, Robert H.I. Andtbacka and colleagues published the results of a Phase III study evaluating the effectiveness of T-VEC in melanoma patients (preliminary study results were presented at the American Society of Clinical Oncology (ASCO) Annual Meetings in 2013 and 2014) [1, 2]. The study involved 436 patients with grade IIIB to IV unresectable melanoma. The melanoma lesions had to be feasible for direct (or under ultrasound control) injection of the tumors, as the drug is administered intratumorally. In the control group, an intratumoral cytokine, namely granulocyte-macrophage colony-stimulating factor (GM-CSF) was administered. The study was open-label, prospective, randomized, multicenter, and international. Patients were recruited in 64 centers. Ultimately, the study drug (T-VEC) was administered in 291 patients and the comparator (GM-CSF) in 127 patients.

The primary endpoint of the study was the durable response rate (DRR; defined as a continuous objective response for at least 6 months) to treatment. Secondly, the objective response rate (ORR), overall survival (OS), and (time to) complete response (CR) were assessed. The study showed an advantage of T-VEC over control drug in terms of local response (DRR 16% for T-VEC, 2% for GM-CSF; ORR: 26% and 6%, respectively). The results also suggested an improvement in OS in the T-VEC arm (median OS was 23.3 months versus 18.9 months, for the T-VEC and comparator group, respectively, $p = 0.051$) [3]. In the final analysis of the study published in 2019, the results were even slightly better, and prolonged survival was shown in the T-VEC group (median OS was 24.5 months for patients who received T-VEC, and 18.9 months for patients who received GM-CSF, $p = 0.0439$). It is also worth noting that about 17% of patients treated with T-VEC achieved durable CR—a median of response time was not reached in 4 years follow-up [4]. Efficacy was the most marked aspect in the population of patients in stage IIIB, IIIC, or IVM1a, i.e., in patients without visceral metastases. Based on the results of this study, T-VEC has been approved in the United States, European Union and Switzerland, and Australia, to treat patients with unresectable stage IIIB–IV melanoma with one or more injectable (sub)cutaneous, or nodal lesions.

Mechanism of Action, Mode of Administration, and Adverse Events

T-VEC is a genetically modified herpes simplex virus type 1. Due to genetic modifications, the virus lost its affinity for the nervous system but gained the ability to selectively multiply in tumor cells. The replication process eventually leads to lysis of infected tumor cells. At the same time, a cytokine coding sequence, namely granulocyte-macrophage colony-stimulating factor (GM-CSF), was built into the viral genome. The cytokine is produced during the replication process and released when the cancer cell breaks down. The release of GM-CSF has a multidirectional effect on immune response, and its most important effects in terms of anticancer effectiveness are activation of macrophages to secrete other cytokines (such as IL-6, IL- 12, and TNF-α) and maturation of antigen-presenting cells (dendritic cells). These mechanisms induce the tumor-specific T cell response [5]. Activation of the local immune response is further enhanced by the release of tumor-specific antigens during the breakdown of the tumor cells, thus T-VEC may also trigger systemic effects.

T-VEC vials should be transported and stored frozen at a temperature of $-90\,^{\circ}$C to $-70\,^{\circ}$C. Before injection, the vials should be thawed ($\pm$30 min, at room temperature) until liquid. After thawing, vials cannot be refrozen. T-VEC is administered intratumorally, either directly or under the control of radiological imaging techniques (usually ultrasound). Before treatment, the target lesion(s) should be measured, as it determines the required volume of T-VEC (up to a maximum of 4 mL per treatment visit, based on lesion size) (Table 13.1). The recommended initial T-VEC dose is at a concentration of 10^6 plaque-forming units (PFU)/mL (as dose-limiting local reactions occurred in seronegative patients at 10^7 PFU/mL). The second T-VEC treatment is injected 3 weeks after the initial dose and subsequently administered every 2 weeks, at a concentration of 10^8 PFU/mL. After injection, injection sites

Table 13.1 T-VEC dosing schedule, including injection volumes based on lesion size (according to: Kevin J Harrington et al. [6])

Treatment visit	Dose concentration (PFU/mL)	Selection of lesions to be injected	Injection volume based on lesion size	
			Lesion size (longest diameter)	Injection volume
Initial	10^6 (one million)	Inject largest lesion(s) first	>5 cm >2.5–5 cm >1.5–2.5 cm >0.5–1.5 cm ≤0.5 cm	Up to 4 mL Up to 2 mL Up to 1 mL Up to 0.5 mL Up to 0.1 mL
		Prioritize injection of remaining lesions based on lesion size until maximum injection volume is reached		
Second	10^8 (100 million)	Inject any new lesions (lesions may have developed since initial treatment)		
		Prioritize injection of remaining lesions based on lesion size until maximum injection volume is reached		
Allsubsequentvisits	10^8 (100 million)	Inject any new lesions (lesions may have developed since initial treatment)		
		Prioritize injection of remaining lesions based on lesion size until maximum injection volume is reached		

PFU plaque-forming units

should be covered with occlusive dressings for at least 1 week, to prevent (potential) viral transmission. Treatment should be continued for a minimum of 6 months if effective, or until complete (pathologically confirmed) remission of lesions [6].

Treatment with T-VEC injections is usually well tolerated. Reported adverse events (AEs) include chills, fatigue, influenza-like illness, pyrexia, and inflammation at the injection site (Fig. 13.2). These AEs occur in the majority of patients, but their severity usually does not exceed grade 2 according to Common Terminology Criteria for Adverse Events (CTCAE). The most frequently reported

Fig. 13.2 Erasmus Medical Center case of in-transit melanoma patient treated with T-VEC: inflammation at the injection site

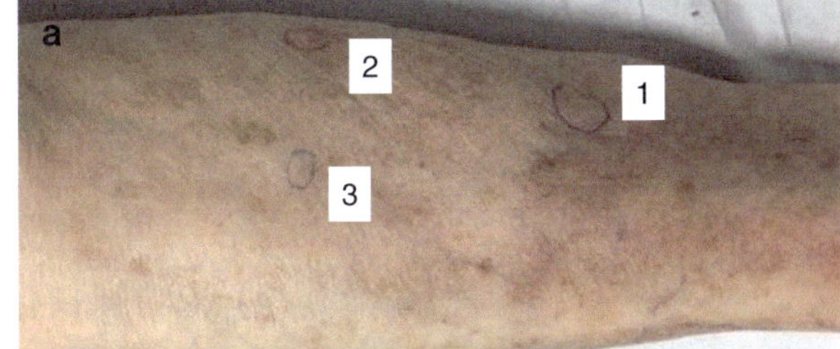

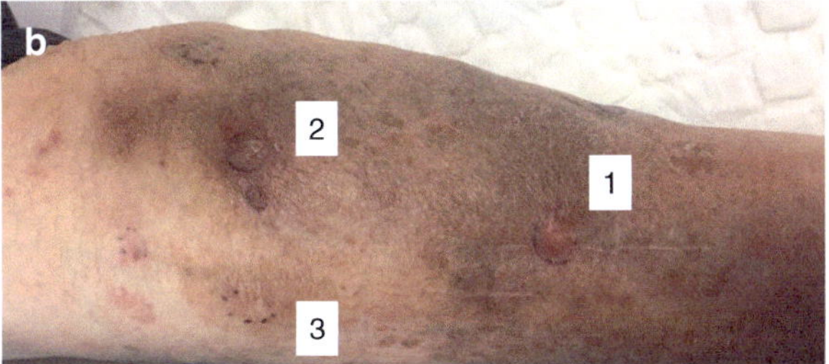

Fig. 13.3 Erasmus Medical Center patient after therapy with T-VEC: vitiligo

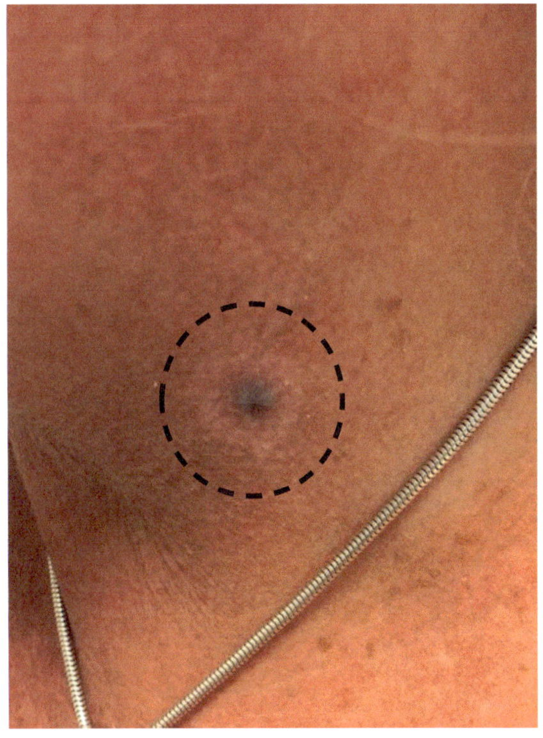

immune-related grade 1/2 AE is vitiligo (Fig. 13.3). Grade 3/4 AEs occur in the minority of patients (~10%), of which cellulitis is the most the most common complication and is observed in approximately 2% of patients [4].

Clinical Efficacy and Further Studies

Currently, T-VEC is administered at the outpatient clinic in dedicated melanoma centers across the world. After the clinical diagnosis of locoregional recurrence of melanoma, patients are here discussed within a multidisciplinary tumor board. Although the drug has only recently become available, the first reports evaluating the effectiveness of T-VEC in everyday clinical practice, have been published. Although these studies describe retrospective analyses of small groups of melanoma patients treated with T-VEC, the results are promising. The studies imply that the effectiveness of T-VEC is even higher than has been described during previous clinical trials (up to 40% response to treatment, most of them durable), with good tolerability and relatively low toxicity [7–11]. This suggests that proper selection of patients (by a multidisciplinary team) and treatment with T-VEC in experienced centers, validates this drug as a beneficial option for modern therapy of advanced melanoma. T-VEC has also been used in the setting of patients with a primary acral melanoma (Fig. 13.4) [12]. The mixed mechanism of action (the activity of replicable virus and alteration of the local immune response) ensures that the drug does not act only at the injection sites. After replication, the virus can infect surrounding tissues, resulting in regression of non-injected lesions. This applies to both superficial lesions and, to a lesser extent, visceral metastases. An attempt to assess this phenomenon was made by Howard L. Kaufman and colleagues, in a study published in 2016. The study included patients who were treated with T-VEC in a phase II trial ($N = 50$) who had both injected and uninjected lesions. In the case of directly injected nodules, the ORR was 67% (including 46% CRs). For non-injected superficial nodules (mainly metastases to the skin, subcutaneous tissue, and superficial lymph nodes) response was observed in 41% of cases (including 30% of complete responses). See Fig. 13.5 for an example from daily clinical practice. The study also included 12 patients with at least one visceral metastasis (most commonly located in the lungs and liver), with 32 visceral lesions in total. Remission of all visceral lesions was observed in 2 out of 12 patients (17%). Out of 32 visceral lesions, 4 lesions (13%) decreased in size, and 3 lesions (9%) completely disappeared [13].

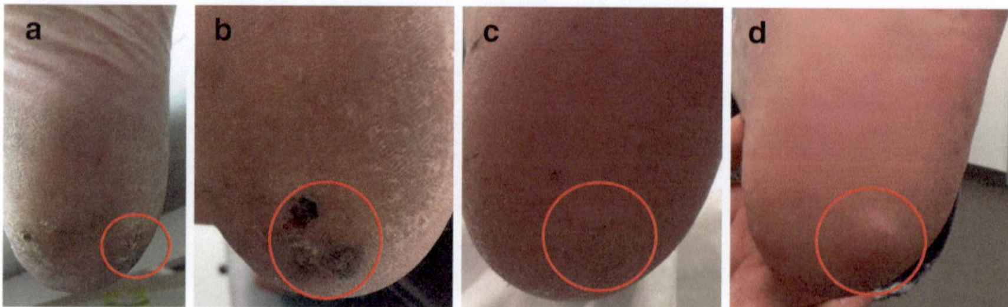

Fig. 13.4 Erasmus Medical Center case of patient treated with T-VEC due to acral melanoma

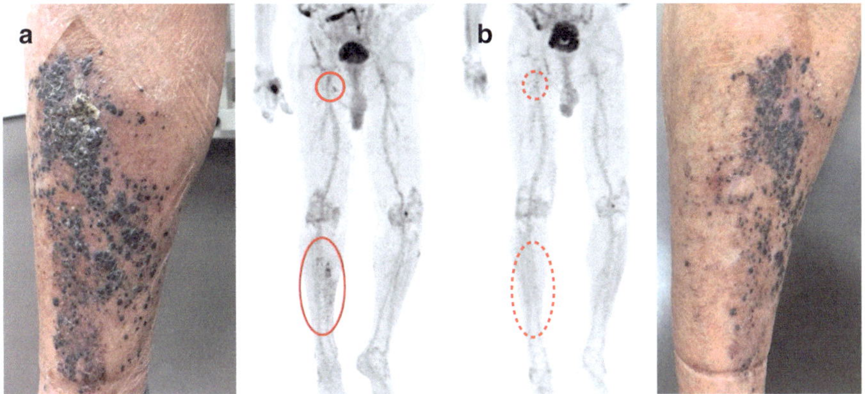

Fig. 13.5 T-VEC's success in (un)injected lesions

The development of systemic checkpoint inhibitors (CPIs), namely anti-CTLA-4 or anti-PD-1 and molecular-targeted therapy (BRAF/MEK-inhibitors) has significantly improved outcomes in advanced melanoma patients. Yet, patients can develop resistance to these systemic agents, which resulted in a search for alternative treatment strategies. It is believed that some of the failures of CPI treatment correspond to an insufficient cellular response within the tumor. T-VEC has the potential to reverse resistance to CPIs after melanoma relapse, by altering the local immune response [14]. In addition, T-VEC injection leads to an increased number of activated CD8+ tumor infiltrating lymphocytes and effector CD8+ T cells, which may improve the effectiveness of CPI treatment [15]. The oncolytic activity of the virus may be blocked by the expression of inhibitory receptors, including cytotoxic T-lymphocyte-associated protein 4 (CTLA-4) and programmed cell death protein 1 (PD-1). By blocking these receptors, the effectiveness of T-VEC may be increased [16]. Therefore, there are theoretical reasons for combining T-VEC with CPI. In 2016, the results of a phase I study evaluating the combination of Ipilimumab and T-VEC in patients with stage IIIb-IV unresectable melanoma ($N = 19$ patients) were published. For both drugs, standard dosing was used (i.e., 3 mg/kg for Ipilimumab, and up to 4 mL per T-VEC treatment). The safety profile of the combination was assessed as tolerable, however, it should be noted that grade 3 or 4 toxicity occurred in 26.3% of patients. Most side effects resulted from the use of Ipilimumab. The ORR in the study was 50%, with a DRR of 44% [17]. Due to the introduction to the clinical practice of the second generation of CPIs (anti PD-1, such as Pembrolizumab), with higher efficacy than ipilimumab and with a more favorable safety profile, studies on the combination of T-VEC and pembrolizumab are currently underway (NCT02263508, NCT04068181) [18]. The first trial to determine safety and tolerability (phase Ib) of the combination T-VEC with molecular-targeted therapy (dabrafenib/ trametinib) is being conducted at this moment.

Although still in its infancy, the effectiveness of T-VEC in the treatment of injectable locoregional melanoma may indicate a role in the neoadjuvant setting, or as an induction therapy of lesions not feasible for radical resection. Its use could lead to a reduction of unresectable lesions, and ultimately allow radical surgical treatment. The use of T-VEC in the neoadjuvant setting has already been evaluated. In 2019, at the European Society for Medical Oncology (ESMO) Annual Meeting, R. Dummer presented the results of the preoperative use of T-VEC in patients with injectable, potentially resectable, advanced melanoma. The control group consisted of patients who underwent surgery alone. A total of 150 patients participated in the study. Among patients receiving T-VEC, 29.5% remained free of relapse after 2 years, compared with 16.5% in the surgery group. In addition, $a \sim 10\%$ improvement in overall survival (OS) was observed after 2 years (88.9% and 77.4%, respectively, $p = 0.05$) [19].

The summary of trials reporting on the use of T-VEC for injectable lesions in monotherapy, neoadjuvant therapy, and in combination with systemic therapy is presented in Table 13.2.

The use of T-VEC in patients with an impaired immune system, e.g., patients with autoimmune disorders and/or e.g., organ transplant recipients receiving immunosuppressants, has not been evaluated in clinical trials, as these immuno-compromised patients were not included. Physicians are apprehensive for flare-up of autoimmune symptoms or (acute) transplant rejection in these immunocom-promised patients. Paradoxically, these patients have a higher risk of developing (skin) cancer, among which melanoma, and safe therapeutic options are urgently needed [20, 21]. The robustness of systemic immune response caused by T-VEC, and its effect on immunocompromised patients is still unknown. Successful experimental use of T-VEC has been described in two transplant patients (heart, kidney) who were diagnosed with locally advanced melanoma not eligible for PD-1 inhibitors [22, 23]. Although evidence is limited, the possibility of treatment with T-VEC in immunocompromised patients must not be denied in advance, but should be discussed within a multidisciplinary team, assessing the risks and benefits.

Table 13.2 Trials reporting on the use of T-VEC for injectable lesions; monotherapy, neoadjuvant therapy, and in combination with systemic therapy

	NCT number (status)	Phase	Study design
Monotherapy	N/A (Completed)	I	First administration of T-VEC in patients—a study of its safety, biodistribution and biological activity. Dose escalation study: 106 pfu/mL, 107 pfu/mL, 108 pfu/mL
	NCT02014441 (Completed)	II	Multicenter, single-arm trial to evaluate the biodistribution and shedding of T-VEC. Safety analysis by using blood and urine samples, and swabs from injected lesions, exterior of dressings, oral mucosa, and the anogenital area
	NCT00289016 (Completed)	II	Multicenter, open-label, single-arm trial to evaluate the efficacy, safety and immunogenicity of T-VEC
	NCT02366195 (Active, not recruiting)	II	Multicenter, open-label, single arm study to evaluate the correlation between ORR and baseline intratumoral CD8+ cell density in patients treated with T-VEC [TVEC-325]
	NCT00769704 (Completed)	III	Multicenter, open-label, randomized trial: patients were randomized (2:1) to receiving intratumoral T-VEC or subcutaneous recombinant GM-CSF [OPTiM]
Neoadjuvant	NCT02211131 (Active, not recruiting)	II	Multicenter, open-label, randomized trial assessing the efficacy and safety of T-VEC neoadjuvant plus surgery versus surgery alone
Combination therapy	NCT01740297 (Active, not recruiting)	Ib	Multicenter, open-label, randomized trial: patients were randomized to receive either T-VEC in combination with Ipilimumab compared to Ipilimumab alone
		II	
	NCT02263508 (Active, not recruiting)	Ib	Multicenter, open-label, randomized trial: patients were randomized to receive either T-VEC in combination with pembrolizumab compared to pembrolizumab alone [MASTERKEY-265/ KEYNOTE-034]
		III	
	NCT03088176 (Recruiting)	Ib	Open-label, single-arm study of T-VEC in combination with dabrafenib and trametinib in primary or recurrent BRAF mutant melanoma
	NCT04068181 (Recruiting)	II	Multicenter, open-label, single-arm study of T-VEC in combination with pembrolizumab [MASTERKEY-115]

(continued)

Table 13.2 (continued)

	Stages of melanoma	Number of melanoma subjects	Objectives and endpoints	Treatment-emergents AEs (usually grade 1–2)
Monotherapy	Refractory (sub)cutaneous metastases from malignant melanoma	$N = 9$	Safety and efficacy: • Well tolerated: local inflammation/erythema, flu-like symptoms • Tolerability improved with initial administration of 106 pfu/ml • ORR in 1 patient, SD in 2 patients	
	Unresectable, IIIB–IVM1c	$N = 60$	T-VEC can be administered safely to patients with advanced melanoma and is unlikely to be transmitted to close contacts with appropriate use of occlusive dressings.	• Chills (65%) • Fatigue (57%) • Nausea, headache (45%)
	Unresectable, IIIC–IV	$N = 50$	Efficacy and immunogenicity • ORR 26% (8 CR, 5 PR), after 2–12 months of treatment • Directly injected lesions: ORR 67% (46%CR) • Responses in 41% of uninjected lesions (subcutaneous, nodal and visceral), at a median of 23 (non-visceral) vs. 51 weeks (visceral)	Safety: • Fever (52%) • Chills (48%) • Fatigue (32%) • Nausea (30%)
	Unresectable, IIIB–IVM1c	$N = 112$	T-VEC increases CD8+ tumor-infiltrating lymphocytes, granzyme B+ effector CD8+ T cells, memory CD8+ T cells, and CD8+ T cells expressing checkpoint markers PD-1 and CTLA-4 but not macrophages	• Pyrexia (47%) • Chills (27%) • Influenza-like illness (25%)
	Unresectable, IIIB–IV	$N = 437$	Efficacy (T-VEC vs. GM-CSF): • Median OS 23.3 vs. 18.9 months [unstratified HR 0.79, $p = 0.0494$] • DRR 19.0% vs. 1.4% [unadjusted OR 16.6, $p <.0.0001$] • ORR 31.5% (16.9%CR) vs. 5.7% (0.7%CR), median time to CR was 8.6 months	T-VEC vs. GM-CSF • Fatigue (51% vs. 37%) • Chills (50% vs. 8%) • Pyrexia (40% vs. 11%) • Influenza-like illness (34% vs. 9%) • Nausea (34% vs. 21%) Among T-VEC-treated patients, AEs decreased over time to 10%, 8%, 8%, 5% and 7%, respectively.

Neoadjuvant	Resectable, IIIB–IVM1a	$N = 150$	Efficacy (neoadjuvant T-VEC plus surgery vs. surgery alone) • 2-year RFS: 29.5% vs. 16.5% [HR 0.75, $p = 0.07$] • 2-year OS 88.9% vs. 77.4% [HR 0.49, $p = 0.050$] • In T-VEC group: increased intratumoral CD8+ cell density [$p < 0.001$] and PD-L1 [$p \leq 0.05$]	Not assessed
Combination therapy	Unresectable, IIIB–IV	$N = 19$	Tolerability and efficacy: • No DLTs observed, 26.3% grade 3–4 toxicity • ORR: 50% ($N = 9$), DRR 44% ($N = 8$) • 18-months PFS: 50%, OS: 67% ($N = 12$)	
		$N = 198$	Efficacy (T-VEC + Ipilimumab vs. Ipilimumab alone): *NB No injectable lesions required* • ORR: 39% vs. 18% [OR 2.9, $p = 0.002$]. • Visceral response: 52% vs. 23%	T-VEC + Ipilimumab vs. Ipilimumab alone: • Fatigue (59% vs 42%) • Chills (53% vs 3%)) • Diarrhea (42% vs 35%) Incidence of grade ≥ 3 AEs was 45% and 35%, respectively.
	Unresectable, IIIB–IVM1c	$N = 21$	Tolerability and efficacy: • No DLTs observed, 33% ($N = 7$) grade 3–4 toxicity • ORR: 62% (7 CR, 6 PR), median time to response was 17 weeks	
		$N = 713$	Enrolling, estimated primary completion date: July 2022	
	Unresectable, IIIB–IVM1c	$N \approx 20$[a]	Enrolling, estimated primary completion date: June 2021	
	Unresectable/Metastatic IIIB–IVM1d (in patients who have progressed on prior anti-PD-1 based therapy)	$N \approx 100$[a]	Enrolling, estimated primary completion date: May 2021	

AEs adverse events, *CR* complete response[b], *DLTs* dose-limiting toxicities (treatment-related non-laboratory grade $\geq$4 AE, grade $\geq$4 immune-mediated dermatitis or endocrinopathy, and grade $\geq$3 immune-mediated AE of any other type), *DRR* durable response rate (objective response lasting $\geq$ 6 months). *GM-CSF* granulocyte-macrophage colony-stimulating factor, *HR* hazard ratio, *NCT* national clinical trial, *OS* overall survival, *OR* odds ratio, *ORR* objective response rate[b], *PFS* progression-free survival, *PR* partial response[b], *RFS* recurrence-free survival, *SD* stable disease[b], *T-VEC* talimogene laherparepvec

[a]Target number

[b]As measured by modified response evaluation criteria in solid tumors (RECIST) criteria, patients can have CR, PR, SD, or progressive disease

Summary

The use of intralesional T-VEC, a relatively new oncolytic virotherapy, in patients with unresectable locoregional melanoma is an effective and well-tolerated treatment. By adequately selecting patients who might benefit from T-VEC, as discussed within a multidisciplinary tumor board in experienced and dedicated melanoma centers, T-VEC's success rates are increasing. Although it is easy to administer, the use of T-VEC does present some (logistical) challenges for centers providing the treatment; the drug requires transport and storage in a deep-frozen state, and, despite changes in the regulatory environment regarding genetically modified organisms (GMOs), regulations are still stringent in some countries, as it is a live virus. Depending on respective national legislations, this may impose additional obligations on the treatment center, related to safety checks, training of personnel, etc. Nevertheless, monotherapy with T-VEC is currently one of the standard options for local treatment of locoregional recurrence of melanoma [24]. Early reports and interim results show that T-VEC in the neoadjuvant setting as well as in combination with systemic immunotherapy is promising. Further research and long-term treatment results are needed to determine the exact position of T-VEC in the overall treatment regimen for advanced melanoma.

References

1. Andtbacka RHI, Collichio FA, Amatruda T, Senzer NN, Chesney J, Delman KA, et al. OPTiM: a randomized phase III trial of talimogene laherparepvec (T-VEC) versus subcutaneous (SC) granulocyte-macrophage colony-stimulating factor (GM-CSF) for the treatment (tx) of unresected stage IIIB/C and IV melanoma. J Clin Oncol. 2013;31(18_suppl):LBA9008-LBA.
2. Kaufman HL, Andtbacka RHI, Collichio FA, Amatruda T, Senzer NN, Chesney J, et al. Primary overall survival (OS) from OPTiM, a randomized phase III trial of talimogene laherparepvec (T-VEC) versus subcutaneous (SC) granulocyte-macrophage colony-stimulating factor (GM-CSF) for the treatment (tx) of unresected stage IIIB/C and IV melanoma. J Clin Oncol. 2014;32(15_suppl):9008a-a.
3. Andtbacka RH, Kaufman HL, Collichio F, Amatruda T, Senzer N, Chesney J, et al. Talimogene laherparepvec improves durable response rate in patients with advanced melanoma. J Clin Oncol. 2015;33(25):2780–8.
4. Andtbacka RHI, Collichio F, Harrington KJ, Middleton MR, Downey G, hrling K, et al. Final analyses of OPTiM: a randomized phase III trial of talimogene laherparepvec versus granulocyte-macrophage colony-stimulating factor in unresectable stage III-IV melanoma. J Immunother Cancer. 2019;7(1):145.
5. Kaufman HL, Ruby CE, Hughes T, Slingluff CL Jr. Current status of granulocyte-macrophage colony-stimulating factor in the immunotherapy of melanoma. J Immunother Cancer. 2014;2:11.
6. Harrington KJ, Michielin O, Malvehy J, Pezzani Gruter I, Grove L, Frauchiger AL, et al. A practical guide to the handling and administration of talimogene laherparepvec in Europe. Onco Targets Ther. 2017;10:3867–80.
7. Franke V, Berger DMS, Klop WMC, van der Hiel B, van de Wiel BA, Ter Meulen S, et al. High response rates for T-VEC in early metastatic melanoma (stage IIIB/C-IVM1a). Int J Cancer. 2019;145(4):974–8.

8. Louie RJ, Perez MC, Jajja MR, Sun J, Collichio F, Delman KA, et al. Real-world outcomes of talimogene laherparepvec therapy: a multi-institutional experience. J Am Coll Surg. 2019;228(4):644–9.

9. Masoud SJ, Hu JB, Beasley GM, JHt S, Mosca PJ. Efficacy of talimogene laherparepvec (T-VEC) therapy in patients with in-transit melanoma metastasis decreases with increasing lesion size. Ann Surg Oncol. 2019;26(13):4633–41.

10. Mohr P, Haferkamp S, Pinter A, Weishaupt C, Huber MA, Downey G, et al. Real-world use of talimogene laherparepvec in German patients with stage IIIB to IVM1a melanoma: a retrospective chart review and physician survey. Adv Ther. 2019;36(1):101–17.

11. Perez MC, Zager JS, Amatruda T, Conry R, Ariyan C, Desai A, et al. Observational study of talimogene laherparepvec use for melanoma in clinical practice in the United States (COSMUS-1). Melanoma Manag. 2019;6(2):MMT19.

12. Franke V, Smeets PMG, van der Wal JE, van Akkooi ACJ. Complete response to talimogene laherparepvec in a primary acral lentiginous melanoma. Melanoma Res. 2020;30(6):548–51.

13. Kaufman HL, Amatruda T, Reid T, Gonzalez R, Glaspy J, Whitman E, et al. Systemic versus local responses in melanoma patients treated with talimogene laherparepvec from a multi-institutional phase II study. J Immunother Cancer. 2016;4:12.

14. Frohlich A, Niebel D, Fietz S, Egger E, Buchner A, Sirokay J, et al. Talimogene laherparepvec treatment to overcome loco-regional acquired resistance to immune checkpoint blockade in tumor stage IIIB-IV M1c melanoma patients. Cancer Immunol Immunother. 2020;69(5):759–69.

15. Ribas A, Dummer R, Puzanov I, VanderWalde A, Andtbacka RHI, Michielin O, et al. Oncolytic virotherapy promotes intratumoral T cell infiltration and improves anti-PD-1 immunotherapy. Cell. 2017;170(6):1109–19 e10.

16. Dummer R, Hoeller C, Gruter IP, Michielin O. Combining talimogene laherparepvec with immunotherapies in melanoma and other solid tumors. Cancer Immunol Immunother. 2017;66(6):683–95.

17. Puzanov I, Milhem MM, Minor D, Hamid O, Li A, Chen L, et al. Talimogene laherparepvec in combination with ipilimumab in previously untreated, unresectable stage IIIB-IV melanoma. J Clin Oncol. 2016;34(22):2619–26.

18. Chiu M, Armstrong EJL, Jennings V, Foo S, Crespo-Rodriguez E, Bozhanova G, et al. Combination therapy with oncolytic viruses and immune checkpoint inhibitors. Expert Opin Biol Ther. 2020;20(6):635–52.

19. Dummer R, Gyorki DE, Hyngstrom J, Berger A, Conry R, Demidov L, et al. Primary 2-year (yr) results of a phase II, multicenter, randomized, open-label trial of efficacy and safety for talimogene laherparepvec (T-VEC) neoadjuvant (neo) treatment (tx) plus surgery (surg) vs surg in patients (pts) with resectable stage IIIB-IVM1a melanoma. Ann Oncol. 2019;30(Supplement 5):v903.

20. Dahlke E, Murray CA, Kitchen J, Chan AW. Systematic review of melanoma incidence and prognosis in solid organ transplant recipients. Transplant Res. 2014;3:10.

21. Spain L, Higgins R, Gopalakrishnan K, Turajlic S, Gore M, Larkin J. Acute renal allograft rejection after immune checkpoint inhibitor therapy for metastatic melanoma. Ann Oncol. 2016;27(6):1135–7.

22. Ressler J, Silmbrod R, Stepan A, Tuchmann F, Cicha A, Uyanik-Unal K, et al. Talimogene laherparepvec (T-VEC) in advanced melanoma: complete response in a heart and kidney transplant patient. A case report. Br J Dermatol. 2019;181(1):186–9.

23. Schvartsman G, Perez K, Flynn JE, Myers JN, Tawbi H. Safe and effective administration of T-VEC in a patient with heart transplantation and recurrent locally advanced melanoma. J Immunother Cancer. 2017;5:45.

24. Trager MH, Geskin LJ, Saenger YM. Oncolytic viruses for the treatment of metastatic melanoma. Curr Treat Options in Oncol. 2020;21(4):26.

Part IV
Future of Melanoma Immunotherapy

Chapter 14
Perspectives of Immunotherapy in Advanced Melanoma: Combinations and Sequencing

A. M. Di Giacomo, Elisabetta Gambale, and Michele Maio

Immunotherapy: The Fourth Pillar of Cancer Treatment

Therapeutic intervention with monoclonal antibodies (mAb) that target immune checkpoint(s) inhibitors (ICI) is a novel and rapidly evolving anticancer strategy that is providing meaningful clinical efficacy in a proportion of cancer patients with different tumor histotypes [1]. The prototype approach of this therapeutic modality relies on the inhibition of negative signals delivered by cytotoxic T lymphocyte-associated protein (CTLA)-4 expressed on activated T lymphocytes. Ipilimumab, the first anti-CTLA-4 mAb approved by regulatory agencies, has profoundly changed the therapeutic landscape of patients with cutaneous metastatic melanoma (MM), significantly improving their survival. However, objective clinical responses with ipilimumab are limited, and only ~20% of patients achieve long-term disease control [2]. Since these initial results, an improved understanding of the molecular mechanisms regulating

A. M. Di Giacomo (✉) M. Maio
Department of Oncology, Center for Immuno-Oncology, Medical Oncology and Immunotherapy, University Hospital of Siena, Siena, Italy

NIBIT Foundation Onlus, Genova, Italy

University of Siena, Siena, Italy
e-mail: a.m.digiacomo@ao-siena.toscana.it

E. Gambale
Department of Oncology, Center for Immuno-Oncology, Medical Oncology and Immunotherapy, University Hospital of Siena, Siena, Italy

University of Siena, Siena, Italy
e-mail: elisabetta.gambale@ao-siena.toscana.it

P. Rutkowski, M. Mandalà (eds.), *New Therapies in Advanced Cutaneous Malignancies*, https://doi.org/10.1007/978-3-030-64009-5_14

host's immune response to tumor has led to the expansion of the repertoire of checkpoint signaling pathways; among these, one of the most crucial is the programmed cell death-1 (PD-1) pathway.

Immunomodulatory mAb against PD-1, like nivolumab and pembrolizumab, have significantly increased the survival of MM, with ~40% of subjects achieving a long-term survival [3]. However, despite these unprecedented results, a significant proportion of MM patients fail to respond to ICI therapy either upfront (primary resistance) or after an initial benefit (acquired/secondary resistance) [1]. Therefore, identifying new mechanism(s) underlying treatment failure and designing novel therapeutic combinations and/or sequences to overcome primary and acquired resistance are mandatory to improve the overall efficacy of ICI therapy.

Resistance to ICI Therapy and Rationale for PD-1-Based Combinations

First-line therapy with anti-PD-1 mAb nivolumab and pembrolizumab has significantly improved the survival of MM patients [3]. Unfortunately, 40–65% of MM patients treated with anti-PD-1 mAb develop a primary or acquired resistance to PD-1 therapy. The mechanisms leading to resistance to PD-1 inhibition can occur at any phase of the cancer immunity cycle, are multifactorial, and can be overlapping in an individual patient. Among others they can include (1) alterations in the antigen-processing pathway; (2) lack of tumor antigen expression; (3) loss of Human Leukocyte Antigen (HLA) expression; and (4) constitutive expression by tumor cells of the ligands for Immune Checkpoints (IC) [e.g., PD-1 ligand (PD-L1)]. Besides these mechanisms, neoplastic cells can utilize immune-evasive strategies to prevent T-cell trafficking and infiltration into tumors, including overexpression of vascular endothelial growth factor (VEGF) that downregulates T-cell adhesion to the endothelium, and upregulation of endothelin B receptor, controlling T-cell trafficking through the tumor and lymph nodes. Additionally, the expression of a specific subset of genes, called the innate anti-PD-1 resistance signature or IPRES, has been identified as a mechanism of primary resistance. IPRES is associated with the transition of melanoma cells to a mesenchymal subtype, a reversion back to a more stem cell-like phenotype [4]. Upregulation of these genes may be produced by inflammation in the tumor microenvironment (TME), driving increased tumor plasticity, and angiogenesis. Other factors driving resistance to PD-1 therapy are tumor cell extrinsic and involve the TME [4]. Indeed, the migration of immunosuppressive cells into the TME can inhibit local immune cells from exerting their effector functions. Furthermore, increased numbers of regulatory T cells (Treg) and of myeloid-derived suppressor cells (MDSC), mediated by indoleamine 2,3-dioxygenase (IDO) that is expressed in a wide range of human cancers, have all been linked to primary resistance to immunotherapy. The expression of IC (including PD-1 and CTLA-4) at the surface of these immune suppressive cells provides them with the ability to inhibit local T-cell activation directly. Additionally, immunosuppressive mediators produced by Treg and MDSC, including Interleukin (IL)-10 and Transforming Growth Factor (TGF)-β, can enhance the establishment of a local network of immunosuppressive cells in the TME. For instance, TGF-β can induce differentiation of neutrophils into a pro-tumor, "N2-like" phenotype, thereby limiting the anticancer activity of N1-like neutrophils. Similarly, IL-10 and TGF-β can polarize monocytes to protumor M2-like tumor-associated macrophages (TAM), which, among their immune-suppressive actions, can also fight with local dendritic cells (DCs) for tumor antigens and consequently inhibit T-cell priming [4].

Most of the factors responsible of primary resistance drive also the occurrence of acquired immune escape. In this regard, truncating mutations in JAK 1 and 2 were recently shown to result in a lack of responsiveness to Interferon (IFN)-γ in tumor cells and consequently in a secondary resistance to ICI [4]. Alterations of JAK1 and JAK2 were also found to correlate with tumor relapse, providing initial evidence that acquired resistance to ICI therapy may involve substantial alteration and evolution of cancer cells and immune cells in the TME [4]. Furthermore, the loss of beta-2-microglobulin (B2M) expression observed in melanoma cell lines from patients treated with immunotherapy, resulted in a loss of Major Histocompatibility Complex (MHC) class I expression, and thus in a subsequent decrease in recognition by CD8+ T cells [4]. Notably, other immune IC pathways, such as lymphocyte activation gene 3 (LAG-3) and T-cell immunoglobulin and mucin domain 3 (TIM-3), have also been revealed to interfere with the effector activity of T cells, resulting in acquired resistance to immunotherapy (Table 14.1) [4].

Table 14.1 Mechanisms of resistance to ICI therapy

Phase of immunity cancer cycle	Mechanisms of resistance	Contributing factors
Antigen presentation and T-cell activation	Insufficient antigen presentation and recognition	Low tumor mutational burden Lack of neoantigen recognition Loss of B2M Loss of MHC class I Loss of function of transporters associated with antigen-processing (TAP) proteins
T-cell trafficking and tumor infiltration	Absence of T cells from TME	VEGF overexpression Upregulation of endothelin B receptor
T-cell killing activity within TME	Presence of immunosuppressive molecules within the TME	Expression of IPRES Induction of IDO Upregulation of PD-L1 Upregulation of Tregs Upregulation of MDSCs Upregulation of immune-checkpoint markers (LAG-3, TIM-3)

TME tumor microenvironment, *B2M* beta-2-microglobulin, *MHC* major histocompatibility complex, *VEGF* vascular endothelial growth factor, *IDO* indoleamine 2,3-dioxygenase, *IPRES* innate anti-PD-1 resistance signature, *Tregs,* regulatory T cells, *MDSCs* myeloid-derived suppressor cells, *LAG-3* lymphocyte activation gene 3, *TIM-3* T-cell immunoglobulin and mucin domain 3

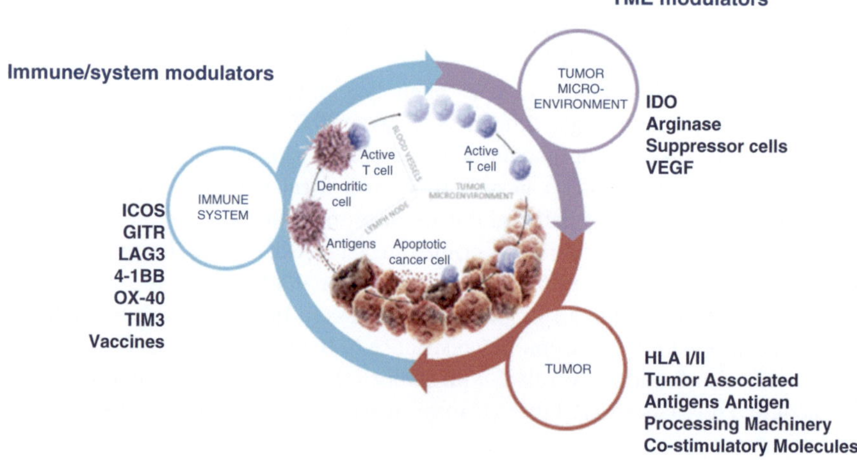

Fig. 14.1 The future of immunotherapy: targeting and modulating multiple compartments. The initiation of a successful antitumor immune response requires (1) effective antigen presentation and T-cell activation, (2) T-cell trafficking and tumor infiltration, and (3) T-cell killing activity within the tumor microenvironment. The mechanisms triggering both primary and acquired resistance to PD-1 inhibition can happen at any phase of cancer immunity cycle. Potential therapeutic strategies targeting immune system, tumor, and TME can be utilized at each stage of the cancer immune cycle to overcome immunotherapy resistance. *ICOS* inducible T-cell co-stimulatory, *GITR* glucocorticoid-induced TNFR family-related gene, *LAG-3* lymphocyte activation gene 3, *TIM-3* T-cell immunoglobulin and mucin domain 3, *IDO* indoleamine 2,3-dioxygenase, *VEGF* vascular endothelial growth factor, *HLA* human leukocyte antigen

All these recent insights into the mechanisms of ICI resistance support the investigation into novel combination strategies, using multiple treatment modalities such as new IC agonist/antagonists, TME modulators, targeted agents, and epigenetic drugs (Fig. 14.1; Table 14.2).

Combinations or Sequencing with Anti-CTLA-4 mAbs

The rational to combine an anti-CTLA-4 and an anti-PD-1/PD-L1 mAb stems from their non-redundant functional activity, acting at different sites and at different stages of T-cell activation: CTLA-4 on naïve T cells typically in the lymph nodes; PD-1 on antigen-experienced T cells, primarily in peripheral tissues [5]. From preclinical experiences to early-phase studies, combination therapy has shown to be more effective than monotherapy in terms of melanoma control by increasing T-cell infiltration and the presence of effector T cells in the TME; also INF-γ and other pro-inflammatory cytokines were upregulated in the course of combination therapy,

Table 14.2 Selected immunotherapy combination trials in melanoma[a]

Trial number	Trial name	Status
Dual monoclonal antibody therapies		
NCT02599402 (CheckMate 401)	Nivolumab Combined with Ipilimumab Followed by Nivolumab Monotherapy as First-Line Treatment for Patients with Advanced Melanoma	Active, not recruiting
NCT03470922	A Study of Relatlimab Plus Nivolumab Versus Nivolumab Alone in Participants with Advanced Melanoma	Recruiting
Anti-PD-1 in combination with oncolytic viral therapy		
NCT04068181 (Masterkey-115)	Talimogene Laherparepvec with Pembrolizumab in Melanoma Following Progression on Prior Anti-PD-1 Based Therapy	Recruiting
Anti-PD-1/PD-L1 in combination with BRAF and MEK inhibitors		
NCT02224781	Dabrafenib and Trametinib Followed by Ipilimumab and Nivolumab or Ipilimumab and Nivolumab Followed by Dabrafenib and Trametinib in Treating Patients with Stage III–IV BRAFV600 Melanoma	Recruiting
NCT03625141 (TRICOTEL)	A Study Evaluating the Safety and Efficacy of Cobimetinib Plus Atezolizumab in BRAFV600 Wild-Type Melanoma with Central Nervous System Metastases and Cobimetinib Plus Atezolizumab and Vemurafenib in BRAFV600 Mutation-Positive Melanoma with Central Nervous System Metastases	Recruiting
Anti-PD-1 in combination with co-stimulatory molecules and cytokines		
NCT02253992	An Investigational Immuno-therapy Study to Determine the Safety of Urelumab Given in Combination with Nivolumab in Solid Tumors and B-Cell Non-Hodgkin's Lymphoma	Completed
NCT02528357 (ENGAGE-1)	GSK3174998 Alone or with Pembrolizumab in Subjects with Advanced Solid Tumors	Completed
NCT02554812 (JAVELIN Medley)	A Study of Avelumab In Combination with Other Cancer Immunotherapies in Advanced Malignancies	Recruiting
NCT02723955 (INDUCE-1)	Dose Escalation and Expansion Study of GSK3359609 in Participants with Selected Advanced Solid Tumors	Recruiting
NCT02983045 (PIVOT-02)	A Dose Escalation and Cohort Expansion Study of NKTR-214 in Combination with Nivolumab and Other Anti-Cancer Therapies in Patients with Select Advanced Solid Tumors	Active, not recruiting
NCT03635983	A Study of NKTR-214 Combined with Nivolumab vs Nivolumab Alone in Participants with Previously Untreated Inoperable or Metastatic Melanoma	Recruiting
Immune-checkpoint inhibitors and TME modulators		
NCT03589651	INCMGA00012 in Combination with Other Therapies in Patients with Advanced Solid Tumors	Recruiting
NCT03459222	An Investigational Study of Immunotherapy Combinations in Participants with Solid Cancers That Are Advanced or Have Spread	Recruiting

(continued)

Table 14.2 (continued)

Trial number	Trial name	Status
NCT02903914	Arginase Inhibitor INCB001158 as a Single Agent and in Combination with Immune Checkpoint Therapy in Patients with Advanced/Metastatic Solid Tumors	Recruiting
Epigenetic-based combinations		
NCT04250246 (NIBIT-ML1)	A Study of NIVO Plus IPI and Guadecitabine or NIVO Plus IPI in Melanoma and NSCLC Resistant to Anti-PD1/PDL1	Not yet recruiting
NCT02437136 (ENCORE-601)	Ph1b/2 Dose-Escalation Study of Entinostat with Pembrolizumab in NSCLC with Expansion Cohorts in NSCLC, Melanoma, and Colorectal Cancer	Active, not recruiting

TME tumor microenvironment, *NSCLC* non-small cell lung cancer
[a]As of Jul 26, 2020. Source: clinicaltrials.gov

with the creation of an inflammatory rather than immunosuppressive TME. Furthermore, blockade of both molecules supports the expansion of tumor-infiltrating CD8(+) T cells; however, at variance with PD-1 blockade, CTLA-4 targeting triggers a powerful CD4(+) effector T-cell response via the expansion of an Inducible T-cell co-stimulator (ICOS) + T helper (Th)1-like CD4 subset, therefore sustaining long-term antitumor immune responses [5]. All these lines of evidence suggested that combination therapies may act in a complementary or even synergistic fashion, and this hypothesis was confirmed by the higher response rates and improved survival of cancer patients treated with the combination of PD-1 and CTLA-4 blockers [6]. More in detail, the combination of nivolumab and ipilimumab has been investigated as sequential and combination approaches in MM, in several clinical trials.

In the phase II CheckMate 064 study, patients with unresectable stage III or IV MM were randomized to receive a sequential induction treatment with nivolumab followed by ipilimumab (Cohort A) or ipilimumab followed by nivolumab (Cohort B). Following induction treatment, both cohorts received nivolumab until progression or unacceptable toxicity. Objective Response Rate (ORR) at week 25 was higher in the nivolumab–ipilimumab group vs the ipilimumab–nivolumab group (41.2% vs 20%), with a lower progression rate (38.2% vs 60%). Notably, the group receiving nivolumab followed by ipilimumab exhibited a greater 12-month overall survival rate compared with the group treated with ipilimumab followed by nivolumab (76%; 95% CI 64–85 vs 54%; 42–65). Treatment-related grade 3–4 Adverse Events (AEs) occurred in 50.0% in the nivolumab–ipilimumab group and in 42.9% in the ipilimumab–nivolumab group [7]. Given the similar results in terms of clinical outcomes and toxicity, sequential treatment does not appear to offer any significant improvement over concurrent combination therapy. However, it should be noted that the study design was not optimal, with a different time interval between sequential treatments (2 weeks for Cohort A and 3 weeks for Cohort B), thus not answering the question of the optimal sequence [7].

In the phase III, randomized CheckMate 067 study, 945 treatment-naïve cutaneous and mucosal melanoma MM patients were randomly assigned 1:1:1 to receive ipilimumab (3 mg/kg), nivolumab (1 mg/kg), or ipilimumab *plus* nivolumab (3 mg/ kg + 1 mg/kg). The long-term follow-up of the study has shown a median overall survival (OS) of more than 60.0 months in the nivolumab *plus* ipilimumab group, 36.9 months in the nivolumab group, and 19.9 months in the ipilimumab group. Overall survival at 5 years was 52% in the nivolumab *plus* ipilimumab group and 44% in the nivolumab group, as compared with 26% in the ipilimumab group. Median progression-free survival (PFS) was 11.5 months (95% CI, 8.7–19.3) for nivolumab *plus* ipilimumab, 6.9 months (95% CI, 5.1–10.2) for nivolumab, and 2.9 months (95% CI, 2.8–3.2) in the ipilimumab arm. Progression-free survival rate at 5 years was 36% in the nivolumab *plus* ipilimumab group, 29% in the nivolumab group, and 8% in the ipilimumab group. The rate of objective response among treated patients was 58% in the nivolumab *plus* ipilimumab group, 45% in the nivolumab group, and 19% in the ipilimumab group. The median duration of response had not been reached in the nivolumab *plus* ipilimumab and nivolumab groups and was 14.4 months in the ipilimumab group, with ongoing responses at 5 years in 62%, 61%, and 40% of the patients with a response, in nivolumab *plus* ipilimumab, nivolumab, and ipilimumab groups, respectively. The duration of response was sustained across stratification subgroups (according to BRAF muta- tion status, PD-L1 status, and metastasis stage). These long-term data clearly showed that patients with MM treated with nivolumab, delivered either as mono- therapy or in combination with ipilimumab, continued to show superior OS, PFS, and response rates compared with those on ipilimumab. Combination therapy was more toxic with grade 3 or worse AEs in 59% of patients, compared with 21% for nivolumab and 28% for ipilimumab; however, managing patients with established safety guidelines, AEs usually resolved within 3–4 weeks. Notably, the 5-year sur- vival rate was similar between patients who discontinued nivolumab *plus* ipilim- umab due to treatment-related adverse events and the overall population [8]. These data suggest that combined treatment elicited higher rates of toxicity than either monotherapies, but that benefit from dual therapy was conferred even despite dis- continuation of treatment.

A separate consideration deserves mucosal melanoma. Although objective response rate was lower than in the overall population, limited short-term data indicated clinical benefit with nivolumab *plus* ipilimumab, nivolumab, and ipili- mumab in patients with mucosal melanoma [9]. In detail, a pooled analysis, that included also data from CheckMate 067, reported, among mucosal melanoma patients who received nivolumab monotherapy, a median PFS of 3.0 months (95% CI, 2.2–5.4 months, with ORR of 23.3% (95% CI, 14.8%–33.6%). Median PFS in patients treated with nivolumab combined with ipilimumab was 5.9 months (95% CI, 2.8 months to not reached), with ORR of 37.1% (95% CI, 21.5%–55.1%). The incidence of grade 3 or 4 treatment-related adverse events was 8.1% for nivolumab monotherapy and 40.0% for combination therapy [9]. Thus, nivolumab combined with ipilimumab seemed to have greater efficacy than either agent alone also in mucosal melanoma and, although the activity was lower than in cutaneous melanoma, the safety profile was similar between the two subtypes. The 5-year outcomes of mucosal melanoma patients treated in CheckMate 067 were also recently reported, confirming that patients with mucosal melanoma treated with nivolumab *plus* ipilimumab have more favorable survival outcomes than those treated with nivolumab or ipilimumab alone. However, the 5-year analysis showed that patients with mucosal melanoma in the CheckMate 067 had poorer long-term efficacy vs ITT [10].

In order to define the optimal dosage of the combination of ipilimumab *plus* nivolumab, clinical trials have explored a lower dose of ipilimumab that would possibly have lower toxicity rates. Regarding this evidence, the phase IIIb/IV CheckMate 511 study has investigated the combination of nivolumab 3 mg/kg *plus* ipilimumab 1 mg/kg. In part 1 of the study, MM patients received either nivolumab 3 mg/kg *plus* ipilimumab 1 mg/kg (NIVO3 + IPI1) or nivolumab 1 mg/kg *plus* ipilimumab 3 mg/kg (NIVO1 + IPI3) once every 3 weeks for four doses [11]. Patients who discontinued combination therapy as a result of toxicity did not enter the maintenance phase (part 2 of the study) in which nivolumab was administered at a flat dose of 480 mg once every 4 weeks until disease progression or unacceptable toxicity. At a minimum follow-up of 12 months, incidence of treatment-related grade 3–5 AEs was 34% with NIVO3 + IPI1 versus 48% with NIVO1 + IPI3 ($P = 0.006$). In descriptive analyses, ORR was 45.6% in the NIVO3 + IPI1 group and 50.6% in the NIVO1 + IPI3 group, with complete responses in 15.0% and 13.5% of patients, respectively. Median PFS was 9.9 months in the NIVO3 + IPI1 group and 8.9 months in the NIVO1 + IPI3 group. Median OS was not reached in either group [11]. The CheckMate 511 study met its primary end point, demonstrating a significantly lower incidence of treatment-related grade 3–5 AEs with NIVO3 + IPI1 versus NIVO1 + IPI3. Descriptive analyses showed that there were no significant differences between the groups for any efficacy end point, even if a longer follow-up may help to better characterize clinical efficacy outcomes [11].

Based on these results, the combination of ipilimumab and nivolumab is an effective strategy in MM, though the identification of the right patient, dosage, and duration of treatment remains a challenge.

Role of ICI Combination in Brain Metastases

Although melanoma brain metastases are the third-most common origin of metastases to the brain after lung and breast cancers, melanoma shows the highest level of cerebral tropism of all cancer types. Brain metastases affect 25% of patients at diagnosis of advanced melanoma, and up to 75% of melanoma patients have brain metastases at the time of death [12]. In light of this evidence, the American Joint Committee on Cancer (AJCC) has acknowledged the negative impact of brain metastases on the prognosis of patients with MM in its latest eighth edition staging system, by defining this subgroup as M1d. Moreover, until recently, most of the systemic chemotherapeutic agents had limited activity on brain metastases, due to their acknowledged limitation to effectively cross the blood–brain barrier (BBB). In light of this notion and of their association with a poorer prognosis, patients with brain metastases were generally excluded from clinical trials with chemotherapeutic agents in the past, and also from the initial studies with ICI. Nevertheless, in the last years, the better comprehension of the interactions between the immune system and the TME in brain metastases has led to recognize the TME of brain metastases as one of the most important factors responsible for response or resistance to treatment. TME is the environment around a tumor and it is composed of neoplastic and non-neoplastic cells (i.e., endothelial cells, pericytes, fibroblasts, and immune cells) [13]. It was reported that the alteration in the pericyte subpopulation in brain metastases causes a remodeling of the BBB favoring a great infiltration of multiple immune suppressive cell types from the peripheral circulation, thus contributing to resistance to therapy. Additionally, it was shown that brain-metastasizing melanoma cells can promote astrocytes to express the pro-inflammatory cytokine IL-23, which induces the production of matrix metalloproteinase-2 (MMP-2) that enhances the degradation of the extracellular matrix, thus promoting the extravasation and consequent spreading of tumor cells in the brain [13]. Moreover, the recruitment of type 2 TAM, MDSC, T-reg, and cancer-associated fibroblasts (CAF), with their pro-tumorigenic features, reduced the expression of co-stimulatory molecules (i.e., CD80, CD86, CD40) involved in T-cell activation, resulting thereby in an impairment of antigen presentation, and deregulation of the homeostasis of the brain microenvironment [13]. In this highly immune-suppressive TME, tumor-infiltrating lymphocytes (TIL) are poorly represented and functionally impaired. About this latter evidence, different studies reported a downregulation of T-cell activity in brain metastases, resulting from tumor-induced T-cell exhaustion. Indeed, PD-1 expression was detected on >60% of TIL, although the correlation with clinical outcomes has yet to be fully understood. In light of this evidence and based on the upcoming clinical results, the use of immunotherapeutic agents should be encouraged also in patients with brain metastases [13].

The initial clinical evidence of ICI activity used in combination with other therapeutic agents in MBM was generated in the Italian Network for Tumor Biotherapy (NIBIT)-M1 study [14]. In this phase II trial, 86 patients with MM were assigned to receive ipilimumab at 10 mg/kg combined with fotemustine; among the 20 patients who had asymptomatic brain metastases at study enrollment, the immune-related Disease Control Rate (ir-DCR) was 50%, as compared with 46.5% in the whole population. Notably, the 3-year survival rate was 27.8% in patients with brain metastases and 28.5% in the whole population, suggesting for a long-term clinical benefit also in patients with asymptomatic brain metastases [15]. A more recent follow-up of this study has shown that 5 complete regressions of brain disease were obtained, with a duration of brain complete response (CR) of 16, 28, 39, 80+, 94+ months; notably, the 2 patients still alive, in the absence of subsequent treatment, had achieved a CR both intra- and extra-cranial [13]. In light of these intriguing clinical data and of available results showing the therapeutic efficacy of ipilimumab combined with nivolumab in melanoma, the multicenter, phase III, randomized, open-label NIBIT-M2 study (NCT02460068), sponsored by the NIBIT Foundation, was activated. This three-arm study was designed to assess the OS of previously untreated metastatic melanoma patients with asymptomatic brain metastases who received fotemustine, its combination with ipilimumab, or the combination of ipilimumab and nivolumab. In this study, 76 patients with active, untreated, and asymptomatic brain metastases were randomly assigned to ARM A (fotemustine), ARM B (ipilimumab *plus* fotemustine), or ARM C (nivolumab *plus* ipilimumab). With a median follow-up of 39 months, median OS was 8.5 months for ARM A, 8.2 months for ARM B, and 29.2 months for ARM C. The ir-ORR was 0%, 19.2%, and 44.4% in ARMs A, B, and C, respectively [16].

Other two studies have recently investigated the dual blockade of CTLA-4 and PD-1 molecules in MBM. The phase II, single-arm, CheckMate 204 study enrolled patients into two cohorts: those with asymptomatic brain metastases (cohort A) and those with neurologic symptoms (cohort B). In both cohorts, patients received nivolumab (1 mg/Kg) *plus* ipilimumab (3 mg/Kg) every 3 weeks for up to four doses, followed by nivolumab (3 mg/kg) every 2 weeks until progression of unacceptable toxic effects. Among the 94 asymptomatic enrolled patients, the intracranial and extracranial ORR were 55% and 50%, respectively, with a global ORR of 51%, and with 90% ongoing objective responses at a relatively short median duration of follow-up of 14 months [17]. An updated analysis of cohort A (with a follow-up of 20.6 months) reported an intracranial and extracranial ORR of 54% and 49%, respectively, with a global ORR of 51%, among the 101 evaluable patients; the 18-month survival rate was 75%. In cohort B, at a median follow-up of 5.2 months, intracranial ORR was 16.7%, with a 6-month survival rate of 66%. The safety profile of the regimen was similar to that reported in patients with melanoma who do not have brain metastases [18].

In line with these results are those from the Australian Brain Collaboration (ABC) study, a phase II, prospective trial enrolling 3 cohorts of patients with asymptomatic or symptomatic brain metastases. Patients with no prior local brain treatment were randomized to receive nivolumab 1 mg/kg *plus* ipilimumab 3 mg/kg followed by nivolumab 3 mg/kg (Cohort A) or nivolumab 3 mg/kg (Cohort B), whereas patients with brain metastases progressed after local therapy, or who had neurological symptoms or leptomeningeal spreading disease were enrolled in non-randomized cohort C (nivolumab 3 mg/kg). At a median follow-up of 17 months, the intracranial ORR was 46%, 20%, and 6% in Cohorts A, B, and C, respectively, with complete intracranial response in 17%, 12%, and 0% patients in each cohort. Among patients enrolled in Cohort A, those with treatment-naïve brain disease achieved a 56% ORR while it was 16% in BRAF mutant patients pretreated with BRAF and MEK inhibitors [19]. In a more recent analysis with a median follow-up of 34 months, the intracranial ORR in Cohorts A, B, and C were 51%, 20%, and 6%, respectively, with complete intracranial response in 26%,16%, and 0% patients in each cohort. The 24-month intracranial PFS rate was 49% in Cohort A, 15% in Cohort B, and 6% in Cohort C, with a 24-month survival rate of 63%, 51%, and 19% in Cohorts A, B, and C, respectively [20]. Consistent with the safety results from CheckMate 204 study, treatment-related grade 3/4 adverse events in Cohorts A, B, and C were 54%, 20%, and 13%, respectively, with no treatment-related deaths [19]. Altogether, these results supported the safety and tolerability of nivolumab utilized alone or in combination with ipilimumab in MM patients with brain metastases.

Notably, a recent systematic literature review and meta-analysis suggested that combined immunotherapy increased long-term OS and PFS of MM patients with brain metastases, compared with anti-PD1 mAb monotherapy or targeted therapy [21]. Taken together, consistent with those reported in extracranial disease, available data show a considerable efficacy and with a good safety profile of combination therapy with CTLA-4 *plus* PD-1 in melanoma patients with brain metastases, that should now represent the standard of care in this clinical setting. Furthermore, several ongoing clinical trials are exploring novel combinations also with radiotherapy in this subset of melanoma patients.

Combinations with Other ICI

The increasing knowledge about inhibitory molecules whose mechanisms may act within the TME has led to the development of new therapeutic agents that could have complementary functions to those of approved immunotherapeutic agents. Currently, multiple clinical trials are underway examining the activity and safety of combined immunotherapies, in particular using an anti-PD-1 mAb in combination with agents that target novel emerging checkpoints. Among these, ICI directed at lymphocyte-activation gene 3 (LAG-3), a cell surface molecule expressed on Teff and Tregs, are among the most deeply investigated. At least 60 clinical trials are presently ongoing targeting LAG-3 both alone and in combination with other immune checkpoints, in melanoma and other different tumor types. Specifically, LAG-3 is an additional immune checkpoint pathway known primarily to be expressed on exhausted T cells which have less potent effector functions [22]. It may downregulate T-cell responses via interaction with MHC-II on DC. As result of continuous melanoma antigen expression, LAG-3 expression on T cells is increased, thereby inhibiting T-cell action and reducing IFN-γ production within the TME under the influence of PD-1 co-stimulation [22]. Moreover, in vivo studies in murine cancer models have shown that when expressed at high levels, concomitant LAG-3/PD-1 expression is mostly restricted to infiltrating TILs [23]. This may indicate that a combined immunotherapy targeting LAG-3 and PD-1 may elicit tumor-specific responses, avoiding nonspecific or self-antigen-specific immune responses, possibly improving safety profile as compared with PD-1 and CTLA-4 blockade combination. Indeed, preclinical evidence, suggesting that LAG-3 has a synergistic activity with anti-CTLA-4 or anti-PD-1 mAbs, is driving its clinical development [24]. Immuno-modulating mAbs targeting LAG-3 is being tested in several clinical trials, and new combinations of anti-LAG-3 and anti-PD-1 mAbs have shown encouraging activity in fighting PD-1 resistance. In detail, preliminary results from the ongoing phase 1/2a study which is testing the combination ofanti-LAG-3 mAb relatlimab with nivolumab (NCT01968109) have shown encouraging initial clinical activity in patients who were refractory to a previous anti-PD-1/PD-L1 therapy. Furthermore, this combination showed a good safety profile, comparable with nivolumab monotherapy, with uncommon grade 3/4 AEs. Moreover, the combination therapy can increase objective response rates from 5% to 18% in patients with LAG-3-positive tumors [25]. In light of these results, the ongoing phase 2/3 CA224-047 (NCT03470922) clinical trial will hopefully assess efficacy and safety of relatlimab with nivolumab versus nivolumab monotherapy as first-line treatment in advanced melanoma.

Additionally, TIM-3, a co-inhibitory receptor expressed on T cells, has both inhibitory and activating properties. It induces T-cell apoptosis, anergy, and exhaustion through the interaction with galectin-9 on immune cells [26]. Since TIM-3 has been established as an exhaustion marker in cancer, it can represent an interesting immunotherapy target. The combination of TIM-3/PD-1 blockade led to superior tumor regression than single-agent PD-1 blockade in murine cancer models and the combination of anti-TIM-3 plus anti-PD-1 mAbs is currently being investigated in phase I/II trials (NCT02817633, NCT02608268) [26].

B7–H3 (CD276) is a receptor of the CD28 (a co-stimulatory molecule) and B7 (a co-inhibitory molecule) family molecules found on Antigen-Presenting Cells (APCs). B7–H3 has found to be over-expressed in melanoma, favoring tumor growth and conferring resistance to apoptosis induction [26]. Enoblituzumab, a first in class mAb targeting B7–H3, has been tested in phase I trials in combination with pembrolizumab in refractory cancers (NCT02475213) and also with ipilimumab (NCT02381314) [26]. Final results of these studies are awaited.

V-domain Ig suppressor of T-cell activation (VISTA) is a PD-L1 homolog and a co-inhibitory receptor of the B7 family, expressed primarily within the hematopoietic compartment (MDSCs, TAMs, and DCs) and on leukocytes such as naïve T cells. VISTA may contribute to the suppression of effector T-cell (T-eff) responses and T-reg induction via interaction with its ligand V-Set and immunoglobulin domain containing 3 (VSIG-3). VSIG-3 can inhibit T-cell function and, in the presence of T-Cell Receptor (TCR) signaling, it may impair T-cell proliferation via the VSIG-3/VISTA pathway. Preclinical experience has indicated that VISTA blockade with a monoclonal antibody (13F3) enhanced effector T-cell response within the TME through the production of cytokines such as IFN-y and TNF-alpha. Concurrent blockade of VISTA and PD-1 checkpoints is emerging as a therapeutic option, therefore the small oral molecule antagonist CA-170 electively targets PD-L1/2 and VISTA has been investigated in a phase Idose escalation trial (NCT02812875) in advanced hematologic and solid tumors, with acceptable safety [26].

Combinations with Oncolytic Viral Therapy

Oncolytic virus therapy is an antitumor approach that utilizes native or genetically modified viruses that selectively replicate within cancer cells. Even if its mechanism of action is not completely understood, oncolytic viruses seem to mediate anticancer activity through the combination of two distinct mechanisms of action: a direct cancer cell lysis resulting from the selective viral replication within neoplastic cells and indirect induction of systemic antitumor immune response [27]. Moreover, immunosuppressive TME, such as in melanoma, is ideal for viral replication. Upon infection with an oncolytic virus, cancer cells initiate an antiviral response that leads to the upregulation of reactive oxygen species (ROS) and the initiation of antiviral cytokine production. ROS and cytokines, specifically type I IFNs, are released from the infected cancer cell and stimulate immune cells [i.e., APCs, CD8(+) T cells, and natural killer (NK) cells] [27]. Subsequently, the virus causes oncolysis, that triggers the release of viral progeny, pathogen-associated molecular patterns (PAMPs), danger-associated molecular pattern signals (DAMPs), and tumor-associated antigens (TAAs), including neo-antigens [27]. The release of viral progeny propagates the infection with the oncolytic virus, but, on the other hand, the PAMPs (consisting of viral particles) and DAMPs (comprising host cell proteins) stimulate the immune system by triggering activating receptors such as Toll-like receptors (TLRs). In the context of the resulting immune-stimulatory environment, TAAs and neo-antigens are released recognized by APCs. Altogether, these events result in the activation of immune responses against virally infected cancer cells, as well as de novo immune responses against TAAs/neo-antigens displayed on un-infected cancer cells [27].

Talimogene laherparepvec (T-VEC) is a herpes simplex virus type 1 derived oncolytic immunotherapy [28]. Preclinical studies have shown that T-VEC elicits antitumor activity by selectively replicating within cancer cells and thereby destroying them, as well as through the release of TAAs and the production of granulocyte-macrophage colony-stimulating factor (GM-CSF), which enhances antitumor immune response.

T-VEC was approved in the United States in 2015 for the local treatment of unresectable MM with cutaneous, subcutaneous, and nodal recurrent lesions, based on data from the phase III, open-label, randomized OPTiM, trial [25]. In this study, intratumoral administration of T-VEC was compared with subcutaneous administration of GM-CSF in patients with stage IIIB–IVM1 melanoma. Overall response rates were 31.5% and 6.4%, with a median OS of 23.3 and 18.9 months (hazard ratio 0.79; $p = 0.0494$) for T-VEC and GM-CSF, respectively. With grade 3–4 events in less than 2% of the 436 treated patients, the durable response rate (>6 months) was higher with T-VEC (19%) than GM-CSF (1.4%). Talimogene laherparepvec efficacy was more marked in stage IIIB–IVM1a melanoma [28].

Moreover, in the OPTiM study T-VEC has considerable local immune activity, with intralesional administration resulting in responses (regression ≥50%) in 64% of injected lesions. A 50% reduction in tumor size was also seen in 34% of non-injected, non-visceral lesions and in 15% of visceral lesions, indicating that T-VEC also induces systemic antitumor immunity and response. While activity was observed at distant metastases, it has been hypothesized that combining T-VEC with other systemic immunotherapies may further enhance the activity of both agents. It has been also shown that TVEC contributes to anti-PD1 mAb activity by augmenting the inflammatory state of the TME, which results in the increased homing and activation of tumor-reactive T cells [29]. Promoting the influx of T cells into the tumor is extremely important for patients with low intratumoral TILs, thus limiting response to PD-1 blockade [29]. Indeed, intratumoral administration of single-agent T-VEC resulted in increased levels of circulating and tumor-infiltrating T cells [29]. In light of this evidence, the complementary mechanism of action of talimogene supports its use in combination with different immunomodulatory agents within clinical trials.

Along this line, T-VEC was evaluated in combination with pembrolizumab in the phase Ib part of the MASTERKEY-265 clinical trial [30]. Pembrolizumab was administered intravenously at 200 mg every 2 weeks, after the third dose of T-VEC [30]. This sequential treatment was associated with a confirmed ORR of 57% and a confirmed CR rate of 24% [30]. In a follow-up efficacy analysis after a median follow-up of 38.6 months, ORR was 67% with a CR rate increased to 43% [31]. As previously reported, an increase in circulating cytotoxic T cells as well as an upregulation of PD-1 on these cells was observed after T-VEC monotherapy administration, suggesting a priming effect of T-VEC on the immune response during the subsequent pembrolizumab therapy [30]. Additional data from the MASTERKEY-265 clinical trial might confirm the role of this strategy in advanced melanoma. Furthermore, clinical studies combining T-VEC with BRAF and MEK inhibitors in BRAF-mutated advanced melanoma (NCT03088176), or with pembrolizumab, following progression on prior anti-PD-1-based therapy (NCT04068181) are recruiting. Finally, a trial of T-VEC with or without radiotherapy (NCT02819843) is currently ongoing, and T-VEC will be also tested in neoadjuvant setting in combination with nivolumab for resectable early metastatic (stage IIIB/C/D–IV M1a) melanoma with injectable disease (NIVEC) (NCT04330430).

Combinations with BRAF and MEK Inhibitors

BRAF and MEK inhibitors as well as ICI have significantly improved treatment outcomes of patients with BRAF-mutant melanoma. Although BRAF and MEK inhibitors are associated with a higher ORR as compared with immunotherapy, acquired resistance results in relapse within months, with a median progression-free survival of 11.5 months [32]. However, preclinical and translational data have shown that BRAF and MEK inhibition has an immune-modulating effect, augmenting antitumor immunity [32]. For instance, BRAF inhibition alone (vemurafenib) or BRAF+MEK inhibition (dabrafenib+trametinib) are associated with increased tumor infiltration by CD8(+) lymphocytes and consequently with tumor shrinkage and increased necrosis in posttreatment biopsies [32]. Furthermore, BRAF inhibition or BRAF+MEK inhibition are correlated with an enhanced expression of melanoma antigens at least in the first weeks after treatment initiation. Moreover, a decrease in immunosuppressive cytokines like IL-6 and IL-8 and an increase in markers of T-cell cytotoxicity were observed [32]. Intriguingly, BRAF V600E mutation downregulates the expression of IFN-α-receptor-1 (IFNAR-1), while BRAF inhibition upregulates the expression of most of the HLA class I antigen-processing machinery components, enhancing thereby the recognition of melanoma cells by relative T cells.

Regarding the potential overlapping efficacy from combined BRAF and immune checkpoint inhibitor, evidences from patients treated with BRAF inhibitors showed increased expression PD-1 and its ligand, PD-L1, suggesting potential benefit from this combinatorial approach. Of note, some preclinical experiences have also reported the efficacy of the triple combination therapy with dabrafenib, trametinib, and anti-PD1 in increasing the expression of melanoma antigens and MHC, as well as of the global immune-related gene upregulation in tumors with BRAF V600E mutation. Interestingly, the amount of circulating MDSCs, which repress antitumor immunity, decreased in response to vemurafenib [32].

Taken together, these findings support a combinatorial approach in BRAF-mutated melanoma by the testing of triple combination of BRAF and MEK inhibitors with immunotherapy. Notably, the combination of the BRAF inhibitor vemurafenib and the anti-CTLA-4 ipilimumab was associated with an unacceptable rate of grade 3–4 hepatitis, which led to subsequent discontinuation of the phase I study [33]. Similarly, a phase I trial with dabrafenib and ipilimumab was prematurely closed due to the occurrence of severe colitis in three patients [34]. In contrast, early-phase studies have shown promising anti-melanoma activity and manageable safety profile with combinations of BRAF-inhibitors, MEK-inhibitors, and anti-PD-1 leading thereby to develop phase II and III clinical trials [35].

In detail, Keynote-022 study is a double-blind, randomized, phase II study, comparing the efficacy of pembrolizumab *plus* dabrafenib and trametinib with dabrafenib and trametinib *plus* placebo, in patients with BRAF V600 E/K mutant melanoma. Initial results at a 9-month follow-up demonstrated improved PFS in the triplet group, 16.0 months, compared with 10.3 months in the doublet group (hazard ratio, 0.66; $P = 0.043$) without reaching statistical significance [32]. A more recent analysis (with a follow-up of 24 months) reported a median PFS of 16.9 (95% CI, 11.3–27.9) months with pembrolizumab and 10.7 (95% CI, 7.2–16.8) months with placebo (hazard ratio, 0.53; 95% CI, 0.34–0.83), with a survival rate at 24 months of 63.0% and 51.7% with pembrolizumab and placebo, respectively [36]. Of note, the combination of dabrafenib, trametinib, and pembrolizumab has led to higher rates of grade 3/4 AEs than would be expected for targeted therapy alone. Indeed, grade 3/4 treatment-related AEs occurred in 58.3% of patients in the triplet group and 26.7% in the doublet group. The most common adverse events were pyrexia, increased transaminase level, and rash. One patient receiving triplet therapy died of pneumonitis [35].

The COMBI-i phase III trial investigating dabrafenib, trametinib, and the anti-PD-1 agent PDR001 in patients with advanced BRAF V600 mutant melanoma has yielded encouraging preliminary results. Indeed, a first analysis, with a median follow-up of 15.2 months, of part 1 and part 2 reported a DCR of 94% and a CR rate of 33% [37]. The full results of these trials are eagerly awaited.

Furthermore, IMspire150 is a randomized, double-blind, phase 3 study testing the efficacy of atezolizumab *plus* vemurafenib and cobimetinib compared with vemurafenib and cobimetinib *plus* placebo, in previously untreated BRAFV600E/K mutant advanced melanoma patients. The primary endpoint PFS was significantly prolonged with atezolizumab compared with placebo (15.1 vs 10.6 months; hazard ratio 0.78; p = 0–025), while overall response rates in the atezolizumab (66%) and control groups (65%) were similar. Moreover, the prevalence of treatment-related grade 3 or 4 AEs was 182 (79%) of 230 in the atezolizumab arm and 205 (73%) of 281 in the placebo arm [38].

All these data suggest that the combination of anti-PD-1 mAb with BRAF and MEK inhibitors as first-line therapy in patients with advanced BRAFV600-mutant melanoma induced durable response with an encouraging PFS. Although triplet therapy led to a higher incidence of grade 3/4 treatment-related adverse events, most resolved with treatment interruption or dose reduction. In light of these results, the Food and Drug Administration (FDA) has recently approved the combination of atezolizumab with cobimetinib and vemurafenib for patients with BRAF V600 mutation-positive unresectable or MM.

However, the role of the triple combination of PD-1/PD-L1 *plus* BRAF and MEK inhibitors in the rapidly evolving melanoma treatment scenario will have to be established, mainly due to the increasing use of combined CTLA-4–PD-1 therapy. Ongoing trials [i.e., Immuno-CobiVem (NCT02902029), SECOMBIT (NCT02631447), DREAMseq (NCT02224781), and part 3 of COMBI-i)] will certainly advise the better therapeutic algorithm with regard to optimal combination or sequencing for the first-line treatment of BRAF-mutated MM [38].

Combinations with Co-stimulatory Molecules and Cytokines

T-cell activation is controlled by two sets of signals mediated by TCR and T-cell co-signaling receptors. Positive (co-stimulatory) and negative (co-inhibitory) signals from T-cell co-signaling receptors regulated T-cell function in response to TCR stimulation. Several studies have shown that activating T-cell co-stimulatory receptors, such as OX40, CD137 (4-1BB), and ICOS, can enhance T cell-mediated antitumor immunity. Thus, they emerged as novel targets for immunotherapeutic strategies.

CD137 and OX40 are members of the tumor necrosis factor receptors (TNFR) super family, expressed on T and NK cell surface and they act through a complex interplay of cytolytic T lymphocytes, helper T cells, regulatory T cells, dendritic cells, and vascular endothelium in tumors. Their stimulation promotes a high antitumoral immunity in a variety of murine tumor models. Furthermore, preclinical evidence suggests that combining agonist mAbs specific for TNFR members with conventional cancer therapies or additional immunotherapeutic agents may be particularly effective. Indeed, T-cell responses elicited by tumor antigens released through immunogenic tumor cell death are enhanced by these immunostimulatory agonist mAbs. Combinations with other immunomodulatory mAbs such as CTLA-4 and PD-1 are under investigation and seem to be promising [39].

More in detail, the clinical development of the anti-CD137 mAb urelumab started in 2005. Urelumab was evaluated as a monotherapy in two studies, CA186-001 (NCT00309023) and CA186-006 (NCT00612664). In December 2008, urelumab development program was put on hold due to the occurrence of two hepatotoxicity-related deaths. Subsequent detailed analysis of the clinical safety data showed that urelumab dose was the most important factor contributing to the development of the reported severe immune-related liver inflammation. Thus, in February 2012, the urelumab clinical development program was restarted with CA186-011 study (NCT01471210) to investigate monotherapy doses <1 mg/kg and it has been established that the optimal dosage seems to be 0.1 mg/kg every 3 weeks. Afterwards, a clinical trial was conducted that combined urelumab at this dose with nivolumab (NCT02253992) and its results are awaited [40].

In addition, early-phase clinical trials evaluating agonist antibodies targeting the OX40 pathway alone or in combination with ICI in cancer patients are ongoing. Among these, ENGAGE-1 (NCT02528357) is testing the combination of OX40 agonist mAb and pembrolizumab, JAVELIN Medley (NCT02554812) is investigating the combination of OX40 agonist mAb and avelumab, while INDUCE-1 study is testing the combination of OX40 agonist mAb and an anti-ICOS receptor agonist mAb (NCT02723955).

ICOS is a member of the CD28 superfamily that is expressed on activated T cells and regulates a lot of T-cell functions, including effector T-cell activation, interactions with B cells, and Treg infiltration. Additionally, preclinical work reports that an ICOS agonistic aptamer enhances the efficacy of anti-CTLA-4 therapy against melanoma in vivo. Thus, ICOS agonist mAbs are currently tested in early-phase clinical trials alone and in combination with ICI, in solid tumors [41].

Lastly, cytokines are soluble proteins acting as strong but complex mediators of immune activation. Due to the discovery of their potent antitumor activities in animal models, some of the earliest immunotherapeutic strategies have involved exogenous administration of interferon and IL-2. Both drugs exhibited only modest efficacy and produced significant toxicity, limiting their clinical value [42]. However, a renovated interest in the antitumor properties of cytokines has led to an exponential increase in the clinical studies that investigate the safety and efficacy of cytokine-based drugs, not only as monotherapy, but also in combination with other immunomodulatory drugs. These second-generation drugs under clinical development include known molecules with novel mechanisms of action, new targets, and fusion proteins that increase half-life and target cytokine activity to the TME or to the expected effector immune cells [42]. They could represent key molecules to overcome primary and acquired resistance mechanisms to anti-PD(L)-1 immunotherapies in light of their power to expand and reactivate effector NK and T lymphocytes, and promote tumor infiltration by lymphocytes, as well as due to their persistence in the TME. In this scenario, cytokines are being investigated in combination with other immunotherapeutic agents, mainly with anti-PD-1 and anti-PD-L1 mAbs.

We here report initial data about ICOS agonists and, among second-generation IL-2, about bempegaldesleukin (NKTR-214), a pegylated (PEG)-IL-2 designed to improve safety profile as recently reported in the phase I/II trial PIVOT-02 [43].

ICOS Agonists

In light of the demonstrated efficacy of CTLA-4 and PD-1 antagonists in blocking inhibitory pathways, great interest surrounds the targeting of T-cell co-stimulatory molecules, such as ICOS. ICOS is a co-stimulatory immune checkpoint expressed on activated T cells. Its ligand, ICOSL, is widely expressed on APCs and somatic cells, including cancer cells in the TME. ICOS and ICOSL expression is linked to the release of cytokines, induced by activation of the immune response. ICOS and ICOSL binding promotes either antitumor T-cell responses when activated in Th1, CD4(+) and CD8(+) cells, or pro-tumor responses when triggered in Tregs. Thus, mAbs targeting this pathway are being tested for cancer immunotherapy [41]. In preclinical studies, ICOS agonistic mAbs enhance the efficacy of anti-CTLA-4. ICOS knockout mice do not respond well to anti-CTLA-4 indicating that ICOS signaling is required for successful antitumor responses, possibly mediated by effector T cells. Hence, concomitant CTLA-4 and ICOS stimulation had a superior antitumor effect in comparison with anti-CTLA-4 alone. Interestingly, ICOS (+) T cells were described to be increased posttreatment with ipilimumab and to correlate with clinical responses in terms of DCR and OS in MM patients. Thus, changes in the number of circulating ICOS(+), CD4(+), and CD8(+) T cells assessed at baseline and during treatment with ipilimumab may be considered as early biomarkers of clinical response [44]. Even though ICOS alone seems to be less active in comparison with other pathways targeted by immunotherapeutic agents, especially due to the predominance of CD4(+) Tregs, the combination of ICOS agonistic mAbs and anti-CTLA-4 or PD-1/PD-L1 mAbs might have the potential to generate robust synergistic effects [41, 44]. The first-in-human, INDUCE-1 trial (NCT02723955), is testing an ICOS agonist mAb administered alone (part 1) or in combination (chemotherapy or pembrolizumab or an anti-OX40 mAb or dostarlimab, a novel anti-PD-1, or dostarlimab plus an anti-TIM-3 mAb or a bifunctional fusion protein targeting TGF-β and PD-L1) (part 2) in patients with advanced solid tumors, including melanoma. The study has shown promising results in terms of tolerability, safety profile, and clinical activity. The most frequent treatment-related AEs were fatigue (15%), fever (8%), transaminitis (5%, representing also the most frequent grade 3–4 AE) and diarrhea (3%).One dose-limiting grade 3 pneumonitis occurred, no related deaths were reported [45]. Final analysis of the INDUCE trial and additional data from new ongoing clinical trials evaluating the combination with the anti-CTLA-4 mAb tremelimumab (e.g., NCT03693612) or with an anti-PD1 mAb (e.g., NCT04128696) will confirm the role of this strategy.

PEG-IL-2

IL-2 represents a key cytokine in promoting the expansion of NK cells and T lymphocytes [42].The administration of this cytokine at high doses is currently approved by the FDA for the treatment of metastatic Renal Cell Carcinoma (RCC) and MM [42]. However, the systemic administration of this cytokine at the recommended dose is associated with high-grade toxicity, which often includes grade 3 and 4 adverse events. Along this line, second-generation IL-2-based drugs, with improved pharmacokinetic and pharmacodynamic profiles, are being developed [42]. Improvement of the pharmacokinetic profile is achieved through covalent binding of IL-2 to Conjugating Polyethylene Glycol (PEG) molecules that increases the half-life in circulation. IL-2 is recognized by three types of receptor complex expressed on NK and T lymphocytes: low-, medium-, and high-affinity IL-2 receptor, that are highly expressed on Treg cells. Therefore, the high-affinity IL-2 receptor shifts IL-2 activity toward the expansion of Treg cells and reduces the bioavailability of the cytokine that can stimulate antitumor effector NK and T lymphocytes [42]. Several of the second-generation IL-2-based compounds, designed to avoid binding to the high-affinity IL-2 receptor, were tested within clinical trials. Among these, bempegaldesleukin (NKTR-214) is composed of a recombinant IL-2 and multiple molecules of PEG. Directed PEGylation generates an inactive cytokine with a long half-life in circulation; the PEG groups are progressively released, yielding IL-2 molecules with double or single PEGylation that can interact with the medium affinity- but not with the high-affinity IL-2 receptor [42]. Improvement of the pharmacodynamic properties is reached by using biotechnology modifications to reduce binding to the high-affinity IL-2 receptor, while maintaining binding to the medium-affinity IL-2 receptor to increase the amount of cytokine available to stimulate NK and T cells. NKTR-214 has undergone dose-escalation studies and has also been used in combination with nivolumab, with encouraging response rates in immunotherapy-naive melanoma, RCC or non-small-cell lung cancer (NSCLC) patients [43]. Indeed, results of the phase I/II PIVOT-02 (NCT02983045) study, that investigated NKTR-214 combined with nivolumab, are very promising, remarkably for treatment-naive melanoma patients, with a ORR and DCR of 63.6% and 90.9%, respectively, without signals of overlapping or unexpected toxicity [43]. Moreover, part 3 and part 4 of the PIVOT-02 trial have investigated the combination of NKTR-214 with nivolumab plus ipilimumab. Furthermore, an ongoing phase III study (NCT03635983) is testing the efficacy, safety, and tolerability of NKTR-214, when combined with nivolumab versus nivolumab given alone in patients with previously untreated unresectable or metastatic melanoma. NKTR-214 is also being evaluated in clinical trials in combination with pembrolizumab (NCT03138889). Final results of these trials are awaited.

ICI in Combinations with TME Modulators

Growing data are providing evidence that TME is critical for the efficacy of immunotherapy. TME consists of nonmalignant cells such as immune cells (e.g., myeloid cells, including macrophages, MDSC, DCs, and neutrophils), cells of mesenchymal origin (e.g., fibroblasts, myofibroblasts, mesenchymal stromal cells), and vascular cells (e.g., endothelial cells and pericytes) which create a tumor-promoting milieu, producing multiple factors including reactive oxygen species (ROS), cytokines (IL-10, TGF-β), PD-L1, as well as IDO and arginase [46].

IDO is an enzyme that often overexpresses in tumor, with special interest in immuno-oncology because of the immunosuppressive effects that result from its role in tryptophan catabolism [46].

An additional pathway that plays an important role in the regulation of immune cell reactivity is arginine metabolism, mediated by arginase and responsible for impairment of T-cell functions. Inhibition of also arginase could represent another target to improve the efficacy of cancer immunotherapy [47].

Finally, Toll-Like Receptors (TLRs) are a family of pattern-recognition receptors. They recognize molecules that are broadly shared by pathogens but distinguishable from host molecules, collectively referred to as PAMPs, thereby inducing potent innate and adaptative immune response. TLRs are widely expressed on TME immune cells, including monocytes, DCs, macrophages, etc. Activation of TLRs on DCs stimulates maturation of the APC, induction of inflammatory cytokines and the subsequent priming of naive T cells for adaptive immunity [48, 49]. In light of this evidence, the activation of TLRs is becoming an interesting target for cancer treatment. TLR agonists, administered intratumorally, due to the upregulation of IC genes including IDO-1, PD-L1, and CTLA-4 in injected and uninjected lesions, in combination with ICI, may suppress tumor growth and reshape the TME. Indeed, preclinical experiences have shown the ability of TLR agonists to increase the ratio of M1/M2 macrophages, T-cell clonality, and recruitment of CD8(+) T cells [48, 49]. We describe TLR9 agonists.

Combinations with IDO Inhibitors

IDO is expressed in tumor cells, T-regs, DCs, macrophages, and endothelial cells in the TME. It is an enzyme responsible for the degradation of tryptophan into kynurenine. Depletion of local tryptophan by IDO can induce naive CD4(+) T cells toward differentiation into Treg cells. In addition, IDO produces soluble factors (kynurenine and downstream metabolites) that bind and activate the aryl hydrocarbon receptor (AhR) that can induce Treg cell differentiation and can also induce DCs and macrophages toward an immunosuppressive phenotype [46]. This inducible counter-regulation is helpful when IDO is controlling dangerous inflammation or creating tolerance to apoptotic cells but is highly unfavorable when it is suppressing the immune system's attempted response against cancer [46]. In light of its function, blocking IDO emerged as a potential target to enhance immunity against cancer. Intriguingly, preclinical evidence in a melanoma mouse model reported IDO overexpression after treatment with anti-CTLA-4 and anti-PD-1 mAbs [46]. Moreover, IDO overexpression conferred resistance to anti-CTLA-4 and anti-PD-1 mAbs, promoting thereby tumor growth. This property was found to be reversible by combination treatment with anti-CTLA-4 and IDO inhibitors. Studies conducted in the B16.SIY melanoma mouse model have shown that combinations of CTLA-4 or PD-1/PD-L1 with IDO blockade restored both IL-2 production and CD8(+) T-cell proliferation within the TME, underlying the potential ability of a combinatorial targeting approach. Furthermore, overexpression of isoform 1 (IDO1) is associated with poor patient survival in several tumor types [46]. Despite these findings and the promising antitumor activity shown by the anti-PD-1 inhibitor/IDO inhibitor combination therapy in phase I/II trials, the results of the phase III study (ECHO-301) combining the IDO1-selective inhibitor epacadostat with pembrolizumab did not show improved PFS and OS, in comparison with pembrolizumab alone [50]. Unfortunately, these results have led to the stoppage of the ongoing phase III trials with IDO1 inhibitors in different tumor histotypes [50], despite this failure it should be considered with caution, first of all due to the uncertainty of the appropriate target inhibition. In this regard, no direct evidence exists about the degree of IDO1 inhibition within the tumor, and previous data suggested that a sufficient drug exposure may not have been reached at the dose tested in ECHO-301 [46]. Thus, the optimal dose of epacadostat in combination with a novel anti-PD-1 mAb (retifanlimab) continues to be explored in an ongoing clinical trial (NCT03589651). Furthermore, the evaluation of IDO1 expression was not an eligibility criterion and no subgroups of interest based on clinical features or biomarkers were identified [43]. In light of these limitations and given the potential of IDO1 to enhance immunologic function, it would be desirable to continue to design clinical trials combining an anti-PD-1 inhibitor *plus* IDO1 inhibitors, tailoring them for specific subset of melanoma patients.

TLR 9 Agonists

Among the TLR family, Toll-like receptor 9 (TLR 9) recognizes unmethylated cytosine–phosphate–guanine (CpG) dinucleotide motifs present in bacterial and viral deoxyribonucleic acid (DNA) and synthetic oligodeoxynucleotides and is expressed in endosomal compartments of DCs and B cells. Signaling mediated by TLR 9 triggers cytokine production and release, including interferon (IFN)-α and T helper 1 (Th1)-type cytokines, B-cell proliferation, and upregulation of co-stimulatory molecules. Accordingly, TLR 9 agonists are being widely investigated not only in the treatment of infectious diseases, allergy, asthma, but also in the treatment of cancer [48, 49]. Along this line, IMO-2125 is a synthetic phosphorothioate oligonucleotide that acts as a direct agonist of TLR 9 to stimulate the innate and adaptive immune systems. IMO-2125 induces high levels of IFN-α from DCs along with an array of endogenous cytokines and chemokines. IMO-2125 also induces B-cell proliferation and differentiation and it can activate TLR 9 on B cells and dendritic cells in the TME to initiate and potentiate a Th1-polarized local and systemic immune response when administered by intratumoral injection [48, 49]. In vivo studies in mouse models of colon carcinoma, lymphoma, and melanoma indicate that intratumoral IMO-2125 monotherapy has been shown to produce effects both in injected and uninjected lesions, including antitumor activity associated with an increase in infiltrating CD8(+) T cells, and durable and specific cytotoxic T-cell responses against tumor antigens. Intratumoral administration was more effective than subcutaneous administration. Although intratumoral delivery of pattern recognition receptor agonists like TLR 9 is an effective means of creating an adaptive antitumor immune response, this can still be attenuated by dampening mechanisms such as immunosuppressive tumor-infiltrating regulator T cells and anergic/exhausted tumor-infiltrating or peritumoral cytotoxic T cells [48, 49]. Therefore, combining a TLR 9 agonist with checkpoint inhibitors or other modulators of the immune response to enhance systemic immunity is a compelling strategy. In vivo studies in mouse models have indeed shown that the combination of intratumoral IMO-2125 with either an anti-CTLA-4 or anti-PD-1 antibody results in improved tumor control compared with either agent alone. Preliminary clinical experience is also promising as the combination of IMO-2125 with ipilimumab is well tolerated and shows encouraging clinical activity in the setting of PD-1 refractory melanoma [51]. In detail, clinical trials are currently evaluating IMO-2125 monotherapy or combination with ipilimumab, or pembrolizumab, in previously treated metastatic melanoma patients. A phase 1/2 clinical study in patients with advanced melanoma that is refractory to PD-1 inhibitors (NCT02644967) has investigated intratumoral IMO-2125 in combination with ipilimumab or pembrolizumab in melanoma. At the time of the first analysis, tilsotolimod with ipilimumab was well tolerated and associated with an ORR in 3 out of the 6 evaluable patients, including complete response lasting >21 months [51]. Interestingly, dendritic cell activation, type I interferon response, CD8(+) T-cell proliferation was also reported in responding patients [51]. In light of this evidence, it has been designed the ILLUMINATE 301 trial (NCT03445533), a randomized phase 3 multicenter, open-label study of intratumoral tilsotolimod (8 mg) in combination with ipilimumab (3 mg/kg) versus ipilimumab monotherapy in patients with advanced melanoma who progressed on or after anti-PD-1 therapy [52]. Results of these trials are highly expected.

Combinations with Arginase Inhibitors

Recent studies have also demonstrated that specific enzymes in the TME are able to inhibit the immune response by limiting amino acid availability. Among them, there are two arginase isoforms (ARG1 and ARG2) that catalyze degradation of semi-essential L-arginine to L-ornithine and urea. Besides their fundamental role in the hepatic urea cycle, arginases have been shown to impair T-cell functions [47]. ARG1 is a cytosolic protein, while ARG2 is mostly located in the mitochondria. High arginase levels, either ARG1 or ARG2, have been reported in several cancer types, including breast cancer, NSCLC, head and neck squamous cell carcinoma, RCC, colorectal cancer, skin cancer, and cervical cancer. Arginases are mainly produced by MDSCs that are widely represented in the TME, and the role of ARG1-expressing MDSCs in altering T-cell responses in cancer patients has been well established. Depletion of L-arginine from the microenvironment arrests T-cell cycle progression and inhibits IFN-γ production. Arginase activity also leads to the downregulation of the expression of MHC class II molecules essential for antigen presentation [47]. Inhibitors of arginine degradation are thus being studied as monotherapy or combination with ICI in an early-phase clinical trial (NCT02903914). In detail, this is an open-label phase 1 trial, which has evaluated INCB001158 as a single agent and in combination with pembrolizumab in patients with advanced/metastatic solid tumors, including melanoma. Patients have been enrolled into monotherapy or combination cohorts. Interestingly, this trial has enrolled melanoma patients resistant to anti-PD-1 therapy. Final results of this trial are awaited and might define the role of this combination also in metastatic melanoma treatment.

Epigenetic-Based Combinations

Epigenetic alterations play a crucial role in cancer development and progression. Pharmacologic reversion of such alterations is feasible, and "epigenetic drugs" have demonstrated significant immunomodulatory properties, thus representing a promising strategy to overcome ICI resistance. Both DNA methylation and posttranslational histone modifications have been described to regulate the expression of different molecules of the antigen-processing and presentation machinery (APM), and to impair cellular immunity by modulating Th1 chemokines and IFN-related genes [53].

In detail, epigenetic modifications require the activity of specific cellular enzymes to be generated and maintained: DNA methyl transferases (DNMT) for DNA methylation, and the opposite activities of histone acetyl transferases (HAT)/histone deacetylases (HDAC) and histone methyltransferases (HMT)/histone demethylases in determining the status of histone acetylation and methylation, respectively. Epigenetic gene regulation is finally delivered by the cooperation of promoter DNA methylation, histone deacetylation, and by specific patterns of histone methylation that trigger chromatin condensation leading to gene silencing [53].

Epigenetic alterations are well acknowledged to be used by tumor cells to impair their immunogenicity and immune recognition. The latter occurs through the downregulation, either direct or indirect, of the expression of key molecules required for the efficient interaction of cancer cells with the host's immune system. All steps of antigen processing and presentation, including suppression of TAA expression, generation of intratumor TAA heterogeneity, downregulation of TAP1/2 and chaperone molecules, reduced MHC expression, as well as reduced levels of accessory/co-stimulatory molecules and of surface-exposed stress-induced ligands can be affected by epigenetic silencing. These molecular events finally lead to an increased uptake and immunogenic presentation of tumor antigens by professional APCs, which is compulsory for the induction of antitumor T-cell immune responses [53].

It has also been reported that epigenetic alterations can modulate Th1-type chemokines and IFN-related genes and impair CD8(+) T-cell activation and proliferation and the cytolytic activity of human IFN-γ + T cells, which correlated with decreased antitumor responses and survival of patients with solid tumors [53].

In light of this evidence, different epigenetic drugs that can revert epigenetic modifications are developed and they are currently tested within clinical trials. Among these, the best known are DNMT inhibitors (DNMTi) and HDAC inhibitors (HDACi). However, second-generation DNMTi [e.g., guadecitabine (SGI-110)] has become more recently available, showing a higher in vivo stability and a better safety profile. The significant role of epigenetics in cancer immune escape provides a strong rationale for the use of epigenetic modifiers to improve immunologic targeting of cancer cells and to design novel clinical trials to improve immunotherapy efficacy and overcome ICI resistance. Combined treatment with the CTLA-4-blocking mAb and either first- or next-generation DNMTi5-aza-CdR or guadecitabine, respectively, significantly reduced the growth of poorly immunogenic syngeneic grafts of murine mammary carcinoma and of mesothelioma as compared to single agents [54]. Consistent with these data, combined treatment with the DNMTi 5-azacytidine, the HDACi entinostat, and ICI (anti-PD-1 and anti-CTLA-4 mAb) markedly improved survival and tumor regression in syngeneic mammary (i.e., 4T1) and colorectal (i.e., CT26) carcinoma mouse models [53].

Along this line, based on the preclinical evidence gained on the broad immunomodulatory activity of the DNA hypomethylating agents (DHAs), the proof-of-concept phase 1 NIBIT-M4 combination study has been designed to provide evidence to the immunologic and clinical activity of an epigenetic immune-sequencing strategy with CTLA-4 blockade combined with DHA in metastatic cutaneous melanoma [55].

Epigenetic Immune Remodeling: The NIBIT-M4 Study

The Investigator Initiated Trial (IIT) NIBIT-M4 is a phase Ib study, sponsored by the NIBIT Foundation, that has evaluated for the first time safety, clinical and immunobiologic activities of the epigenetic priming with the second-generation DHAs, guadecitabine, followed by CTLA-4 blockade with ipilimumab in melanoma patients. In detail, patients with unresectable stage III/IV melanoma received escalating doses of guadecitabine at 30, 45, or 60 mg/m^2/day subcutaneously on days 1–5 every 3 weeks, followed by ipilimumab 3 mg/kg intravenously on day 1 every 3 weeks, starting 1 week after guadecitabine, for four cycles. Primary endpoints were safety, tolerability, and Maximum Tolerated Dose (MTD) of treatment; secondary were ir-DCR, ir-ORR, OS, and PFS; exploratory endpoints included the pharmacokinetic profile of guadecitabine and decitabine at cycle 1, day 1, patient-wise genome-wide DNA methylation and RNA sequencing, and analysis of the tumor immune contexture, using neoplastic samples obtained by surgical removal at baseline, week 4, and week 12. Nineteen melanoma patients were treated; 84% had grade 3/4 adverse events, and neither dose-limiting toxicities nor overlapping toxicities were observed [55]. Treatment-related AEs of any grade were observed in 18

(95%) patients, and grade 3 or 4 events in 15 (79%) patients [55]. The most common treatment-related AEs of any grade were myelotoxicity in 17 (89%) patients, and ir-AEs in 12 (63%) patients. Myelotoxicity events were grade 3 or 4 in 79% of cases and were more frequent in patients treated with guadecitabine at 60 mg/m^2/day; no febrile neutropenia was observed. All ir-AEs were grade 1 or 2 and were most commonly skin or gastrointestinal toxicities. No DLTs were observed at any investigated dose of guadecitabine. Treatment-related AEs and ir-AEs were generally manageable and reversible as per protocol management guidelines [55].

The ir-ORR was 26% (95% CI, 10.1–51.4) and the ir-DCR was 42% (95% CI, 21.1–66.0). At a median follow-up of 26.3 months, median PFS was 5.6 months (95% CI, 4.5–6.6) and median OS was 26.2 months (95% CI, 3.5–48.9); 1- and 2-year OS rates were 80% (95% CI, 59.2–100.0) and 56% (95% CI, 29.0–83.0), respectively [54].

Genome-scale analysis of DNA methylation of tumor samples showed a wide demethylating effect of guadecitabine during therapy in comparison with pretreatment levels. RNA sequencing data analysis displayed that immune-related pathways were mainly activated by treatment; frequent activation of pathways related to T-cell function/activation indicated intratumoral enhancement of the T-cell compartment. Even if the relative contributions of guadecitabine and ipilimumab to this finding cannot be unequivocally established, CTLA-4 blockade possibly plays an active role due to its effect on T-cell function. In turn, upregulation of HLA class I molecules described on melanoma cells in the majority of investigated tumor samples supports their specified upregulation, formerly reported in vitro and in syngeneic mouse models with various DHAs, comprising guadecitabine [55].

Tumor contexture analysis has shown an increase in median values of CD8(+) and PD-1(+) T-cell densities in tumor core specimens at week 12, but not at week 4, compared with baseline, suggesting that longer exposure to guadecitabine and ipilimumab may be required to generate high levels of tumor-infiltrating CD8(+) T cells. Notably, median values of CD8(+) and PD-1(+) T-cell densities were higher in responding compared with non-responding [55].

The comprehensive results of the NIBIT-M4 study provide initial support to the efficacy of tumor remodeling by epigenetic drugs in metastatic disease and support the notion that DHA represents ideal "partner drug" to improve the therapeutic efficacy of immune-checkpoint blockade, including their foreseeable role in reverting primary resistance to treatment [55].

Epigenetic and ICI Combination in PD-1/PD-L1-Resistant Patients: The NIBIT-ML1 Study

The lack of adequate therapies for patients resistant to ICI therapy remains a critical unmet need in melanoma and NSCLC patients. Therefore, identifying mechanism(s) underlying treatment failure(s) and designing novel therapeutic approaches to overcome primary/secondary resistance are mandatory to improve the overall efficacy of anti-PD-1 therapy. We have firstly demonstrated the clinical and immunological activity of the combination of ipilimumab *plus* guadecitabine in the NIBIT-M4 study. These results provided a scientific rationale to develop novel immunotherapeutic approaches combining guadecitabine with ICI in patients with primary resistance to anti PD-1/PDL-1 therapy, even due to epigenetic drugs' potential role in reverting resistance to treatment. Along this line, we have hypothesized that priming the tumor with DHA might improve the therapeutic efficacy of CTLA-4 blockade combined with anti-PD-1 in patients with MM and NSCLC resistant to PD-1 treatment; therefore, the NIBIT-ML1 study was designed. The NIBIT-ML1(NCT04250246) is a randomized, phase II study designed according to a two-stage optimal design by Simon, in unresectable Stage III or Stage IV MM (Cohort A) or NSCLC (Cohort B) patients who failed therapy with anti-PD-1/PDL-1. Primary objective of the study was immune(i) ORR according to iRECIST criteria. Secondary objectives included safety, iDCR, PFS, median OS, and survival rate at 1 and 2 years. Exploratory endpoints will investigate immuno-biologic correlates. Following a safety run-in phase in 6 subjects *per* cohort, eligible patients will be randomized to receive guadecitabine *plus* ipilimumab and nivolumab (ARM A) or ipilimumab and nivolumab (ARM B). Sample size will range from 6 to 92 patients *per* cohort [56]. The first patient first visit is foreseen in August 2020.

Additionally, initial evidence of clinical activity of epigenetic drugs in combination with ICI was reported in patients with melanoma and NSCLC who have progressed following treatment with prior PD-1 and PDL-1 blockade. In detail, preliminary results of the ENCORE-601 (NCT02437136), open-label phase Ib/II study evaluating entinostat, a HDACi, (5 mg PO weekly) plus pembrolizumab (200 mg IV Q3W) in patients with unresectable or metastatic melanoma, NSCLC, and colorectal cancer who have progressed to prior PD-1 blockade, CTLA-4 blockade, showed significant clinical activity and acceptable safety profile [57]. The confirmed objective response rate with entinostat plus pembrolizumab was 19%, while grade 3/4 related AEs occurring in >5% of patients included neutropenia, fatigue, and hyponatremia. Five patients (9%) experienced a grade 3/4 immune-related AEs (2 events of rash, 1 each of colitis, pneumonitis, and immune-related hepatitis) [57].

Results from these ongoing clinical trials might define the role of an epigenetic-based immune combination to overcome resistance to anti-PD-1 blockade in melanoma and NSCLC.

Conclusions

The last decade has witnessed a dramatic shift in the care of cancer patients from a focus on cytotoxic therapies toward approaches that enhance antitumor immunity through IC targeting. Immunotherapy with ICI has significantly extended the survival of cancer patients, though a proportion of patients do not achieve durable disease control yet. Therefore, identifying novel mechanism(s) underlying treatment failure(s) and designing new IC-based combinations/sequences to overcome primary/secondary resistance are mandatory to achieve the full potential of cancer immunotherapy. Along this line, given the complexity of the immune activation and the considerable variability in tumor biology across patients and tumor types, the identification of biomarkers to warrant patient selection needs to be further explored.

In summary, combined immunotherapies have undoubtedly shown significant clinical results in cancer patients, but efforts are required to identify the optimal combinations, dosages, and timing of therapy. Ongoing clinical trials will hopefully shed light on the treatment paradigm with regard to the ideal combination and sequencing of immunotherapeutic strategies.

References

1. Topalian SL. Targeting immune checkpoints in cancer therapy. JAMA. 2017;318(17):1647–8. https://doi.org/10.1001/jama.2017.14155.
2. Hodi FS, O'Day SJ, McDermott DF, et al. Improved survival with ipilimumab in patients with metastatic melanoma [published correction appears in N Engl J Med. 2010 Sep 23;363(13):1290]. N Engl J Med. 2010;363(8):711–23. https://doi.org/10.1056/NEJMoa1003466.
3. Larkin J, Minor D, D'Angelo S, et al. Overall survival in patients with advanced melanoma who received nivolumab versus investigator's choice chemotherapy in CheckMate 037: a randomized, controlled, open-label phase III trial. J Clin Oncol. 2018;36(4):383–90. https://doi.org/10.1200/JCO.2016.71.8023.
4. Gide TN, Wilmott JS, Scolyer RA, et al. Primary and acquired resistance to immune checkpoint inhibitors in metastatic melanoma. Clin Cancer Res. 2018;24(6):1260–70. https://doi.org/10.1158/1078-0432.CCR-17-2267.
5. Wei SC, Levine JH, Cogdill AP, et al. Distinct cellular mechanisms underlie anti-CTLA-4 and anti-PD-1 checkpoint blockade. Cell. 2017;170(6):1120–1133.e17. https://doi.org/10.1016/j.cell.2017.07.024.
6. Rotte A. Combination of CTLA-4 and PD-1 blockers for treatment of cancer. J Exp Clin Cancer Res. 2019;38(1):255. https://doi.org/10.1186/s13046-019-1259-z.
7. Weber JS, Gibney G, Sullivan RJ, et al. Sequential administration of nivolumab and ipilimumab with a planned switch in patients with advanced melanoma (CheckMate 064): an open-label, randomised, phase 2 trial [published correction appears in Lancet Oncol. 2016 Jul;17 (7):e270]. Lancet Oncol. 2016;17(7):943–55. https://doi.org/10.1016/S1470-2045(16)30126-7.
8. Larkin J, Chiarion-Sileni V, Gonzalez R, et al. Five-year survival with combined nivolumab and ipilimumab in advanced melanoma. N Engl J Med. 2019;381:1535–46. https://doi.org/10.1056/NEJMoa1910836.
9. D'Angelo SP, Larkin J, Sosman JA, et al. Efficacy and safety of nivolumab alone or in combination with ipilimumab in patients with mucosal melanoma: a pooled analysis. J Clin Oncol. 2017;35(2):226–35. https://doi.org/10.1200/JCO.2016.67.9258.
10. Shoushtari AN, Wagstaff J, Ascierto PA, et al. CheckMate 067: Long-term outcomes in patients with mucosal melanoma. J Clin Oncol. 2020;38(15_suppl):10019. https://doi.org/10.1200/JCO.2020.38.15_suppl.10019.
11. Lebbé C, Meyer N, Mortier L, et al. Evaluation of two dosing regimens for nivolumab in combination with ipilimumab in patients with advanced melanoma: results from the phase IIIb/IV CheckMate 511 trial. J Clin Oncol. 2019;37(11):867–75. https://doi.org/10.1200/JCO.18.01998.

12. Cagney DN, Martin AM, Catalano PJ, et al. Incidence and prognosis of patients with brain metastases at diagnosis of systemic malignancy: a population-based study. Neuro-Oncology. 2017;19(11):1511–21. https://doi.org/10.1093/neuonc/nox077.

13. Di Giacomo AM, Valente M, Cerase A, et al. Immunotherapy of brain metastases: breaking a "dogma". J Exp Clin Cancer Res. 2019;38(1):419. https://doi.org/10.1186/s13046-019-1426-2.

14. Di Giacomo AM, Ascierto PA, Pilla L, et al. Ipilimumab and fotemustine in patients with advanced melanoma (NIBIT-M1): an open-label, single-arm phase 2 trial. Lancet Oncol. 2012;13(9):879–86. https://doi.org/10.1016/S1470-2045(12)70324-8.

15. Di Giacomo AM, Ascierto PA, Queirolo P, et al. Three-year follow-up of advanced melanoma patients who received ipilimumab plus fotemustine in the Italian Network for Tumor Biotherapy (NIBIT)-M1 phase II study. Ann Oncol. 2015;26(4):798–803. https://doi.org/10.1093/annonc/mdu577.

16. Di Giacomo AM, Chiarion-Sileni V, Del Vecchio M, et al. Efficacy of ipilimumab plus nivolumab or ipilimumab plus fotemustine vs fotemustine in patients with melanoma metastatic to the brain: primary analysis of the phase III NIBIT-M2 trial. Accepted as Oral Presentation at ESMO Virtual Congress 2020.

17. Tawbi HA, Forsyth PA, Algazi A, et al. Combined nivolumab and ipilimumab in melanoma metastatic to the brain. N Engl J Med. 2018;379(8):722–30. https://doi.org/10.1056/NEJMoa1805453.

18. Tawbi HA, Forsyth PA, Hodi S, et al. Efficacy and safety of the combination of nivolumab (NIVO) plus ipilimumab (IPI) in patients with symptomatic melanoma brain metastases (CheckMate 204). J Clin Oncol. 2019;37(15):9501–950. https://doi.org/10.1200/JCO.2019.37.15_suppl.9501.

19. Long GV, Atkinson V, Lo S, et al. Combination nivolumab and ipilimumab or nivolumab alone in melanoma brain metastases: a multicentre randomised phase 2 study. Lancet Oncol. 2018;19(5):672–81. https://doi.org/10.1016/S1470-2045(18)30139-6.

20. Long GV, Atkinson VG, Lo S, et al. Long-term outcomes from the randomized phase II study of nivolumab (nivo) or nivo+ ipilimumab in patients (pts) with melanoma brain metastases (mets): anti-PD1 brain collaboration (ABC). Ann Oncol. 2019;30(Suppl_5):v533–63. https://doi.org/10.1093/annonc/mdz255.

21. Rulli E, Legramandi L, Salvati L, et al. The impact of targeted therapies and immunotherapy in melanoma brain metastases: a systematic review and meta-analysis. Cancer. 2019;125(21):3776–89. https://doi.org/10.1002/cncr.32375.

22. He Y, Rivard CJ, Rozeboom L, Yu H, et al. Lymphocyte-activation gene-3, an important immune checkpoint in cancer. Cancer Sci. 2016;107:1193–7. https://doi.org/10.1111/cas.12986.

23. Woo SR, Turnis ME, Goldberg MV, et al. Immune inhibitory molecules LAG-3 and PD-1 synergistically regulate T cell function to promote tumoral immune escape. Cancer Res. 2012;72:917–27. https://doi.org/10.1158/0008-5472.CAN-11-1620.

24. Huang RY, Francois A, Mc Gray AR, et al. Compensatory upregulation of PD-1, LAG-3, and CTLA-4 limits the efficacy of single-agent checkpoint blockade in metastatic ovarian cancer. Onco Targets Ther. 2016;6:e1249561. https://doi.org/10.1080/2162402X.2016.1249561.

25. Ascierto PA, Bono P, Bhatia S, et al. Efficacy of BMS-986016, a monoclonal antibody that targets lymphocyte activation gene-3 (LAG-3), in combination with nivolumab in pts with melanoma. Ann Oncol. 2017;28(Suppl_5):v605–49. https://doi.org/10.1093/annonc/mdx440.

26. Burugu S, Dancsok AR, Nielsen TO. Emerging targets in cancer immunotherapy. Semin Cancer Biol. 2018;52(Pt 2):39–52. https://doi.org/10.1016/j.semcancer.2017.10.001.

27. Manzano C, Clise-Dwyer K, Bover L, et al. Oncolytic adenovirus and tumor-targeting immune modulatory therapy improve autologous cancer vaccination. Cancer Res. 2017;77:3894–907. https://doi.org/10.1158/0008-5472.CAN-17-0468118.

28. Andtbacka RHI, Collichio F, Harrington KJ, et al. Final analyses of OPTiM: a randomized phase III trial of talimogene laherparepvec versus granulocyte-macrophage colony-stimulating

factor in unresectable stage III-IV melanoma. J Immunother Cancer. 2019;7(1):145. https://doi.org/10.1186/s40425-019-0623-z.

29. Liu Z, Ravindranathan R, Kalinski P, et al. Rational combination of oncolytic vaccinia virus and PD-L1 blockade works synergistically to enhance therapeutic efficacy. Nat Commun. 2017;8:14754. https://doi.org/10.1038/ncomms14754.

30. Long GV, Dummer R, Ribas A, et al. Efficacy analysis of MASTERKEY-265 phase 1b study of talimogene laherparepvec (T-VEC) and pembrolizumab (pembro) for unresectable stage IIIB-IV melanoma. J Clin Oncol. 2016;34:15. https://doi.org/10.1200/JCO.2016.34.15_suppl.9568.

31. Long GV, Dummer R, Andtbacka RH, et al. Follow-up analysis of MASTERKEY-265 phase 1b (ph1b) study of talimogene laherparepvec (T-VEC) in combination (combo) with pembrolizumab (pembro) in patients (pts) with unresectable stage IIIB–IV M1c melanoma (MEL). Presented at: SMR 2018, Manchester.

32. Ascierto PA, Dummer R. Immunological effects of BRAF+MEK inhibition. Onco Targets Ther. 2018;7(9):e1468955. https://doi.org/10.1080/2162402X.2018.1468955.

33. Ribas A, Hodi FS, Callahan M, et al. Hepatotoxicity with combination of vemurafenib and ipilimumab [published correction appears in N Engl J Med. 2018;379(22):2185]. N Engl J Med. 2013;368(14):1365–6. https://doi.org/10.1056/NEJMc1302338.

34. Puzanov I, Callahan ML, Linette GP, et al. Phase 1 study of the BRAF inhibitor dabrafenib (D) with or without the MEK inhibitor trametinib (T) in combination with ipilimumab (Ipi) for V600E/K mutation-positive unresectable or metastatic melanoma (MM). J Clin Oncol. 2014;32(Suppl):abstract 2511. https://doi.org/10.1200/jco.2014.32.15_suppl.2511.

35. Ascierto PA, Ferrucci PF, Fisher R, et al. Dabrafenib, trametinib and pembrolizumab or placebo in BRAF-mutant melanoma. Nat Med. 2019;25(6):941–6. https://doi.org/10.1038/s41591-019-0448-9.

36. Ferrucci PF, Ascierto PA, Maio M, et al. Updated survival in patients (pts) with BRAF-mutant melanoma administered pembrolizumab (pembro), dabrafenib (D), and trametinib (T). Presented at: SMR 2019; Salt Lake City.

37. Long GV, Lebbe C, Atkinson V, et al. The anti–PD-1 antibody spartalizumab (S) in combination with dabrafenib (D) and trametinib (T) in previously untreated patients (pts) with advanced BRAF V600–mutant melanoma: updated efficacy and safety from parts 1 and 2 of COMBI-i. J Clin Oncol. 2019;37(15 Suppl):9531. https://doi.org/10.1200/JCO.2019.37.15_suppl.9531.

38. Gutzmer R, Stroyakovskiy D, Gogas H, et al. Atezolizumab, vemurafenib, and cobimetinib as first-line treatment for unresectable advanced BRAF^{V600} mutation-positive melanoma (IMspire150): primary analysis of the randomised, double-blind, placebo-controlled, phase 3 trial. Lancet. 2020;395(10240):1835–44. https://doi.org/10.1016/S0140-6736(20)30934-X.

39. Murciano-Goroff YR, Warner AB, Wolchok JD. The future of cancer immunotherapy: microenvironment-targeting combinations. Cell Res. 2020;30(6):507–19. https://doi.org/10.1038/s41422-020-0337-2.

40. Segal NH, Logan TF, Hodi FS, et al. Results from an integrated safety analysis of urelumab, an agonist anti-CD137 monoclonal antibody. Clin Cancer Res. 2017;23(8):1929–36. https://doi.org/10.1158/1078-0432.CCR-16-1272.

41. Solinas C, Gu-Trantien C, Willard-Gallo K. The rationale behind targeting the ICOS-ICOS ligand costimulatory pathway in cancer immunotherapy. ESMO Open. 2020;5(1):e000544. https://doi.org/10.1136/esmoopen-2019-000544.

42. Berraondo P, Sanmamed MF, Ochoa MC, et al. Cytokines in clinical cancer immunotherapy. Br J Cancer. 2019;120(1):6–15. https://doi.org/10.1038/s41416-018-0328-y.

43. Diab A, Tannir NM, Bentebibel SE, et al. Bempegaldesleukin (NKTR-214) plus nivolumab in patients with advanced solid tumors: phase I dose-escalation study of safety, efficacy, and immune activation (PIVOT-02). Cancer Discov. 2020;10(8):1158–73. https://doi.org/10.1158/2159-8290.CD-19-1510.

44. Di Giacomo AM, Calabrò L, Danielli R, et al. Long-term survival and immunological parameters in metastatic melanoma patients who responded to ipilimumab 10mg/kg within an

expanded access programme. Cancer Immunol Immunother. 2013;62(6):1021–8. https://doi.org/10.1007/s00262-013-1418-6.

45. Hansen AR, Bauer TM, Moreno V, et al. First-in-human study with GSK3359609, an inducible T cell costimulator receptor agonist in patients with advanced, solid tumours: preliminary results from INDUCE-1. Ann Oncol. 2018;29(suppl_8):viii400–41. https://doi.org/10.1093/annonc/mdy288.

46. Labadie BW, Bao R, Luke JJ. Reimagining IDO pathway inhibition in cancer immunotherapy via downstream focus on the tryptophan-kynurenine-aryl hydrocarbon axis. Clin Cancer Res. 2019;25(5):1462–71. https://doi.org/10.1158/1078-0432.CCR-18-2882.

47. Grzywa TM, Sosnowska A, Matryba P, et al. Myeloid cell-derived arginase in cancer immune response. Front Immunol. 2020;11:938. https://doi.org/10.3389/fimmu.2020.00938.

48. Wang D, Jiang W, Zhu F, et al. Modulation of the tumor microenvironment by intratumoral administration of IMO-2125, a novel TLR 9 agonist, for cancer immunotherapy. Int J Oncol. 2018;53(3):1193–203. https://doi.org/10.3892/ijo.2018.4456.

49. Middleton MR, Hoeller C, Michielin O, et al. Intratumoural immunotherapies for unresectable and metastatic melanoma: current status and future perspectives [published online ahead of print, 2020 Jul 27]. Br J Cancer. 2020;123(6):885–97. https://doi.org/10.1038/s41416-020-0994-4.

50. Long GV, Dummer R, Hamid O, et al. Epacadostat plus pembrolizumab versus placebo plus pembrolizumab in patients with unresectable or metastatic melanoma (ECHO-301/KEYNOTE-252): a phase 3, randomised, double-blind study. Lancet Oncol. 2019;20(8):1083–97. https://doi.org/10.1016/S1470-2045(19)30274-8.

51. Uemura MI, Haymaker CL, Murthy R, et al. Intratumoral (i.t.) IMO-2125 (IMO), a TLR 9 agonist, in combination with ipilimumab (ipi) in PD-(L)1 refractory melanoma (RM). J Clin Oncol. 2017;35(7_suppl) https://doi.org/10.1200/JCO.2017.35.7_suppl.136.

52. Butler MO, Robert C, Negrier S, et al. ILLUMINATE 301: a randomized phase 3 study of tilsotolimod in combination with ipilimumab compared with ipilimumab alone in patients with advanced melanoma following progression on or after anti-PD-1 therapy. J Clin Oncol. 2019;37:15. https://doi.org/10.1200/JCO.2019.37.15_suppl.TPS9599.

53. Maio M, Covre A, Fratta E, et al. Molecular pathways: at the crossroads of cancer epigenetics and immunotherapy. Clin Cancer Res. 2015;21(18):4040–7. https://doi.org/10.1158/1078-0432.CCR-14-2914.

54. Covre A, Coral S, Nicolay H, et al. Antitumor activity of epigenetic immunomodulation combined with CTLA-4 blockade in syngeneic mouse models. Onco Targets Ther. 2015;4(8):e1019978. https://doi.org/10.1080/2162402X.2015.1019978.

55. Di Giacomo AM, Covre A, Finotello F, et al. Guadecitabine plus ipilimumab in unresectable melanoma: the NIBIT-M4 clinical trial. Clin Cancer Res. 2019;25(24):7351–62. https://doi.org/10.1158/1078-0432.CCR-19-1335.

56. Di Giacomo AM, Calabrò L, Danielli R, et al. A randomized, multicenter, phase II study of nivolumab combined with ipilimumab and guadecitabine or nivolumab combined with ipilimumab in melanoma and NSCLC patients resistant to anti-PD-1/-PD-L1: the NIBIT-ML1 study. Proceedings from the American Association for Cancer Research; AACR Virtual Annual Meeting 2020. Session VPO.CT07.02 - Virtual Meeting I: Phase II Trials in Progress, Abstract CT270.

57. Sullivan RJ, Moschos SJ, Johnson ML, et al. Abstract CT072: efficacy and safety of entinostat (ENT) and pembrolizumab (PEMBRO) in patients with melanoma previously treated with anti-PD1 therapy. Cancer Res. 2019;79(13 Suppl):CT072. https://doi.org/10.1158/1538-7445.AM2019-CT072.

Part V
Immunological Therapies in Advanced Skin Carcinomas

Chapter 15
Avelumab

Monika Dudzisz-Śledź, Paweł Teterycz, Piotr Rutkowski, and Jurgen C. Becker

Pharmacological Properties and Early Development

Avelumab (formerly known as MSB0010718C, trade name Bavencio, chemical formula $C6374H9898N1694O2010S44$) is a fully human monoclonal antibody of isotype IgG1 directed against ligand for programmed cell death protein 1 (PD-L1, programmed cell death-ligand 1). It is the first inhibitor of the immune system checkpoint registered by the US Food and Drug Administration (FDA) for the treatment of Merkel cell carcinoma (MCC).

The pharmacokinetic properties of avelumab were evaluated in a group of 1629 patients suffering from a variety of different cancers. The dose range administered every 2 weeks was 1 to 20 mg/kg body weight. Steady-state serum drug levels were reached approximately 4–6 weeks after initiation of treatment. Among patients receiving avelumab at a dose of 10 mg/kg body weight, the geometric mean volume of drug distribution was 4.72 l [1]. Avelumab, like other antibodies, is eliminated from the body primarily through the mechanism of proteolytic degradation. Its clearance is 0.59 l/day, and the half-life for 10 mg/kg body weight is 6.1 days. Post hoc analysis of patients treated for MCC showed a decrease in avelumab clearance over time. The average maximum reduction reached 41.7% [with a coefficient of

M. Dudzisz-Śledź (✉) · P. Teterycz · P. Rutkowski
Department of Soft Tissue/Bone Sarcoma and Melanoma, Maria Sklodowska-Curie National Research Institute of Oncology, Warsaw, Poland
e-mail: monika.dudzisz-sledz@pib-nio.pl

J. C. Becker
Translational Skin Cancer Research, German Cancer Consortium (DKTK), Department of Dermatology, University Duisburg-Essen, Essen, Germany

German Cancer Research Center (DKFZ), Heidelberg, Germany

P. Rutkowski, M. Mandalà (eds.), *New Therapies in Advanced Cutaneous Malignancies*, https://doi.org/10.1007/978-3-030-64009-5_15

variation (CV) of 40.0%] [1]. A proportional correlation was observed between avelumab clearance and the patient's body weight. However, this parameter was independent of the patient's age and sex, tumor size, and PD-L1 status. The degree of renal (for patients with glomerular filtration rate equal to or greater than 15 ml/min, calculated according to the Cockroft–Gault formula) or liver (up to bilirubin concentration equal to three times the upper limit of normal) insufficiency did not affect the rate of elimination of this antibody. However, there are no data on the pharmacokinetics of avelumab in patients with severe hepatic impairment [1].

The first preclinical study on the effectiveness of avelumab in modulating immunological anti-tumor activity was done on several human tumor cell lines [2]. It has been shown that the use of this drug in the presence of granulocytes or natural killers (NK) cells leads to lysis of cancer cells. This effect occurred regardless of whether leukocytes from healthy donors or cancer patients were used. It is also worth paying attention to the experiment, which tested avelumab activity against four chordoma cell lines [3]. The chordoma cells were incubated with avelumab either in the presence of NK cells alone or together with CD8+ T cells specific for the Brachyura factor. An increased percentage of tumor cell lysis was observed in both groups, which was boosted by the addition of CD8+ lymphocytes. This experiment shows that the unique mechanism of action of avelumab—consisting of both blocking PD-L1 and the stimulation of antibody-dependent cytotoxicity—may be active in tumors that, like chordoma, are insensitive to existing treatments. The anti-tumor activity of avelumab has been demonstrated not only in cell lines grown in vitro but also in vivo in a mouse model of noninvasive bladder cancer. During therapy, a statistically significant decrease in tumor size was observed, which was also reflected in a significant extension of survival of the animals [4].

The first phase Ia study lasted from January 2013 to October 2014 (NCT01772004). Fifty-three patients were enrolled in this study: four patients received a dose of 1 mg per kg of body weight, 13 patients received 3 mg per kg of body weight, 15 patients received 10 mg per kg of body weight, and 21 patients received 20 mg per kg of body weight. Due to toxicity, dose reduction was required only for one patient who received avelumab in a dose of 20 mg per kg of body weight. In the whole group (53 patients), the safety profile of the studied drug and its pharmacokinetic properties were evaluated. The drug was well tolerated. Only six (11%) patients had serious treatment-related adverse events (TRAE). Three cases of autoimmune reactions, lower abdominal pain, fatigue, and flu-like syndrome occurred in three patients receiving avelumab in a dose of 10 mg per kg of body weight. While, in three out of 21 patients receiving a dose of 20 mg per kg of body weight, one case each of autoimmune reaction, myositis, increase in serum amylase, and dysphonia was reported. During the study, some clinical activity of avelumab was observed—in four patients, there was an objective response to treatment, while in another 30 (57%), stabilization of the disease. The results of the study indicated that avelumab can be administered safely up to a dose of 20 mg/kg body weight. The maximum tolerated dose has not been reached. Due to the pharmacokinetic profile and immunological analysis, a dose of 10 mg/kg body weight given every 2 weeks was chosen for further studies [5].

Activity and Efficacy

The activity and efficacy of avelumab in the treatment of metastatic MCC (mMCC) have been demonstrated in JAVELIN Merkel 200 phase II single-arm study. The analyses of data from this study became the basis for drug registration in this indication (NCT02155647). The JAVELIN Merkel 200 study consisted of two parts: part A, which included patients treated in the second line ($n = 88$), and part B for systemic treatment-naive patients ($n = 116$).

The first published data from part A of this study resulted in registration of avelumab in mMCC. The patients aged at least 18 years with good performance status, that is, ECOG 0-1 (ECOG, an Eastern Cooperative Oncology Group), with mMCC confirmed by histology, whose disease progressed following at least one previous systemic treatment administered due to metastatic disease were eligible for this study. The disease had to be measurable per RECIST v. 1.1 criteria (RECIST, Response Evaluation Criteria in Solid Tumors). The patients had to have adequate bone marrow, renal, and hepatic function. Avelumab was administered at a dose of 10 mg/kg of body weight intravenously every 2 weeks until disease progression or unacceptable toxicity. The primary endpoint was confirmed objective response (CR- complete response or PR- partial response) assessed by an independent review committee according to RECIST 1.1. Efficacy and safety were assessed in all patients who received at least one dose of the study drug (the modified intention-to-treat population). The objective response rate (ORR) was 31.8% (95% confidence interval (CI): 21.9–43.1%; $n = 28$). Eight patients achieved CR (9%), and 20 patients achieved PR (23%). Additionally, in nine patients (10%) SD (stable disease) was observed. The treatment responses had a lasting effect and, at the moment of analysis, they were maintained in 23 (82%) patients. The duration of response (DOR) was at least 6 months in 92% of cases. The median PFS (progression-free survival) was 2.7 months (95% CI: 1.4–6.9), the rate of patients free from disease progression (PD) after 6 months was 40%. The PFS curve reached a plateau. The overall survival (OS) rate after 6 months was 69% (95% CI: 58–78), and the median OS was 11.3 months (95% CI: 7.5–14.0). In 58 of 74 evaluated cases (79%) PD-L1 expression ($\geq$ 1% positive cells) was found, and in 46 out of 77 (60%), the presence of the MCPyV (Merkel cell polyomavirus) was detected. More responses were obtained in patients who had previously undergone only one line of treatment [6].

Updated results with a median follow-up 18 months and 24 months published in 2018, confirmed the efficacy of avelumab described in the original report. Based on the analysis of the data from patients followed up for 29.2 months (24.8–38.1) the median OS was 12.6 months (95% CI: 7.5–17.1), with a 2-year survival rate of 36% (50% survival after 12 and 39% after 18 months). The median treatment duration was 3.9 months (0.5–36.3). The confirmed ORR was 33.0% (95% CI: 23.3–43.8; CR in 11.4% patients) and this remained on the same level as in previously reported analyses. The median DOR was not reached (2.8–31.8 months; 95% CI: 18.0—not reached). The long-term responses determine stable PFS values after 12 (29%), 18

(29%), and 24 months of follow-up (26%). Clinical activity persisted irrespectively of PD-L1 expression status and the presence of MCPyV [7, 8].

As per updated long-term data from patients treated in the second line (JAVELIN Merkel 200 trial, part A) published in 2020, confirmed ORR to avelumab was 33.0% (95% CI: 23.3% to 43.8%). CR was observed in 10 patients (11.4%). Responses were ongoing in 17 of 29 patients who achieved response to treatment (58.6%). Four patients had a continuous response lasting at least 3 years. Among them, one patient with a continuous CR received 88 doses of study drug. DOR was 40.5 months (median; 95% CI: 18.0 months—not estimable). PFS rate at 24 months was 26% (95% CI: 17–36%) and at 36 months, it was 21% (95% CI: 12–32%). OS after ≥44 months of follow-up was 12.6 months (median; 95% CI: 7.5–17.1 months). OS rate at 36 months was 32% (95% CI: 23–42%), and at 42 months, it was 31% (95% CI: 22–41%). Among patients with OS more than 36 months, who had PD-L1 expression status ($n = 22$) assessed, the PD-L1 status was positive in 81.8%. In this study, high tumor mutational burden and high expression of MHC I (major histo-compatibility complex class I) were related to trends for improved OS and ORR. Responses lasting at least 3 years were observed regardless of PD-L1 expression [9].

In 2017, during the annual conference of the American Society of Clinical Oncology (ASCO), the preliminary results of part B of JAVELIN Merkel 200 with avelumab in the first line of treatment of mMCC were presented [10]. In 16 patients, after a follow-up period of at least 3 months, the unconfirmed response rate was 68.8% (95% CI: 41.3–89.0) [10]. The extrapolated survival data published in 2018 suggested a mean survival rate of 49.9 months (6.3; 179.4), with 1 year and 5 years survival rates being 66% and 23%, respectively [11]. The updated results of part B of this trial confirmed that 77.8% (14 out of 18) of treatment responses were maintained and the response duration in 83% cases was longer than 6 months (95% CI: 46–96%) [12].

A further updated analysis after ≥15 months of follow-up from JAVELIN Merkel 200, part B, with a median follow-up of 21.2 months (range, 14.9–36.6) was published in 2019 ($n = 116$). The median treatment duration was 5.5 months (range, 0.5–35.4). Treatment was ongoing in only 26 patients (22.4%) at the data cut-off. The ORR was 39.7% (95% CI: 30.7%–49.2%), 19 patients (16.4%) achieved CR and 27 (23.3%) experienced PR. In patients with PD-L1+ tumors ($n = 21$) ORR was 61.9% (95% CI: 38.4%–81.9%), whereas in the larger subgroup of patients whose tumors did not express PD-L1 ($n = 87$) the ORR was 33.3% (95% CI: 23.6%–44.3%). Median DOR was 18.2 months (95% CI: 11.3 months-not esti-mable). The response lasting at least 6 months was observed in 35 patients. PFS rate at 6 months was 41% (95% CI: 32–50%) and at 12 months was 31% (95% CI: 23–40%). Median OS was 20.3 months (95% CI: 12.4 months-not evaluable). The OS rate at 12 months was 60% (95% CI: 50–68%). In PD-L1+ and PD-L1− sub-groups, 12-month OS rates were 71% (95% CI: 47–86%) and 56% (95% CI: 45–66%), respectively [13].

The efficacy of avelumab in a "real-world setting" was assessed in the expanded access program. Enrolled patients had to have advanced MCC either progressing during or after chemotherapy, may not have been eligible for chemotherapy or clinical trial participation. Of the total 494 patients receiving avelumab, 240 were evaluable for efficacy. The median age was 73 years (range, 23–95), 66.8% of patients were male, 90.9% had an ECOG PS of 0–1. However, the population also included patients who had an ECOG PS 2 or 3, who had brain metastases stable after therapy, or were potentially immunocompromised. Continuation of avelumab beyond radiological progression was permitted in the absence of significant clinical deterioration and based on investigator assessment. The efficacy was assessed based on RECIST 1.1 criteria. The median duration of avelumab treatment was 7.9 months (range, 1.0–41.7). The ORR was 46.7% in the evaluable patients including CR in 22.9% and PR in 23.8% [14].

Currently, a multicenter, phase III, double-blinded, placebo-controlled clinical trial (NCT03271372) is recruiting patients with clinical stage III MCC to evaluate the efficacy of avelumab in the adjuvant treatment after surgery (with or without radiotherapy). The primary endpoint is RFS (relapse-free survival) [15].

Pembrolizumab, anti-PD1 monoclonal antibody, also has been approved for the treatment of metastatic MCC. It is indicated for the treatment of patients with recurrent locally advanced or metastatic Merkel cell carcinoma [16]. This drug has been approved based on KEYNOTE-017 study results (NCT02267603), only in the US. Among the 50 patients with MCC stage IIIB–IVC, the median age was 71 years (with 80% at least 65 years), 68% were male, all had an ECOG PS of 0 or 1, 14% had stage IIIB disease and 86% had stage IV disease, and 84% had prior surgery and 70% had prior radiation therapy. In 64%, the tumor was MCPyV(+). The ORR was 56% (CR 24%, PR 32%; 95% CI: 41.3–70.0%), the ORR in the patients in the group MCPyV(+) was 59%, while in those in the group MCPyV(−), it was 53%, with a median follow-up of 14.9 months (range 0.4–36.4 months).The DOR was not reached. Among the 28 patients with responses, 96% had a response duration of more than 6 months, and 54% had a response duration of more than 12 months. The PFS ratio after 24 months was 48.3%, with a median PFS of 16.8 months. OS rate after 24 months was 68.7%, and the median OS was not reached. The presence of polyomavirus did not correlate with ORR, PFS, or OS. Some trend for better results concerning PFS and OS was observed in patients with PD-L1 expression [17, 18].

Nivolumab, another anti-PD1 monoclonal antibody was tested in a neoadjuvant setting for resectable MCC. In the CheckMate 358 (NCT02488759), phase I/II study, dedicated to the assessment of safety and efficacy of avelumab in patients with virus-associated solid tumors, 39 patients with resectable MCC (stage IIA-IV) were enrolled. The patients received nivolumab in a dose of 240 mg intravenously on days 1 and 15. The surgery was scheduled for day 29. The evaluation of the response was based on radiological and pathological examination. The tumor biopsies before the treatment administration to assess tumor mutational burden, expression of PD-L1 and MCPyV status were done. 7.7% of patients treated with avelumab ($n = 3$) were not operated due to disease progression ($n = 1$) or toxicity ($n = 2$). TRAEs of any grade were reported in 46.2% of patients ($n = 18$), TRAEs G3 and G4 were observed in 7.7% of patients ($n = 3$). There were no unexpected toxicities reported in this patient group. Thirty-six patients underwent surgery. The pathologic complete response (pCR) was achieved in 47.2% of patients who underwent surgery ($n = 17$). Thirty-three of operated patients were evaluable by radiology imaging. In 54.5% of them ($n = 18$) the tumor reductions by at least 30% were reported. The responses did not depend on TMB, PD-L1, and MCPyV status. No tumor relapse among patients with pCR was observed. With a median follow-up of 20.3 months, median RFS and OS were not achieved. There was a significant correlation between RFS and pCR, as well as the radiological response at the surgical stage [19].

The safety and efficacy of nivolumab were also assessed in advanced MCC in the CheckMate 358 study. Nivolumab was administered in a group of 25 patients with MCC. The ORR rate in response evaluable patients ($n = 22$) was 68% after the 26-week follow-up period (range 5–35 weeks), and it was larger in patients who had not been systemically treated previously (71%, $n = 14$), in comparison with those who had been previously treated (63%, 1 or 2 lines of previous treatment, $n = 8$) [20].

Currently, a multicenter randomized phase III trial (ADMEC-O, NCT02196961) is testing the efficacy of nivolumab applied at a fixed dose of 480 mg by IV infusion every 4 weeks for up to 1 year in patients with all clinical stages MCC which had been rendered no evidence of disease by surgery and/or radiation therapy, that is, in an adjuvant setting. There is 2:1 randomization favoring nivolumab treatment over observation. The primary endpoint is RFS (relapse-free survival) [21].

The results of clinical trials with immunotherapy in advanced MCC are summarized in Table 15.1.

Table 15.1 Summary of clinical trials in line 1 and line 2 treatments in advanced MCC

Drug (study)	Treatment line	Target	n	Previous systemic treatment	ORR	mPFS	mOS
Pembrolizumab (NCT02267603)	1.	PD-1	50	No	56%	16.8 months	Not reached
Avelumab (NCT02155647) JAVELIN Merkel 200 part B	1.	PD-L1	116	No	39.7%	4.1 months	20.3 months
Avelumab (NCT02155647) JAVELIN Merkel 200 part A	2.	PD-L1	88	Yes	33%	2.7 months	12.6 months
Nivolumab (NCT02488759) CheckMate-358	1. 2.	PD-1	14 8	No Yes	71% 63%	Not reached	Not reached

Toxicity Profile

In the JAVELIN Merkel 200, avelumab therapy was generally well-tolerated.

In the part A of the study as per analysis published in 2016, five grade 3 treatment-related adverse events occurred in four (5%) patients: lymphopenia in two patients, blood creatine phosphokinase increase in one patient, aminotransferase increase in one patient, and blood cholesterol increase in one patient. There were no treatment-related grade 4 AEs or treatment-related deaths. Serious treatment-related adverse events were reported in five patients (6%): enterocolitis, infusion-related reaction, aminotransferases increased, chondrocalcinosis, synovitis, and interstitial nephritis ($n = 1$ each) [6]. In the subsequent analyses published for part A of the study, the tolerance profile of avelumab was consistent with those previously published. In 67 patients (76.1%) treatment-related AEs were observed and in ten patients (11.4%) they were at least G3. In 20 patients (22.7%) immune-related adverse events were observed. No treatment related deaths occurred [7, 8]. As per updated analysis from JAVELIN Merkel 200 part A, published in 2020, after ≥ 36 months of follow-up, any grade AEs were reported in 86 of 88 patients (97.7%). There were 65 grade ≥ 3 (73.9%) observed. TRAEs of any grade occurred in 68 patients (77.3%). Those patients included six additional patients in comparison to a safety analysis done after 10 months. The most commonly reported TRAEs ($>10\%$) were fatigue in 25% of patients ($n = 22$), diarrhea in 12.5% of patients ($n = 11$), and nausea in 12.5% of patients ($n = 11$). In 11.4% of patients, TRAEs grade of at least 3 were reported ($n = 10$). The following TRAEs occurring in at least one patient were observed: increased blood creatine phosphokinase ($n = 3$; 3.4%) and lymphopenia ($n = 2$; 2.3%). Nineteen patients (21.6%) experienced an immune related adverse event (irAE). Four (4.5%) irAE were grade at least 3: increased transaminases, increased alanine aminotransferase, autoimmune disorder, and hypothyroidism. IRRs were reported in 19 patients (21.6%). None of IRRs were grade ≥ 3. Eight patients (9.1%) required treatment discontinuation due to TRAEs. No deaths related to treatment were reported. Two of the thirteen patients who received at least 52 doses of avelumab and were treated for at least 2 years discontinued treatment due to a TRAE (immune-related colitis and suspected immune-related thrombocytopenia) [9].

As per analysis from part B of the JAVELIN Merkel 200 study, published in 2017, the safety of the therapy was evaluated in 29 patients. TRAEs at least grade 3 occurred in five patients (17.2%), and this was the reason for the termination of the treatment (two patients with infusion-related reaction, one patient each with increased activity of aspartate aminotransferase and alanine aminotransferase, cholangitis, paraneoplastic syndrome) [10]. According to the next updated analysis, in eight patients in total, there were reported G3 AEs related to the immunology system (20.5%) [12]. Based on the abstract presented in 2019 during SITC (Society for Immunotherapy of Cancer) conference, treatment-related adverse events (TRAEs) of any grade occurred in 94 patients (81.0%), including grade ≥ 3 TRAEs in 21 (18.1%). No treatment-related deaths occurred [13].

The safety data from expanded access program are limited as safety events were likely under-reported because data were reported at the treating physician's discretion, and many patients had no evaluable data beyond the 3 months. The most frequently reported AEs related to avelumab were infusion-related reaction ($n = 9$), fever ($n = 7$), fatigue ($n = 6$), rash ($n = 4$), asthenia ($n = 4$), abdominal pain (3), chills (3), and dyspnea (3) [15].

Adverse reactions in patients treated with avelumab as monotherapy in clinical study JAVELIN Merkel 200 and from a phase I study JAVELIN Solid Tumor are listed in Table 15.2, based on the summary of product characteristics.

The incidence of immune-related adverse reactions under avelumab is described in the Summary of Product Characteristics (last update in October 2020) and is based on 1738 patients treated in the above-mentioned trials:

- Immune-related pneumonitis developed in 1.2% of patients. Of these patients, there was one patient with a fatal outcome, one patient with Grade 4, and five patients with Grade 3 pneumonitis. The median time to onset of immune-related pneumonitis was 2.5 months (range: 3 days to 11 months). The median duration was 7 weeks (range: 4 days to more than 4 months). All patients with immune-related pneumonitis were treated with corticosteroids and 17 of them received

Table 15.2 Adverse reactions in patients treated with avelumab as monotherapy in clinical study JAVELIN Merkel 200 and from a phase I study JAVELIN Solid Tumor are presented by system organ class and frequency. Frequencies are defined as: very common ($\geq$1/10); common ($\geq$1/100 to <1/10); uncommon ($\geq$1/1000 to <1/100); rare ($\geq$1/10,000 to <1/1000); very rare (<1/10,000). Within each frequency grouping, adverse reactions are presented in the order of decreasing seriousness) [1]

Frequency	Adverse reactions
Blood and lymphatic system disorders	
Very common	Anemia
Common	Lymphopenia
Uncommon	Thrombocytopenia, eosinophilia[a]
Immune system disorders	
Uncommon	Drug hypersensitivity, hypersensitivity anaphylactic reaction, Type I hypersensitivity
Endocrine disorders	
Common	Hypothyroidism[b]
Uncommon	Adrenal insufficiency[b], hyperthyroidism[b], thyroiditis[b], autoimmune thyroiditis[b], adrenocortical insufficiency acute[b], autoimmune hypothyroidism[b], hypopituitarism[b]
Metabolism and nutrition disorders	
Very common	Decreased appetite
Uncommon	Diabetes mellitus[b], Type 1 diabetes mellitus[b]
Nervous system disorders	
Common	Headache, dizziness, neuropathy peripheral
Uncommon	Myasthenia gravis[c], myasthenic syndrome[c], Guillain–Barré syndrome[b]
Eye disorders	
Uncommon	Uveitis[b]
Cardiac disorders	

Table 15.2 (continued)

Frequency	Adverse reactions
Rare	Myocarditis[b]
Vascular disorders	
Common	Hypertension, hypotension
Uncommon	Flushing
Respiratory, thoracic, and mediastinal disorders	
Very common	Cough, dyspnea
Common	Pneumonitis[b]
Gastrointestinal disorders	
Very common	Nausea, diarrhea, constipation, vomiting, abdominal pain
Common	Dry mouth
Uncommon	Colitis[b], autoimmune colitis[b], enterocolitis[b], ileus
Rare	Pancreatitis[b]
Hepatobiliary disorders	
Uncommon	Autoimmune hepatitis[b], acute hepatic failure[b], hepatic failure[b], hepatitis[b]
Skin and subcutaneous tissue disorders	
Common	Rash[b], pruritus[b], rash maculo-papular[b], dry skin
Uncommon	Rash pruritic[b], erythema[b], rash generalized[b], psoriasis[b], rash erythematous[b], rash macular[b], rash papular[b], dermatitis exfoliative[b], erythema multiforme[b], pemphigoid[b], pruritus generalized[b], eczema, dermatitis
Musculoskeletal and connective tissue disorders	
Very common	Back pain, arthralgia
Common	Myalgia
Uncommon	Myositis[b]
Renal and urinary disorders	
Uncommon	Tubulo-interstitial nephritis[b]
General disorders and administrative site conditions	
Very common	Fatigue, pyrexia, edema peripheral
Common	Asthenia, chills, influenza like illness
Uncommon	Systemic inflammatory response syndrome[b]
Investigations	
Very common	Weight decreased
Common	Gamma-glutamyltransferase increased, blood alkaline phosphatase increased, amylase increased, lipase increased, blood creatinine increased
Uncommon	Alanine aminotransferase (ALT) increased[b], aspartate aminotransferase (AST) increased[b], blood creatine phosphokinase increased[b], transaminases increased[b]
Injury, poisoning, and procedural complications	
Very common	Infusion-related reaction

[a]Reaction only observed from study JAVELIN Merkel 200 (Part B) after the data cut-off of the pooled analysis, hence frequency estimated

[b]Immune-related adverse reaction based on medical review

[c]Adverse reactions occurred in estimated 4,000 patients exposed to avelumab monotherapy beyond the pooled analysis

high-dose corticosteroids. Pneumonitis has resolved in 57% of the patients at the time of data cut-off [1].

- Immune-related hepatitis developed in 0.9% of patients, in two patients with a fatal outcome. The median time to onset of hepatitis was 3.2 months (range: 1 week to 15 months). The median duration was 2.5 months (range: 1 day to more than 7.4 months). Avelumab was discontinued in 0.5% of patients due to the hepatitis. Almost all patients received high-dose corticosteroids for a median of 14 days (range: 1 day to 2.5 months). Hepatitis has resolved in 56% at the time of data cut-off [1].
- Immune-related colitis developed in 1.5% patients, in 0.4% with Grade 3. The median time to onset of colitis was 2.1 months (range: 2 days to 11 months). The median duration was 6 weeks (range: 1 day to more than 14 months). Avelumab was discontinued in 0.5% of patients due this AE. All patients with immune-related colitis were treated with corticosteroids and 58% of them received high-dose corticosteroids for a median of 19 days (range: 1 day to 2.3 months). Colitis resolved in 70% patients at the time of data cut-off [1].
- Immune-related thyroid disorders occurred in 6% of patients: 90 patients with hypothyroidism, seven with hyperthyroidism, and four with thyroiditis. In three cases up to Grade 3. The median time to onset of thyroid disorders was 2.8 months (range: 2 weeks to 13 months). The median duration was not estimable (range: 1 day to more than 26 months). Avelumab was discontinued in 0.1% of patients for this reason. Thyroid disorders resolved in only 7% of the patients at the time of data cut-off [1].
- Immune-related adrenal insufficiency developed in 0.5% of patients. In one case reaching Grade 3, the median time to onset of this AE was 2.5 months (range: 1 day to 8 months). The median duration was not estimable (range: 2 days to more than 6 months). Avelumab was discontinued in two of these patients. All patients with immune-related adrenal insufficiency were treated with high-dose systemic corticosteroids ($\geq$40 mg 15 prednisone or equivalent) followed by a taper. Adrenal insufficiency has resolved in only one patient with corticoid treatment at the time of data cut-off [1].
- Type 1 diabetes mellitus without an alternative etiology occurred in two patients both with Grade 3 leading to permanent discontinuation of avelumab [1].
- Immune-related nephritis occurred in one patient receiving avelumab leading to permanent discontinuation of avelumab [1].
- Immune-related pancreatitis and myocarditis have been observed in avelumab treated patients with a very low frequency (less than 0.1%).

Of the above described 1738 patients, 1627 were evaluable for treatment-emergent anti-drug antibodies (ADA) of which 96 (5.9%) tested positive. In ADA positive patients, there may be an increased risk for infusion-related reactions (about 40% and 25% in ADA ever-positive and ADA never-positive patients, respectively). Based on data available, including the low incidence of immunogenicity, the impact of ADA on pharmacokinetics, efficacy, and safety is uncertain, while the impact of neutralizing antibodies (nAb) is unknown [1].

Fertility studies have not been conducted with avelumab [1]. Preclinical studies evaluated the effect of avelumab on the reproductive organs of the crab-eating macaque (Cynomolgus monkey). After three months of weekly drug administration, no significant morphological changes were found in either male or female reproductive organs [20]. However, the effect of the drug on animal reproductive performance has not been evaluated. The effect of avelumab on pregnancy has not been studied in animal models. There are no data on the use of the drug in pregnant women. Nevertheless, due to the central role of the PD1/PD-L1 pathway in the development of placental and fetal immune tolerance in pregnant women, it is expected that the use of avelumab may significantly increase the risk of miscarriage or stillbirth [22].

Summary of Approval and Regulatory Indications

In March 2017, FDA approved avelumab for the treatment of adults and pediatric patients 12 years and older with metastatic Merkel cell carcinoma (MCC) irrespective of prior therapy. In September 2017, EMA approved avelumab as monotherapy for the treatment of adult patients with metastatic Merkel cell carcinoma. The recommended dose of avelumab as monotherapy is 800 mg administered intravenously over 60 min every 2 weeks. Treatment should continue according to the recommended schedule until disease progression or unacceptable toxicity. Patients have to be premedicated with an antihistamine and with paracetamol before the first four infusions of Bavencio. If the fourth infusion is completed without an infusion-related reaction, premedication for subsequent doses should be administered at the discretion of the physician. Dose escalation or reduction is not recommended. Dosing delay or discontinuation may be required based on individual safety and tolerability, the detailed management of immune-related adverse events, including infusion-related reactions, is described in the summary of product characteristics. No dose adjustment is needed for older patients. No dose adjustment is needed for patients with mild or moderate renal impairment and there are insufficient data in patients with severe renal impairment for dosing recommendations. No dose adjustment is needed for patients with mild hepatic impairment and there are insufficient data in patients with moderate or severe hepatic impairment for dosing recommendations. The safety and efficacy of avelumab in children and adolescents below 18 years of age have not been established [1, 23].

References

1. Bavencio, Summary of product characteristics. October 2020. https://www.ema.europa.eu/en/documents/product-information/bavencio-epar-product-information_en.pdf
2. Boyerinas B, Jochems C, Fantini M, et al. Antibody-dependent cellular cytotoxicity activity of a novel anti-PD-L1 antibody avelumab (MSB0010718C) on human tumor cells. Cancer Immunol Res. 2015;3:1148–57.

3. Fujii R, Friedman ER, Richards J, et al. Enhanced killing of chordoma cells by antibody-dependent cell-mediated cytotoxicity employing the novel anti-PD-L1 antibody avelumab. Oncotarget. 2016;7:33498–511.

4. Vandeveer AJ, Fallon JK, Tighe R, et al. Systemic immunotherapy of non-muscle invasive mouse bladder cancer with avelumab, an anti-PD-L1 immune checkpoint inhibitor. Cancer Immunol Res. 2016;4:452–62.

5. Heery CR, O'Sullivan-Coyne G, Madan RA, et al. Avelumab for metastatic or locally advanced previously treated solid tumours (JAVELIN Solid Tumor): a phase 1a, multicohort, dose-escalation trial. Lancet Oncol. 2017;18:587–98.

6. Kaufman HL, Russel J, Hamid O, et al. Avelumab in patients with chemotherapy-refractory metastatic Merkel cell carcinoma: a multicentre, single-group, open-label, phase 2 trial. Lancet Oncol. 2016;17(10):1374–85.

7. Nghiem P, Bhatia S, Scott Brohl A, et al. Two-year efficacy and safety update from JAVELIN Merkel 200 part A: a registrational study of avelumab in metastatic Merkel cell carcinoma progressed on chemotherapy. J Clin Oncol. 2018;36(15-suppl):9507.

8. Kaufman HL, Russel JS, Hamid O, et al. Updated efficacy of avelumab in patients with previously treated metastatic Merkel cell carcinoma after ≥1 year of follow-up: JAVELIN Merkel 200, a phase 2 clinical trial. J Immunother Cancer. 2018;6(1):7.

9. D'Angelo SP, Bhatia S, Brohl AS, et al. Avelumab in patients with previously treated metastatic Merkel cell carcinoma: long-term data and biomarker analyses from the single-arm phase 2 JAVELIN Merkel 200 trial. J Immunother Cancer. 2020;8(1):e000674.

10. D'Angelo SP, Russel J, Hassel JC, et al. First-line (1L) avelumab treatment in patients (pts) with metastatic Merkel cell carcinoma (mMCC): preliminary data from an ongoing study. J Clin Oncol. 2017;35(15-suppl):9530.

11. Bullement A, D'Angelo S, Amin A, et al. Predicting overall survival in patients (pts) with treatment-naive metastatic Merkel cell carcinoma (mMCC) treated with avelumab. J Clin Oncol. 2018;36(15-suppl):e21620.

12. D'Angelo SP, Russell J, Lebbé C, et al. Efficacy and safety of first-line avelumab treatment in patients with stage IV metastatic Merkel cell carcinoma: a preplanned interim analysis of a clinical trial. JAMA Oncol. 2018;4(9):e180077.

13. D'Angelo SP, Lebbé C, Mortier L, et al. First-line avelumab treatment in patients with metastatic Merkel cell carcinoma: primary analysis after ≥15 months of follow-up from JAVELIN Merkel 200, a registrational phase 2 trial. SITC 2019, p 362

14. Walker JW, Lebbé C, Grignani G, et al. Efficacy and safety of avelumab treatment in patients with metastatic Merkel cell carcinoma: experience from a global expanded access program. J Immunother Cancer. 2020;8(1):e000313.

15. Bhatia S, Brohl A, Brownell I, et al. ADAM trial: a multicenter, randomized, double-blinded, placebo-controlled, phase 3 trial of adjuvant avelumab (anti-PD-L1 antibody) in Merkel cell carcinoma patients with clinically detected lymph node metastases; NCT03271372. J Clin Oncol. 2018;36(15-suppl):TPS9605.

16. Pembrolizumab (Keytruda) injection for intravenous use, prescribing information.

17. Nghiem PT, Bhatia S, Lipson EJ, et al. PD-1 blockade with pembrolizumab in advanced Merkel-cell carcinoma. N Engl J Med. 2016;374(26):2542–52.

18. Nghiem P, Bhatia S, Lipson E, et al. Durable tumor regression and overall survival in patients with advanced Merkel cell carcinoma receiving pembrolizumab as first-line therapy. J Clin Oncol. 2019;37(9):693–702.

19. Topalian SL, Bhatia S, Kudchadkar RR, et al. Nivolumab (Nivo) as neoadjuvant therapy in patients with resectable Merkel cell carcinoma (MCC) in CheckMate 358. J Clin Oncol. 2018;36(15-suppl):9505.

20. Topalian SL, Bhatia S, Hollebecque A, et al. Abstract CT074: Non-comparative, open-label, multiple cohort, phase 1/2 study to evaluate nivolumab (NIVO) in patients with virus-associated tumors (CheckMate 358): Efficacy and safety in Merkel cell carcinoma (MCC). Cancer Res. 2017;77(13-suppl):CT074.

21. Adjuvant therapy of completely resected merkel cell carcinoma with immune checkpoint blocking antibodies vs observation (ADMEC-O). https://clinicaltrials.gov/ct2/show/NCT02196961
22. Guleria I, Khosroshahi A, Ansari MJ, et al. A critical role for the programmed death ligand 1 in fetomaternal tolerance. J Exp Med. 2005;202:231–7.
23. Bavencio (avelumab) injection for intravenous use, prescribing information.

Chapter 16
Cemiplimab

Monika Dudzisz-Śledź and Piotr Rutkowski

Pharmacological Properties and Early Development

Cemiplimab (REGN2810) is a high-affinity, highly potent, fully human, hinge-stabilized IgG4 monoclonal antibody that potently blocks PD-1/PD-L1 functional interaction. It was generated using VelocImmune mice containing human immuno-globulin gene segments. Cemiplimab binds to PD-1 with high affinity and specificity, inhibits PD-1 binding to PD-L1 and PD-L2 ligands. This antibody does not induce antibody-dependent cell-mediated cytotoxicity (ADCC) or complement-dependent cytotoxicity (CDC) and blocks PD-1/PD-L1 inhibitory signals and promotes T-cell activation in vitro [1].

Concentration data were collected in 548 patients with various solid tumors, including 178 patients with CSCC (cutaneous squamous cell carcinoma) treated with cemiplimab. At dosing regimens of 1 mg/kg to 10 mg/kg every 2 weeks (Q2W) and 350 mg every 3 weeks (Q3W), kinetics of cemiplimab were linear and dose proportional. The exposures to cemiplimab achieved with the doses of 350 mg Q2W and 3 mg/kg Q2W are similar. Steady-state exposure is achieved after approximately 4 months of treatment. Cemiplimab is expected to degrade to small peptides and individual amino acids. Clearance of cemiplimab is linear at doses of 1 mg/kg to 10 mg/kg Q2W. Cemiplimab clearance after the first dose is approximately 0.33 l/day. The total clearance appears to decrease by approximately 35% over time, resulting in a steady state clearance (CLss) of 0.21 l/day; the decrease in CL is not considered clinically relevant. The within dosing interval half-life at steady state is 19.4 days [2].

M. Dudzisz-Śledź (✉) · P. Rutkowski
Department of Soft Tissue/Bone Sarcoma and Melanoma, Maria Sklodowska-Curie National Research Institute of Oncology, Warsaw, Poland
e-mail: monika.dudzisz-sledz@pib-nio.pl

P. Rutkowski, M. Mandalà (eds.), *New Therapies in Advanced Cutaneous Malignancies*, https://doi.org/10.1007/978-3-030-64009-5_16

The effect of renal impairment on the exposure of cemiplimab was evaluated by a population PK analysis in patients with mild (CLcr 60 to <89 ml/min; $n = 197$), moderate (CLcr 30 to <60 ml/min; $n = 90$), or severe (CLcr <30 ml/min; $n = 4$) renal impairment. No clinically important differences in the exposure of cemiplimab were found between patients with renal impairment and patients with normal renal function. Cemiplimab has not been studied in patients with CLcr <25 ml/min [2].

In the first-in-human phase 1 study (NCT02383212), cemiplimab pharmacokinetic parameters were similar to monotherapy or in combination with hfRT and/or CPA. Cemiplimab concentrations in serum increased in a close to dose-proportional manner. Cemiplimab half-life after the first dose was approximately 12 days and steady state was reached after 4 months of treatment [3, 4].

The effect of hepatic impairment on the exposure of cemiplimab was evaluated by population PK analysis. In patients with mild hepatic impairment, no clinically important differences in the exposure of cemiplimab were found compared to patients with normal hepatic function. Cemiplimab has not been studied in patients with moderate or severe hepatic impairment [1].

Cemiplimab was assessed in the first-in-human phase 1 study (NCT02383212). This was an open-label, multicenter, dose escalation, and cohort expansion study of cemiplimab in patients with advanced solid tumors. The main purpose of this study was to assess the safety, tolerability, dose-limiting toxicities (DLT), antitumor activity, and pharmacokinetics of cemiplimab as monotherapy and in combination with hypofractionated radiotherapy (hfRT) and/or chemotherapy-cyclophosphamide (CPA). Patients were enrolled in 1 of 10 possible cohorts in the dose escalation study within traditional 3 + 3 design. Between February 2015 and March 2016, 60 patients were enrolled in the dose-escalation part of this study, with six patients enrolled into each of the 10 dose escalation cohorts. Patients received cemiplimab 1, 3, or 10 mg/kg Q2W by intravenous infusion over 30 min for up to six 56-day treatment cycles, for a total of up to 48 weeks of treatment or until disease progression, unacceptable toxicity, withdrawal of consent, or other reasons defined in the study protocol. There was a posttreatment follow-up period of up to 24 weeks. In hfRT cohorts, patients received either 30 Gy (6 Gy daily × 5, every day) or 27 Gy (9 Gy daily × 3, every other day) starting 1 week after the first dose of cemiplimab. In CPA cohorts, low-dose (200 mg/m^2) CPA was administered intravenously 1 day prior to each of the four doses of cemiplimab in cycle 1. The treatment related adverse events were assessed based on the National Cancer Institute Common Terminology Criteria for Adverse Events (NCI-CTCAE, v. 4.03). Tumor assessments were done by investigators, every 8 weeks, based on Response Evaluation Criteria in Solid Tumours v. 1.1 (RECIST 1.1) [3, 4].

Cemiplimab demonstrated a safety profile comparable with profile of other anti–PD-1 agents in patients with advanced solid tumors.

Maximum tolerated dose (MTD) was not reached in the escalation part of this study. No dose limiting toxicities (DLTs) were reported. The median duration of follow-up was 19.3 weeks (range 2.3–84.3). Treatment emergent adverse events (TEAE) of any grade (G) were reported in 58 patients (96.7%). 30 patients (50.0%)

experienced TEAEs G ≥ 3. 15 patients (25.0%) experienced serious TEAEs of any G. Two patients (3.3%) discontinued treatment due to G ≥ 3 TEAEs (increased bilirubin, anti-HuD associated paraneoplastic limbic encephalitis). The most common TEAEs of any G were fatigue (45.0%), nausea (36.7%), and vomiting (25.0%). G ≥ 3 TEAEs that occurred in more than one patient were lymphopenia ($n = 6$, 10.0%), anemia ($n = 5$, 8.3%), increased aspartate aminotransferase (AST) ($n = 4$, 6.7%), hyponatremia and increased blood alkaline phosphatase (ALP) (each $n = 3$, 5.0%), hyperglycemia, increased alanine aminotransferase (ALT), and hyperbilirubinemia (each $n = 2$, 3.3%). 32 patients (53.3%) experienced immune-related adverse events (irAE) with 4 (6.7%) grade ≥ 3 irAEs. The most common irAEs of any G were arthralgia ($n = 6$, 10.0%), hypothyroidism ($n = 5$, 8.3%), and maculo-papular rash ($n = 5$, 8.3%).

A total of 49 patients was evaluable for anti-drug antibodies (ADA) assessments. The ADA incidence rate was low ($n = 1$; 2.0%).

The objective response rate (ORR) was 15.0% [95% CI: 7.1–26.6), 22.2% (95% CI: 6.4–47.6) for patients treated with cemiplimab monotherapy and 20.8% (95% CI: 7.1–42.2) for patients treated with cemiplimab in combination with hfRT. Two patients experienced complete response (CR), seven patients achieved partial response (PR), and 24 patients had stable disease (SD). No response was observed in patients treated with CPA. The durable disease control rate (DCR) for all patients was 30.0% (95% CI: 18.8–43.2). Duration of response (DOR) was ≥12 months in 6 of 9 responding patients (66.7%). The median progression free survival (PFS) was 3.6 (1.9–4.0) months and median overall survival (OS) was 23.5 (11.0–not evaluable) months.

In the dose-escalation portion of the phase 1 study of cemiplimab (NCT02383212), a deep and durable response was observed in a patient with advanced CSCC [5]. This patient with recurrent cheek CSCC underwent many surgeries, received radiation therapy, was heavily pretreated with systemic drugs including chemotherapy and cetuximab and required emergent decompression of cervical spinal cord with C4-C5 anterior corpectomy and C4-C6 posterior laminectomy due to invasive CSCC at C4-C5 vertebral bodies, before enrollment into this study. He was treated within the study with cemiplimab in a dose 1 mg/kg Q2W iv. He has experienced an ongoing CR persisting during follow-up after treatment (16+ months).

Activity and Efficacy

Cemiplimab has shown substantial antitumor activity in patients with locally advanced (laCSCC) and metastatic cutaneous squamous cell carcinoma (mCSCC).

Cempilimab activity in laCSCC and mCSCC has been proven in open label, phase 2, single arm clinical trial. This pivotal study (NCT02760498) was done across 25 outpatient clinics. Eligible patients were participants aged ≥18 years with histologically confirmed laCSCC or mCSCC and an ECOG PS 0–1. Tumor response was assessed every 8 weeks. The primary endpoint was ORR, defined as the proportion of patients with complete or partial response, according to independent central review as per RECIST 1.1 for radiological scans and WHO criteria for medical photography. Analyses were done as per the intention-to-treat (ITT) principle. This study included three groups of patients with advanced CSCC. Group 1 (GP1) contained patients with metastatic disease and group 2 (GP2) had patients with locally advanced disease, in both groups, patients received 3 mg/kg of cemiplimab Q2W. In group 3 (GP3), patients with metastatic disease received 350 mg of cemiplimab Q3W [6–8].

In 2018, the combined analysis of the results of the phase 1 study for expansion cohorts of patients with CSCC ($n = 26$) and the results of the primary analysis of the pivotal phase 2 study for cohort of patients with mCSCC ($n = 59$) was published (NCT02383212, NCT02760498). The expansion cohorts of the phase 1 study involved adult patients with laCSCC (not eligible for surgery) or mCSCC. In both studies, the patients received an intravenous dose of cemiplimab (3 mg per kilogram of body weight) Q2W and were assessed for a response every 8 weeks. The data cut-off points were October 2, 2017, for the expansion cohorts of the phase 1 study and October 27, 2017, for the metastatic-disease cohort of the phase 2 study. Cemiplimab has shown similar efficacy for the treatment of mCSCC and laCSCC. The response rate in the group of 75 patients with mCSCC (59 patients with mCSCC from phase 2 study, and 16 patients with mCSCC from phase 1 study who met the criteria for metastatic disease used in phase 2 study) was 47% (95% CI: 35–59) [9].

The analysis after 12-month follow-up from GP1 has confirmed the efficacy of cemiplimab in mCSCC ($n = 59$). The data cut-off date was Sep 20, 2018. The median duration of follow-up was 16.5 months (range: 1.1–26.6). ORR by central review was 49.2% (95% CI: 35.9–62.5), 10 CRs and 19 PRs have been achieved. Median DOR has not been reached. The longest DOR at data cut-off was 21.6 months and was still ongoing. Observed DOR exceeded 12 months in 22/29 pts (75.9%) with response. Durable DCR, defined as CR + PR + SD for ≥16 weeks, was 62.7% (95% CI: 49.1–75.0). Median observed time to response was 1.9 months (range: 1.7–9.1). Median PFS was 18.4 months (95% CI: 7.3–not evaluable) and median OS has not been reached [6].

The analysis for GP2 published in 2020 confirmed the efficacy of cemiplimab in laCSCC ($n = 78$). At the time of data cut-off the median duration of study follow-up was 9.3 months. An objective response was observed in 34 (44%; 95% CI 32–55) of 78 patients. The best overall response was 10 patients with CR (13%) and 24 (31%) with PR. DCR was 79%. Among all patients, median PFS and median OS had not been reached at data cut-off. 48 (62%) of the 78 patients enrolled had samples available for tumor PD-L1 status assessment at baseline. Expression was assessed as the percentage of tumor cells with detectable PD-L1 membrane staining (tumor proportion score, TPS). An objective response was observed in 6 (35%) of the 17 patients with PD-L1 TPS of less than 1% and in 17 (55%) of the 31 patients with PD-L1 TPS at least 1%. Objective responses were observed in patients regardless of baseline PD-L1 TPS. Tumor mutational burden (TMB) was assessed in the DNA samples extracted from the formalin-fixed paraffin embedded tumor biopsies with the ana-lytically validated TruSight Oncology 500 to detect single nucleotide variants, insertions and deletions, copy number alterations in 500 genes, and a selected set of gene rearrangements and was calculated as the total number of somatic single nucleotide variants and insertions and deletions in the coding regions of targeted genes per megabase of analyzed genomic sequence. 50 (64%) of the 78 patients enrolled had pretreatment tumor samples available for the analysis of TMB. Median TMB was 74 mutations per megabase among 21 patients who responded to treat-ment and 29 mutations per megabase among 29 patients who did not respond. Among 29 patients with durable disease control median TMB was 65. The analysis of association of TMB has shown that TMB is not predictive biomarker in laCSCC [8].

The primary analysis from GP3 ($n = 56$) with median follow-up 8.1 months and long-term outcome from GP1 ($n = 59$) with median follow-up 16.5 months were published by Rischin et al. [10]. ORR based on central review was 41.1% (95% CI: 28.1%–55.0%) in GP3, 49.2% (95% CI: 35.9%–62.5%) in GP1, and 45.2% (95% CI: 35.9%–54.8%) in both groups combined. Based on investigator assessments ORR was 51.8% (95% CI: 38.0%–65.3%) in GP3, 49.2% (95% CI: 35.9%–62.5%) in GP1, and 50.4% (95% CI: 41.0%–59.9%) in both groups combined. DCR based on central review was 64.3% (95% CI: 50.4%–76.6%) in GP3, 71.2% (95% CI: 57.9%–82.2%) in GP1, and 67.8% (95% CI: 58.5%–76.2%) in both groups com-bined. The durable DCR (defined as CR + PR + SD for $\geq$ 105 days) per central review was 57.1% (95% CI: 43.2%–70.3%) in GP3, 61.0% (95% CI: 47.4%–73.5%) in GP1, and 59.1% (95% CI: 49.6%–68.2%) in both groups combined. Median PFS, OS and DOR have not been reached. Median TMB in patients with response from GP3 was 61.4 and in patients with response from GP1 was 53.2 mutations per megabase. Median TMB in patients without response from GP3 and GP1 was 13.7 and 19.4 mutations per megabase, respectively [10].

The updated analysis published in May 2020, with the data cut-off October 11, 2019, confirmed the efficacy of cemiplimab in advanced CSCC [11]. Eventually 193 patients were enrolled into the study, 128 patients were treatment-naive and 65 patients were previously treated with anti-cancer systemic therapy. ORR per inves-tigator assessment was 57.8% (95% CI: 48.8–66.5) among treatment-naïve patients and 47.7% (95% CI: 35.1–60.5) among previously treated patients. The observed time to response was 2 months for 41 (46.1%) patients, 2–4 months for 29 (32.6%) patients, 4–6 months for eight (9.0%) patients, and >6 months for 11 (12.4%) patients. Median DOR has not been reached (1.8–34.2 months). In patients with response to treatment estimated proportion of patients with ongoing response at 24 months was 76.0% (95% CI: 64.1–84.4). Median OS has not been reached and estimated OS at 24 months was 73.3% (95% CI: 66.1–79.2). The duration of follow-up and ORR based on investigator assessment for the whole study popula-tion and for each cohort are presented in Table 16.1.

In 2020, the post hoc exploratory analysis of quality of life (QoL) from phase 2 clinical trial (NCT02760498) has been published. The QoL was examined using the EORTC cancer specific 30-item HRQL questionnaire (QLQ-C30). The QLQ-C30

Table 16.1 Updated results from phase 2 study [11]

	All patients (n = 193)	GP1 (n = 59)	GP2 (n = 78)	GP3 (n = 56)
Median duration of follow-up (range), in months	15.7 (0.6–36.1)	18.5 (1.1–36.1)	15.5 (0.8–35.0)	17.3 (0.6–26.3)
ORR per investigator assessment	54.4% (95% CI: 47.1–61.6)	50.8% (95% CI: 37.5–64.1)	56.4% (95% CI: 44.7–67.6)	55.4% (95% CI: 41.5–68.7)

was completed by patients at baseline and day 1 of each treatment cycle. At baseline the reported scores indicated moderate to high levels of functioning and low symptom burden. There was a clinically meaningful improvement in pain score observed from baseline to cycle 5, other items remained stable or showed a trend toward improvement (global health status, physical function, role function, emotional function, social function, fatigue, insomnia). Similar findings were observed on individual symptoms (dyspnea, nausea/vomiting, diarrhea, constipation, appetite loss) and in each treatment group. The health-related quality of life (HRQL) in most patients was either improved or maintained [12].

The efficacy of cemiplimab has been confirmed in clinical practice. The retrospective analysis of data from 247 patients with CSCC treated with cemiplimab 3 mg per kg Q2W in 45 French sites has been published in 2020. Among the patients included in this analysis 37% had laCSCC, 36% had regional disease, and 27% had mCSCC. 26% of patients were immunocompromised. 72% of patients was in good PS (0–1). Half of the patients received cemiplimab in first line treatment. The median follow-up was 12 months. Median number of cemiplimab infusions was 10 (0–35). The best response rate among 188 patients who received more than 1 infusion of cemiplimab was 50% (CI 95%: 43–57), 40 patients achieved CR, and 54 patients experienced PR. DCR was 60%. Median PFS was 11 months. Median OS and DOR were not reached [13].

Toxicity Profile

In the phase 2 study (NCT02760498), all patients who received at least one dose of cemiplimab were assessed for safety. Safety assessment was done from the first study dose up to 105 days after the last study dose. Laboratory tests, i.e., blood chemistry and hematology, were done before each study drug dose and 30 days after the last dose. The severity of adverse events was graded according to the NCI-CTCAE v. 4.03 [6–8].

In the first analysis from the mCSCC cohort from phase 2 study published in 2018, the most common AEs were diarrhea (in 27% of the patients), fatigue (24%), nausea (17%), constipation (15%), and rash (15%). Four patients (7%) discontinued treatment due to AE. AEs of G3 or higher that occurred in more than one patient were cellulitis, pneumonitis, hypercalcemia, pleural effusion, and death. 21 serious

AEs were reported (36%), 17 at least G3 (29%). Four AEs of any G led to treatment discontinuation and three were associated with an outcome of death [9].

The data reported in 2019 for GP1 indicated that there were no new safety signals. The most common TEAEs (all G, G ≥ 3) were diarrhea (28.8%, 1.7%), fatigue (25.4%, 1.7%), and nausea (23.7%, 0%). Based on investigator assessment G ≥ 3 immune-related adverse events occurred in 13.6% of patients [6].

As per the updated analysis for GP2 from the phase 2 study published in 2020 no new safety signals were reported in comparison to previous reports of cemiplimab or other anti-PD-1 agents [8]. Most of reported TRAE were G1 or G2. In the group of 78 patients with locally advanced CSCC G3–4 TEAEs occurred in 34 (44%) of 78 patients. The most common were hypertension in six (8%) patients and pneumonia in four (5%) patients. One (1%) of the 78 patients required dose reduction due to arthralgia G2, that was considered related to study treatment. Six (8%) of the 78 patients discontinued treatment due to the following TEAE: G4 pneumonia and G4 pneumonitis in one patient; G3 hepatitis, G3 increased ALT, G3 increased AST, and G3 increased ALP in the second patient; and the following in each of the remaining four patients: G4 pneumonitis, G3 proctitis, G3 encephalitis, and G1 arthralgia. Serious TEAE occurred in 23 (29%) of 78 patients. In seven (9%) patients serious TEAE were considered treatment related. The most common was pneumonitis in three (4%) patients. G ≥ 3 irAEs, occurred in eight (10%) of the 78 patients. Two of 78 patients (3%) had TEAE that resulted in death. One was due to infectious pneumonia that was assessed as unrelated to study treatment by the investigator and one occurred 10 days after the onset of aspiration pneumonia and was assessed as related to study drug.

In the long-term follow-up, the most common TEAEs by any G were fatigue (34.7%), diarrhea (27.5%), and nausea (23.8%). The most common G ≥ 3 TEAEs were hypertension (4.7%), anemia, and cellulitis (each 4.1%) [11].

Based on cemiplimab summary of product characteristics the safety of cemiplimab has been evaluated in 591 patients with advanced solid malignancies, including 219 patients with advanced CSCC. Immune-related adverse reactions (irARs) occurred in 20.3% of patients treated with cemiplimab including G5 (0.7%), G4 (1.2%) and G3 (6.3%). IrARs led to permanent treatment discontinuation in 4.4% of patients. The most common irARs were hypothyroidism (7.1%), pneumonitis (3.7%), immune-related skin adverse reactions (2.0%), hyperthyroidism (1.9%), and hepatitis (1.9%). Serious ARs were reported in 8.6% patients and led to permanent discontinuation of cemiplimab in 5.8% of patients. Severe cutaneous ARs (SCARs), including Stevens-Johnson syndrome (SJS) and toxic epidermal necrolysis (TEN) have been reported in patients treated with cemiplimab (Table 16.2).

The selected adverse reactions based on safety of cemiplimab in 591 patients in uncontrolled clinical studies are summarized in Table 16.3.

The following clinically significant, immune-related adverse reactions occurred at an incidence of less than 1% of 591 patients treated with cemiplimab. The events were Grade 3 or less unless stated otherwise [2]:

Nervous system disorders: Meningitis (Grade 4), paraneoplastic encephalomyelitis (Grade 5), Guillain-Barre syndrome, central nervous system inflammation,

Table 16.2 Adverse reactions in patients treated with cemiplimab [2]

System organ class preferred term	G1–5 (Frequency category)	G 1–5 (%)	G3–5 (%)
Immune system disorders			
Infusion-related reaction	Common	4.1	0
Sjogren's syndrome	Uncommon	0.5	0
Immune thrombocytopenic purpura	Uncommon	0.2	0
Vasculitis	Uncommon	0.2	0
Solid organ transplant rejection[a]	Not known	–	–
Endocrine disorders			
Hypothyroidism	Common	9.6	0
Hyperthyroidism	Common	2.7	0
Type 1 diabetes mellitus[b]	Uncommon	0.7	0.7
Adrenal insufficiency	Uncommon	0.5	0.5
Hypophysitis	Uncommon	0.5	0.5
Thyroiditis	Uncommon	0.2	0
Nervous system disorders			
Paraneoplastic encephalomyelitis	Uncommon	0.2	0.2
Chronic inflammatory demyelinating polyradiculoneuropathy	Uncommon	0.5	0
Encephalitis	Uncommon	0.5	0.5
Meningitis[c]	Uncommon	0.5	0.5
Guillain-Barre syndrome	Uncommon	0.2	0.2
Central nervous system inflammation	Uncommon	0.2	0
Neuropathy peripheral[d]	Uncommon	0.5	0
Myasthenia gravis	Uncommon	0.2	0
Eye disorders			
Keratitis	Uncommon	0.5	0
Cardiac disorders			
Myocarditis[e]	Uncommon	0.5	0.5
Pericarditis[f]	Uncommon	0.5	0.5
Respiratory, thoracic and mediastinal disorders			
Pneumonitis	Common	5.9	2.3
Dyspnoea[g]	Common	2.6	0.3
Gastrointestinal disorders			
Diarrhea[h]	Very common	13.2	0.5
Stomatitis	Common	2.4	0
Hepatobiliary disorders			
Hepatitis[i]	Common	1.4	1.4
Skin and subcutaneous skin disorders			
Rash[j]	Very common	23.3	1.4
Pruritus[k]	Very common	12.3	0

System organ class preferred term	G1–5 (Frequency category)	G 1–5 (%)	G3–5 (%)
Musculoskeletal and connective tissue disorders			
Arthralgia	Common	5.0	0
Musculoskeletal pain[l]	Common	4.1	0.5
Arthritis[m]	Common	1.4	0.5
Muscular weakness	Uncommon	0.9	0
Polymyalgia rheumatica	Uncommon	0.5	0
Myositis[g]	Rare	< 0.1	< 0.1
Renal and urinary disorders			
Nephritis	Uncommon	0.5	0
General disorders and administration site conditions			
Fatigue[n]	Very common	21.5	0.9
Investigations			
Alanine aminotransferase increased	Common	5.5	0.5
Aspartate aminotransferase increased	Common	5.0	0.9
Blood alkaline phosphatase increased	Common	2.7	0
Blood creatinine increased	Common	1.8	0

[a]Post-marketing event
[b]Type 1 diabetes mellitus is a composite term that includes diabetes mellitus, diabetic ketoacidosis, and type 1 diabetes mellitus
[c]Meningitis is a composite term that includes meningitis and meningitis aseptic
[d]Neuropathy peripheral is a composite term that includes neuropathy peripheral and neuritis
[e]Myocarditis is a composite term that includes autoimmune myocarditis and myocarditis
[f]Pericarditis is a composite term that includes autoimmune pericarditis and pericarditis
[g]Frequency was based on 2184 patients in ongoing clinical studies across multiple cancer types
[h]Diarrhea is a composite term that includes diarrhea and colitis
[i]Hepatitis is a composite term that includes hepatitis and autoimmune hepatitis
[j]Rash is a composite term that includes rash maculo-papular, rash, dermatitis, rash generalized, dermatitis bullous, drug eruption, erythema, pemphigoid, psoriasis, rash erythematous, rash macular, rash pruritic, and skin reaction
[k]Pruritus is a composite term that includes pruritus and pruritus allergic
[l]Musculoskeletal pain is a composite term that includes back pain, musculoskeletal pain, myalgia, neck pain, and pain in extremity
[m]Arthritis is a composite term that includes arthritis and polyarthritis
[n]Fatigue is a composite term that includes fatigue and asthenia

chronic inflammatory demyelinating polyradiculoneuropathy, encephalitis, myasthenia gravis, neuropathy peripheral.

Cardiac Disorders: Myocarditis, pericarditis

Immune system disorders: Immune thrombocytopenic purpura

Vascular disorders: Vasculitis

Musculoskeletal and connective tissue disorders: Arthralgia (1.4%), arthritis, muscular weakness, myalgia, polymyalgia rheumatica, Sjogren's syndrome

Table 16.3 The selected adverse reactions based on safety of cemiplimab in 591 patients in uncontrolled clinical studies (GC, corticosteroid) [2]

irAR	Number of AR	Grades at least 3	Discontinuation due to this AR	Median time to onset (range)	Median duration (range)	Patients treated with GC	Duration of GC, median (range)	Resolution at the data cut-off
Pneumonitis	22/591 (3.7%)	G3–6 (1.0%); G4–2 (0.3%); G5–2 (0.3%)	11/591 (1.9%)	3.8 months (7 days to 18 months)	21.5 days (5 days to 6.5 months)	18 (high dose GC)	8.5 days (1 day to 5.9 months)	14/22 (63.6%)
Diarrhea or colitis	7/591 (1.2%)	G3–2 (0.3%)	1/591 (0.2%)	3.8 months (15 days to 6.0 months)	30 days (4 days to 8.6 months)	4 (high dose GC)	29 days (19 days to 2.0 months)	4/7 (57.1%)
Hepatitis	11/591 (1.9%)	G3–9 (1.5%); G4–1 (0.2%); G5–1 (0.2%)	5/591 (0.8%)	1.0 month (7 days to 4.2 months)	15 days (8 days to 2.7 months)	10 (high dose GC)	10.5 days (2 days to 1.9 months)	8/11 (72.7%)
Hypothyroidism	42/591 (7.1%)	G3–1 (0.2%)	0/591	4.2 months (15 days to 18.9 months)	No data	No data	No data	No data
Hyperthyroidism	11/591 (1.9%)	G3–1 (0.2%)	0/591	1.9 months (28 days to 14.8 months)	No data	No data	No data	No data
Adrenal insufficiency	3/591 (0.5%)	G3–1 (0.2%)	0/591	11.5 months (10.4 months to 12.3 months)	No data	1	No data	No data
Hypophysitis	1/591 (0.2%)	G3–1	No data	No data	No data	No data	No data	No data
Type 1 diabetes mellitus	4/591 (0.7%)	G3–1 (0.2%); G4–3 (0.5%)	1/591 (0.2%)	2.3 months (28 days to 6.2 months)	No data	No data	No data	No data
Skin reactions	12/591 (2.0%)	G3–6 (1.0%)	2/591 (0.3%)	1.5 months (2 days to 10.9 months)	4.4 months (14 days to 9.6 months)	9 (high dose GC)	16 days (7 days to 2.6 months)	6/12 (50%)
Nephritis	3/591 (0.5%)	G3–2 (0.3%)	1/591 (0.2%)	1.8 months (29 days to 4.1 months)	18 days (9 days to 29 days)	2 (high dose GC)	1.5 months (16 days to 2.6 months)	3/3 (100%)

Eye disorders: Keratitis

Gastrointestinal disorders: Stomatitis

Endocrine: Thyroiditis

Infusion-related reactions (IRR) occurred in 54 of 591 patients (9.1%) including 1 (0.2%) patient with G3 reaction and led to treatment discontinuation of cemiplimab in 2 (0.3%) patients. The most common symptoms of IRR were nausea, pyrexia, vomiting, abdominal pain, chills, and flushing. All patients recovered from IRR.

1.1% of patients developed treatment-emergent antibodies, with about 0.2% exhibiting persistent antibody responses. No neutralizing antibodies have been observed. There was no evidence of an altered pharmacokinetic or safety profile with anti-cemiplimab antibody development.

No studies have been done to test the potential of cemiplimab for carcinogenicity or genotoxicity. Animal reproduction studies have not been conducted.

In the French study published by Hober et al. [13] TRAEs were reported in 49 patients (26%). The most common were fatigue, hypothyroidism, and cholestasis. G3-G4 TRAEs were reported in 18 patients (9%). 10 patients discontinued therapy due to TRAE. No treatment-related deaths were reported [13].

Summary of Approval and Regulatory Indications

Cemiplimab as monotherapy is indicated for the treatment of adult patients with metastatic or locally advanced cutaneous squamous cell carcinoma who are not candidates for curative surgery or curative radiation. The drug has been approved in United States in September 2018 and in Europe in July 2019. The recommended dose is 350 mg cemiplimab, every 3 weeks, administered as an intravenous infusion over 30 min. Treatment may be continued until disease progression or unacceptable toxicity. No premedication is required. No dose reductions are recommended. Dosing delay or discontinuation may be required based on individual safety and tolerability. Recommended modifications to manage adverse reactions are provided in the summary of product characteristics. No dose adjustment is recommended for older patients. No dose adjustment is recommended for patients with renal impairment and patients with mild hepatic impairment. Cemiplimab has not been studied in patients with moderate or severe hepatic impairment. The safety and efficacy of cemiplimab in children and adolescents below the age of 18 years have not been established [2, 14].

References

1. Burova E, Hermann A, Waite J, et al. Characterization of the anti-PD-1 antibody REGN2810 and its antitumor activity in human PD-1 knock-in mice. Mol Cancer Ther. 2017;16:861–70.
2. Libtayo, cemiplimab, summary of product characteristics. December 2020. https://www.ema.europa.eu/en/documents/product-information/libtayo-epar-product-information_en.pdf.

3. Papadopoulos KP, Owonikoko TK, Johnson ML, et al. REGN2810: A fully human anti-PD-1 monoclonal antibody, for patients with unresectable locally advanced or metastatic cutaneous squamous cell carcinoma (CSCC) – Initial safety and efficacy from expansion cohorts (ECs) of phase I study. J Clin Oncol. 2017;35(suppl):abstr. 9503.

4. Papadopoulos KP, Johnson ML, Lockhart AC, et al. First-in-human study of cemiplimab alone or in combination with radiotherapy and/or low dose cyclophosphamide in patients with advanced malignancies. Clin Cancer Res. 2020;26(5):1025–33.

5. Falchook GS, Leidner R, Stankevich E, et al. Responses of metastatic basal cell and cutaneous squamous cell carcinomas to anti-PD1 monoclonal antibody REGN2810. J Immunother Cancer. 2016;4:70.

6. Guminski AD, Lim AML, Khushalani NI, et al. Phase 2 study of cemiplimab, a human monoclonal anti-PD-1, in patients (pts) with metastatic cutaneous squamous cell carcinoma (mCSCC; Group 1): 12-month follow-up. J Clin Oncol. 2019;37(suppl):abstr. 9526.

7. Migden MR, Khushalani NI, Chang ALS, et al. Primary analysis of Phase 2 results of cemiplimab, a human monoclonal anti-PD-1, in patients (pts) with locally advanced cutaneous squamous cell carcinoma (laCSCC). J Clin Oncol. 2019;37(suppl):abstr. 6015.

8. Migden MR, Khushalani NI, Chang ALS, et al. Cemiplimab in locally advanced cutaneous squamous cell carcinoma: results from an open-label, phase 2, single-arm trial. Lancet Oncol. 2020;21(2):294–305.

9. Migden MR, Rischin D, Schmults CD. PD-1 blockade with cemiplimab in advanced cutaneous squamous-cell carcinoma. N Engl J Med. 2018;379:341–51.

10. Rischin D, Migden MR, Lim AM, et al. Phase 2 study of cemiplimab in patients with metastatic cutaneous squamous cell carcinoma: primary analysis of fixed-dosing, long-term outcome of weight-based dosing. J Immunother Cancer. 2020;8(1):e000775. https://doi.org/10.1136/jitc-2020-000775.

11. Rischin D, Khushalani NI, Schmults CD, et al. Phase II study of cemiplimab in patients (pts) with advanced cutaneous squamous cell carcinoma (CSCC): longer follow-up. J Clin Oncol. 2020;38(suppl 15):10018.

12. Migden MR, Rischin D, Sasane M, et al. Health-related quality of life (HRQL) in patients with advanced cutaneous squamous cell carcinoma (CSCC) treated with cemiplimab: Post hoc exploratory analyses of a phase II clinical trial. J Clin Oncol. 2020;38(suppl):abst. 10033.

13. Hober C, Fredeau L, Pham Ledard A, et al. 1086P Cemiplimab for advanced cutaneous squamous cell carcinoma: Real life experience. Annals of Oncology. 2020;31:S737.

14. Cemiplimab (Libtayo) injection, for intravenous use, prescribing information.

Chapter 17
Perspectives of Immunotherapy in Non-Melanoma Skin Cancers

Marco Rubatto, Paolo Fava, Gianluca Avallone, Andrea Agostini, Luca Mastorino, Martina Merli, Simone Ribero, and Pietro Quaglino

Non-Melanoma Skin Cancer: Definition of the Disease Group and Implications for Treatment

Non-melanoma skin cancers (NMSCs) represent the most common form of cancer in Caucasians, with continuing increase in incidence worldwide [1]. Traditionally, this term referred mainly to skin tumours deriving from keratinocytes, thus including basal cell carcinoma (BCC) and cutaneous squamous cell carcinoma (cSCC), which represent from an epidemiological point of view, the most frequent subtypes. However, as a broad interpretation, NMSCs refer to all kind of tumours that primarily arise in the skin and are not melanoma. In this view, NMSCs represent a wide and heterogeneous group of diseases including a great variety of skin tumours characterised by different origins, clinical features, disease courses and prognoses. Indeed, besides BCC and cSCC, we can consider as part of this group Merkel cell carcinoma (MCC) (Fig. 17.1), dermatofibrosarcoma protuberans, adnexal carcinoma, atypical fibroxanthoma, soft tissue sarcomas including angiosarcoma and particularly Kaposi sarcoma, and primary cutaneous lymphoma.

From an epidemiological point of view, BCC is the most common form and represents the most frequent malignant tumour types in humans, followed by cSCC. On the other hand, other NMSCs such as Merkel cell carcinoma or primary cutaneous lymphoma are very rare even if for all these diseases, the incidence is rapidly increasing. In the majority of cases, affected people are elderly and cutaneous sites of development are represented by the head and neck area (BCC, cSCC and MCC). This body site links the clinic with the pathogenesis. Three main pathogenetic

M. Rubatto · P. Fava · G. Avallone · A. Agostini · L. Mastorino · M. Merli · S. Ribero
P. Quaglino (✉)
Department of Medical Sciences, Dermatologic Clinic, University of Turin Medical School, Turin, Italy
e-mail: pietro.quaglino@unito.it

P. Rutkowski, M. Mandalà (eds.), *New Therapies in Advanced Cutaneous Malignancies*, https://doi.org/10.1007/978-3-030-64009-5_17

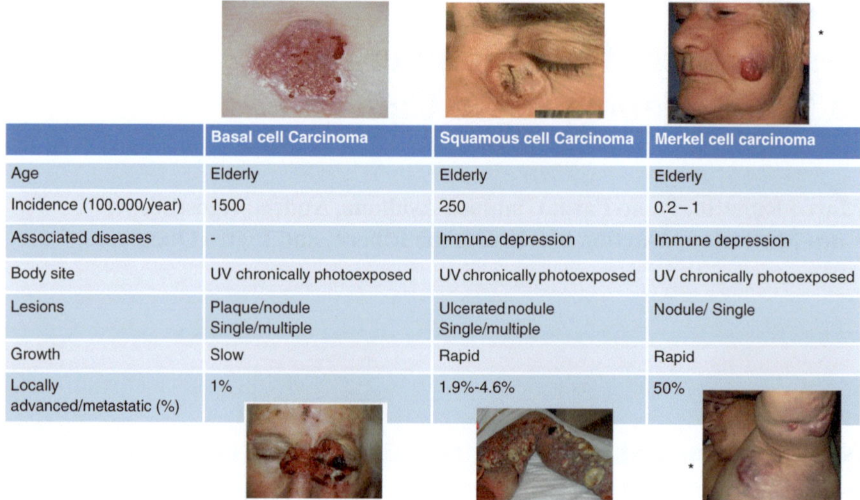

	Basal cell Carcinoma	Squamous cell Carcinoma	Merkel cell carcinoma
Age	Elderly	Elderly	Elderly
Incidence (100.000/year)	1500	250	0.2 – 1
Associated diseases	-	Immune depression	Immune depression
Body site	UV chronically photoexposed	UV chronically photoexposed	UV chronically photoexposed
Lesions	Plaque/nodule Single/multiple	Ulcerated nodule Single/multiple	Nodule/ Single
Growth	Slow	Rapid	Rapid
Locally advanced/metastatic (%)	1%	1.9%-4.6%	50%

Fig. 17.1 The main demographic, clinical and disease course features of BCC, SCC and MCC (asterisk, courtesy of Dr. Franco Picciotto, AOU Città della Salute e della Scienza, Torino)

factors are present in specific subtypes of NMSC. The most important and shared by BCC, cSCC and MCC is constituted by Ultraviolet (UV)-chronic irradiation. The second is represented by the presence of virus as co-factor (HHV-8 for Kaposi sarcoma, Merkel cell polyoma virus for MCC and papillomavirus for some kind of cSCC particularly those arising on mucosal sites and in immune-suppressed patients). As third factor, immune suppression characteristically increases the risk of developing these tumours, as demonstrated by the largely shared evidence that cSCC are most common in transplanted patients and that about 20% of MCC develop in patients with onco-haematological diseases, treated by chemotherapy, organ-transplant recipients and patients undergoing immune-suppressive regimens for autoimmune diseases.

Significant differences can be found between these diseases according to disease course and survival. As to cSCC, even if more than 90% of patients are disease-free after surgery at a 5-year follow-up, a percentage of patients ranging from 1.9% to 4.6% develop disease recurrence or progression, the majority of whom in the first 2 years after the initial intervention. The term of advanced cSCC refers indeed to these cases which can be further sub-divided into two groups: locally advanced cSCC and metastatic. The first group of patients show a local progression, which per definition is no longer amenable to surgery or radiation therapy [2]. Even if there is no exact agreement on which cSCC are considered advanced, it is clear that specific characteristics contribute to this appearance beyond the dimensions (generally more than T2) including a critical site (e.g. periocular region), depth of invasion, multiple lesions and previous repeated relapses. It can be considered that roughly advanced CSS can represent 5% of the total CSS population [3]. Even if the disease-specific survival is favourable as overall (93.6% at 10 year) [4], the survival of advanced cases is poor. According to a French collaborative study [5], the median progression-free survival (PFS) after the first line of systemic treatment in the pre-check point inhibitors era is 6 months, and the associated median overall survival (OS) is 18.3 months.

BCC is more frequent overall than cSCC even if it is characterised by a very indolent disease course, with only 1% of cases developing advanced disease. The possibility of metastatic disease in these cases is anecdotic (less than 200 cases reported in the literature). Median OS for metastatic BCC patients treated with vismodegib is 33.4 months according to the data of the Erivance study [6].

MCC is characterised by a highly aggressive disease course, as more than half the patients show metastatic disease at the initial diagnosis [7]. According to AIRTUM data, survival at 1 year after initial diagnosis is 85%, and it drops to 57% after 5 years from diagnosis [8]. Survival of metastatic patients in the era pre-check point inhibitors is poor with 18% at 5 years for distant metastatic disease [9, 10].

Rationale for the Use of Immunotherapy in NMSC

The treatment of NMSC is based on surgery which represents the first line therapy. A wide local excision is recommended. For MCC, sentinel node biopsy and completion dissection is required. Radiotherapy represents a treatment of choice in cases not amenable to surgery but also it is used a consolidation after surgery in high-risk cSCC (peri-neural invasion), and routinely used in MCC both on T and N if involved by disease. Chemotherapy was usually deserved to locally advanced or metastatic patients, however with low activity particularly in terms of response duration. Moreover, chemotherapy is weighted by frequently severe side effects particularly relevant in this subset of elderly patients.

Immunotherapy with check-point inhibitors (ICI) (namely anti-PD-1 or anti-PDL-1) has now become part of our therapeutic armamentarium in these patients, on the basis of the relevant results achieved by multicentre trials even if due to the rarity of these diseases (MCC) or the rarity of advanced cases (BCC and cSCC) together with the absence of a well-recognised standard treatment of care, no randomised clinical study is available. At the moment in Italy two drugs are approved and reimbursed by the national health system (avelumab for MCC and cemiplimab for cSCC).

The rationale for the application of immunotherapy in NMSC is based on three group of factors: molecular, pathologic and clinical (Fig. 17.2).

Tumour mutational burden (TMB) measures the quantity of somatic mutations found in a tumour and has been attributed to both endogenous factors and environmental damage. Defective DNA replication/repair or exogenous stimuli, including UV radiation, tobacco smoking, alcohol, and chemicals, cause biased accumulation of somatic mutations, which result in corresponding signatures in specific tumours. A number of clinical trials have revealed that TMB is correlated with the rate of response to anti-PD-1/PD-L1 blockade [11]. Both BCC and cSCC show a marked

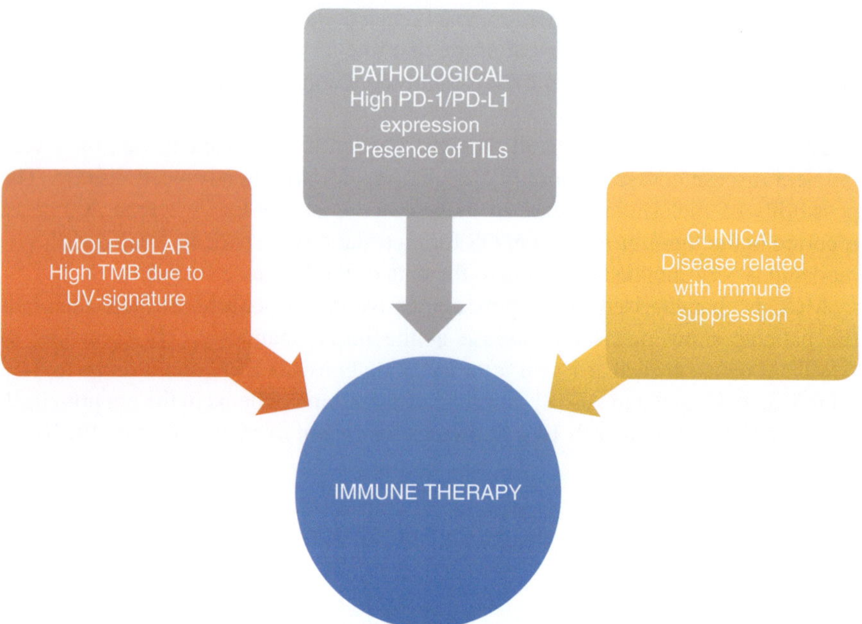

Fig. 17.2 The rationale for the use of immune therapy in NMSC. *TMB* tumour mutational burden, *TIL* tumour-infiltrating lymphocytes, *UV* ultraviolet

UV-signature, thus it is conceivable that these cancers exhibit the highest TMB among all other cancer types. In a work in which the DNA of 100,000 human tumours was analysed and in which the tumour mutational burden was studied, it was evident that the BCC and cSCC rank at the top of the ranking with a higher mutation rate (47.3 mutations/Mb for BCC and 45.2 for cSCC). The mutational load of cSCCs is the second highest of all human cancers. At a median rate of approximately 45 mutations/Mb, this rate suggests that PD-1 inhibitors could have activity against cSCC. TMB values are also similar for virus-negative MCC which shows the same UV-signature. The increased expression of neo-antigens which is associated with a high TMB, which likely results in higher levels of tumour neo-antigens that may be targets for the immune system. Viral antigens in virus-positive MCC are also strongly immunogenic [12].

As a second point, from a clinical perspective, the mentioned high incidence of NMSC, in particular cSCC and MCC, with conditions of immune suppression as well as the poor disease course of these cases highlights the relevance of the host immune response in the development and evolution of these diseases.

As a third point, from a pathological point of view, these tumours are characterised by a significant expression of the PD-1/PDL-1 axis both in tumour cells and microenvironment in the immune infiltrate. In an analysis of 67 MCC specimens, tumour cells expressed PD-L1 in 49% of cases, whilst tumour-infiltrating lymphocytes PD-L1 expression were observed in 55% of patients [13]. In another study,

PD-L1 was found to be expressed in the tumour microenvironment in half the cases; considering the cases with moderate-to-high intensity of tumour-infiltrating lymphocytes, 100% of cases stained positive for PD-L1 tumour expression [14]. Similarly, in a study on biopsy specimens in cSCC and lung adenocarcinoma, PD-1 and CD8 Tumour-infiltrating lymphocytes (TILs) were more frequently distributed in SCC than in lung cancer and the density of TILs was a favourable prognostic indicator in cSCC. Moreover, PD-L1 levels had prognostic clinical relevance in as much as patients with a tumour microenvironment type characterised by high expression of both PD-L1 and TILs had the longest survival [15]. Also concerning cutaneous T-cell lymphoma, it has been shown that specific subtypes of these diseases express PD-1 at high levels [16].

Even if immune environment plays a major role in both BCC and cSCC, probably cSCC presents a higher immunogenicity than BCC in spite of its higher TMB. This theory could also explain the higher incidence of cSCC in immune-suppressed and transplant patients. The biological features in BCC associated with this difference include a reduced infiltration by CD4 and particularly CD8 T cells with increased T-regs, the expression of immunosuppressive Th2 cytokines and interleukin-10 and the reduced antigen presentation due to major histocompatibility complex type 1 (MHC-I)down-regulation [17].

Immunotherapy with Anti-PD-1/PD-L1 Blockade in NMSC: Clinical Results

cSCC

The first medication for cSCC, a breakthrough therapy, was the PD-1 inhibitor cemiplimab (REGN2810), which was approved in 2018 by the US Food and Drug Administration (FDA) for use in patients with locally advanced or metastatic disease who are not candidates for curative surgery or curative radiation. The approved dose was 350 mg intravenously over 30 min every 3 weeks. The drug has been approved also by European Medicines Agency (EMA), and it is actually reimbursed in Italy for the same indications.

The approval is based on the results of combined data from phase I (for expansion cohorts of patients with locally advanced or metastatic cSCC; $n = 26$) and pivotal phase II (only patients with metastatic disease; $n = 59$) open-label, multicentre trial. Cemiplimab was given intravenously at a dose of 3 mg per kilogram of body weight) every 2 weeks. In the phase 2 study, the primary end-point was the overall response rate (ORR), as assessed by independent central review. The majority of patients had prior surgery and radiation, and inclusion into the study required a multidisciplinary evaluation regarding lack of suitability for further surgery and radiation. In the expansion cohorts of the phase 1 study, a response to cemiplimab was observed in 13 of 26 patients (50%), whilst in the metastatic-disease cohort of the phase 2 study, a 47% response rate was achieved. The data showed a 50% best ORR, with over 60% achieving durable disease control, defined as disease control for >105 days. Serious adverse effects accounted for less than 10% of adverse events. The most common adverse events observed in the published data, in descending order of frequency, included diarrhoea (27% of patients), fatigue (24%), nausea (17%), constipation (15%), and rash (15%). Hypothyroidism, alanine aminotransferase, and pneumonitis were all observed in 8% of patients [3].

The second study on cemiplimab was published recently [18]. It was an open-label, phase 2, single-arm trial performed in Australia, Germany and the USA which enrolled 78 patients with histologically confirmed locally advanced cSCC treated with cemiplimab 3 mg/kg intravenously over 30 min every 2 weeks for up to 96 weeks. The primary end-point was objective response. An objective response was observed in 34 (44%) of 78 patients, with 13% of patients with complete response. Disease control was achieved in 79% of patients and durable disease control (defined as lasting more than 105 days) in 63% of patients. The response characteristics were represented by a short time of induction (median: 1.9 months; range: 1.9–3.7) and a long duration (median not reached; 68% of responses lasting for > = 6 months; 87% of patients maintaining the response at 12 months). PFS at 1 year was 58%, whilst OS 93%.

In a post-hoc subgroup analysis exploring the different reasons why patients were not considered candidates for curative surgery, the response to cemiplimab was 50% in patients with substantial local invasion that precluded complete resection, 57% in patients with cSCC lesions in anatomically challenging locations for which surgery would result in severe deformity or dysfunction, whilst only 24% in patients with cSCC in the same location after 2 or more surgical procedures and disease relapsed. Treatment activity was not dependent on PD-L1 tumour expression at baseline whilst it was associated with the tumour mutational burden, as patient who both achieved a response and a clinical benefit showed higher mutation values.

During 2020 American Society of Clinical Oncology (ASCO) Congress, the updated results at 3-year follow-up of the EMPOWER-CSCC (NCT02760498) were shown [19]. The EMPOWER-CSCC study includes the two cohorts of the phase II trial plus a third cohort of 53 patients with metastatic cSCC treated with the flat dose of 350 mg every 3 weeks, for a total of 200 patients available. Median duration of follow-up for all patients was 15.7 months. The results of this study confirmed the previous data. On a total of 193 patients evaluable, the objective response rate (ORR) was 46.1% with 16.1% complete responses; clinical benefit was achieved in 72.5%. The median time to response was 2.1 months, even if the time to obtain complete response is 11 months. The study reports also the percentages of responses achieved during time: 46% within the first 2 months, 32% from the 2nd to the 4th and 9% from the 4th to the 6th; only 13% of responses were developed after the 6th month of treatment. These data provide significant guidance in the clinical practice for the duration of treatment in not responding patients. At 2 years, the estimated percentage of patients with ongoing response was 69.4%. No differences in ORR was found between locally advanced and metastatic disease patients. The median

PFS was 18.4 months, the median OS not reached, estimated 73.3% at 2-years. Grade ≥ 3 treatment-related adverse events were reported in 33 (17.1%) patients, with the most common being pneumonitis ($n = 5$, 2.6%), autoimmune hepatitis ($n = 3$; 1.6%), anaemia, colitis, and diarrhoea (all $n = 2$; 1.0%). No new adverse events resulting in death were reported compared to previous reports. The study reported also an analysis of the quality of life, showing an improvement in global health status/health-related quality of life (HRQL) observed as early as cycle 3 with clinically meaningful improvement seen by cycle 12.

Another PD-1 inhibitor, pembrolizumab, is currently being tested in a multicentre study for cCSCC (ClinicalTri- als.gov identifier NCT03284424). The Keynote-629 study was a phase II trial enrolling 2 cohorts of patients, the recurrent/metastatic ($n = 105$) and the locally advanced ($n = 50$), with primary end-point ORR. The results presented at ESMO 2019 are available for the recurrent/metastatic cohort showing 34.3% ORR with 52.4% disease control rate. The clinical activity was superior in patients who received pembrolizumab at first line with respect to those already pre-treated [20].

Given the similarities between PD-1 inhibitors, it is likely that different drugs within this class will have activity against cSCCs. Long-term outcomes remain to be determined, but PD-1 inhibitors have already led to improved outcomes in many cSCC patients.

BCC

Anti-PD-1/PD-L1 therapies did not yet achieve regulatory approvals for BCC. The largest endeavour is a phase II trial of cemiplimab in advanced BCC patients relapsed after hedgehog inhibitors [21, 22]: the trial is currently in progress with no finalised results.

The largest series reported is a proof-of-principle, non-randomised, open-label study of pembrolizumab with or without vismodegib in 16 patients with advanced BCC treated with pembrolizumab monotherapy or pembrolizumab in combination with vismodegib [23]. The ORR for the total cohort was 38%, with higher responses in patients treated with pembrolizumab monotherapy than in the combined therapy group (44 vs. 29%).

There are also reported anecdotal cases with positive results.

Ikeda et al. reported a patient with metastatic BCC progressed albeit treated with vismodegib, sonidegib and cytotoxic chemotherapy, who achieved a near complete remission with nivolumab. The biologic rationale for the off-label use of anti PD-1 has been the high TMB and the amplification of chromosome 9p24.1 (the locus for PD-L1, PD-L2 and JAK2) described in this tumour. This structural anomaly has been found in the majority of patients with classical Hodgkin lymphoma (HL) [24]. In a pivotal study, HL responded to nivolumab with an ORR of 87% in a group of 23 relapsed/refractory HL patients (NCT01592370). Another case is provided by Delaitre et al., with the successful treatment of a nasal ulcerated BCC with pembrolizumab, administered for a locally advanced inoperable cSCC [25]. Fischer et al. also reported a case of near-complete response to pembrolizumab after failure with hedgehog inhibitors [26].

In the literature, it has also been shown that BCC can have biological features enabling the escape from the immune surveillance and explaining the lack of response to immunotherapy as shown in some cases. For example, Sabbatino et al. described a case of a woman treated with nivolumab for a lung squamous cell carcinoma and with an ulcerated nodular BCC of the nose appeared after 18 cycles of immunotherapy. The immunohistochemical study revealed a PD-L1 expression <1% on both tumour and immune cells, and no expression of MHC-1 and β2-microglobulin on tumour cells could be found. Besides, in the immune cell infiltrate there was a low number of activated cytotoxic T cells [18].

The use of immunotherapy seems to be useful in syndromic forms such as Gorlin-Goltz syndrome. Moreira et al. reported the case of a man with more than 50 basal cell carcinomas not responding to several lines of treatment (surgery, imiquimod, retinoids, itraconazole, and vismodegib). Hence, therapy with pembrolizumab was initiated with a good clinical response after four infusions [27].

Thanks to the spread of immunotherapy in oncology, it is possible to study its effects on NMSC. In a study of Zhao et al., the authors compared the incidence of BCC and SCC in patients with metastatic melanoma in treatment with anti PD-1, BRAF inhibitor monotherapy or dabrafenib and trametinib combination therapy, with a control group. All the subjects had similar risk factors for NMSC. It was highlighted that the incidence of BCCs in the group on anti PD-1 was significantly lower than the one in the control group (2.4% vs. 19.4%; $p < 0.001$). No statistically significant differences were found among the other two groups [28].

MCC

Treatment recommendations for MCC depend on stage and disease extension. Localised MCC is treated with surgical resection and/or radiotherapy. In the case of metastatic disease, chemotherapy was used (cisplatin with or without etoposide or combination of cyclophosphamide, adriamycin, and vincristine). Although associated with high initial rates of response, response duration was low and treatment was associated with a high incidence of toxicities with a clinical impact in this elderly patient population [29]. FDA-approved anti-PD-1/PD-L1 drugs are pembrolizumab and avelumab.

To date, the largest study of ICI in MCC is a phase II trial with the anti-PD-L1 blocker avelumab in 88 patients progressed on chemotherapy (Javelin Merkel 200 study). The primary end-point was ORR by independent review. After a median follow-up of 40.8 months, the ORR was 33% with complete response in 11.4% and the median duration of response was 40.5 months. The time for response induction was short, with a median of 6.1 weeks and 75.9% of responses were observed at the first evaluation 6 weeks after the beginning of treatment [30]. In the updated results, the median overall survival (OS) was 12.6 months. The activity was higher in patients less heavily pre-treated and was similar in virus positive or negative patients. The study reports also an exploratory biomarker analysis showing that high TMB (≥ 2 non-synonymous somatic variants per megabase) and high MHC class I expression (30% of tumours with highest expression) were associated with trends for improved ORR and OS. Moreover, PD-L1 tumour expression was found to be associated with long-term survival [31]. Grade ≥ 3 treatment-related adverse events occurred in 11.4% of patients, 21.6% of patients developed an immune-related adverse event.

In a recently published experience with avelumab from an expanded access program, 494 patients received the drug and 240 were evaluable. The ORR was 46.7%, with 22.9% complete response, and the disease control rate was 71.2%, thus confirming the results of the Javelin trial in this real-world setting [32].

The results of the study with pembrolizumab confirmed those achieved with avelumab supporting the relevance of considering immunotherapy as first line. The Keynote-017 study is a multicentre phase II trial which enrolled patients with advanced MCC naïve to systemic therapy to receive pembrolizumab for up to 2 years [33]. Among 50 patients, the ORR was 56% with 24% complete response rate. The median response duration was not reached (range 5.9 to 36.4+ months). The 24-month progression-free survival (PFS) and OS rates were 48.3% and 68.7%, respectively. Tumour viral status did not correlate with ORR, PFS, or OS, whilst there was a trend towards improved activity in PD-L1 positive patients. Grade 3 or greater treatment-related adverse events occurred in 28% of patients.

The CheckMate 358 study was a phase I/II study enrolling virus-associated cancer types. A total of 25 metastatic MCC were included and treated with nivolumab. The ORR was 64% with 73% in the 15 treatment-naïve patients. Median time to response was 2 months. There are also published experience with ICI as neo-adjuvant treatment. In the phase I/II CheckMate 358 study of virus-associated cancer types, patients should receive nivolumab 240 mg on days 1 and 15 and then surgery on day 29. 39 patients with resectable MCC were included after receiving 1 or 2 nivolumab doses, 36 of whom underwent surgery with evidence of pathologic complete response in 47.2%. Relapse-free survival after surgery significantly correlated with pathological complete response and radiographic response [34].

Cutaneous Lymphoma

Cutaneous T-cell lymphomas (CTCL) are a family of primary extranodal lymphoid disorders that originate from the malignant transformation of post-thymic skin-homing T cells. Mycosis fungoides (MF) is the most common form of CTCL, characterised by an aberrant and excessive proliferation of CD4 T cells in the skin. Clinically, MF is typically characterised by skin patches, plaques, or tumours, with an indolent behaviour and without extracutaneous involvement. Sézary syndrome (SS) is an aggressive subtype of CTCL defined by the presence of erythroderma, generalised superficial lymphadenopathy, and a high burden of circulating malignant T cells (Sézary Cells) [35]. Although early-stage MF have an indolent course, advanced stages and SS are affected by a poor survival [36, 37]. Both MF and SS are considered immunogenic neoplasms that can elicit an immune response as confirmed by the presence of high numbers of CD8 cytotoxic T cells along with dermal dendritic cells in early MF lesions [38]. However, by the production of several cytokines (such as IL4, IL-5, and IL-10) MF/SS cells are capable to induce a TH2 immune environment that reduce the TH1 driven anti-tumour CD8 cytotoxic response. Moreover, these neoplasms are characterised by increased expressions of PD-1, PD-1 ligand, and CTLA-4 [39, 40].

On these biological bases, several clinical studies are exploring ICI treatment in MF/SS patients.

In a phase I, open-label, dose-escalation, cohort-expansion basket trial enrolling 81 patients, 13 heavily pre-treated MF patients received nivolumab. The ORR was 15%. Drug-related adverse events occurred in 63% of patients, most of them grade 1 or 2; duration of responses ranged up to 81 weeks [41].

In a phase II clinical trial, pembrolizumab was administered to 24 heavily pre-treated and advanced-stage MF/SS patients. Nine out of 24 patients (38%) responded (two complete responses and eight partial responses), interestingly eight patients achieved durable responses. Immune-related adverse events led to treatment discontinuation in four patients. A transient worsening of erythroderma and pruritus was observed in 53% of patients with SS, however not resulting in treatment discontinuation [42].

An European Organisation for Research and Treatment of Cancer (EORTC) phase II trial of atezolizumab (anti-PD-L1) in the treatment of stage IIb–IV with advanced CTCL (NCT03011814) patients relapsed/refractory is ongoing. Another phase 1/2 clinical trial is evaluating the PD-L1 inhibitor durvalumab in patients with advanced CTCL.

Overall, the results of these preliminary are encouraging particularly in terms of response duration even if anti-PD1 blockade seems to give less favourable results in CTCL with respect to other solid tumours or haematological malignancies.

Immunotherapy with Anti-PD1/PD-L1 Blockade in NMSC: A Comprehensive Scenario

Figure 17.3 shows together and summarises the main clinical results with ICI in the different disease subtypes of NMSC. Despite the clinical differences in the disease course, some major features can be highlighted across the different subtypes.

The percentage of responses range between 33% and 56%; usually the time to response is short and the response is characterised by a potentially long duration.

The treatment is generally well tolerated which is a very important issue in elderly patients, with grade 3 or more adverse events in a minority of patients

Ref	Drug	Trial	Disease status/ stage	No. of pts	RR	Time to response (median)	Response duration	PFS	OS	Side effects (% grade III/IV)	Predictive factors
D'angelo, 2020, Kaufman2018	Avelumab	Javelin Merkel 200 Phase II	Merkel Metastatic	88	33%	6.1wks	40.5 mo (median)	21% (3-yr)	12.6 mo (median)	11.4%	PD-L1,TMB
Nghiem, 2019	Pembrolizumab	Keynote-017	Merkel Advanced untreated	50	56%	2.8mo	Not reached	48.3% (2-yr)	68.7% (2-yr)	28%	PD-L1
Khodadoust, 2020	Pembrolizumab	Phase II	CTCL, Advanced stage	24	38%	-	> 58 wks	-	-	4/24 tx discont-inuation	Not related to PD-L1
Migden 2018-2020, Rischin, 2020	Cemiplimab	EMPOWER -CSCC phase II	cSCC, locally advanced and metastatic	193	46.1%	2.1mo	69.4% (2years)	18.4 mo (median)	73.3% (2-years)	17.1%	TMB, not related to PD-L1

Fig. 17.3 Comparison of the results of the main studies using anti-PD-1/PD-L1 in NMSC. *RR* response rate, *CTCL* cutaneous T-cell lymphoma, *cSCC* cutaneous squamous cell carcinoma

(11–28%). PD-L1 tumour expression shows a different predictive value according to the disease subtype: it is associated with higher clinical activity in MCC but not in cSCC, whilst in both tumours the TMB is related with the response.

Ongoing Trials and Future Perspectives

Regarding NMSC, in addition to further studies related to the "classics" anti PD-1 and anti-PDL1 [43, 44], there has been an increasing interest in the "next generation" ICI, both systemic and intra-lesional [45, 46]. The term "next generation" implies that in addition to the inhibitory effect that PD1-PD-L1 interaction has on the immune response, the tumour microenvironment contains several other inhibitory factors expressed by T-cell including LAG3, TIM3 and TIGIT. Among these new ICIs, Talimogene laherparepvec (T-VEC) which is a herpes simplex virus type 1 genetically modified to produce G-CSF to stimulate localised immune response, is currently under study (NCT03458117) for all major NMSCs (MCC, BCC and cCSCC).

Several ongoing studies investigating MCC [47] evaluate the efficacy of nivolumab in association with surgery or radiotherapy, whether in monotherapy or in combination with daratumumab (anti CD38 antibody) or Ipilimumab (anti-CTLA-4 antibody). Two clinical trials are currently assessing the effects of IL-15 superagonist in conjunction with pembrolizumab (NCT04234113) and avelumab (NCT03853317). IL-15 seems to increase the number of CD8+ and Nk cells enhancing the innate immune response. Additionally, there are a series of ongoing trials related to the "next generation" immunotherapy, such as the monoclonal antibodies antagonists of TIM3, a protein expressed by CD-8+ T-cell that promotes the shutdown of the cellular T response (NCT036520077). Another option are the antagonists of LAG-3 (Relatamib in association with nivolumab in the CheckMate 358) and TIGIT (NCT03628677), expressed by CD8+, CD4+ and NK cells, with a similar function to PD-1. Further studies are investigating the efficacy of Toll-Like Receptors Agonists (TLRs) intralesional therapy alone, such as Glucopyranosil lipid A in stable emulsion (GLA-SE) (NCT02035657), or in association with ICI (NCT03684785). As far as the best prognosis of MCC with a high level of NK cell population is concerned, Neukoplast-based innate immune cell therapy (i.e. NK cells infusion) appears promising (NCT0246557). Finally, other immune-mediated treatments such as Adoptive T-cell Immunotherapy, specific for MCPyV virus positive MCC, and T-cell co-stimulation, with anti-GITR (Glucocorticoid-induced TNF receptor) (NCT03126110) and antiOX40 (also studied for SCC) (NCT03894618) agonistic antibodies in association with classic ICI, are currently being studied.

With regard to BCC [48], the association between pembrolizumab and vismodegib, investigated in the Phase II study NCT02690948, does not show better results than pembrolizumab in monotherapy. Another trial is investigating cemiplimab (NCT03132636), whose efficacy had only been proven by anecdotal data collected until now. Two clinical trials studying pembrolizumab and ipilimumab with nivolumab in patients with advanced BCC are ongoing (NCT02834013 and NCT02693535).

Ongoing trials on cSCC involve not only the well-known cemiplimab in various therapy regimens but also anti-PD-1/PD-L1 [49], including the recently introduced molecule cosibelimab which has been investigated in a Phase I "Basket" study including cSCC and MCC (NCT03212404). Relatively to pembrolizumab, there are current association studies with intra-lesional therapy involving TLR agonists such as AST-008 (NCT03684785) and viral-derived oncolytic therapies such as MG1-MAGEA3 vaccine derived from Maraba Virus (NCT03773744). Advanced cases of NMSC are problematic to manage but multi-disciplinary collaboration between dermatologists, medical oncologists, surgeons and radiation oncologists is the best solution for the patient. It is so critical because high-risk patients, most of the time, need more than one type of treatment to manage in a better way their disease in the long-term, for ongoing monitoring for recurrence, and to handle treatment adverse effects.

For a better understanding of the majority of the key aspects of immunotherapy against tumours we need additional researches. These difficult and problematic questions include:

1. Response rates can be additionally improved by combining different immunotherapies or mixing immunotherapy with other treatment modality;
2. Chance of response can be predicted ahead of immunotherapy start so that patients can be chosen to maximise potential benefits of immunotherapy while avoiding adverse effects in patients with low probability of response.
3. Immunotherapies should be used for leading the way of treatments (including as neoadjuvant therapy);
4. The usage of immune-stimulating therapies for cancer in patients with co-morbid conditions such as multiple myeloma or chronic lymphocytic leukaemia, without worsening their disease.

It is probable that these doubts will be solved in the coming years through ongoing studies that are currently on the way.

References

1. Rogers HW, Weinstock MA, Feldman SR, Coldiron BM. Incidence estimate of nonmelanoma skin cancer (keratinocyte carcinomas) in the U.S. population, 2012. JAMA Dermatol. 2015;151(10):1081–6. https://doi.org/10.1001/jamadermatol.2015.1187.
2. Soura E, Gagari E, Stratigos A. Advanced cutaneous squamous cell carcinoma: how is it defined and what new therapeutic approaches are available? Curr Opin Oncol. 2019;31(5):461–8. https://doi.org/10.1097/CCO.0000000000000566.
3. Migden MR, Rischin D, Schmults CD, et al. PD-1 blockade with cemiplimab in advanced cutaneous squamous-cell carcinoma. N Engl J Med. 2018;379(4):341–51. https://doi.org/10.1056/NEJMoa1805131.

4. Eigentler TK, Leiter U, Häfner HM, Garbe C, Röcken M, Breuninger H. Survival of patients with cutaneous squamous cell carcinoma: results of a prospective cohort study. J Invest Dermatol. 2017;137(11):2309–15. https://doi.org/10.1016/j.jid.2017.06.025.

5. Chapalain M, Baroudjian B, Dupont A, et al. Stage IV cutaneous squamous cell carcinoma: treatment outcomes in a series of 42 patients. J Eur Acad Dermatol Venereol. 2020;34(6):1202–9. https://doi.org/10.1111/jdv.16007.

6. Sekulic A, Migden MR, Basset-Seguin N, et al. Long-term safety and efficacy of vismodegib in patients with advanced basal cell carcinoma: final update of the pivotal ERIVANCE BCC study [published correction appears in BMC Cancer. 2019 Apr 18;19(1):366]. BMC Cancer. 2017;17(1):332. https://doi.org/10.1186/s12885-017-3286-5.

7. Calder KB, Smoller BR. New insights into merkel cell carcinoma. Adv Anat Pathol. 2010;17(3):155–61. https://doi.org/10.1097/PAP.0b013e3181d97836.

8. www.registri-tumori.it

9. Schadendorf D, Lebbé C, Zur Hausen A, et al. Merkel cell carcinoma: epidemiology, prognosis, therapy and unmet medical needs. Eur J Cancer. 2017;71:53–69. https://doi.org/10.1016/j.ejca.2016.10.022.

10. Lemos BD, Storer BE, Iyer JG, et al. Pathologic nodal evaluation improves prognostic accuracy in Merkel cell carcinoma: analysis of 5823 cases as the basis of the first consensus staging system. J Am Acad Dermatol. 2010;63(5):751–61. https://doi.org/10.1016/j.jaad.2010.02.056.

11. Yarchoan M, Hopkins A, Jaffee EM. Tumor mutational burden and response rate to PD-1 inhibition. N Engl J Med. 2017;377(25):2500–1. https://doi.org/10.1056/NEJMc1713444.

12. Chalmers ZR, Connelly CF, Fabrizio D, et al. Analysis of 100,000 human cancer genomes reveals the landscape of tumor mutational burden. Genome Med. 2017;9(1):34. https://doi.org/10.1186/s13073-017-0424-2.

13. Lipson EJ, Vincent JG, Loyo M, et al. PD-L1 expression in the Merkel cell carcinoma microenvironment: association with inflammation, Merkel cell polyomavirus and overall survival. Cancer Immunol Res. 2013;1(1):54–63. https://doi.org/10.1158/2326-6066.CIR-13-0034.

14. Lipson EJ, Vincent JG, Loyo M, et al. PD-L1 expression in the Merkel cell carcinoma microenvironment: association with inflammation, Merkel cell polyomavirus and overall survival. Cancer Immunol Res. 2013;1(1):54–63. https://doi.org/10.1158/2326-6066.CIR-13-0034.

15. Chen L, Cao MF, Zhang X, et al. The landscape of immune microenvironment in lung adenocarcinoma and squamous cell carcinoma based on PD-L1 expression and tumor-infiltrating lymphocytes. Cancer Med. 2019;8(17):7207–18. https://doi.org/10.1002/cam4.2580.

16. Cetinözman F, Jansen PM, Vermeer MH, Willemze R. Differential expression of programmed death-1 (PD-1) in Sézary syndrome and mycosis fungoides. Arch Dermatol. 2012;148(12):1379–85. https://doi.org/10.1001/archdermatol.2012.2089.

17. Hall ET, Fernandez-Lopez E, Silk AW, Dummer R, Bhatia S. Immunologic characteristics of nonmelanoma skin cancers: implications for immunotherapy. Am Soc Clin Oncol Educ Book. 2020;40:1–10. https://doi.org/10.1200/EDBK_278953.

18. Sabbatino F, Marra A, Liguori L, et al. Resistance to anti-PD-1-based immunotherapy in basal cell carcinoma: a case report and review of the literature. J Immunother Cancer. 2018;6(1):126. https://doi.org/10.1186/s40425-018-0439-2.

19. Migden MR, Khushalani NI, Chang ALS, et al. Cemiplimab in locally advanced cutaneous squamous cell carcinoma: results from an open-label, phase 2, single-arm trial. Lancet Oncol. 2020;21(2):294–305. https://doi.org/10.1016/S1470-2045(19)30728-4.

20. Grob JJ, Gonzalez R, Basset-Seguin N, et al. Pembrolizumab monotherapy for recurrent or metastatic cutaneous squamous cell carcinoma: a single-arm phase II trial (KEYNOTE-629) [published online ahead of print, 2020 Jul 16]. J Clin Oncol. 2020;38(25):2916–25. https://doi.org/10.1200/JCO.19.03054.

21. Lewis KD, Fury MG, Stankevich E, et al. 1240TiPPhase II study of cemiplimab, a human monoclonal anti-PD-1, in patients with advanced basal cell carcinoma (BCC) who experienced progres-sion of disease on, or were intolerant of prior hedgehog pathway inhibitor (HHI) therapy. Ann Oncol. 2018;29(suppl_8):79.

22. Stein JE, Brothers P, Applebaum K, et al. A phase 2 study of nivolumab (NIVO) alone or plus ipilimumab (IPI) for patients with locally advanced unresectable (laBCC) or metastatic basal cell carcinoma (mBCC). J Clin Oncol. 2019;37:TPS9595.80.
23. Chang ALS, Tran DC, Cannon JGD, et al. Pembrolizumab for advanced basal cell carcinoma: an investigator-initiated, proof-of-concept study. J Am Acad Dermatol. 2019;80(2):564–6. https://doi.org/10.1016/j.jaad.2018.08.017.
24. Ikeda S, Goodman AM, Cohen PR, et al. Metastatic basal cell carcinoma with amplification of PD-L1: exceptional response to anti-PD1 therapy. NPJ Genom Med. 2016;1:16037. https://doi.org/10.1038/npjgenmed.2016.37.
25. Delaitre L, Martins-Héricher J, Truchot E, et al. Régression de carcinomes basocellulaire et épidermoïde cutanés sous pembrolizumab [Regression of cutaneous basal cell and squamous cell carcinoma under pembrolizumab]. Ann Dermatol Venereol. 2020;147(4):279–84.
26. Fischer S, Hasan Ali O, Jochum W, Kluckert T, Flatz L, Siano M. Anti-PD-1 therapy leads to near-complete remission in a patient with metastatic basal cell carcinoma. Oncol Res Treat. 2018;41(6):391–4. https://doi.org/10.1159/000487084.
27. Moreira A, Kirchberger MC, Toussaint F, Erdmann M, Schuler G, Heinzerling L. Effective anti-programmed death-1 therapy in a SUFU-mutated patient with Gorlin-Goltz syndrome. Br J Dermatol. 2018;179(3):747–9. https://doi.org/10.1111/bjd.16607.
28. Zhao CY, Hwang SJE, Anforth R, et al. Incidence of basal cell carcinoma and squamous cell carcinoma in patients on antiprogrammed cell death-1 therapy for metastatic melanoma. J Immunother. 2018;41(7):343–9. https://doi.org/10.1097/CJI.0000000000000237.
29. Nghiem P, Kaufman HL, Bharmal M, Mahnke L, Phatak H, Becker JC. Systematic literature review of efficacy, safety and tolerability outcomes of chemotherapy regimens in patients with metastatic Merkel cell carcinoma. Future Oncol. 2017;13(14):1263–79. https://doi.org/10.2217/fon-2017-0072.
30. Kaufman HL, Russell JS, Hamid O, et al. Updated efficacy of avelumab in patients with previously treated metastatic Merkel cell carcinoma after ≥1 year of follow-up: JAVELIN Merkel 200, a phase 2 clinical trial. J Immunother Cancer. 2018;6(1):7. https://doi.org/10.1186/s40425-017-0310-x.
31. D'Angelo SP, Russell J, Lebbé C, et al. Efficacy and safety of first-line avelumab treatment in patients with stage IV metastatic merkel cell carcinoma: a preplanned interim analysis of a clinical trial. JAMA Oncol. 2018;4(9):e180077. https://doi.org/10.1001/jamaoncol.2018.0077.
32. Walker JW, Lebbé C, Grignani G, et al. Efficacy and safety of avelumab treatment in patients with metastatic Merkel cell carcinoma: experience from a global expanded access program. J Immunother Cancer. 2020;8(1):e000313. https://doi.org/10.1136/jitc-2019-000313.
33. Nghiem P, Bhatia S, Lipson EJ, et al. Durable tumor regression and overall survival in patients with advanced merkel cell carcinoma receiving pembrolizumab as first-line therapy. J Clin Oncol. 2019;37(9):693–702. https://doi.org/10.1200/JCO.18.01896.
34. Topalian SL, Bhatia S, Amin A, et al. Neoadjuvant nivolumab for patients with resectable merkel cell carcinoma in the CheckMate 358 trial. J Clin Oncol. 2020;38(22):2476–87. https://doi.org/10.1200/JCO.20.00201.
35. Willemze R, Cerroni L, Kempf W, et al. The 2018 update of the WHO-EORTC classification for primary cutaneous lymphomas [published correction appears in Blood. 2019 Sep 26;134(13):1112]. Blood. 2019;133(16):1703–14. https://doi.org/10.1182/blood-2018-11-881268.
36. Jawed SI, Myskowski PL, Horwitz S, Moskowitz A, Querfeld C. Primary cutaneous T-cell lymphoma (mycosis fungoides and Sézary syndrome): part II Prognosis, management, and future directions. J Am Acad Dermatol. 2014;70(2):223.e1–242. https://doi.org/10.1016/j.jaad.2013.08.033.
37. Wong HK, Mishra A, Hake T, Porcu P. Evolving insights in the pathogenesis and therapy of cutaneous T-cell lymphoma (mycosis fungoides and Sezary syndrome). Br J Haematol. 2011;155(2):150–66. https://doi.org/10.1111/j.1365-2141.2011.08852.x.

38. Goteri G, Filosa A, Mannello B, et al. Density of neoplastic lymphoid infiltrate, CD8+ T cells, and CD1a+ dendritic cells in mycosis fungoides. J Clin Pathol. 2003;56(6):453–8. https://doi. org/10.1136/jcp.56.6.453.
39. Querfeld C, Leung S, Myskowski PL, et al. Primary T cells from cutaneous T-cell lymphoma skin explants display an exhausted immune checkpoint profile. Cancer Immunol Res. 2018;6(8):900–9. https://doi.org/10.1158/2326-6066.CIR-17-0270.
40. Cetinözman F, Jansen PM, Vermeer MH, Willemze R. Differential expression of programmed death-1 (PD-1) in Sézary syndrome and mycosis fungoides. Arch Dermatol. 2012;148(12):1379–85. https://doi.org/10.1001/archdermatol.2012.2089.
41. Lesokhin AM, Ansell SM, Armand P, et al. Nivolumab in patients with relapsed or refractory hematologic malignancy: preliminary results of a phase Ib study. J Clin Oncol. 2016;34(23):2698–704. https://doi.org/10.1200/JCO.2015.65.9789.
42. Khodadoust MS, Rook AH, Porcu P, et al. Pembrolizumab in relapsed and refractory mycosis fungoides and sézary syndrome: a multicenter phase II study. J Clin Oncol. 2020;38(1):20–8. https://doi.org/10.1200/JCO.19.01056.
43. Choi FD, Kraus CN, Elsensohn AN, et al. Programmed cell death 1 protein and programmed death-ligand 1 inhibitors in the treatment of nonmelanoma skin cancer: a systematic review. J Am Acad Dermatol. 2020;82(2):440–59. https://doi.org/10.1016/j.jaad.2019.05.077.
44. Patrinely JR, Dewan AK, Johnson DB. The role of anti-PD-1/PD-L1 in the treatment of skin cancer. BioDrugs. 2020;34(4):495–503. https://doi.org/10.1007/s40259-020-00428-9.
45. Wilken R, Criscito M, Pavlick AC, Stevenson ML, Carucci JA. Current research in melanoma and aggressive nonmelanoma skin cancer. Facial Plast Surg. 2020;36(2):200–10. https://doi. org/10.1055/s-0040-1709118.
46. Bobrowicz M, Zagozdzon R, Domagala J, Vasconcelos-Berg R, Guenova E, Winiarska M. Monoclonal antibodies in dermatooncology-state of the art and future perspectives. Cancers (Basel). 2019;11(10):1420. https://doi.org/10.3390/cancers11101420.
47. Babadzhanov M, Doudican N, Wilken R, Stevenson M, Pavlick A, Carucci J. Current concepts and approaches to merkel cell carcinoma. Arch Dermatol Res. 2020; https://doi.org/10.1007/s00403-020-02107-9.
48. Niebel D, Sirokay J, Hoffmann F, Fröhlich A, Bieber T, Landsberg J. Clinical management of locally advanced basal-cell carcinomas and future therapeutic directions. Dermatol Ther (Heidelb). 2020;10(4):835–46. https://doi.org/10.1007/s13555-020-00382-y.
49. Varra V, Smile TD, Geiger JL, Koyfman SA. Recent and emerging therapies for cutaneous squamous cell carcinomas of the head and neck. Curr Treat Options Oncol. 2020;21(5):37. https://doi.org/10.1007/s11864-020-00739-7.

Part VI
Mechanism of Resistance to Therapy

Chapter 18
Mechanisms of Resistance to Targeted Therapies in Skin Cancers

Anna M. Czarnecka, Michał Fiedorowicz, and Ewa Bartnik

Melanoma-Targeted Therapies Resistance Overview

BRAF (v-Raf murine sarcoma viral oncogene homolog B) protooncogene mutations are detected in 50–60% of metastatic melanoma patients and 7–10% of all cancers. In 80–90% of cases, a missense *V600E* mutation is present, where the wild-type amino acid in position 600—valine (V)—is replaced by glutamic acid (E) [1, 2]. Other known substitutions are 7.7% V600K (lysine), 1% V600R (arginine), 0.3% V600L (leucine), and 0.1% V600D (aspartic acid) [3]. Mutations in other *BRAF* gene positions are found in <1% metastatic melanoma cases. The discovery of this mutation led to the development of specific inhibitors of mutated BRAF protein (BRAFi), including vemurafenib, dabrafenib, and encorafenib [4–6]. To increase

A. M. Czarnecka (✉)
Department of Soft Tissue/Bone, Sarcoma and Melanoma, Maria Sklodowska-Curie National Research Institute of Oncology, Warsaw, Poland

Department of Experimental Pharmacology, Mossakowski Medical Research Institute, Polish Academy of Sciences, Warsaw, Poland
e-mail: am.czarnecka@pib-nio.pl

M. Fiedorowicz
Small Animal Magnetic Resonance Imaging Laboratory, Mossakowski Medical Research Institute, Polish Academy of Sciences, Warsaw, Poland

Interinstitute Laboratory of New Diagnostic Applications of MRI, Nalecz Institute of Biocybernetics and Biomedical Engineering, Polish Academy of Sciences, Warsaw, Poland
e-mail: mfiedorowicz@imdik.pan.pl

E. Bartnik
Faculty of Biology, Institute of Genetics and Biotechnology, University of Warsaw, Warsaw, Poland

Institute of Biochemistry and Biophysics, Polish Academy of Sciences, Warsaw, Poland
e-mail: ebartnik@igib.uw.edu.pl

© The Author(s), under exclusive license to Springer Nature Switzerland AG 2021
P. Rutkowski, M. Mandalà (eds.), *New Therapies in Advanced Cutaneous Malignancies*, https://doi.org/10.1007/978-3-030-64009-5_18

BRAFi efficacy, overcome resistance development resulting from paradoxical MAPK pathway activation, mitogen-activated protein kinase kinase (MEK)-targeted drugs—MEK inhibitors (MEKi) were developed subsequently—cobimetinib, trametinib, and binimetinib [7–9]. Nowadays, BRAFi and MEKi are used in clinical practice as combinations of vemurafenib with cobimetinib, dabrafenib with trametinib, and encorafenib with binimetinib. Routine clinical use of BRAFi and MEKi therapies has resulted in dramatic improvements in progression-free survival (PFS) and overall survival (OS) time in patients with *BRAF*-mutated advanced melanoma in the last 5 years [9–14].

Physiologically, *BRAF* mutations are important as wild-type BRAF protein is active as a dimer, but protein with the V600E mutation is active as a monomer. Such gain of activity by the monomers is possible because of the substitution of nonpolar valine (V) by phosphomimetic negatively charged glutamic acid (E) at position 600 (V600E). Amino acid substitution blocks BRAF kinase in an activated conformation and induces the downstream mitogen-activated protein kinase (MAPK)–extracellular signal-regulated kinase (ERK) signaling pathway. This pathway is primarily responsible for cell proliferation and survival [15, 16] and is also the main hub of primary and acquired resistance to the used therapy. Up to 15–20% of *BRAF* mutant cases do not respond to BRAFi/MEKI and are primarily resistant [17–19]. The majority of patients initially respond to BRAFi/MEKi treatment with a selected group of patients with an immune-related gene signature being favorable in terms of response. At the same time, patients with upregulated cell cycle-related genes are in the unfavorable group and are resistant to BRAFi/MEKi treatment [20, 21].

Primary resistance to targeted therapies results mostly from tumor tissue heterogeneity with specific genomic or epigenetic abnormalities in selected melanoma cells. Secondary resistance develops in consequence of tumor suppressor loss and/or activation of additional protooncogenes upon treatment. A specific role in resistance development is attributed to the tumor microenvironment, intratumoral hypoxia, and cell–cell interactions including immunological deregulation. BRAFi/MEKi-resistant melanoma cells have upregulated expression of receptor tyrosine kinases (RTKs), including epidermal growth factor receptor (EGFR), insulin growth factor 1 receptor (IGF1R), platelet-derived growth factor receptor α and β (PDGFR α and PDGFRβ), or fibroblast growth factor receptor-3 (FGFR-3) [22]. Analyses of BRAFi/MEKi-resistant cells and tissues have revealed a repetitive pattern of mutations and amplifications, including these (1) in the RAS/RAF/MEK/ERK pathway, *i.e. N-RAS* and *K-RAS* mutations, *BRAF* amplifications/mutations, *MAP2K1* mutations, and *MAP2K2* mutations; (2) in the PI3K pathway genes including *PIK3CA, PTEN*, and *PIK3R1*, or (3) the TGF pathway. At the same time, mutations in *PTEN, NF1, MITF*, and Homeobox D8 *(HOXD8)* cause resistance to BRAFi/MEKi [17, 23–26]. Mechanistically, the primary cause of BRAFi/MEKi resistance is the reactivation of the inhibited MAPK signaling pathway. This phenomenon was detected in 80% of BRAFi-resistant tumors. Reactivation of BRAF/MEK signaling in the presence of an inhibitor often results from the deregulation of BRAF protein activity—due to secondary mutations, alternative splicing, or its overexpression. In other cases, activation of alternative pathways is responsible for melanoma cell survival and proliferation under BRAFi/MEKi. Hyperactivity of upstream signaling from N-RAS, C-RAF, COT, as well as NF1 loss were all reported to activate the MAP/ERK pathway [27, 28]. Activation of the MAPK/ERK pathway on BRAFi treatment has been shown to result from the presence of BRAFV600E amplification, expression of BRAFV600E splice variants, as well as activating mutations in *MAP2K1* or *MAP2K2* [22]. On the other hand, BRAFi resistance may develop by phosphoinositide 3-kinase (PI3K)—protein kinase B (AKT)—mechanistic target of rapamycin kinase (mTOR) pathway hyperactivation. Mutations in *AKT1, AKT3, PIK3CA, PIK3CG, PIK3R2,* or *PHLPP1*, as well as *PTEN* loss, were shown to induce PI3K signaling. In fact, there is a network cross-talk between the MAP/ERK pathway and the mTOR pathway, microphthalmia-associated transcription factor (MITF) signaling, as well as c-Jun *N*-terminal kinase (JNK) and Wnt/β-catenin pathways. Network interactions are *per se* responsible for inducing activity downstream of ERK (extracellular signal-regulated kinase) during BRAFi/MEKi therapy [16, 29–32]. In particular, c-Jun and protein kinase C (PKC) were shown as the main drivers of BRAFi resistance [33], while p-21-activated kinase (PAK) is mostly responsible for MEKi therapy resistance [34].

Melanoma Tumor Microenvironment and BRAFi/MEKi Resistance

In general, research on drug resistance is mainly focused on the genome, proteome, and metabolome of tumor cells. However, disease progression and resistance to targeted BRAFi/MEKi therapies in melanoma, and other malignancies, are known to develop not only as a result of genomic or epigenetic abnormalities in tumor cells, but the tumor microenvironment is also important. Cell–cell interactions are a complicated phenomenon, encompassing among other interactions between the tumor cells and the stroma [35–37]. Recent research has identified the role of intratumoral macrophages and fibroblasts in the development of resistance to RAS–RAF–MAPK–ERK pathway inhibitors in melanoma. Most recent data suggest that within the tumor, the BRAFi-sensitive phenotype of metastatic melanoma cells may be shifted toward resistant phenotype by BRAFi-resistant melanoma cells secreting PDGFRβ in extracellular vesicles [38].

Cancer-associated fibroblasts (CAFs) or actually intratumoral melanoma-associated fibroblasts (MAFs) have been shown to facilitate melanoma progression and to mediate therapeutic escape from BRAF inhibition. CAFs were discovered in the tumor niche and differ from normal skin fibroblasts by upregulated expression of vimentin, α-smooth-muscle actin (SMA), fibroblast activation protein-1 (FAP1), as well as PDGFR and TGFβ signaling [27]. Physiologically, there is a cross-talk between melanoma cells and MAFs. In the presence of fibroblasts, neighboring melanoma cells acquire a dedifferentiated and aggressive mesenchymal phenotype. After treatment with BRAFi, melanoma cells maintain a high level of phosphorylated ribosomal S6 protein (pS6) and active mTOR signaling if they are in cell–cell contact with MAFs [39]. mTOR activation in melanoma cells leads to phosphorylation and activation of ribosomal protein S6 kinase p70 and of the eukaryotic protein-binding factor 4E 1E and promotes the utilization of nutrients from the microenvironment, protein synthesis, and melanoma cell growth [40]. Melanoma cells also respond to growth factors and cytokines secreted by fibroblasts. These molecules - including TGF-β and VEGF - promote melanoma cell survival and growth [27]. MAFs secrete multiple proinvasive factors in the tumor niche that act in a paracrine manner [41]. Primary and acquired resistance to BRAFi is induced by hepatocyte growth factor (HGF) secreted by MAFs. It was shown that vemurafenib directly activates the fibroblasts to secrete HGF by paradoxical stimulation of the MAP–ERK pathway [41]. HGF is a pleiotropic factor that promotes melanoma cell growth, morphogenesis, and mobility [42]. HGF binds to the cMET protooncogene (receptor) on the surface of melanoma cells, activates both MAPK/ERK and PI3K/AKT signaling pathways and as a result induces melanoma cell proliferation [43, 44]. HGF also downregulates the expression of pro-apoptotic genes and in a feedback loop induces *RAS* expression. As a result, in melanoma HGF finally promotes invasion and angiogenesis [43–45]. MAFs secrete also neuregulin 1 (NRG1) that stimulates the receptor tyrosine kinase 3 (erbB-3, HER3) pathway and limits RAF inhibition [46]. A specific phenomenon was reported for aging fibroblasts which is important for melanoma therapy resitance. Aging fibroblasts were reported as more invasive. This is important due to age-related melanoma occurrence. Aging fibroblasts were shown to express and secrete frizzled related protein 2 (sFRP2)—a β-catenin inhibitor. sFRP2 downregulates microphthalmia-associated transcription factor (MITF) and apurinic/apyrimidinic endonuclease (APE1) expression rendering melanoma cells more resistant to targeted therapies such as vemurafenib [47].

Fibroblasts in contact with melanoma cells also secrete extracellular matrix components. Stiff calcified ECM is built in large part by MAFs. ECM-induced integrin signaling promotes the development of BRAFi resistance. Laminin IV secreted by MAFs facilitates migration and thus metastasis of melanoma cells [48, 49]. BRAFi may paradoxically hyperactivate MAP-ERK pathway in fibroblasts. Such BRAFi-activated fibroblasts deregulate extracellular matrix of the tumor niche. As a result integrin β1 and focal adhesion kinase (FAK; protein tyrosine kinase 2, PTK2) signaling in the melanoma cell is activated. Upon this interaction, melanoma cells induce ERK signaling and escape BRAFi [50]. Moreover, MAFs secrete cellular communication network factor 2 (CTGF, also known as CCN2 or connective tissue growth factor). This matricellular protein promotes integrin-mediated signaling through direct binding to a variety of integrins, including integrin beta-1 (ITGB1) on melanoma cells [51]. These CCN2 expressing MAFs also express alpha integrin (ITGA11), prolyl endopeptidase FAP, and collagen alpha-1(I) chain (COL1A1) and are therefore profibrotic. Fibrotic microenvironment promotes vasculogenic mimicry, neovascularization, and metastasis to the lungs [52, 53]. Downregulation of CCN2-induced signalling in melanoma cells diminishes their ability to invade through collagen and reduces expression of periostin—ECM protein that promotes invasion and metastasis [54].

In the reciprocal interaction, factors secreted by melanoma cells stimulate MAFs in a paracrine manner. Vemurafenib-resistant melanoma cells release TGF-β. TGF-β promotes fibroblast differentiation that results in an increase in α-smooth muscle actin (α-SMA) expression, fibronectin secretion, and deposition in ECM. TGF-β induced fibroblasts release also neuregulin (NRG) [41]. MAFs that undergo differentiation, in turn, increase the expression of extracellular matrix (ECM) molecules. ECM protein secretion is significant for further BRAFi/MEKi resistance development as a tumor niche that is rich in ECM proteins accelerates the development of resistance, as described above [41]. In fact, BRAFi treatment promotes overexpression of ECM proteins in melanoma cells, including collagen alpha-1(I) chain (COL1A1) and fibronectin 1 (FN1), which then positively affects the recruitment of MAFs and remodeling of F-actin [41]. Adhesion of melanoma cells to fibronectin is also critical in the amplification of fibroblast-derived HGF, and NRG-mediated PI3K/AKT signaling in these cells. For that reason, combined BRAF/PI3K inhibition is expected to overcome fibroblast-mediated BRAFi/MEKi resistance, as shown in xenograft models [41].

Tumor-infiltrating mononuclear inflammatory cells that are macrophages, effector T cells, and regulatory T cells for many years have been suggested to regulate BRAFi response and impact the survival of melanoma patients [55]. Tumor stroma cells with proven role BRAFi/MEKi resistance are macrophages—referred as to tumor-associated macrophages (TAMs). TAMs are activated M2 macrophages that, in the melanoma tumor niche, express a variety of anti-inflammatory factors and build an immune-suppressive microenvironment. Polarization of macrophages to CD163+ M2 phenotype is induced by exosome-derived growth factors and interleukins released by melanoma cells, other macrophages, and T-regulatory cells. The tyrosine-protein kinase receptor UFO (AXL), C-mer proto-oncogene tyrosine kinase (MERTK), and colony-stimulating factor 1 receptor (CSF1R) signaling pathways are known to favor M2 phenotypes [56]. In paracrine mode, macrophages that express CSF1 receptor respond to CSF secreted by melanoma cells, which also stimulate resistance in an autocrine manner in melanoma cells [27]. In turn, macrophages in the melanoma niche, secrete the melanoma-stimulating molecules: angiotensin, cyclooxygenase-2 (COX-2), interferon-gamma (IFN-γ), and interleukin 1-beta (IL-1β) and as a result support melanoma growth and metastatic spread [57]. A high number of high intratumoral CD163[+] macrophages correlate with BRAFi resistance [58]. Moreover, BRAFi themselves stimulate macrophages in the tumor. In macrophages activation induces the production of vascular endothelial growth factor A (VEGF-A), which stimulates not only angiogenesis in the tumor but also macrophage survival, tumor immune escape. All these procesess induce melanoma tumor growth [59, 60]. At the same time, MEKi stimulates bidirectional melanoma-TAM signaling via RTKs including AXL and MER Proto-Oncogene, Tyrosine Kinase (MERTK) and their ligands—growth arrest-specific 6 (GAS6) and protein S (PROS1) [56]. Moreover, intratumoral macrophages secrete tumor necrosis factor alpha (TNFα), which promotes nuclear factor kappa beta (NF-kβ)-dependent- MITF expression in melanoma cells. At the same time, TNFα also blocks apoptosis in melanoma cells with inhibited BRAF protein [61, 62]. Moreover, BRAFi paradoxically activates the MAPK/ERK pathway in macrophages that secrete VEGF as a result. VEGF in paracrine mode stimulates melanoma cells. For dabrafenib and vemurafenib, it was proven that macrophages do not disturb the G2/M phase in melanoma cells, but protect melanoma cells from BRAFi-induced apoptosis and induce angiogenesis in the tumor [63].

Deregulation of Melanocyte Differentiation as BRAFi Resistance Mechanism

BRAFV600E-mutated melanoma is characterized by deregulated melanocyte-inducing transcription factor (MITF, melanogenesis-associated transcription factor or microphthalmia-associated transcription factor) expression and activity [64]. In melanoma tissues, *MITF* loss was shown to be a predictor of early resistance to BRAFi and is also a frequent event in acquired BRAFi resistance [65]. Amplification of the *MITF* gene was demonstrated in 10% of cases in the Melanoma Genome Project group study, and this amplification was noted in all melanoma subtypes [66]. Overexpression of MITF was shown to decrease the therapeutic effect of BRAFi [67, 68] as well as MEKi [69] due to the prosurvival functions of MITF. On the other hand, the downregulation of MITF was shown to promote an invasive phenotype, as MITF regulates phenotype switching [70]. In fact, both overexpression and loss of MITF may contribute to BRAFi resistance [64, 71]. *MITF* expression distinguishes melanoma cells in the proliferative from those in the invasive state, as it is a prosurvival factor. Melanoma cells actually undergo phenotype switching from proliferative to invasive states which depend on MITF (and Wnt) signaling [47]. Different levels of expression of *MITF* result in differently deregulated physiology of melanoma cells. High (normal) MITF levels promote melanocyte differentiation, while moderate *MITF* expression drives melanoma cell proliferation and downregulated low *MITF* expression promotes invasion [71].

Melanocyte-inducing transcription factor is a key regulator of melanocyte development and physiology, including exit and maintenance of their postmitotic state. MITF binds to DNA as a homodimer or heterodimer with Transcription Factor EB (TFEB) or Transcription Factor Binding To IGHM Enhancer 3 (TFE3). Moreover, MITF stimulates cAMP pathway signaling in the melanoma cell [67]. MITF, by its target genes, controls cell metabolism and DNA repair, as well as melanocyte survival, differentiation, and proliferation or senescence [72]. MITF regulates melanoma cell proliferation and differentiation by cell cycle inhibition. MITF binds the INK4A promoter and activates transcription and p16^{Ink4a} protein expression. The p16^{Ink4a} induces retinoblastoma protein (pRb) hypophosphorylation and arrest cell cycle [73]. MITF exerts its functions through regulating the expression of multiple genes: *TYRP1* (tyrosinase-related protein 1), *GPNMB* (transmembrane glycoprotein NMB), *TYR* (tyrosinase), *BCL2* (B-cell lymphoma 2), or *CDK2*. The regulatory actions of MITF are exerted through several types of posttranslational modifications: ubiquitination, sumoylation, and phosphorylation that affect the function of

MITF. Among those, MITF sumoylation was shown to affect cell senescence and melanoma development [74]. MITF downregulation is also correlated with the upregulation of AXL. Low *MITF*/high *AXL* expression results with enhanced drug resistance. Even though such an expression pattern can be observed in cells unexposed to BRAF inhibitors, the low MITF/high *AXL* pattern increases upon progression [65, 75].

Epithelial–Mesenchymal Transition in Melanoma BRAF/ MEKi Resistance

Upon BRAFi/MEKi treatment, melanoma cells undergo a morphology change relevant to epithelial-to-mesenchymal transition (EMT). This phenomenon has recently been linked to therapy resistance [76]. In EMT, melanoma increases its invasiveness, and melanoma cells become motile. Upon EMT melanoma cells lose apical-basolateral polarization, basement membrane integrity, and cell–cell adhesion and become migratory and downregulate apoptosis. Such cells overexpress N-cadherin, vimentin, fibronectin, matrix metalloproteinases (MMPs), and selected integrins (i.e., A5B1). EMT arises when BRAF-inhibited melanoma cells undergo kinase switching and activate RAF isoforms other than BRAF. After kinase switching melanoma cells activate downstream RAS/RAF/MEK/ERK signaling. RAS/ RAF/MEK/ERK, PI3K/AKT/mTOR, TGF-β, and Wnt/β-catenin pathways promote the mesenchymal phenotype. In fact, it is ERK that has been shown to stabilize pro-mesenchymal transcription factors. ERK-mediated phosphorylation inhibits the degradation of pro-mesenchymal transcription factors—Snail, Slug, Zeb1, and Twist. Snail represses E-cadherin expression and the epithelial phenotype [77–79]. Dabrafenib-resistant melanoma cells show, in addition to the re-activation of MAPK/ERK signaling, CD20 and CD90 (mesenchymal marker) expression upregulation, and E-cadherin (epithelial marker) expression downregulation and translocation of Oct4 from the cytoplasm to the nucleus [80].

Various RTKs and intracellular signaling pathways can mediate phenotype switching and promote EMT by mechanisms different from BRAF/MAPK-dependent regulation of EMT. TGF-β is also an inducer of EMT, due to its role in extracellular matrix remodeling and in cell phenotype regulation. Wnt activation, rather than acting *via* the classical Wnt pathway in EMT events, transmits the signal through the protein kinase C (PKC) pathway. In fact, MAPK sensitive and resistant melanoma cells may be distinguished by the expression of 15 proteins. The highest discriminatory potential is for polymerase I and transcript release factor (PTRF also known as Cavin1) and insulin-like growth factor-binding protein 7 (IGFBP 7), which were shown to promote EMT, TGF β signaling, cell migration and the ability to form 3D spheres [81]. Besides melanoma cell direct interactions, MAFs are also involved in EMT, as they deposit prometastatic ECM and release proinvasive factors promoting EMT [41]. On the other hand, melanoma cells undergoing EMT, with high β-catenin expression, inhibit inflamed immunogenic tumor phenotype. Melanoma cells with high β-catenin expression actually inhibit T-cell infiltration, excluding CD8+ effector T cells, FOXP3+ regulatory T cells but also CD103+ cells from the tumor microenvironment [82, 83]. This further downregulates antitumor response as CD103$^+$ dendritic cells (DCs) enhance the clinical response to BRAF blockade because they are priming tumor-specific CD8$^+$ T cells if present [84].

Deregulated Membrane Signaling in BRAFi-Resistant Melanoma Cells

Resistant melanoma cells have upregulated levels of receptor tyrosine kinases (RTKs), including epidermal growth factor receptor (EGFR), platelet-derived growth factor receptor B (PDGFRB), insulin growth factor 1 receptor (IGF1R), or TGFβ receptor 1 (TGFBR1). High expression of the RTK receptors on the surface of melanoma cells is correlated with acquired BRAFi resistance both *in vitro* and *in vivo*. In BRAFi-resistant melanoma cell lines and in resistant tumor samples, upregulation of EGFR expression was reported. Overexpression of EGFR in melanoma is known to derive from demethylation of *EGFR* regulatory DNA elements. Epidermal growth factor receptor (EGFRErbB-1; HER1), a transmembrane protein with receptor tyrosine kinase activity responding to epidermal growth factor family (EGF family) ligands, is involved in autocrine growth of melanoma cells [85]. EGFR signaling activates the PI3K/AKT pathway. As a result, resistant melanoma cells show high spontaneous migration and invasion with highly increased activity of matrix metallopeptidases (MMPs)—MMP2, MMP9, and MMP14 [86]. PI3K/AKT signaling prevents apoptosis and favors melanoma cell survival. After EGFR activation, the complex formed by the Grb2 and Sos proteins binds the adaptor protein Shc. This binding causes conformational changes in the Sos protein, which then recruits and activates Ras-GDP. Subsequently, downstream MAPK–ERK kinase phosphorylates specific transcription factors such as TS Like-1 protein Elk1 and C-myc, inducing melanoma cell proliferation [87]. It was also confirmed that EGFR overexpression induces BRAFi resistance without ERK activation in a MAPK-independent pathway [88]. Hyperactivation of the EGFR-SRC family kinase-signal transduction and subsequent activator of transcription 3 (STAT3) pathway signaling was reported [22]. EGF signaling promotes BRAFi resistance and induces melanoma invasion by Src pathways. Inhibition of the EGF receptor and Src re-sensitizes BRAFi-resistant melanoma cells to vemurafenib [70]. RTK pathways are also interconnected as downregulation of sex determining region Y-box 10 (SOX10) activity described in some melanomas promotes TGF-β signaling, which in turn increases EGFR expression and the activity of the receptor of the platelet-derived growth factor (PDGFRB) [17, 89].

BRAFi-Resistant Melanoma Cell Growth and Division

The RAS–RAF–MEK–ERK signal transduction pathway regulates the transcription of genes involved in cell growth, division, and differentiation. This signal transduction pathway is activated by growth factors, hormones, and cytokines, which interact with a membrane receptor with tyrosine kinase activity (RTK), leading to its phosphorylation, which in turn transfers the signal to a protein from the RAS (rat sarcoma) family of proteins. RAF and ERK are serine-threonine protein kinases, and MEK is a serine-tyrosine-threonine kinase. The signal is transduced by the phosphorylation of successive proteins (Ras–Raf–MEK–ERK), and the final targets are more than 50 transcription factors, including c-Myc and CREB [90]. Deregulation at each of the pathway steps may contribute to BRAFi/MEKi resistance. Modifications or mutation downstream of BRAF can occur, including *MEK* mutations that make this kinase constitutively active. Such mutations subsequently activate ERK. Activated ERK migrates to the nucleus where it phosphorylates and thus activates the targeted transcription factors [91]. The MAP/ERK pathway interacts with other pathways, such as MITF described earlier, but also with Wnt/β-catenin, c-Jun *N*-terminal kinase (JNK), and mechanistic target of rapamycin (mTOR). A complicated network of interactions maintains ERK activity despite BRAFi/MEKi. The network of resistance-related signaling pathways is complex. JUN and PKC were recently identified as key players in BRAFi resistance [33], while p-21-activated kinase (PAK) was reported as pivotal for BRAFi/MEKi combination resistance [34].

The Role of RAS

The MAPK/ERK pathway may also be activated due to secondary mutations in the *RAS* gene. Mutated Ras hyperactivates a RAF family protein (ARAF, BRAF, and CRAF—rapidly accelerated fibrosarcoma proteins), which in turn phosphorylates and activates MEK (mitogen-activated protein kinase kinases MEK1 and MEK2 also known as MAP2K1 and 2, or MAPKK 1 and 2), and MEK phosphorylates and activates the mitogen-activated protein kinase (MAPK/ERK). Hyperactivated RAS may phosphorylate the ARAF and CRAF proteins, which compensates for BRAF inhibition and promotes cell division via MAP/ERK signaling. In melanoma cells, *ARAF* or *CRAF* may be overexpressed, while BRAF is blocked, as described in the following. Some mutations have been described such as NRAS p.Q61K and KRAS p.K117N activating CRAF [92]. The mutated RAS protein after binding GTP does not dissociate to the inactive form bound to GDP and is permanently activated. The mutated protein - bound to GTP - also promotes BRAFV600E dimerization and reactivation of the MAP/ERK signal transduction pathway in this manner. In general, deregulated RAS in melanoma leads to resistance to BRAFi treatment. RAS hyperactivation may also lead to the formation of BRAFV600E dimers and signal transduction [25, 93, 94].

Another protein belonging to the Ras superfamily of small GTP-binding proteins and affecting BRAFi/MEKi resistance is RAC1. The *RAC1* gene (Rac family small GTPase 1, other names: cell migration-inducing gene 5 protein, Ras-related C3 botulinum toxin substrate 1, Ras-like protein TC25, P21-Rac1) encodes a GTPase that regulates cell differentiation, adhesion, mobility, and cell cycle [95]. The P29S mutation in the *RAC1* gene is found in 20% of BRAFi-resistant patients [23, 96]. Mutated Rac1 activates the c-Fos serum response element-binding transcription factor (SRF)/myocardin related transcription factor A (MRTF) pathway as well as serine/threonine-protein kinase PAK and AKT. In consequence, EMT is observed [97], as well as cell proliferation and metastatic spread [96].

The Role of RAS Regulators

Loss of a functional *PTEN* gene is observed in 10–35% of melanoma cases and is one of the most common causes of resistance to BRAF inhibitors [98, 99]. Lack of PTEN protein activity results in constitutive activation of the PI3K/AKT signaling pathway and cell growth, proliferation, and inhibition of apoptosis. The *PTEN* (phosphatase and tensin homolog) gene is a suppressor gene—the protein it encodes, phosphatidylinositol-3,4,5-trisphosphate 3-phosphatase (PTEN, MMAC1), is involved in cell cycle regulation. PTEN catalyzes PIP3 dephosphorylation in the 3′ position of the inositol ring, which inhibits the PI3K/AKT signal transduction pathway and as a result blocks cellular proliferation [100]. Inhibition of apoptosis in the case of *PTEN* loss is induced through the BIM (BCL2L11) protein [98].

The *NF1* gene was found to be the third most frequently mutated in melanoma after *BRAF* and *NRAS* [101]. NF-1 loss of function contributes to one of the mechanisms of BRAFi resistance in melanoma. The resultant constitutive activation of the MAPK/ERK signaling pathway is not suppressed by BRAFi [102]. The *NF1* gene encodes neurofibromin (also called neurofibromatosis-related protein NF-1) that is a member of the GTPase activating group of proteins. Neurofibromin regulates cell proliferation, differentiation, and survival. It is a negative regulator of RAS, the first protein of the MAPK signal transduction pathway—neurofibromin inactivates RAS–GTP by catalyzing the hydrolysis of RAS–GTP to RAS–GDP. In melanocytes, neurofibromin also regulates melanogenesis, and *NF1* loss results in enhanced production of melanin [103]. The absence of functional neurofibromin results in enhancement of several signaling pathways, including not only MAPK/ERK but also AKT/PI3K, and subsequently promotes melanoma cell proliferation and cell survival [104]. Suppression or loss of neurofibromin is a frequent event in cases treated with BRAFi/MEKi. Mutations in the *NF1* gene play a significant role in acquiring resistance to BRAF inhibitors [105].

The Role of RAF

BRAF protein function may also be reactivated through numerous mechanisms in BRAFi-resistant cells. In BRAFi-resistant melanoma, upstream reactivation of MAK/ERK signal transduction from the cell membrane may be caused by activation of ARAF and CRAF kinases in the place of BRAF—so-called kinase switching [106]. Kinase switching causes reactivation of signal transduction via the MAP/ERK pathway [107]. Vemurafenib was even described to bind to stabilized BRAF-CRAF heterodimers, thus reactivate the MAPK pathway. This potentiates the resistance in BRAF wild-type tumors, where in cells, the expression of CRAF was shown to be higher. This is the so-called paradoxical activating role of the BRAF inhibitor [90].

A frequent event is the amplification of the mutated *BRAF* allele. *BRAF*$^{V600E/K}$ amplification has been reported in about 13–20% of patients [99, 108]. Amplification results in overexpression of the BRAF protein. As a result, the administered dose of the BRAF inhibitor is insufficient to inhibit the activity of the abundant protein. BRAF amplification results in ERK signaling reactivation [109] and contributes to limiting the effectiveness of the treatment [110, 111]. This leads to inhibitor resistance, which is described as dose dependent as it can be overcome *in vitro* by higher doses of a BRAFi such as vemurafenib [24]. BRAF protein overload may also lead to spontaneous dimerization of the mutated BRAFV600E proteins, which also activates ERK signaling [99, 108].

Another BRAFi resistance mechanism is dependent on splicing. Splicing variants of *BRAF* may form dimers regardless of RAS signaling, thus abrogating the effects of BRAF inhibitors, which only act on BRAFV600E monomers. Splicing variants of BRAF are found in approximately 13–30% of resistant melanomas [108, 112, 113]. Splicing variant p61BRAFV600E has been described in patients with secondary resistance to vemurafenib. The alternative splicing BRAF isoforms result from mutations or epigenetic changes [114, 115].

The Role of MEK

First of all, RAS–RAF–MEK–ERK may become activated by mutations in genes encoding the MEK1/MEK2 proteins (mitogen-activated protein kinase 1/2). This reactivation of the MEK protein signaling downstream of BRAF abrogates the effects of BRAF inhibition as an initiation of the signal at the level of BRAF is no longer necessary for activation of final target genes [17]. MAPK signaling reactivation was found in up to 70% of melanoma cases upon disease progression [69]. Primary MAP2K1 (dual-specificity mitogen-activated protein kinase kinase 1 (MAP2K1, CFC3, MAPKK1, MEK1, MKK1)) and MAPK1 (mitogen-activated protein kinase 1, MAPK1, or ERK2) mutations are found in only 5.38% and 1.77%

melanoma cases, respectively, and were often inclusion criteria for patients in clinical trials with MEK inhibitors (MEKi) [116]. Little is reported on MEK-related resistance to BRAFi/MEKi therapy. MEK1C121S mutation was shown to increase MAP kinase activity and induce resistance to both RAF and MEK inhibitors [26]. Recently, secondary mutations in both MEK1 and MEK2 have been found in 7% of BRAFi-resistant melanomas. Known activating MEK1 mutations include Q56P, E203K, C121S, and K57E, whereas MEK2 mutations include E207K and Q60P [18, 99].

The Role of MAP-ERK Regulators

Multiple phosphatases and kinases regulate the MAP-ERK pathway and, if mutated, amplified or loss enable propagation of abnormal signaling. One most widely described is a mitogen-activated protein kinase kinase kinase 8 (*MAP3K8, COT* — cancer Osaka thyroid oncogene). The *MAP3K8* gene encodes the MAP3K8 proto-oncogene protein, also called as EST, ESTF, MEKK8, TPL2, Tpl-2, c-COT, and AURA2. Wild-type MAP3K8 protein phosphorylates MEK and activates the MAPK/ERK signal transduction pathway [117]. MAP3K8 activates MEK-dependent signaling and activates ERK without upstream RAF signaling. Overexpression of COT protein maintains proliferation during BRAFi treatment [99, 118, 119]. Administration of BRAFi in cases with primarily upregulated *MAP3K8* further increases the expression of this protein and as a result stimulates proliferation of melanoma cells [118, 119]. Mutations in *MAP3K8* are present in about 1.5% of all melanoma cases [120]. The usage of MEK and EKR inhibitors has been suggested as a strategy to overcome MAP3K8-related melanoma BRAFi resistance [121].

At the same time, the loss of function of dual-specificity phosphatase 4 (DUSP4) was reported to be correlated with BRAFi/MEKi resistance. These phosphatases dephosphorylate phosphoserine/threonine and phosphotyrosine residues in target kinases and render them inactive. If wild type and active, it inactivates ERK1 and ERK2, and therefore, loss of DUSP4 deregulates inhibition of signaling from BRAF [122]. Furthermore, DUSP phosphatase is also regulated. Block of proliferation 1 (BOP1), a ribosomal biogenesis factor, is a gene and the loss of which results in BRAFi resistance. BOP1 loss/downregulation results in the downregulation of DUSP4 and dual-specificity phosphatase 6 (DUSP6) expression. Lack of regulatory phosphatases results in the activation of MAP kinase signaling. Downregulation of BOP1 was reported in vemurafenib-resistant melanoma cells. These cells had significantly upregulated MAP kinase signaling and a high level of phosphorylated ERK1/2 [123].

BRAFi/MEKi-Resistant Melanoma Cell Proliferation

The Role of the PI3K/AKT/mTOR Pathway

Melanoma cell proliferation and quiescence are regulated by PI3K/AKT/mTOR pathway. This pathway also promotes melanoma cell survival in stress conditions. Activated AKT signaling provides a growth advantage and promotes metastatic spread and angiogenesis in melanoma [45]. Mutations leading to an increase in PI3K/AKT pathway activity have been identified in 22% melanomas with acquired resistance to BRAF inhibitors. An increase in AKT protein expression has been demonstrated several days after administering a BRAF inhibitor [69].

During treatment with BRAFi/MEKi, there is a strong selection pressure for cells with increased PI3K/AKT pathway activity, so cells continue to divide. The PI3K/AKT signal transduction pathway communicates with the ERK pathway, and therefore, inhibition of one of these two pathways can increase the activity of the other one. The blockage of ERK signaling leads to adaptive overactivity of PI3K/ AKT, which compensates for BRAF inactivation and results in acquired BRAFi resistance [69, 124, 125]. Moreover, activating mutations in PI3K and AKT promote signaling in the AKT pathway, and again increase antiapoptotic signals and upregulate key genes involved in proliferation. Actually activated AKT phosphorylates 9000 substrate proteins, including MDM-2 (murine double minute-2), p21 (p21 cyclin-dependent kinase inhibitory protein, Cip1), XIAP (X-linked inhibitor of apoptosis), ASK1 (apoptotic signal kinase 1), Bim (B cell leukemia/lymphoma-2 interacting mediator of cell death), Bad (B cell leukemia/lymphoma-2 associated death agonist), or Foxo3a (forkhead box O3) [126]. These mutations allow the survival and replication of melanoma cells during BRAFi treatment and are responsible for acquired resistance [17, 125, 127].

The Role of Cyclins and Kinases

CCND1 amplification has been observed in 20–38% melanoma cases resistant to BRAFi [128–130]. The *CCND1* (*BCL1*) gene encodes **cyclin D1** (also called B-cell lymphoma 1 protein), a key protein of the cell cycle and G1/S phase transition [131]. In cells with *CCND1* gene amplification, cyclin D1 expression is high, and as a consequence, BRAF inhibition is not sufficient to inhibit proliferation [131]. Cyclin D1 overexpression is sufficient to induce melanoma BRAFi resistance, but cyclin D1 and CDK4 concurrently overexpressed potentiate this phenomenon [131], because cyclin D1 regulates proliferation by binding to CDK4 and CDK6. The cyclin–cyclin-dependent kinase doublet activates the retinoblastoma protein (pRb) and promotes cell cycle progression [130].

Epigenetic Abnormalities Leading to BRAFi/MEKi Resistance

Epigenetic mechanisms contribute to BRAFi resistance. Epigenetic events promote an EMT and progenitor-like phenotype [132]. DNA methylation (presence/transfer of methyl groups covalently bound to cytosine bases) is catalyzed by DNA methyl-transferases (DNMTs). In particular, in CpG sites (dinucleotide sequence with a cytosine base preceding a guanine base with a phosphodiester bond shared between these two dinucleotides) are usually methylated. CpG islands, regions rich in CG dinucleotides, are present mostly at gene promoter regions and remain unmethyl-ated in normal cells. In malignant cells, the pattern of methylation is changed—globally, DNA methylation is usually decreased (hypomethylation) with some site-specific hypermethylation [132]. The role of methylation in melanoma and BRAFi resistance is still not clear. The combination of BRAFi and MEKi increases histone deacetylase 8 (HDAC8) expression, and this mechanism induces a drug-resistant phenotype [133]. Other players in melanoma resistance are KDM5A (lysine demethylase 5A) demethylation of H3K4, KDM1B (lysine (K)-specific demethylase 1B), KDM5A (lysine demethylase 5A), KDM5B (lysine demethylase 5B) demethylation of H3K4, KDM6A (lysine demethylase 6A), KDM6B (lysine (demethylase 6B) demethylation of H3K27, KDM6B demethylation of H3K27, EZH2 methylation of H3K27 and TADA2B (transcriptional adapter 2-beta), and TADA1 acetylation of histones H3 and H4 [134]. Histone modifications rather than changes in DNA methylation in melanoma contribute to drug resistance [135]. Histone modifications are driven by histone-modifying enzymes, including histone demethylases and histone deacetylases (HDACs) [136]. Downregulation of HAT1 (histone acetyltransferase 1) was observed in vemurafenib-resistant melanoma cells and resulted in high MAP kinase activity and ERK1/2 phosphorylation [123]. Exposure of melanoma cells to BRAFi/MEKi induces the upregulation of histone methyltransferases (SETDB1 and SETDB2) [135] as well as overexpression of his-tone demethylases (KDM6A, KDM6B, KDM1B, JARID1A, JARID1B) [137–139]. MAPKi-resistant melanoma cells have reduced expression of histone deacetylase SIRT6 that activates the AKT pathway [140].

The Role of Mitochondria in Melanoma Resistance to BRAF Inhibitors

The role of mitochondria in cancer has been analyzed and described for quite a long time, and many different strategies have been proposed to target mitochondria or mitochondrial metabolism in various types of neoplasms. Hanahan and Weinberg [141] described the "deregulation of cellular bioenergetics" as a hallmark of cancer, and mitochondria have been the subject of numerous studies with the idea of utiliz-ing their properties to attack, but also to understand, cancer [142, 143].

In order to design better drugs for treating melanoma, the mechanisms leading to resistance to currently used therapeutics have to be understood, and this is difficult, as the phenomenon of resistance is complex. Melanomas exhibit primary or acquired resistance to BRAF inhibitors (BRAFi), but this sentence is an oversimplification of the problem as both the use of the word melanomas and primary and secondary resistance are not as simple as they appear.

BRAFi acts only on cells with a *BRAF* mutation, but not on cells with wild-type *BRAF*. In general, melanomas are not homogeneous, and they may be a mixture of *BRAF* wild-type (WT) and *BRAF* mutant cells, the *BRAF* WT cells are resistant to BRAF inhibitors, and moreover, BRAFi can activate the wild-type protein. Secondary resistance develops in *BRAF* mutant cells as a result of mutations, non-mutational (e.g., epigenetic) events, and changes in the tumor microenvironment [144].

The population of melanoma cells is also not homogeneous with respect to their metabolism and the functioning of their mitochondria. Even though Warburg's idea that tumors only perform aerobic glycolysis is no longer in force, some tumor cells are more glycolytic than others, whereas some rely more on mitochondrial respiration [145], but all appear to have functional mitochondria. Among the cells of the tumor, there is a subpopulation with slow-cycling mitochondria, which is associated with resistance to targeted therapies [144], as the targeted inhibitors act mainly on rapidly proliferating cells. The slow cells can undergo expansion, and surprisingly, they are highly aggressive and invasive and appear to be stem-cell like. These cells are defined by the expression of JAR1D1B, a histone H3K4 demethylase. They are capable of increasing their rate of mitochondrial biogenesis and of oxidative phosphorylation [145], but this requires autophagy.

Microphthalmia-associated transcription factor (MITF) is a key regulator of melanoma cells, determining their proliferation. Its activity is complex, but briefly high levels can confer resistance to BRAFi. Interestingly, inhibition of this transcription factor by a compound called Icariside II led to overcoming BRAFi (vemurafenib) resistance in two melanoma cell lines; this was accompanied by an increase in reactive oxygen species (ROS) production by mitochondria. Both apoptosis and autophagy were enhanced in the cell lines in the presence of Icariside II [146].

Autophagy is a process of recycling damaged cell parts, and mitophagy is the only process allowing for the elimination of damaged/dysfunctional mitochondria and reutilizing their components for new organelles. It appears that in BRAF-driven tumors, not only in melanoma, autophagy is crucial for the proper functioning of mitochondria. The inhibition of autophagy, together with inhibition of BRAF, has thus been proposed as a method of circumventing BRAFi resistance [145].

Attacking mitochondria has proved successful in a number of experiments, indicating that their role in melanoma development is indeed important. Inhibition of mitochondrial respiration in a mouse model of melanoma by the well-known substance beta-sitosterol caused inhibition of mitochondrial complex I and prevented metastases to the brain in mice. In the same paper, vemurafenib resistance was found to be abrogated by sitosterol [147]. Interestingly, in the same paper, the authors analyzed almost 200 human brain metastases from various cancers and found the highest expression of complex I in melanoma metastases, but both in BRAF WT and BRAF mutant tumors.

Another substance used in addressing the problem of BRAFi resistance is metformin—one of the most widely used drugs in type II diabetes, with over 120 million patients treated worldwide [148]. Its main action is inhibition of mitochondrial complex I, also induces endoplasmic reticulum stress, and inhibits mammalian target of rapamycin complex I (mTORC1). It induces both apoptosis and autophagy in melanoma cells (the induction of autophagy is in contrast to previously discussed results); it has been tried in numerous clinical trials with BRAFi, but so far there are no encouraging results.

The interactions of BRAFi with mitochondria are complex, and it would be beyond the scope of this review to try to pinpoint the reasons for the observed inconsistencies, but there are interesting data on the effects of vemurafenib on mitochondria in BRAF-mutated human melanoma cells. Mitochondria maintain a delicate balance between fission and fusion in cells, and vemurafenib appears to cause a hyperfused phenotype, with increased phosphorylation. Complex I inhibition with rotenone enhanced vemurafenib activity [149].

Zhang et al. [150] (with an excellent comment by Luo, Puigserver [151]) investigated the role of mitochondria in resistance to vemurafenib. Again a slow-growing population was found, which was resistant to the drug but could give rise to rapidly growing cells. They were—or some of them were—characterized by the expression of the histone methylase JAR1D1B. The problem seems to be that the slow-growing cells resist inhibition by vemurafenib, but are capable of changing their growth and their oxidative phosphorylation/glycolysis ratios to evade inhibition by BRAFi.

Metabolic Abnormalities and Their Significance for Resistance to Targeted Therapies in Melanoma

BRAF mutations are known to affect the metabolism of melanoma cells dramatically. The most prominent metabolic alterations are the upregulation of glycolysis and suppression of oxidative phosphorylation [152]. One result of this metabolic shift is a higher level of glycolysis intermediates that may promote cancer progression. Some of these intermediates, like succinate, α-ketoglutarate, fumarate, 2-hydroxyglutarate, besides their "basic" metabolic function, promote cancer progression through epigenetic mechanisms or posttranslational protein modifications [153]. Another result of the melanoma "metabolic shift" is that melanoma cells, in normoxic conditions, metabolize up to 80% of glucose into lactate, and in hypoxic conditions, the rate of glucose to lactate transformation is even higher [154]. The metabolic shift and metabolic flexibility of melanoma cells seem to contribute to the aggressiveness of this type of tumor and also to the development of BRAFi resistance [155].

The specific proteins that contribute to melanoma metabolic shift and plasticity are BRAF, AKT, p14ARF, MYC, NRAS, PTEN, and PIK3CA [152]. Activation of the RAS/RAF/MEK/ERK pathway promotes a shift toward glycolytic metabolism. Constitutive activation of the MAPK signaling pathway increases the transcription of hypoxia inducible factor 1α (HIF1α), which also results in the upregulation of glycolytic metabolism [156]. BRAF mutations were also shown to drive the metabolic alterations in melanoma cells. The presence of the *BRAFV600E* mutation upregulates the expression of HIF1α [157]. Additionally, MYC overexpression induced by activation of the MAPK pathway may also increase glycolysis rate. MYC regulates *inter alia* the glucose transporter 1 (GLUT1) and lactate dehydrogenase (LDH). High GLUT1 expression was shown to correlate with poor prognosis, while lower GLUT1 expression was shown to correlate with better overall survival in melanoma patients [158, 159].

In vivo monitoring of metabolic activity of the skin, cancers seems an interesting direction for monitoring of drug resistance and for testing new therapeutic approaches. Widely used 18F-fluorodeoxyglucose positron emission tomography (PET) indicated higher glucose turnover in melanoma and may be useful for the detection of metastasis. The value of this approach was recently reviewed by Ayati, Sadeghi [160]. However, it would be desirable to monitor not only glucose uptake but also lactate production as lactate levels were shown to correlate with poorer prognosis in melanoma [152]. One technique that allows monitoring of lactate production is 13C magnetic resonance imaging combined with administration of hyperpolarized 13C-labeled tracers, in particular 13C-pyruvate that is quickly taken up by cells and metabolized to a few easily detectable products. Hyperpolarized 13C-pyruvate was recently shown in an animal melanoma model to be useful as a metabolic marker of response to BRAFi [161]. Moreover, it seems that this approach might be useful for detecting BRAFi resistance according to the in vitro results described in this study.

The data on specific alterations in skin cancers other than melanoma are very scarce. Basal cell carcinoma was shown to possess a specific metabolic signature as determined by magic angle spinning 1H NMR spectroscopy [162]. Higher levels of glycine and alanine were observed, indicating enhanced glycolysis. This study also detected elevated choline levels, a frequently observed phenomenon in cancers, indicating enhanced turnover of lipid membranes. However, in contrast to melanoma, the level of lactate was low, probably as a result of slow proliferation in this type of skin cancer. Another recent study in eyelid basal cell carcinoma revealed changes in glycine and creatine levels, but in this study that focused on a relatively small group of patients, the other metabolites were unchanged [163]. In squamous cell carcinoma, elevated expression of glucose transporter GLUT-1 was observed. In this tumor, elevated lactate levels were shown to correlate with shorter overall survival and a higher risk of tumor recurrence after radiotherapy [164]. Immunohistochemical analysis of paraffin-embedded primary cutaneous Merkel cell carcinoma specimens demonstrated expression of HIF-1α in all slices, and HIF-1α expression was more pronounced at the invading edges of the tumors. The downstream factors of HIF-1α: GLUT-1, MCT4, and CAIX were expressed in a vast majority of the samples (81–100% depending on the protein tested) [165]. This may suggest that metabolic abnormalities similar to those observed in melanoma would also be present in Merkel cell carcinoma.

Mechanisms of Resistance to Hedgehog Pathway Inhibitors in Basal Cell Carcinoma

The hedgehog pathway is associated with the regulation of embryonic development in a large number of species and is highly conserved. It also plays a role in differentiated adult cells, promoting the proliferation of stem cells or the transition of the hair follicle from the resting to the growth phase [166]. It also plays a role in the development of several cancers, in particular in basal cell carcinoma (BCC) [167]. Somatic alterations in the components of the Hedgehog (Hh) signaling pathway occur in a vast majority of cases, 85%, according to Bonilla, Parmentier [168]. These mutations occur mostly in the Patched-1 gene (or protein patched homolog 1; *PTCH1*; 73%), Smoothened (*SMO*; 20%), and less frequently in *SUFU* (8%). Amplification of transcription factor genes *GLI1*, *GLI2* genes are present in 8% of cases [168]. The *PTCH1* gene encodes a transmembrane protein that is a receptor for sonic hedgehog; when sonic hedgehog binds PTCH1, another component of the hedgehog pathway, smoothened is released and promotes cell proliferation through GLI transcription factors. Inactivating mutations in *PTCH1* lead to constitutive activation of the hedgehog pathway independent of the presence of the ligand [169].

Current FDA-approved drugs targeting the hedgehog pathway affect either SMO or GLI. Arsenic trioxide targets GLI transcription factors, but it was shown to also affect several other molecular targets. The two other drugs, vismodegib and sonidegib, suppress signaling resulting from *PTCH1* or *SMO* mutations by targeting SMO [169]. Vismodegib has approval for primary and metastatic BCCs, while sonidegib has approval for primary BCC. Tumors were found to develop resistance to drugs that target the hedgehog pathway, both approved and in development. Primary resistance to SMA inhibitors seems to be a result of variant genes downstream to SMO [170]. In particular, mutations in *SUFU* (suppressor of fused) were reported [171].

Secondary resistance to SMA inhibitor therapy seems to be mostly driven by *SMO* mutations in the drug-binding domain. SMO mutations were found in 15–33% untreated BCC and 69–77% vismodegib-resistant tumors after the therapy [172, 173]. The SMO mutations, such as D473, H231, W281, Q477, V321, I408, and C469, occurred inside the drug-binding pocket/domain or in its close vicinity. These mutations were only present in vismodegib-resistant tumors [172, 173]. Other mutations outside the drug-binding site may result in SMO instability, reduced affinity for the antagonist, or increase SMO activity. Less frequent molecular mechanisms of SMO inhibitor resistance might be deregulation at the level of GLI2 or SUFU proteins [173]. Gain-of-function mutations of Zinc finger protein Gli2, as well as *PTCH1* copy number loss, allow for uninhibited upregulation of the HH signaling [173]. Wnt pathway was shown as hyperactivated in vismodegib-resistant cells [174]. Moreover, intratumoral fibroblasts (and adipocytes) were suggested to contribute to the decreased drug delivery to the tumor. At the same time, a local immunosuppressive environment with abundant Foxp3$^+$ Treg cells in the tumors was shown to promote BCC growth under vismodegib treatment. CD8$^+$ T lymphocytes and macrophages are also more abundant in vismodegib-resistant BCCs [175].

Conclusions

Melanoma cells become resistant to BRAFi after several months of therapy. Multiple mechanisms have been identified to result in resistance to targeted therapies in melanoma and basal cell carcinoma. However, more data have been reported on melanoma, in maybe hypothesized that similar cellular processes are deregulated in response to therapy in skin cancers. Cancerous cell plasticity, as well as the intratumoral microenvironment, promotes survival under drug-induced stress.

Neoplastic cells under treatment pressure often undergo epithelial–mesenchymal transition with deregulated expression of α-smooth muscle actin (SMA), N-cadherin, vimentin, and fibronectin and become more resistant to targeted therapies and metastasize more easily [39, 78, 86]. Recent research has identified the role of intratumoral fibroblasts and macrophages to promote melanoma cell survival and proliferation. Fibroblasts, most of all, stimulate melanoma cells in a paracrine manner, while macrophages promote an immunosuppressive environment that inhibits anticancer response. For melanoma cells, in fact, the most common pathomechanism of BRAFi/MEKi resistance is the reactivation of the BRAF/MEK transduction pathway. Deregulation of *BRAF* gene expression results in the development of BRAFi resistance as overexpression of mutated BRAFV600E protein results in BRAFi inefficiency. An increased number of copies of the BRAFV600E protein in the cell—resulting from transcription and translation of multiple copies of the gene—favors BRAFV600E dimerization and results in reactivation of the ERK pathway [108, 109]. Moreover, the splicing variant of BRAFV600E, like p61BRAFV600E, can form dimers independently of RAS, making BRAF inhibitors ineffective as they only block monomeric BRAFV600E [112, 113]. Activation of BRAF signaling may also result from activating mutations in the *RAS* gene [17], which are pro-proliferative as mutated RAS–GTP becomes constitutively active, increases BRAFV600E dimerization, and reactivates the ERK pathway [29].

Overexpression of the COT protein, probably due to gene amplification or hitherto unidentified mechanisms, can reactivate MEK in the presence of BRAF inhibition, stimulating ERK signaling and development of resistance to BRAFi [118, 119]. Activation of alternative RAFs, ARAF and CRAF, induces BRAFi resistance as all RAF isoforms are capable of downstream ERK activation. Moreover, BRAFi inhibits tumor growth by inhibiting ERK, and this in turn inhibits the negative feedback inhibition of ERK on RAS, which partially restores RAS activity, leading to the formation of BRAFV600E dimers induced by RAF [29]. Activating mutations in *MEK1/MEK2* make blocking of BRAF ineffective as MEK reactivation means that the MAPK/ERK pathway can still transduce the signal below BRAF, regardless of its inhibition [18, 99]. Finally, reactivation of MAP/ERK pathway-dependent transcription factors may result from downstream ERK activation and loss of the inhibitory function of ERK kinase [29].

Melanoma cell proliferation may also be promoted by the PI3K–AKT–mTOR pathway that may also become activated. Actually blocking ERK signaling may lead to adaptive PI3K/AKT activity, which compensates for BRAF inhibition and promotes resistance. Active AKT pathway provides anti-apoptotic signals and increases proliferation providing melanoma cell survival. With BRAF blocked, tumor cells can overexpress RTK, leading to permanent PI3K/AKT signaling. Activation of receptor tyrosine kinases (RTK) is another mechanism of resistance—the PI3K/AKT pathway is activated by growth factors, which bind RTKs [22]. In BRAFi-resistant melanoma cells with BRAF mutation, PDGFRbeta and IGFR1 overexpression were reported to causes PI3K–AKT–mTOR pathway reactivation. In other resistant cases, overexpression and/or hyperactivity of EGFR was reported [176]. Upregulation of the PI3K/AKT/mTOR signaling axis results also from mutations in *AKT1*, *AKT3*, *PIK3CA*, *PIK3CG*, *PIK3R2*, or *PHLPP1* genes [22]. Such activating mutations in the *PI3K/AKT* genes induce AKT phosphorylation and signaling, which increases anti-apoptotic signaling and increases the expression of key proliferation genes, providing the cell with survival signals independent of BRAF [16, 86].

The presence of the BRAFi resistance-related mutations leads to several metabolic abnormalities both in the melanoma cells and in the tumor microenvironment, the most prominent one is upregulation of glycolysis and downregulation of oxidative phosphorylation. These alterations seem to have a great impact on the melanoma BRAFi resistance and could be potentially important therapeutic targets. Another target could be mitochondria, but their role in the resistance to BRAFi is complex, and their behavior can be different in different tumor cells. While the effect on specific mutations related to BRAFi resistance is relatively well characterized in melanoma, the data concerning metabolic alterations and their significance for resistance to targeted therapies in other skin cancers are very limited. This is a potential new important research area crucial for the effective treatment and for overcoming the drug resistance in these cancers. Data from experimental animal models that will involve advanced in vivo metabolic imaging methods would be especially valuable in this aspect. Moreover, they seem to have a translation potential for the monitoring of the metabolic alterations in patients and for the monitoring of the efficacy of the future and present therapies in suppressing the metabolic alterations in these cancers. The phenomena which are responsible for resistance have not been determined in 41.7% of patient samples [92].

Little is known on the resistance mechanism of hedgehog inhibitors used in BCC. It was reported that the majority of vismodegib resistance cases are caused by mutations in SMO that limit drug binding or increase basal SMO activity. Mutations in downstream genes like SUFU may also contribute to the resistance. At the same time, *GLI2* gain of function mutations, *PTCH1* copy number loss, and *PTEN* loss of function also were reported in resistant cells [173]. As melanoma cells surviving

BRAFi treatment, BCC vismodegib-resistant cells undergo EMT and/or are activated by intratumoral fibroblasts. Resistant tumors are also characterized by immunosuppressive microenvironment due to signaling from macrophages and T regulatory cells [175]. More research is needed to understand the complex molecular pathology of HH-signaling resistance.

References

1. Davies H, et al. Mutations of the BRAF gene in human cancer. Nature. 2002;417(6892):949–54.
2. Zaman A, Wu W, Bivona TG. Targeting oncogenic BRAF: past, present, and future. Cancers (Basel). 2019;11(8):1197.
3. Cheng L, et al. Molecular testing for BRAF mutations to inform melanoma treatment decisions: a move toward precision medicine. Mod Pathol. 2018;31(1):24–38.
4. Hauschild A, et al. Dabrafenib in BRAF-mutated metastatic melanoma: a multicentre, open-label, phase 3 randomised controlled trial. Lancet. 2012;380(9839):358–65.
5. Rutkowski P, et al. The outcomes of Polish patients with advanced BRAF-positive melanoma treated with vemurafenib in a safety clinical trial. Contemp Oncol (Pozn). 2015;19(4):280–3.
6. Kozak K, Rutkowski P. Why do we need a new BRAF-MEK inhibitor combination in melanoma? Oncol Clin Pract. 2019;15:115–9.
7. Jagodzińska-Mucha P, Rutkowski P. Encorafenib in combination with binimetinib — a new therapeutic option with a favourable safety profile in the treatment of patients with advanced BRAF mutation-positive melanoma. Oncol Clin Pract. 2020;16(2):75–82.
8. Grob JJ, et al. Comparison of dabrafenib and trametinib combination therapy with vemurafenib monotherapy on health-related quality of life in patients with unresectable or metastatic cutaneous BRAF Val600-mutation-positive melanoma (COMBI-v): results of a phase 3, open-label, randomised trial. Lancet Oncol. 2015;16(13):1389–98.
9. Kozak K, et al. Summary of experience of melanoma patients treated with BRAF/MEK inhibitors according to Polish National Drug Reimbursement Program Guidelines. Oncol Clin Pract. 2020;16(3):109–15.
10. Pasquali S, et al. Systemic treatments for metastatic cutaneous melanoma. Cochrane Database Syst Rev. 2018;2:CD011123.
11. Larkin J, et al. An open-label, multicentre safety study of vemurafenib in patients with BRAF(V600)-mutant metastatic melanoma: final analysis and a validated prognostic scoring system. Eur J Cancer. 2019;107:175–85.
12. Hauschild A, et al. Long-term outcomes in patients with BRAF V600-mutant metastatic melanoma receiving dabrafenib monotherapy: Analysis from phase 2 and 3 clinical trials. Eur J Cancer. 2020;125:114–20.
13. Robert C, et al. Five-year outcomes with dabrafenib plus trametinib in metastatic melanoma. N Engl J Med. 2019;381(7):626–36.
14. Rutkowski P, Świtaj T. Treatment of BRAF+ melanoma in light of current drug programs. Oncol Clin Pract. 2017;13(6):275–80.
15. Ribas A, Flaherty KT. BRAF targeted therapy changes the treatment paradigm in melanoma. Nat Rev Clin Oncol. 2011;8(7):426–33.
16. Czarnecka AM, et al. Targeted therapy in melanoma and mechanisms of resistance. Int J Mol Sci. 2020;21(13):4576.
17. Griffin M, et al. BRAF inhibitors: resistance and the promise of combination treatments for melanoma. Oncotarget. 2017;8(44):78174–92.
18. Patel H, et al. Current advances in the treatment of BRAF-mutant melanoma. Cancers (Basel). 2020;12(2):482.

19. Kozak K, et al. Podsumowanie doświadczeń w stosowaniu inhibitorów BRAF/MEK u chorych na czerniaka w ramach dostępnych programów lekowych. Oncol Clin Pract. 2020.
20. Lewis KD, et al. Impact of depth of response on survival in patients treated with cobimetinib +/− vemurafenib: pooled analysis of BRIM-2, BRIM-3, BRIM-7 and coBRIM. Br J Cancer. 2019;121(7):522–8.
21. Larkin JMG, et al. Clinical predictors of response for coBRIM: A phase III study of cobimetinib (C) in combination with vemurafenib (V) in advanced BRAF-mutated melanoma (MM). J Clin Oncol. 2016;34(15_suppl):9528.
22. Caporali S, et al. Targeting the PI3K/AKT/mTOR pathway overcomes the stimulating effect of dabrafenib on the invasive behavior of melanoma cells with acquired resistance to the BRAF inhibitor. Int J Oncol. 2016;49(3):1164–74.
23. Van Allen EM, et al. The genetic landscape of clinical resistance to RAF inhibition in metastatic melanoma. Cancer Discov. 2014;4(1):94–109.
24. Shi H, et al. Melanoma whole-exome sequencing identifies (V600E)B-RAF amplification-mediated acquired B-RAF inhibitor resistance. Nat Commun. 2012;3:724.
25. Nazarian R, et al. Melanomas acquire resistance to B-RAF(V600E) inhibition by RTK or N-RAS upregulation. Nature. 2010;468(7326):973–7.
26. Wagle N, et al. Dissecting therapeutic resistance to RAF inhibition in melanoma by tumor genomic profiling. J Clin Oncol. 2011;29(22):3085–96.
27. Almeida FV, et al. Bad company: Microenvironmentally mediated resistance to targeted therapy in melanoma. Pigment Cell Melanoma Res. 2019;32(2):237–47.
28. Kozar I, et al. Many ways to resistance: how melanoma cells evade targeted therapies. Biochim Biophys Acta Rev Cancer. 2019;1871(2):313–22.
29. Bartnik E, Fiedorowicz M, Czarnecka AM. Mechanisms of melanoma resistance to treatment with BRAF and MEK inhibitors. Nowotwory. J Oncol. 2019;69(3–4):133–41.
30. Kakadia S, et al. Mechanisms of resistance to BRAF and MEK inhibitors and clinical update of US Food and Drug Administration-approved targeted therapy in advanced melanoma. Onco Targets Ther. 2018;11:7095–107.
31. Lim SY, Menzies AM, Rizos H. Mechanisms and strategies to overcome resistance to molecularly targeted therapy for melanoma. Cancer. 2017;123(S11):2118–29.
32. Chen G, Davies MA. Targeted therapy resistance mechanisms and therapeutic implications in melanoma. Hematol Oncol Clin North Am. 2014;28(3):523–36.
33. Titz B, et al. JUN dependency in distinct early and late BRAF inhibition adaptation states of melanoma. Cell Discov. 2016;2:16028.
34. Lu H, et al. PAK signalling drives acquired drug resistance to MAPK inhibitors in BRAF-mutant melanomas. Nature. 2017;550(7674):133–6.
35. Tape CJ, et al. Oncogenic KRAS regulates tumor cell signaling via stromal reciprocation. Cell. 2016;165(4):910–20.
36. Buczek M, et al. Resistance to tyrosine kinase inhibitors in clear cell renal cell carcinoma: from the patient's bed to molecular mechanisms. Biochim Biophys Acta. 2014;1845(1):31–41.
37. Kaminska K, et al. The role of the cell-cell interactions in cancer progression. J Cell Mol Med. 2015;19(2):283–96.
38. Vella LJ, et al. Intercellular resistance to BRAF inhibition can be mediated by extracellular vesicle-associated PDGFRbeta. Neoplasia. 2017;19(11):932–40.
39. Seip K, et al. Fibroblast-induced switching to the mesenchymal-like phenotype and PI3K/mTOR signaling protects melanoma cells from BRAF inhibitors. Oncotarget. 2016;7(15):19997–20015.
40. Karbowniczek M, et al. mTOR is activated in the majority of malignant melanomas. J Invest Dermatol. 2008;128(4):980–7.
41. Fedorenko IV, et al. BRAF inhibition generates a host-tumor niche that mediates therapeutic escape. J Invest Dermatol. 2015;135(12):3115–24.
42. Matsumoto K, et al. Hepatocyte growth factor/MET in cancer progression and biomarker discovery. Cancer Sci. 2017;108(3):296–307.

43. Blum D, LaBarge S, Reproducibility Project B. Cancer, registered report: tumour micro-environment elicits innate resistance to RAF inhibitors through HGF secretion. elife. 2014;3:e04034.
44. Straussman R, et al. Tumour micro-environment elicits innate resistance to RAF inhibitors through HGF secretion. Nature. 2012;487(7408):500–4.
45. Porta C, Paglino C, Mosca A. Targeting PI3K/Akt/mTOR signaling in cancer. Front Oncol. 2014;4:64.
46. Capparelli C, et al. Fibroblast-derived neuregulin 1 promotes compensatory ErbB3 receptor signaling in mutant BRAF melanoma. J Biol Chem. 2015;290(40):24267–77.
47. Kaur A, et al. sFRP2 in the aged microenvironment drives melanoma metastasis and therapy resistance. Nature. 2016;532(7598):250–4.
48. Li G, et al. Function and regulation of melanoma-stromal fibroblast interactions: when seeds meet soil. Oncogene. 2003;22(20):3162–71.
49. Flach EH, et al. Fibroblasts contribute to melanoma tumor growth and drug resistance. Mol Pharm. 2011;8(6):2039–49.
50. Hirata E, et al. Intravital imaging reveals how BRAF inhibition generates drug-tolerant micro-environments with high integrin beta1/FAK signaling. Cancer Cell. 2015;27(4):574–88.
51. Huang R, Rofstad EK. Integrins as therapeutic targets in the organ-specific metastasis of human malignant melanoma. J Exp Clin Cancer Res. 2018;37(1):92.
52. Leask A. A centralized communication network: recent insights into the role of the cancer associated fibroblast in the development of drug resistance in tumors. Semin Cell Dev Biol. 2020;101:111–4.
53. Hutchenreuther J, et al. Activation of cancer-associated fibroblasts is required for tumor neo-vascularization in a murine model of melanoma. Matrix Biol. 2018;74:52–61.
54. Hutchenreuther J, et al. CCN2 expression by tumor stroma is required for melanoma metastasis. J Invest Dermatol. 2015;135(11):2805–13.
55. Massi D, et al. The status of PD-L1 and tumor-infiltrating immune cells predict resistance and poor prognosis in BRAFi-treated melanoma patients harboring mutant BRAFV600. Ann Oncol. 2015;26(9):1980–7.
56. Wang SJ, et al. Efficient blockade of locally reciprocated tumor-macrophage signaling using a TAM-avid nanotherapy. Sci Adv. 2020;6(21):eaaz8521.
57. Wang H, et al. Pro-tumor activities of macrophages in the progression of melanoma. Hum Vaccin Immunother. 2017;13(7):1556–62.
58. Massi D, et al. The density and spatial tissue distribution of CD8(+) and CD163(+) immune cells predict response and outcome in melanoma patients receiving MAPK inhibitors. J Immunother Cancer. 2019;7(1):308.
59. Atzori MG, et al. Role of VEGFR-1 in melanoma acquired resistance to the BRAF inhibitor vemurafenib. J Cell Mol Med. 2020;24(1):465–75.
60. Ria R, et al. Angiogenesis and progression in human melanoma. Dermatol Res Pract. 2010;2010:185687.
61. Ruffell B, Coussens LM. Macrophages and therapeutic resistance in cancer. Cancer Cell. 2015;27(4):462–72.
62. Gray-Schopfer VC, et al. Tumor necrosis factor-alpha blocks apoptosis in melanoma cells when BRAF signaling is inhibited. Cancer Res. 2007;67(1):122–9.
63. Wang T, et al. BRAF inhibition stimulates melanoma-associated macrophages to drive tumor growth. Clin Cancer Res. 2015;21(7):1652–64.
64. Amaral T, et al. MAPK pathway in melanoma part II-secondary and adaptive resistance mechanisms to BRAF inhibition. Eur J Cancer. 2017;73:93–101.
65. Müller J, et al. Low MITF/AXL ratio predicts early resistance to multiple targeted drugs in melanoma. Nat Commun. 2014;5(1):5712.
66. Hayward NK, et al. Whole-genome landscapes of major melanoma subtypes. Nature. 2017;545(7653):175–80.

67. Johannessen CM, et al. A melanocyte lineage program confers resistance to MAP kinase pathway inhibition. Nature. 2013;504(7478):138–42.
68. Smith MP, et al. Inhibiting drivers of non-mutational drug tolerance is a salvage strategy for targeted melanoma therapy. Cancer Cell. 2016;29(3):270–84.
69. Shi H, et al. Acquired resistance and clonal evolution in melanoma during BRAF inhibitor therapy. Cancer Discov. 2014;4(1):80–93.
70. Li FZ, et al. Phenotype switching in melanoma: implications for progression and therapy. Front Oncol. 2015;5:31.
71. Levy C, Khaled M, Fisher DE. MITF: master regulator of melanocyte development and melanoma oncogene. Trends Mol Med. 2006;12(9):406–14.
72. Goding CR, Arnheiter H. MITF-the first 25 years. Genes Dev. 2019;33(15–16):983–1007.
73. Loercher AE, et al. MITF links differentiation with cell cycle arrest in melanocytes by transcriptional activation of INK4A. J Cell Biol. 2005;168(1):35–40.
74. Leclerc J, Ballotti R, Bertolotto C. Pathways from senescence to melanoma: focus on MITF sumoylation. Oncogene. 2017;36(48):6659–67.
75. Konieczkowski DJ, et al. A melanoma cell state distinction influences sensitivity to MAPK pathway inhibitors. Cancer Discov. 2014;4(7):816–27.
76. Liu S, et al. miR-200c/Bmi1 axis and epithelial-mesenchymal transition contribute to acquired resistance to BRAF inhibitor treatment. Pigment Cell Melanoma Res. 2015;28(4):431–41.
77. McCubrey JA, et al. Mutations and deregulation of Ras/Raf/MEK/ERK and PI3K/PTEN/Akt/mTOR cascades which alter therapy response. Oncotarget. 2012;3(9):954–87.
78. Pearlman RL, et al. Potential therapeutic targets of epithelial-mesenchymal transition in melanoma. Cancer Lett. 2017;391:125–40.
79. Richard G, et al. ZEB1-mediated melanoma cell plasticity enhances resistance to MAPK inhibitors. EMBO Mol Med. 2016;8(10):1143–61.
80. Cordaro FG, et al. Phenotype characterization of human melanoma cells resistant to dabrafenib. Oncol Rep. 2017;38(5):2741–51.
81. Paulitschke V, et al. Proteomic identification of a marker signature for MAPKi resistance in melanoma. EMBO J. 2019;38(15):e95874.
82. Massi D, et al. Baseline beta-catenin, programmed death-ligand 1 expression and tumour-infiltrating lymphocytes predict response and poor prognosis in BRAF inhibitor-treated melanoma patients. Eur J Cancer. 2017;78:70–81.
83. Wei CY, et al. Downregulation of RNF128 activates Wnt/beta-catenin signaling to induce cellular EMT and stemness via CD44 and CTTN ubiquitination in melanoma. J Hematol Oncol. 2019;12(1):21.
84. Salmon H, et al. Expansion and activation of CD103(+) dendritic cell progenitors at the tumor site enhances tumor responses to therapeutic PD-L1 and BRAF inhibition. Immunity. 2016;44(4):924–38.
85. Staibano S, et al. Epidermal growth factor receptor (EGFR) expression in cutaneous melanoma: a possible role as prognostic marker. Melanoma Res. 2004;14(2):S26.
86. Wang J, et al. Epigenetic changes of EGFR have an important role in BRAF inhibitor-resistant cutaneous melanomas. J Invest Dermatol. 2015;135(2):532–41.
87. Seshacharyulu P, et al. Targeting the EGFR signaling pathway in cancer therapy. Expert Opin Ther Targets. 2012;16(1):15–31.
88. Kwong LN, et al. Co-clinical assessment identifies patterns of BRAF inhibitor resistance in melanoma. J Clin Invest. 2015;125(4):1459–70.
89. Sun C, et al. Reversible and adaptive resistance to BRAF(V600E) inhibition in melanoma. Nature. 2014;508(7494):118–22.
90. Kim A, Cohen MS. The discovery of vemurafenib for the treatment of BRAF-mutated metastatic melanoma. Expert Opin Drug Discov. 2016;11(9):907–16.
91. Bezniakow N, Gos M, Obersztyn E. The RASopathies as an example of RAS/MAPK pathway disturbances - clinical presentation and molecular pathogenesis of selected syndromes. Dev Period Med. 2014;18(3):285–96.

92. Luebker SA, Koepsell SA. Diverse mechanisms of BRAF inhibitor resistance in melanoma identified in clinical and preclinical studies. Front Oncol. 2019;9:268.
93. Corcoran RB, Settleman J, Engelman JA. Potential therapeutic strategies to overcome acquired resistance to BRAF or MEK inhibitors in BRAF mutant cancers. Oncotarget. 2011;2(4):336–46.
94. Romano E, et al. Identification of multiple mechanisms of resistance to vemurafenib in a patient with BRAFV600E-mutated cutaneous melanoma successfully rechallenged after progression. Clin Cancer Res. 2013;19(20):5749–57.
95. Nguyen LK, Kholodenko BN, von Kriegsheim A. Rac1 and RhoA: networks, loops and bistability. Small GTPases. 2018;9(4):316–21.
96. Watson IR, et al. The RAC1 P29S hotspot mutation in melanoma confers resistance to pharmacological inhibition of RAF. Cancer Res. 2014;74(17):4845–52.
97. Lionarons DA, et al. RAC1(P29S) induces a mesenchymal phenotypic switch via serum response factor to promote melanoma development and therapy resistance. Cancer cell. 2019;36(1):68–83.e9.
98. Paraiso KH, et al. PTEN loss confers BRAF inhibitor resistance to melanoma cells through the suppression of BIM expression. Cancer Res. 2011;71(7):2750–60.
99. Tian Y, Guo W. A review of the molecular pathways involved in resistance to BRAF inhibitors in patients with advanced-stage melanoma. Med Sci Monit. 2020;26:e920957.
100. Aguissa-Toure AH, Li G. Genetic alterations of PTEN in human melanoma. Cell Mol Life Sci. 2012;69(9):1475–91.
101. Krauthammer M, et al. Exome sequencing identifies recurrent mutations in NF1 and RASopathy genes in sun-exposed melanomas. Nat Genet. 2015;47(9):996–1002.
102. Whittaker SR, et al. A genome-scale RNA interference screen implicates NF1 loss in resistance to RAF inhibition. Cancer Discov. 2013;3(3):350–62.
103. Allouche J, et al. In vitro modeling of hyperpigmentation associated to neurofibromatosis type 1 using melanocytes derived from human embryonic stem cells. Proc Natl Acad Sci U S A. 2015;112(29):9034–9.
104. Peltonen S, Kallionpaa RA, Peltonen J. Neurofibromatosis type 1 (NF1) gene: beyond cafe au lait spots and dermal neurofibromas. Exp Dermatol. 2017;26(7):645–8.
105. Maertens O, et al. Elucidating distinct roles for NF1 in melanomagenesis. Cancer Discov. 2013;3(3):338–49.
106. Molina JR, Adjei AA. The Ras/Raf/MAPK pathway. J Thorac Oncol. 2006;1(1):7–9.
107. Fedorenko IV, Paraiso KH, Smalley KS. Acquired and intrinsic BRAF inhibitor resistance in BRAF V600E mutant melanoma. Biochem Pharmacol. 2011;82(3):201–9.
108. Johnson DB, et al. Acquired BRAF inhibitor resistance: a multicenter meta-analysis of the spectrum and frequencies, clinical behaviour, and phenotypic associations of resistance mechanisms. Eur J Cancer. 2015;51(18):2792–9.
109. Corcoran RB, et al. BRAF gene amplification can promote acquired resistance to MEK inhibitors in cancer cells harboring the BRAF V600E mutation. Sci Signal. 2010;3(149):ra84.
110. Villanueva J, et al. Acquired resistance to BRAF inhibitors mediated by a RAF kinase switch in melanoma can be overcome by cotargeting MEK and IGF-1R/PI3K. Cancer Cell. 2010;18(6):683–95.
111. Spagnolo F, et al. BRAF-mutant melanoma: treatment approaches, resistance mechanisms, and diagnostic strategies. Onco Targets Ther. 2015;8:157–68.
112. Pupo GM, et al. Clinical significance of intronic variants in BRAF inhibitor resistant melanomas with altered BRAF transcript splicing. Biomark Res. 2017;5:17.
113. Vido MJ, et al. BRAF splice variant resistance to RAF inhibitor requires enhanced MEK association. Cell Rep. 2018;25(6):1501–1510.e3.
114. Poulikakos PI, et al. RAF inhibitor resistance is mediated by dimerization of aberrantly spliced BRAF(V600E). Nature. 2011;480(7377):387–90.
115. Luco RF, et al. Epigenetics in alternative pre-mRNA splicing. Cell. 2011;144(1):16–26.

116. Consortium APG. AACR project GENIE: powering precision medicine through an international consortium. Cancer Discov. 2017;7(8):818–31.
117. Sanchez JN, Wang T, Cohen MS. BRAF and MEK inhibitors: use and resistance in BRAF-mutated cancers. Drugs. 2018;78(5):549–66.
118. Sharma V, et al. Registered report: COT drives resistance to RAF inhibition through MAP kinase pathway reactivation. elife. 2016;5:e11414.
119. Johannessen CM, et al. COT drives resistance to RAF inhibition through MAP kinase pathway reactivation. Nature. 2010;468(7326):968–72.
120. Potentially actionable MAP3K8 alterations are common in spitzoid melanoma. Cancer Discov. 2019;9(5):574.
121. Lehmann BD, et al. Identification of targetable recurrent MAP3K8 rearrangements in melanomas lacking known driver mutations. Mol Cancer Res. 2019;17(9):1842–53.
122. Hugo W, et al. Non-genomic and immune evolution of melanoma acquiring MAPKi resistance. Cell. 2015;162(6):1271–85.
123. Gupta R, et al. Loss of BOP1 confers resistance to BRAF kinase inhibitors in melanoma by activating MAP kinase pathway. Proc Natl Acad Sci U S A. 2019;116(10):4583–91.
124. Mendoza MC, Er EE, Blenis J. The Ras-ERK and PI3K-mTOR pathways: cross-talk and compensation. Trends Biochem Sci. 2011;36(6):320–8.
125. Shi H, et al. A novel AKT1 mutant amplifies an adaptive melanoma response to BRAF inhibition. Cancer Discov. 2014;4(1):69–79.
126. Madhunapantula SV, Mosca PJ, Robertson GP. The Akt signaling pathway: an emerging therapeutic target in malignant melanoma. Cancer Biol Ther. 2011;12(12):1032–49.
127. Das Thakur M, Stuart DD. Molecular pathways: response and resistance to BRAF and MEK inhibitors in BRAF(V600E) tumors. Clin Cancer Res. 2014;20(5):1074–80.
128. Wilson MA, et al. Copy number changes are associated with response to treatment with carboplatin, paclitaxel, and sorafenib in melanoma. Clin Cancer Res. 2016;22(2):374–82.
129. Harris AL, et al. Targeting the cyclin dependent kinase and retinoblastoma axis overcomes standard of care resistance in BRAF (V600E) -mutant melanoma. Oncotarget. 2018;9(13):10905–19.
130. Manzano JL, et al. Resistant mechanisms to BRAF inhibitors in melanoma. Ann Transl Med. 2016;4(12):237.
131. Smalley KS, et al. Increased cyclin D1 expression can mediate BRAF inhibitor resistance in BRAF V600E-mutated melanomas. Mol Cancer Ther. 2008;7(9):2876–83.
132. Khaliq M, Fallahi-Sichani M. Epigenetic mechanisms of escape from BRAF oncogene dependency. Cancers (Basel). 2019;11(10):1480.
133. Emmons MF, et al. HDAC8 regulates a stress response pathway in melanoma to mediate escape from BRAF inhibitor therapy. Cancer Res. 2019;79(11):2947–61.
134. Strub T, Ballotti R, Bertolotto C. The "ART" of epigenetics in melanoma: from histone "alterations, to resistance and therapies". Theranostics. 2020;10(4):1777–97.
135. Al Emran A, et al. Distinct histone modifications denote early stress-induced drug tolerance in cancer. Oncotarget. 2018;9(9):8206–22.
136. Chan JC, Maze I. Nothing is yet set in (Hi)stone: novel post-translational modifications regulating chromatin function. Trends Biochem Sci. 2020;45(10):829–44.
137. Roesch A, et al. A temporarily distinct subpopulation of slow-cycling melanoma cells is required for continuous tumor growth. Cell. 2010;141(4):583–94.
138. Ravindran Menon D, et al. A stress-induced early innate response causes multidrug tolerance in melanoma. Oncogene. 2015;34(34):4448–59.
139. Roesch A, et al. Overcoming intrinsic multidrug resistance in melanoma by blocking the mitochondrial respiratory chain of slow-cycling JARID1B(high) cells. Cancer Cell. 2013;23(6):811–25.
140. Strub T, et al. SIRT6 haploinsufficiency induces BRAF(V600E) melanoma cell resistance to MAPK inhibitors via IGF signalling. Nat Commun. 2018;9(1):3440.
141. Hanahan D, Weinberg RA. Hallmarks of cancer: the next generation. Cell. 2011;144(5):646–74.

142. Weinberg SE, Chandel NS. Targeting mitochondria metabolism for cancer therapy. Nat Chem Biol. 2015;11(1):9–15.
143. Dong L, Neuzil J. Targeting mitochondria as an anticancer strategy. Cancer Commun (Lond). 2019;39(1):63.
144. Ahmed F, Haass NK. Microenvironment-driven dynamic heterogeneity and phenotypic plasticity as a mechanism of melanoma therapy resistance. Front Oncol. 2018;8:173.
145. Strohecker AM, White E. Targeting mitochondrial metabolism by inhibiting autophagy in BRAF-driven cancers. Cancer Discov. 2014;4(7):766–72.
146. Liu X, et al. Icariside II overcomes BRAF inhibitor resistance in melanoma by inducing ROS production and inhibiting MITF. Oncol Rep. 2020;44(1):360–70.
147. Sundstrøm T, et al. Inhibition of mitochondrial respiration prevents BRAF-mutant melanoma brain metastasis. Acta Neuropathol Commun. 2019;7(1):55.
148. Jaune E, Rocchi S. Metformin: focus on melanoma. Front Endocrinol (Lausanne). 2018;9:472.
149. Ferraz LS, et al. Targeting mitochondria in melanoma: interplay between MAPK signaling pathway and mitochondrial dynamics. Biochem Pharmacol. 2020;178:114104.
150. Zhang G, et al. Targeting mitochondrial biogenesis to overcome drug resistance to MAPK inhibitors. J Clin Invest. 2016;126(5):1834–56.
151. Luo C, Puigserver P, Widlund HR. Breaking BRAF(V600E)-drug resistance by stressing mitochondria. Pigment Cell Melanoma Res. 2016;29(4):401–3.
152. Avagliano A, et al. Metabolic plasticity of melanoma cells and their crosstalk with tumor microenvironment. Front Oncol. 2020;10:722.
153. Ryan DG, et al. Coupling Krebs cycle metabolites to signalling in immunity and cancer. Nat Metab. 2019;1(1):16–33.
154. Ratnikov BI, et al. Metabolic rewiring in melanoma. Oncogene. 2017;36(2):147–57.
155. Ruocco MR, et al. Metabolic flexibility in melanoma: a potential therapeutic target. Semin Cancer Biol. 2019;59:187–207.
156. Luís R, Brito C, Pojo M. Melanoma metabolism: cell survival and resistance to therapy. Adv Exp Med Biol. 2020;1219:203–23.
157. Kumar SM, et al. Mutant V600E BRAF increases hypoxia inducible factor-1α expression in melanoma. Cancer Res. 2007;67(7):3177–84.
158. Koch A, et al. Glucose transporter isoform 1 expression enhances metastasis of malignant melanoma cells. Oncotarget. 2015;6(32):32748–60.
159. Yan S, et al. Diagnostic and prognostic value of ProEx C and GLUT1 in melanocytic lesions. Anticancer Res. 2016;36(6):2871–80.
160. Ayati N, et al. The value of (18)F-FDG PET/CT for predicting or monitoring immunotherapy response in patients with metastatic melanoma: a systematic review and meta-analysis. Eur J Nucl Med Mol Imaging. 2020;
161. Acciardo S, et al. Metabolic imaging using hyperpolarized (13) C-pyruvate to assess sensitivity to the B-Raf inhibitor vemurafenib in melanoma cells and xenografts. J Cell Mol Med. 2020;24(2):1934–44.
162. Mun JH, et al. Discrimination of basal cell carcinoma from normal skin tissue using high-resolution magic angle spinning 1H NMR spectroscopy. PLoS One. 2016;11(3):e0150328.
163. Huang J, et al. Metabolic signature of eyelid basal cell carcinoma. Exp Eye Res. 2020;198:108140.
164. Wilkie MD, et al. Metabolic signature of squamous cell carcinoma of the head and neck: consequences of TP53 mutation and therapeutic perspectives. Oral Oncol. 2018;83:1–10.
165. Toberer F, et al. Metabolic reprogramming and angiogenesis in primary cutaneous Merkel cell carcinoma: expression of hypoxia-inducible factor-1α and its central downstream factors. J Eur Acad Dermatol Venereol. 2020;
166. Paladini RD, et al. Modulation of hair growth with small molecule agonists of the hedgehog signaling pathway. J Invest Dermatol. 2005;125(4):638–46.
167. Katoh M. Genomic testing, tumor microenvironment and targeted therapy of Hedgehog-related human cancers. Clin Sci (Lond). 2019;133(8):953–70.

168. Bonilla X, et al. Genomic analysis identifies new drivers and progression pathways in skin basal cell carcinoma. Nat Genet. 2016;48(4):398–406.
169. Carpenter RL, Ray H. Safety and tolerability of sonic hedgehog pathway inhibitors in cancer. Drug Saf. 2019;42(2):263–79.
170. Basset-Seguin N, Sharpe HJ, de Sauvage FJ. Efficacy of hedgehog pathway inhibitors in basal cell carcinoma. Mol Cancer Ther. 2015;14(3):633–41.
171. Sun Q, et al. Clues to primary vismodegib resistance lie in histology and genetics. J Clin Pathol. 2020;0:1–3.
172. Atwood SX, et al. Smoothened variants explain the majority of drug resistance in basal cell carcinoma. Cancer Cell. 2015;27(3):342–53.
173. Sharpe HJ, et al. Genomic analysis of smoothened inhibitor resistance in basal cell carcinoma. Cancer Cell. 2015;27(3):327–41.
174. Biehs B, et al. A cell identity switch allows residual BCC to survive Hedgehog pathway inhibition. Nature. 2018;562(7727):429–33.
175. Lefrancois P, et al. In silico analyses of the tumor microenvironment highlight tumoral inflammation, a Th2 cytokine shift and a mesenchymal stem cell-like phenotype in advanced in basal cell carcinomas. J Cell Commun Signal. 2020;14(2):245–54.
176. Chan XY, et al. Role played by signalling pathways in overcoming BRAF inhibitor resistance in melanoma. Int J Mol Sci. 2017;18(7):1527.

Chapter 19
Mechanisms of Resistance to Immunotherapy in Cutaneous Melanoma

Andrea Anichini and Roberta Mortarini

Introduction

The neoantigen load of a tumor, predicted on the basis of the tumor mutational burden [1], i.e., the total number of nonsynonymous mutations in the coding regions of the genes, and the immune-related gene expression profile of the pre-therapy lesion, captured by the Ayers 18 gene "IFN-γ signature" [2], represent today two of the best predictors of response to immune checkpoint blockade (ICB) in different solid tumors, including melanoma [3]. These two metrics are indicators, respectively, of the potential immunogenicity of the tumor and of the actual development of a spontaneous immune response prior and independently from immunotherapy. However, as shown initially by Spranger et al. [4], the tumor mutational burden (TMB) and the immune-related, "IFN-γ gene signature" of a tumor are largely independent biological processes, a finding that has several far-reaching implications. First, it means that a tumor with a high TMB is not necessarily characterized also by a high "IFN-γ signature" profile and vice versa [4]. In other words, strong tumor immunogenicity is not a necessary, nor a sufficient condition to promote development of a spontaneous adaptive immune response that can always be reactivated by immunotherapy. Second, as shown by Cristescu et al. [3] only a fraction of all cancer patients, in any histology, are expected to have tumors with both a high TMB and a high "immune-related gene expression profile" (GEP). This TMB^{HI}/GEP^{HI} fraction, in the instance of advanced cutaneous melanoma, one of the most immunogenic human tumors, is thought to represent about 40% of the cases [3] and should in principle be the most favorable condition for the efficacy of immunotherapy. In agreement, among melanoma patients receiving anti-PD-1 treatment, those whose

A. Anichini (✉) · R. Mortarini
Department of Research, Human Tumors Immunobiology Unit, Fondazione IRCCS Istituto Nazionale dei Tumori, Milan, Italy
e-mail: andrea.anichini@istitutotumori.mi.it; roberta.mortarini@istitutotumori.mi.it

P. Rutkowski, M. Mandalà (eds.), *New Therapies in Advanced Cutaneous Malignancies*, https://doi.org/10.1007/978-3-030-64009-5_19

tumors fall in the "TMB^{HI}/GEP^{HI}" subset experienced the highest objective response rates (57%), compared to the TMB^{HI}/GEP^{Lo} (42%), TMB^{Lo}/GEP^{Hi} (35%), and TMB^{Lo}/GEP^{Lo} (1%) subsets [3].

Taken together, these findings indicate that there must be several resistance mechanisms that prevent achievement of clinical benefit not only in a high fraction of patients who already developed antitumor immunity (TMB^{Lo}/GEP^{Hi}), or that have a strongly immunogenic tumor (TMB^{Hi}/GEP^{Lo}), but even in the most favorable TMB^{HI}/GEP^{HI} subset. Indeed, immunotherapy failure is thought to be shaped by a heterogeneous spectrum of primary (intrinsic) and secondary (adaptive) immunotherapy resistance mechanisms that will be reviewed in this chapter. Most of these mechanisms have been discovered over the past 5 years and several of them have been identified for the first time by investigating tissues from melanoma patients treated with ICB. These mechanisms can be tumor intrinsic or be mediated by different cellular components of the microenvironment. They contribute to explain why immunotherapy may fail even when tumor immunogenicity or previous immune response could instead suggest that immune checkpoint blockade should work. Resistance mechanisms can impact on all the steps of the cancer immunity cycle [5], including the production of chemokines that regulate recruitment at tumor site of dendritic cells, T cells, myeloid cells, and immunosuppressive cells, the production of key cytokines (such as type I and type II IFN) that bridge innate and adaptive immunity, the stage of antigen presentation and T cell cross-priming by professional antigen-presenting cells, the balance between T cell differentiation to effector stage or toward functional exhaustion and the recognition of tumor cells by therapy re-activated T cells. To simplify the description, the remarkable heterogeneity of the currently known resistance mechanisms has been reduced by identifying two large groups that will be discussed in sequence in this chapter. The first group includes all the mechanisms that share one of three triggering processes: aneuploidy, transcriptional programs of resistance, and master immunoregulatory genes. The second group includes the heterogeneous mechanisms that hit at different levels one of two key immunological processes. The first, type I and type II IFN signaling, is at the beginning of the generation of the response. The other one, the role of HLA molecules in tumor cell recognition by T cells, is at the end of the immunological circuit of adaptive immunity.

Tumor Aneuploidy Promotes Immunotherapy Resistance

Aneuploidy, also known as a somatic copy number alteration (SCNA), is a common feature of human tumors [6]. As shown by Davoli and colleagues [7], when aneuploidy becomes extensive ("chromosomal chaos") such as when tumors have a markedly abnormal number of chromosomes or of chromosomal segments, due to massive amplification or deletion events, then these tumors display a specific immune-related microenvironment profile that predisposes to immunotherapy resistance. Interestingly, in the Davoli study, in 8 out of 12 tumors investigated, but not in melanoma, high SCNA was positively correlated with TMB, suggesting that high tumor immunogenicity may be counteracted by SCNA that promotes an immunosuppressive tumor microenvironment. When these authors investigated the type of immune cells present in the microenvironment, depending on the SCNA levels, they found that tumors with high SCNA values were depleted of immune cells required for effective development of protective adaptive immunity. This was indicated by reduction in expression of genes encoding cytolytic factors, IFN-γ pathway and chemokines, and genes associated with M1-polarized macrophages. Most importantly, low tumor aneuploidy was a better predictor of patients' survival after anti-CTLA-4 therapy compared to TMB, although a combination of SCNA and TMB improved prediction.

The role of SCNA in determining immunotherapy resistance has been confirmed in a subsequent study in the setting of sequential anti-CTLA-4 -->anti-PD-1 treatment in melanoma patients [8]. These authors found a higher burden of copy number losses in pre-anti-CTLA-4 lesions from "double non responders" (i.e., patients who progressed while on anti-CTLA-4 therapy and subsequently progressed also after anti-PD-1 treatment) compared to pre-therapy lesions from single therapy responders (anti-CTLA-4). Re-analysis of an independent dataset of patients treated with anti-CTLA-4 revealed also that both SCNA and TMB contribute to response and resistance. In fact, the $TMB^{Hi}/SCNA^{Lo}$ subset contained a higher proportion of responders compared to the $TMB^{Lo}/SCNA^{Hi}$ subset. Similarly, a higher proportion of nonresponders were found in the $TMB^{Lo}/SCNA^{Hi}$ compared to the $TMB^{Hi}/SCNA^{Lo}$ subset.

Transcriptional Signatures Expressed in Neoplastic Cells Shape Resistance to Immunotherapy

A key notion emerging from studies aiming at deciphering mechanisms of primary resistance is that nonresponding patients can have tumors characterized by constitutive activation of gene programs or master genes that induce one or more of three main effects: (a) prevent development of adaptive immunity often by suppressing T cell recruitment; (b) promote development of a microenvironment characterized by immunosuppressive immune subsets; and (c) induce a dysfunctional program of exhaustion in T cells.

Hugo et al. [9] obtained the first evidence that primary resistance to ICB can be a gene program expressed in melanoma cells of nonresponding patients. These authors found that melanoma lesions of nonresponding patients expressed a transcriptomic profile (named IPRES signature) characterized by co-enriched "gene modules" including epithelial–mesenchymal transition (EMT) genes (AXL, ROR2, WNT5A, LOXL2, TWIST2, TAGLN, FAP), immunosuppressive genes (IL10, VEGFA, VEGFC), chemokine genes involved in recruitment of myeloid cells (CCL2, CCL7, CCL8, CCL13), and genes involved in wound healing and angiogenesis such as VEGFA, the latter being a molecule with a known immuno-suppressive function, i.e., suppression of dendritic cell maturation [10]. These results suggested that this transcriptional profile of resistance is in fact a single program where cellular dedifferentiation (captured by the EMT signature) is coupled to and/or drives activation of genes that may recruit suppressive myeloid cells (the chemokines as CCL2, CCL7, CCL8, CCL13).

Indeed, we know that human melanomas can exist even in vivo as a complex mixture of several distinct differentiation states along a four stages differentiation trajectory [11], where the extreme transcriptional cell states, discovered by Sensi et al. in 2011 [12], are represented by the AXL^{+}/MITF^{-} dedifferentiated and AXL^{-}/MITF^{+}, differentiated tumors. In agreement with the Hugo resistance signature, Tirosh et al. [13] have found that melanomas with a high AXL/MITF expression ratio also shape a specific microenvironment enriched for cell type-specific genes pointing at the presence of cancer-associated fibroblasts (CAFs), T cells, B cells, macrophages, and endothelial cells. This suggests that AXL^{Hi} dedifferentiated tumors have a complex immune-related microenvironment that collectively predisposes to resistance not to response. Moreover, the AXL^{Hi}/MITF^{Lo} program is associated with downregulation of MHC class I antigens [14], contributing to explain failure of immune checkpoint-directed immunotherapy, a therapeutic strategy that strongly relies on tumor recognition by re-activated T cells. Interestingly, the AXL^{Hi}/MITF^{Lo} program is not only associated with resistance to immunotherapy, but also to primary and acquired resistance to multiple targeted drugs [15].

A completely different gene program that impairs response to anti-PD-1 has been discovered by Jerby-Arnon and colleagues in human melanoma and it acts by promoting T cell exclusion [16]. These authors adopted a smart computational strategy based on finding genes, expressed in melanoma cells and that are correlated positively or negatively with T cell signatures (the latter indicating T cell infiltration). They then defined the exclusion program based on genes induced or repressed by malignant cells in "cold" versus "hot" tumors. They found that the resistance program was expressed prior to therapy, but was enhanced after immunotherapy in resistant lesions. They also found that the exclusion program predicts melanoma patient survival in bulk RNA-seq data from TCGA dataset and discriminates progression-free survival after ICB in independent cohorts of melanoma patients.

Gene Signatures of T Cell Exclusion and T Cell Dysfunction Predict Immunotherapy Resistance

Unresponsiveness to ICB may result from lack of antitumor T cells at tumor site (detected either pre-therapy or on-treatment), but it occurs even when there is presence of a population of tumor-associated T cells that have reached a developmental stage of exhaustion that can no longer be reversed by anti-PD-1. The relationship between the activated but pre-exhausted T cells (the T cells that can be reactivated by anti-PD-1) and the fully exhausted T cells (no longer rescued by anti-PD-1) has been recently clarified to be a developmental program controlled by two different transcription factors, TCF-7 and TOX. Briefly, we know that immunotherapy targeting PD-1 works by re-activating a subset of pre-exhausted stem-like TCF7$^+$ T cells that can be found in periphery and tumor site, maintain competence for further differentiation and migrate to tumor tissue upon anti-PD-1 treatment [17]. However, at tumor site, pre-exhausted T cells can proceed to a subsequent and irreversible late stage of T cell exhaustion and these lymphocytes cannot be re-activated by anti-PD-1 [18]. The late stage of T cell exhaustion has been investigated in detail by several groups who have been able to show that it is controlled by an epigenetic program [19], regulated by the transcription factor TOX [20]. This epigenetic program actively suppresses the expression of T cell genes needed to exert effector functions.

Collectively, these findings indicate that a promising way to define mechanisms of resistance is to combine signatures of T cell exclusion and signatures of T cell dysfunction. This is exactly what has been done by Jiang et al. [21] who defined a new signature of PD-1 resistance named TIDE. TIDE was shown to predict melanoma patients' resistance to anti-PD-1 and anti-CTLA-4 therapies, based on pre-treatment lesions, better (by ROC curve analysis) than other ICB response biomarkers including TMB, PD-L1 levels, or the IFN-γ signature.

Master Genes Regulate Immunotherapy Resistance by Promoting T Cell Exclusion

Increasing evidence indicates that T cell exclusion in melanoma, leading to immunotherapy resistance, can be driven not only by transcriptional programs expressed in the tumor or in immune cells, but even by single master genes following their inactivation (PTEN) or constitutive activation (β-catenin, PAK4, SK1, Myosin II). Peng et al. [22] found that loss of PTEN in melanoma is associated with increased production of immunosuppressive factors (VEGFA), of chemokines that recruit myeloid cells (CCL2), with decreased numbers of infiltrating T cells and with reduced response to anti-PD-1 therapy. T cell exclusion in the tumor microenvironment can be achieved in most solid tumors, including melanoma, even by a mechanism that disables production in melanoma cells of a key chemokine that recruits dendritic cells. This is the mechanism, discovered by Gajewski and colleagues [23], centered on constitutively active β-catenin. Mechanistically, they found that active β-catenin signaling in melanoma prevents production of CCL4 by neoplastic cells, a chemokine needed to recruit specific subsets of DCs (CD103$^+$ in mice, CD141$^+$ in humans) at tumor site. This DC subset plays a crucial role in migration of T cells in the tumor tissue. In fact CD141$^+$ DCs, in response to signals from IFN-γ, can produce chemokines as CXCL9 and CXCL10 that recruit T lymphocytes [24]. This mechanism eventually leads to a T cell-poor tumor that is not poised to respond to immunotherapy, as shown recently by the same authors in a study where they found enhanced β-catenin expression associated with secondary resistance to immunotherapy [25].

More recent studies have shed further light on the mechanism of T cell exclusion associated with β-catenin signaling. Abril-Rodrigues and colleagues [26], by investigating pre-therapy and on-treatment lesions from melanoma patients treated with anti-PD-1 found, as expected, that lesions from non-responding patients showed the characteristic features of low T cell and low DC infiltration, as inferred based on cell type-specific signatures. By looking at genes overexpressed in non-responding lesions, characterized by low DC infiltration, they identified PAK4. Interestingly, tumors with enhanced expression of PAK4 also showed evidence for the expression of the previously mentioned Jerby-Arnon exclusion signature. PAK4 is a serine/threonine kinase that phosphorylates β-catenin in the cytoplasm, thus activating its subsequent translocation to the nucleus where it exerts transcriptional functions. In agreement, lesions with high PAK4 expression also expressed CTNNB1 (the gene encoding β-catenin) at high levels. In the majority of cancer types investigated, in addition to melanoma, PAK4 expression was negatively correlated with T cell and dendritic cell infiltration scores (generated by inference from cell type-specific gene signatures).

A further master gene involved in the regulation of immunotherapy resistance is SK1, or sphingosine kinase-1 [27]. Sphingosine kinases are involved in sphingolipid metabolism by inducing phosphorylation of sphingosine to sphingosine-1-phosphate (S1P). The SK type 1 isoform, encoded by the SPHK1 gene is overexpressed in tumors, including melanoma. The authors found that patients with low SPHK1 expression had significantly longer PFS and OS after anti-PD-1 treatment compared to those with high SPHK1. In addition, most patients with high SPHK1 expression did not respond to anti-PD-1 therapy [27]. In vivo models indicated that SK1 silencing increased tumor infiltration by Ki-67$^+$ CD8$^+$ T cells producing IFN-γ and expressing granzyme, while reducing Treg content. Moreover, SK1 silencing downmodulated immunosuppressive molecules (TGFB1, IL-10) and Treg recruiting chemokines (CCL17, CCL22). In these same models SK1 silencing significantly improved anti-tumor efficacy of anti-CTLA-4 and of anti-PD-1. Finally, in melanoma samples, high SPHK1 expression was associated with an immunosuppressive tumor profile as documented by increased expression of genes encoding prostaglandin E2 synthase (PTGES), FOXP3, TGFB1, IL10, IDO1, IDO2, CTLA4, PDCD1, CD274 (encoding PD-L1), PDCD1LG2 (encoding PD-L2), TIGIT, LAG3, and HAVCR2 (encoding TIM-3).

One additional gene, recently implicated in melanoma resistance to immunotherapy is Myosin II, as part of the ROCK-Myosin II pathway, a regulator of invasive activity and metastasis [28]. Non-muscle Myosin II has contractile properties required for cell migration that is controlled among others through Rho kinase (ROCK). The authors focused on these Myosin II functions related to cytoskeletal remodeling in association with therapy resistance. They found that the ROCK-Myosin II pathway was involved in the emergence of resistance not only to MAPK-targeted therapy, but even to anti-PD-1 therapy. They also found that treatment with anti-PD-1 leads to increase expression of several genes in the ROCK-Myosin II pathway suggesting that this pathway is part of an adaptive resistance mechanism. Crucially, high Myosin II was identified in patients non-responding to anti-PD-1 and there was a significant overlap between the ROCK-Myosin II signature and the IPRES PD-1 resistance signature described by Hugo. Finally, they found that ROCK-Myosin II inhibition (by ROCK inhibitors) could improve the efficacy of immunotherapy with anti-PD-1 in immunocompetent mice.

Interferon Pathways in Immunotherapy Resistance

Type I and type II IFNs, the key regulators of the antiviral responses that bridge innate to adaptive immunity [29], play also a central role in spontaneous development and in therapy-induced reactivation of antitumor immunity. Uptake of dying tumor cells, by professional antigen-presenting cells (APCs), leads to intracellular sensing of tumor-derived DNA by the cGAS-STING pathway that subsequently triggers production of Type I IFNs [30]. Type I IFNs in turn promote dendritic cell (DC) maturation, as well as T cell cross-priming by DCs, through a variety of mechanisms. These cytokines drive expression of immunoproteasome subunits that impact on the repertoire of immunogenic peptides being generated for association with HLA class I molecules. Moreover, they increase MHC class I and II as well as costimulatory molecules (CD40, CD80, CD86) expression by DCs [29, 30]. All these activities in principle are necessary for the generation of tumor immunity, nevertheless it has been shown that sustained Type I IFN signaling can also be associated with resistance to PD-1 blockade. As shown by Jacquelot et al. [31], preclinical models involving PD-1-resistant tumors show evidence of sustained IFN-β transcription that induces PD-L1 and NOS2 expression in neoplastic cells and dendritic cells (DC). In these models, NOS2 expression was associated with secondary resistance to PD-1 blockade through increased recruitment of Tregs at tumor site. In agreement with these preclinical data, in melanoma patients treated with the combination of anti-CTLA-4 and anti-PD-1, baseline expression of several Type I IFN genes (IFNA1, IFNA2, IFNA6, IFNA7, IFNA10, IFNA14) was higher in tumor tissue from non-responding subjects compared to responding ones, and pre-therapy lesions of patients who had previously failed to respond to immunotherapy showed enhanced expression of NOS2 transcripts [31].

Type II IFN (IFNγ) is produced by a variety of immune cells belonging to the innate (NK, APCs) and adaptive (T and B) subsets [32] and exerts a large spectrum of key immunoregulatory functions in the context of antitumor immunity. These include inducing the upregulation of MHC class I and II molecules and of the full antigen processing machinery (APM) molecular system, promoting CD4+ polarization toward the TH1 functional profile, and inducing CD8+ differentiation to cytolytic effector stage and macrophages to pro-inflammatory profile. Moreover, IFN-γ plays a specific role in driving the expression of PD-L1 in tumor cells [33], through the JAK1/2—STAT1/3—IRF1 intracellular signaling axis, and of PD-L2 (the latter molecule being modulated also by IFN-β). Crucially, for the generation of spontaneous tumor immunity, and for the response to immunotherapy, IFN-γ has two additional immunoregulatory functions. First, it is a key cytokine stimulating the production by DCs of chemokines such as CXCL9 and CXCL10 that recruit tumor-specific CXCR3$^+$ T cells at tumor site [34]. Second, experimental models of tumor immunotherapy show that T cells reactivated by anti-PD-1 produce IFN-γ, which in turn triggers IL-12 production by DCs at tumor site [35]. IL-12 is the crucial "licensing" signal allowing development of the full cytolytic effector functions of anti-PD-1-reactivated anti-tumor T cells. Therefore, according to this model, anti-PD-1 therapy does not work directly by reactivating functionally impaired T cells, but indirectly, through an IFN-γ–IL-12 axis involving DCs present in the tumor microenvironment. In the light of these central functions for the regulation of the adaptive immune response, it is not surprising that the type II IFN pathway has been implicated in immunotherapy resistance through several mechanisms that include detrimental pathway activation in specific settings or, in contrast, pathway inactivation due to somatic mutations in key components of the intracellular signal transduction module downstream of the IFN-γ receptor.

Pre-clinical and clinical evidence indicates that sustained Type II IFN production paradoxically generates resistance to immunotherapy targeting immune checkpoints if immune treatment is carried out in the condition of low tumor burden (LTB). Pai et al. [36] made a clinical observation linking LTB to resistance to checkpoint blockade that was verified in experimental models leading to define the role of Type II IFN in resistance. These authors stratified cohorts of metastatic melanoma patients treated with monotherapy (anti-PD-1) or combination immune checkpoint blockade (anti-CTLA-4 and anti-PD-1) according to specific baseline tumor size (BTS) cut-offs. By these criteria, patients in the medium and high BTS cohorts showed a higher frequency of visceral metastases and/or elevated LDH values compared to patients in the low BTS cohort. Then they asked: are objective response rates (ORR) significantly different in monotherapy vs combination treatment depending on the BTS cohort? Intriguingly and unexpectedly, ORR were significantly different, but in favor of monotherapy, but only in the low BTS group. These findings were replicated in experimental models of low tumor burden (i.e., by treating mice with ICB in the early stages of tumor growth) showing that combination immunotherapy leads to reduced efficacy of the treatment. Mechanistically, this reduced efficacy was due to increased IFN-γ production in LTB condition, upon combination immune checkpoint blockade. Strong IFN-γ signals then lead to activation-induced cell death (AICD) of tumor-specific T cells.

IFN signaling can lead to immunotherapy resistance even by driving a multigene resistance program that is not explained only by the well-known process of PD-L1 upregulation. By exploiting murine B16 melanoma models, Benci et al. [37] showed that sustained type II interferon signaling promotes STAT1-dependent epigenetic changes leading to increased expression by melanoma cells of multiple ligands for T cell inhibitory receptors. Network analysis of TCGA human melanoma datasets confirmed the central position of STAT1 in linking together modules of interferon-responsive genes (ISG) and of multiple T cell inhibitory receptor ligands.

Acquired resistance to PD-1 blockade in human melanoma can even evolve from somatic mutations that disable key signal transduction molecules downstream of the IFN-γ receptor. Upon binding of IFN-γ to its receptor, signal transduction is initiated by activation of JAK1 and JAK2, resulting in homodimerization and phosphorylation of STAT1, which then migrates to the nucleus where it acts as a transcription factor. Not surprisingly, loss of function mutations of JAK1/2 have been found to be associated with both primary [38] and acquired [39] resistance to anti-PD-1 in melanoma patients. These mutations induce loss of responsiveness to IFN-γ in tumor cells, impairing antigen presentation (no upregulation of MHC molecules in response to IFN-γ) and abolishing the antiproliferative effect of this cytokine on neoplastic cells. As investigated in detail by Sucker et al. [40], development of JAK1/2 mutations in melanoma cells also leads to emergence of T cell-resistant tumor clones characterized by downmodulation of HLA class I and APM components. Loss of IFN-γ pathway genes is also involved in melanoma resistance to anti-CTLA-4 therapy [41]. In a small set ($n = 12$) of non-responding patients to anti-CTLA-4, the tumors were found to harbor frequent genetic changes (most often in the form of copy number alterations, CNA) impacting multiple IFN-γ pathway genes. Strikingly, a total of 184 mutations were found in the 12 nonresponders, whereas only 4 mutations were detected in the responders.

The HLA Antigen Processing and Presentation Pathway in Immunotherapy Resistance

Tumor recognition by T lymphocytes in the setting of immune checkpoint blockade is crucially dependent on expression of HLA molecules on neoplastic cells. Although pre-clinical models indicate a contribution of PD-1[+] NK cells in recognition of low-MHC-I expressing tumors, in the context of anti-PD-1 treatment [42], nevertheless clinical efficacy of immunotherapy is currently thought to be strongly dependent on the antitumor functions of reactivated tumor-specific T cells, belonging mainly but not unique to the CD8[+] subset. These effectors need to recognize HLA–peptide complexes expressed on the surface of tumor cells through their TCRs. Shutting down the expression of histocompatibility molecules, and/or compromising the antigen processing machinery (that generates peptides to be associated with HLA-class I molecules) represent prototypic immune escape mechanisms exploited by human tumors to impair adaptive immunity [43]. In melanoma patients, analysis of the TCGA dataset (i.e., a cohort containing mainly metastatic lesions) indicated an association of shortened survival with low expression of HLA-I antigen processing (LMP2, LMP7, TAP1, TAP2, TAPBP) and presentation (B2M, HLA-A, HLA-B, HLA-C) genes [44]. In agreement, impairing antigen processing and presentation has been found to be the main mechanism that generates primary and acquired resistance to ICB. Initial evidence in anti-CTLA-4-treated melanoma patients [45] indicated a reduction in overall survival in patients with loss of expression of β2M (the light chain of the HLA Class I heterodimer) and of TAP1. TAP1 is one of the two components of the molecular machinery that transports proteasome-generated peptides from the cytosol to the lumen of the endoplasmic reticulum where the peptides are associated with newly synthesized HLA class I molecules [46]. Subsequent larger studies [47] have documented that partial loss (>50% negative of cells) or complete loss of HLA Class I membrane expression on melanoma cells is associated with transcriptional repression of HLA-A, HLA-B, HLA-C, and B2M, and predicts primary resistance to anti–CTLA-4, but not anti–PD-1. The latter results are in conflict with a different study [14] where the authors found that MHC class I downregulation is a hallmark of resistance to PD-1 blockade and is associated with the previously mentioned MITF^{Lo}/AXL^{Hi} dedifferentiated phenotype and with cancer-associated fibroblast signatures.

Several studies have shed light on the spectrum of mechanisms that induce transcriptional silencing of HLA pathway genes leading to immunotherapy resistance. Although some studies have reported rare mutations in HLA pathway genes [39, 47], most of the HLA gene silencing described in the context of immunotherapy resistance is due to a variety of mechanisms that suppress transcription or translation or prevent tumor response to IFN-γ. For example, the embryonic transcription factor DUX4 is reactivated in neoplastic cells and drives transcriptional repression of B2M, HLA-A, HLA-B, and HLA-C genes in most cancer types. DUX4 works by inhibiting HLA gene upregulation induced by IFN-γ. In cohorts of melanoma patients stratified for levels of DUX4 transcriptional activity, highly significant differences were found in progression-free and overall survival upon treatment with anti-CTLA4, where high DUX4 activity was associated with worse clinical outcomes. Silencing of HLA pathway genes, in the context of immunotherapy resistance, can be produced even by mechanisms acting at the mRNA level, after gene transcription. The RNA-binding protein, MEX3B, has been shown to bind the 3′ UTR of HLA-A gene thus destabilizing mRNA stability and compromising MHC protein synthesis and surface expression [48]. In melanoma patients treated with anti-PD-1 expression of MEX3B was higher in nonresponders compared to responders.

Conclusions

There is no doubt that the extreme heterogeneity of the primary and adaptive resistance mechanisms, discovered in cutaneous melanoma, pose a formidable challenge to the development of more effective therapeutic strategies. It does not seem plausible to imagine that a significant fraction of these mechanisms may be successfully counteracted by any single new combination regimen (even those not yet developed), based for example on targeting additional checkpoints, or on introduction of new drugs that target, for example, immunosuppressive cells. It is true that, in principle, some or several of the resistance mechanisms could be counteracted, providing that there is patient-specific prior knowledge on which mechanism to target. For example, pre-clinical evidence has been recently achieved [49] indicating that PD-1 resistance due to genetic defects (JAK1/2 mutations or B2M mutations) can be overcome. In the instance of JAK1/2 mutations resistance could be overcome by adding TLR9 agonists to anti-PD-1. In the instance of B2M mutations reversal of resistance was obtained by activating NK cells and CD4$^+$ cells, through the CD122 preferential interleukin 2 (IL-2) agonist bempegaldesleukin, in association with anti-PD-1 [49]. However, it seems reasonable to predict that translating these pre-clinical studies into patient-tailored treatments will be extremely cumbersome, due to the need for comprehensive profiling of patients' lesions either before treatment or, worse, at the time of development of secondary resistance. Although a large number of new combination immunotherapy regimens are being currently tested in clinical trials, nevertheless several reasons reveal the true dimension of the huge task that lies ahead to break the "glass ceiling" of resistance. First, today, in most instances, even the very factors predisposing to response (TMB and the immune-related profile of the pre-therapy lesions) are completely unknown in most patients. This can be due to a simple reason: lack of availability of surgically removed pre-therapy lesions. This means that even predicting clinical benefit, or likelihood of therapy failure, is almost impossible. Second, a single tumor may express multiple resistance mechanisms at the same time (for example, lack of T cell infiltrate and poor expression of HLA molecules) that cannot be easily targeted with any single strategy. Thus, there is only one way forward. Approaches described in other sections of this book explain how the scientific community is going through this daunting task of overcoming immunotherapy resistance by following the only reasonable and established guidelines: anticipating immunotherapy to earlier clinical stages, introducing immunotherapy in the adjuvant and neoadjuvant settings and slowly, perhaps painfully, but safely, testing new combination immunotherapy regimens in rationally designed controlled clinical trials.

References

1. Alexandrov LB, Nik-Zainal S, Wedge DC, Aparicio SA, Behjati S, Biankin AV, et al. Signatures of mutational processes in human cancer. Nature. 2013;500:415–21.
2. Ayers M, Lunceford J, Nebozhyn M, Murphy E, Loboda A, Kaufman DR, et al. IFN-γ-related mRNA profile predicts clinical response to PD-1 blockade. J Clin Invest. 2017;127:2930–40.
3. Cristescu R, Mogg R, Ayers M, Albright A, Murphy E, Yearley J, et al. Pan-tumor genomic biomarkers for PD-1 checkpoint blockade-based immunotherapy. Science. 2018;362:eaar3593.
4. Spranger S, Luke JJ, Bao R, Zha Y, Hernandez KM, Li Y, et al. Density of immunogenic antigens does not explain the presence or absence of the T-cell-inflamed tumor microenvironment in melanoma. Proc Natl Acad Sci U S A. 2016;113:E7759–68.
5. Chen DS, Mellman I. Oncology meets immunology: the cancer-immunity cycle. Immunity. 2013;39:1–10.
6. Ben-David U, Amon A. Context is everything: aneuploidy in cancer. Nat Rev Genet. 2020;21:44–62.

7. Davoli T, Uno H, Wooten EC, Elledge SJ. Tumor aneuploidy correlates with markers of immune evasion and with reduced response to immunotherapy. Science. 2017;355:eaaf8399.
8. Roh W, Chen PL, Reuben A, Spencer CN, Prieto PA, Miller JP, et al. Integrated molecular analysis of tumor biopsies on sequential CTLA-4 and PD-1 blockade reveals markers of response and resistance. Sci Transl Med. 2017;9:eaah3560.
9. Hugo W, Zaretsky JM, Sun L, Song C, Moreno BH, Hu-Lieskovan S, et al. Genomic and transcriptomic features of response to anti-PD-1 therapy in metastatic melanoma. Cell. 2016;165:35–44.
10. Gabrilovich DI, Chen HL, Girgis KR, Cunningham HT, Meny GM, Nadaf S, et al. Production of vascular endothelial growth factor by human tumors inhibits the functional maturation of dendritic cells. Nat Med. 1996;2:1096–103.
11. Tsoi J, Robert L, Paraiso K, Galvan C, Sheu KM, Lay J, et al. Multi-stage differentiation defines melanoma subtypes with differential vulnerability to drug-induced iron-dependent oxidative stress. Cancer Cell. 2018;33:890–904.
12. Sensi M, Catani M, Castellano G, Nicolini G, Alciato F, Tragni G, et al. Human cutaneous melanomas lacking MITF and melanocyte differentiation antigens express a functional Axl receptor kinase. J Invest Dermatol. 2011;131:2448–57.
13. Tirosh I, Izar B, Prakadan SM, Wadsworth MH II, Treacy D, Trombetta JJ, et al. Dissecting the multicellular ecosystem of metastatic melanoma by single-cell RNA-seq. Science. 2016;352:189–96.
14. Lee JH, Shklovskaya E, Lim SY, Carlino MS, Menzies AM, Stewart A, et al. Transcriptional downregulation of MHC class I and melanoma de-differentiation in resistance to PD-1 inhibition. Nat Commun. 2020;11:1897.
15. Müller J, Krijgsman O, Tsoi J, Robert L, Hugo W, Song C, et al. Low MITF/AXL ratio predicts early resistance to multiple targeted drugs in melanoma. Nat Commun. 2014;5:5712.
16. Jerby-Arnon L, Shah P, Cuoco MS, Rodman C, Su MJ, Melms JC, et al. A cancer cell program promotes T cell exclusion and resistance to checkpoint blockade. Cell. 2018;175:984–97.
17. Sade-Feldman M, Yizhak K, Bjorgaard SL, Ray JP, de Boer CG, Jenkins RW, et al. Defining T cell states associated with response to checkpoint immunotherapy in melanoma. Cell. 2018;175:998–1013.
18. Pauken KE, Sammons MA, Odorizzi PM, Manne S, Godec J, Khan O, et al. Epigenetic stability of exhausted T cells limits durability of reinvigoration by PD-1 blockade. Science. 2016;354:1160–5.
19. Ghoneim HE, Fan Y, Moustaki A, Abdelsamed HA, Dash P, Dogra P, et al. De novo epigenetic programs inhibit PD-1 blockade-mediated T cell rejuvenation. Cell. 2017;170:142–57.
20. Khan O, Giles JR, McDonald S, Manne S, Ngiow SF, Patel KP, et al. TOX transcriptionally and epigenetically programs CD8$^+$ T cell exhaustion. Nature. 2019;571:211–8.
21. Jiang P, Gu S, Pan D, Fu J, Sahu A, Hu X, et al. Signatures of T cell dysfunction and exclusion predict cancer immunotherapy response. Nat Med. 2018;24:1550–8.
22. Peng W, Chen JQ, Liu C, Malu S, Creasy C, Tetzlaff MT, et al. Loss of PTEN promotes resistance to T cell-mediated immunotherapy. Cancer Discov. 2016;6:202–16.
23. Spranger S, Bao R, Gajewski TF. Melanoma-intrinsic β-catenin signalling prevents antitumour immunity. Nature. 2015;523:231–5.
24. Spranger S, Dai D, Horton B, Gajewski TF. Tumor-residing Batf3 dendritic cells are required for effector T cell trafficking and adoptive T cell therapy. Cancer Cell. 2017;31:711–23.
25. Trujillo JA, Luke JJ, Zha Y, Segal JP, Ritterhouse LL, Spranger S, et al. Secondary resistance to immunotherapy associated with β-catenin pathway activation or PTEN loss in metastatic melanoma. J Immunother Cancer. 2019;7:295.
26. Abril-Rodriguez G, Torrejon DY, Liu W, Zaretsky JM, Nowicki TS, Tsoi J, et al. PAK4 inhibition improves PD-1 blockade immunotherapy. Nat Cancer. 2020;1:46–58.
27. Imbert C, Montfort A, Fraisse M, Marcheteau E, Gilhodes J, Martin E, et al. Resistance of melanoma to immune checkpoint inhibitors is overcome by targeting the sphingosine kinase-1. Nat Commun. 2020;11:437.

28. Orgaz JL, Crosas-Molist E, Sadok A, Perdrix-Rosell A, Maiques O, Rodriguez-Hernandez I, et al. Myosin II reactivation and cytoskeletal remodeling as a hallmark and a vulnerability in melanoma therapy resistance. Cancer Cell. 2020;37:85–103.
29. Lee AJ, Ashkar AA. The dual nature of type I and type II interferons. Front Immunol. 2018;9:2061.
30. Vattner RE, Janssen EM. STING, DCs and the link between innate and adaptive tumor immunity. Mol Immunol. 2019;110:13–23.
31. Jacquelot N, Yamazaki T, Roberti MP, Duong CPM, Andrews MC, Verlingue L, et al. Sustained type I interferon signaling as a mechanism of resistance to PD-1 blockade. Cell Res. 2019;29:846–61.
32. Castro F, Cardoso AP, Gonçalves RM, Serre K, Oliveira MJ. Interferon-gamma at the crossroads of tumor immune surveillance or evasion. Front Immunol. 2018;9:847.
33. Garcia-Diaz A, Sanghoon Shin D, Homet Moreno B, Saco J, Escuin-Ordinas H, Abril Rodriguez G, et al. Interferon receptor signaling pathways regulating PD-L1 and PD-L2 expression. Cell Rep. 2017;19:1189–201.
34. Chow MT, Ozga AJ, Servis RL, Frederick DT, Lo JA, Fisher DE, et al. Intratumoral activity of the CXCR3 chemokine system is required for the efficacy of anti- PD-1 therapy. Immunity. 2019;50:1498–512.
35. Garris CS, Arlauckas SP, Kohler RH, Trefny MP, Seth Garren S, Piot C, et al. Successful anti-PD-1 cancer immunotherapy requires T cell-dendritic cell crosstalk involving the cytokines IFN-γ and IL-12. Immunity. 2018;49:1148–61.
36. Pai CS, Huang JT, Lu X, Simons DM, Park C, Chang A, et al. Clonal deletion of tumor-specific T cells by interferon-γ confers therapeutic resistance to combination immune checkpoint blockade. Immunity. 2019;50:477–92.
37. Benci JL, Xu B, Qiu Y, Wu T, Dada H, Twyman-Saint Victor C, et al. Tumor interferon signaling regulates a multigenic resistance program to immune checkpoint blockade. Cell. 2016;167:1540–54.
38. Shin DS, Zaretsky JM, Escuin-Ordinas E, Garcia-Diaz A, Hu-Lieskovan S, Kalbasi A, et al. Primary resistance to PD-1 blockade mediated by *JAK1/2* mutations. Cancer Discov. 2016;7:188–201.
39. Zaretsky JM, Garcia Diaz A, Shin DS, Escuin Ordinas H, Hugo W, Hu-Lieskovan S, et al. Mutations associated with acquired resistance to PD-1 blockade in melanoma. N Engl J Med. 2016;375:819–29.
40. Sucker A, Zhao F, Pieper N, Heeke C, Maltaner R, Stadtler N, et al. Acquired IFNγ resistance impairs anti-tumor immunity and gives rise to T-cell-resistant melanoma lesions. Nat Commun. 2017;8:15440.
41. Gao J, Shi LZ, Zhao H, Chen J, Xiong L, He Q, et al. Loss of IFN-γ pathway genes in tumor cells as a mechanism of resistance to anti-CTLA-4 therapy. Cell. 2016;167:397–404.
42. Hsu J, Hodgins JJ, Marathe M, Nicolai CJ, Bourgeois-Daigneault MC, Trevino TN, et al. Contribution of NK cells to immunotherapy mediated by PD-1/PD-L1 blockade. J Clin Invest. 2018;128:4654–68.
43. McGranahan N, Rosenthal R, Hiley CT, Rowan AJ, Watkins TBK, Wilson GA, et al. Allele-specific HLA loss and immune escape in lung cancer evolution. Cell. 2017;171:1259–71.
44. Such L, Zhao F, Liu D, Thier B, Le-Trilling VTK, Sucker A, et al. Targeting the innate immunoreceptor RIG-I overcomes melanoma-intrinsic resistance to T cell immunotherapy. J Clin Invest. 2020;13:131572. https://doi.org/10.1172/JCI131572.
45. Patel SJ, Sanjana NE, Kishton RJ, Eidizadeh A, Vodnala SK, Cam M, et al. Identification of essential genes for cancer immunotherapy. Nature. 2017;548:537–44.
46. Abele R, Tampè R. Function of the transport complex TAP in cellular immune recognition. Biochim Biophys Acta. 1999;1461:405–19.
47. Rodig SJ, Gusenleitner D, Jackson DG, Gjini E, Giobbie-Hurder A, Jin C, et al. MHC proteins confer differential sensitivity to CTLA-4 and PD-1 blockade in untreated metastatic melanoma. Sci Transl Med. 2018;10:eaar3342.

48. Huang L, Malu S, McKenzie JA, Andrews MC, Talukder AH, Tieu T, et al. The RNA-binding protein MEX3B mediates resistance to cancer immunotherapy by downregulating HLA-A expression. In: Clin Cancer Res, vol. 24; 2018. p. 3366–76.
49. Torrejon DY, Abril-Rodriguez G, Champhekar AS, Tsoi J, Campbell KM, Kalbasi A, et al. Overcoming genetically-based resistance mechanisms to PD-1 blockade. Cancer Discov. 2020;10(8):1140–57. https://doi.org/10.1158/2159-8290.CD-19-1409.

Part VII
Perioperative Therapy of Melanoma

Chapter 20
Neoadjuvant and Adjuvant Therapies of Melanoma

Piotr Rutkowski

Introduction

Surgical intervention is the treatment of choice in melanoma patients. However, the prognosis of patients with melanoma at stages IIC–IV after complete resection of the lesions is heterogenous and disease recurrences occur in 30–70% of high-risk patients of cases. Currently, systemic adjuvant treatment after surgery in high-risk patients is the standard treatment administered with curative intent [1–5]. A novel approach to the treatment of locoregional advanced melanomas is built on systemic preoperative treatment to further reduce the risk of recurrence and increases the cure rate.

Neoadjuvant Treatment

Neoadjuvant therapy has been gaining significance in cases of borderline resectable or locally advanced stage III melanomas. The results of the phase II trials published recently point out that the use of combined preoperative treatment with BRAF and MEK inhibitors (in case of presence of *BRAF* mutation) or immunotherapy with anti-PD-1 alone or in combination with anti-CTLA-4, leads to responses in substantial part of patients and complete pathological remissions are related to better outcomes [6–14].

P. Rutkowski (✉)
Department of Soft Tissue/Bone Sarcoma and Melanoma, Maria Sklodowska-Curie National Research Institute of Oncology, Warsaw, Poland
e-mail: piotr.rutkowski@pib-nio.pl

P. Rutkowski, M. Mandalà (eds.), *New Therapies in Advanced Cutaneous Malignancies*, https://doi.org/10.1007/978-3-030-64009-5_20

The phase II randomized study of Amaria et al. [6] reported the results of neoadjuvant treatment with dabrafenib and trametinib in patients with resectable III and IV stage *BRAF*-mutated melanoma patients (with the exception of the metastases in the brain and bones). Seven patients were randomly selected for a standard surgical intervention with possible standard adjuvant treatment whilst 14 patients for preoperative treatment with dabrafenib with trametinib and then (after resection) for an adjuvant treatment for up to 1 year. The trial was prematurely terminated due to a significantly longer event-free survival (EFS) in the neo−/adjuvant arm in comparison with the standard treatment arm. After a median follow-up of 18.6 months, the rate of patients who survived without any events in the experimental arm (71%; 10/14) was significantly larger than the rate of patients in the arm treated according to standard therapy (0). The median EFS was 19.7 months versus 29 months, respectively ($p < 0.001$). The neo−/adjuvant treatment with dabrafenib with trametinib was well tolerated. A radical surgical intervention in this group was performed in 12 patients and in 7 cases (58%) a complete pathological response was observed, which was also connected with better prognosis.

Similar results were obtained in the II phase trial NeoCombi [7] in which stage IIB-C *BRAF*-mutated patients received dabrafenib with trametinib for 12 weeks before the surgery of metastases and for 40 weeks after resection. The study included 35 patients and in 30 of them (86%) the objective responses to the preoperative treatment according to the RECIST criteria were found, whereas in 17 patients (49%) a pathological complete response (pCR) was observed. The 2-year progression-free survival rate was 43.4% with better results observed in the group of patients with the complete pathological response.

Five other studies evaluated the use of neoadjuvant immunotherapy. The first of them [8] dealt with the administration of preoperative nivolumab (up to 4 doses) in comparison with ipilimumab combined with nivolumab (up to 3 doses) in 23 patients with resectable stage III or IV melanomas. The treatment with a combination of ipilimumab with nivolumab was related to a high response rate (73%; pCR 45%), yet with significant toxicity (73% adverse events [AE] with grade 3/4), on the contrary nivolumab monotherapy lead to fewer responses (25%, pCR 25%), whilst the toxicity was low (8% AE in grade 3/4). The second—OPACIN phase 1b randomized trials tested adjuvant ($n = 10$) versus neoadjuvant ($n = 10$) ipilimumab plus nivolumab at standard doses in macroscopic resectable stage III melanomas except in-transit metastases. Neoadjuvant therapy (2 cycles) induced a high pathological response rate (pRR—78%). Toxicity was high with 90% of grade 3/4 toxicities, which made the standard dose unfeasible for broader testing. None of the patients who achieved a pathological response had relapsed [9, 10], which may suggest that pathologic response may serve as a surrogate marker for durable disease control. At median follow-up time of 36.7 months 3-year relapse-free survival (RFS) rate was 80% in neoadjuvant arm and 60% in adjuvant arm, while the 3-year overall survival (OS) rate was 90% in neoadjuvant arm and 70% in adjuvant arm. RFS data after 2 doses of neoadjuvant immunotherapy seems to be higher when compared to adjuvant anti-PD-1 data in the high-risk macroscopic stage III melanoma patients' population.

The third study—[11, 12] OpACIN-neo trial—evaluated the optimal dosing schedule of the use of neoadjuvant combination of nivolumab and ipilimumab in the randomized fashion:

- In group A: 2 cycles of ipilimumab 3 mg/kg plus nivolumab 1 mg/kg every 3 weeks
- In group B: 2 cycles of ipilimumab 1 mg/kg plus nivolumab 3 mg/kg, every 3 weeks
- In group C: 2 cycles of ipilimumab 3 mg/kg every 3 weeks and then 2 cycles of nivolumab 3 mg/kg every 2 weeks

The study included 86 stage III patients with clinical metastases to loco-regional lymph nodes. Within the first 12 weeks, immune-related adverse events (irAE grade 3–4) were found in 40% of patients in group A, 20% in group B, and 50% in group C. Objective radiological responses were observed in 63% of patients in group A, 57% in group B, and 35% in group C. The dosing schedule tested in arm B: 2 courses IPI 1 mg/kg + NIVO 3 mg/kg has been identified as most favorable schedule. Complete pathogenic responses did not fully correlate with radiological responses and complete pathological responses were observed in patients with radiological evidence of disease. In 57% of patients in group B pCR was confirmed. None of these groups reached the median EFS or RFS. At 18 months, relapses were observed in 1/64 (2%) pathological responders versus 13/21 (62%) of the non-responders. In biomarker analysis the combination of IFN-y signature score and mutational load can identify a group of patients that is less likely to respond to neoadjuvant ipilimumab plus nivolumab.

The next study utilized a single dose of anti-PD-1 agent pembrolizumab administered 3 weeks before surgical removal of tumor in resectable clinical stage III or resectable stage IV melanoma. This study identified a rapid and potent antitumor response and 8 of 27 patients achieved a complete or major pathological response— all remained free of disease. The authors found the correlation between rapid responses and accumulation of exhausted CD8 T cells in the tumor at 3 weeks, as well as they discovered neoadjuvant response immune signature related to clinical benefit to preoperative therapy [13].

The last study utilized different approaches with preoperative injections of oncolytic virus—talimogene laherparepvec (T-VEC) versus surgery in patients with resectable stage IIIB–IVM1a melanoma. The final results showed 2-year RFS and OS improvements in neoadjuvant T-VEC monotherapy + surgery arm compared with surgery alone (RFS per protocol: 50.5% vs. 30.2%, overall HR: 0.75, $P = 0.07$; RFS sensitivity: overall HR: 0.66, $P = 0.038$ and OS 88.9 vs. 77.4%; overall HR: 0.49, $P = 0.050$) [14].

It seems that neoadjuvant immunotherapy (especially with immune checkpoint inhibitors) can be more efficient than adjuvant therapy (what might be connected with the activity of the immune system). In the case of T cell checkpoint blockade, neoadjuvant therapy could induce stronger and broader tumor-specific T cell response. Moreover, it is a short-lasting and cost-effective therapy. This treatment allows also for a better prognostic/predictive evaluation and personalization of post-therapy management, in particular when no complete pathological response is obtained and a patient might require adjuvant treatment (e.g. radiotherapy or

Table 20.1 The most important clinical trials with neoadjuvant clinical trials in locoregional advanced melanomas modified after Menzies et al. [16]

Clinical trials	Treatment	N	pCR (%)	Median RFS (months)	Median follow-up time (months)
Amaria Lancet Oncol 2018 [6]	Dabrafenib/ Trametinib	21	58	19.7	18.6
Long Lancet Oncol 2019 [7]	Dabrafenib/ Trametinib	35	49	23.0	27.0
Amaria Nat Med 2018 [8]	Nivolumab	12	25	NR	
	Ipilimumab +nivolumab	11	45	NR	20
Blank Nat Med 2018 [9]	Ipilimumab+ nivolumab		33	Not reached	32
Blank ESMO 2019 [10]			10	(3-year rate 80%)	36.7
Rozeman Lancet Oncol 2019 [11] ESMO 2019 [12]	Ipilimumab +nivolumab	86	57	Not reached (18-month rate 80%)	8.3
Huang Nat Med 2019 [13]	Pembrolizumab	30	19	NR	18

pCR pathological complete remission, *RFS* relapse-free survival

targeted treatment with BRAF and MEK inhibitors after preoperative immunotherapy) [15]. In the entire studied patient population group with neoadjuvant treatment (Table 20.1), the rate of complete pathological remission was 41% (38% after immunotherapy and 47% after molecular targeted treatment) [16]. Moreover, patients achieving complete remission after immunotherapy seem to have durable response as the memory effect of immune system. This strategy requires further studies and it should be tested in a randomized phase 3 study versus adjuvant therapy.

Systemic Adjuvant Therapy

Currently, systemic adjuvant therapy is a standard treatment in clinical practice for high-risk patients after a radical resection of metastatic regional lymph nodes or distant metastases. The results of recently published clinical trials indicate an improvement in RFS through the use of post-operative immune system checkpoint inhibitors or combined BRAF and MEK inhibitors [1–3, 17].

Interferon

For many years apart from interferon (IFN) no other agents had been effective in the adjuvant treatment of high-risk skin melanomas. Interferon (mainly alfa-2b IFN in monotherapy) used for adjuvant treatment of patients with melanomas (for a highly selected group) leads to (in a repetitive way) prolongation of the relapse-free survival (RFS) in the majority of patients (Table 20.1) [18–21]. However, evidence for the improvement of overall survival (OS) as a result of the use of IFN is much weaker and more controversial. In 10 out of 17 evaluated studies, an improvement in RFS was observed and the recent results of meta-analysis support a decrease of the relative risk of relapse by 17–18% (relative risk [hazard ratio, HR]: 0.82–0.83; $p < 0.0001$) with adjuvant IFN. Evidence for an improvement in OS comes mostly from meta-analyses and translates into an OS improvement of about 3% within 5 years within the entire group of patients. Currently, the use of IFN in adjuvant treatment in all patients with high-risk melanomas is therefore not justified (especially given a significant toxicity of the treatment) and thus becomes the only option in selected patients.

On the basis of the positive results of one of the three studies performed by the Eastern Cooperative Oncology Group (ECOG): ECOG 1684, IFN α-2b administered in high doses was registered in the United States and the European Union for the treatment of melanomas in IIB–III stage, it was registered also in the European Union in low doses for patients in stage II of the disease. The basis for the registration was the prolongation of the overall survival in a 7-year follow-up period; however, it was not confirmed after a longer period of time (12 years). The results of the meta-analyses show that the benefit is confined to patients with an ulcerated primary melanoma, in particular, those with metastases that are not clinically overt (former terminology: micro-metastases), and not with clinically overt metastases (palpable nodes) observed in the enlarged lymph nodes (former terminology: macro-metastases) [20, 21].

Currently, the results of the 18081 trial of the European Organisation for Research and Treatment of Cancer (EORTC), concerning the evaluation of the use of the pegylated IFN in the treatment of stage II ulcerated melanoma patients, showed a similar benefit of IFN (HR 0.69) for RFS as observed in the previous EORTC trials [22]. Unfortunately, this study is underpowered since the recruitment was discontinued due to poor accrual.

The most frequent adverse events of IFN comprise flu-like symptoms, fever, fatigue, neutropenia, hepatoxicity, and depression. The kinetic of toxicities varies the flu-like symptoms decrease whilst others reported adverse events remain unchanged or even increase over time (mainly: fatigue, anorexia, symptoms of depression/anxiety).

Immunotherapy with Immune Checkpoint Inhibitors

In 2015, the positive results of the EORTC 18071 study became available on the use of adjuvant therapy with anti-CTLA-4 antibody (ipilimumab) after lymphadenectomy due to metastases in the regional lymph nodes (stage III) [17]. Nine hundred and fifty one patients were enrolled in the trial and they were randomized to the group with a high dose of ipilimumab 10 mg/kg every 3 weeks for four doses and then every 3 months up to 3 years ($n = 476$) or to the placebo group ($n = 476$). AT the median follow-up period of 2.7 years, 234 recurrences occurred in the group treated with ipilimumab versus 294 with placebo, the median RFS was 26.1 months versus 17.1 months, respectively ($p = 0.0013$). The improvement of RFS concerned both patients with macro- and micro-metastases (definitions according to the TNM classification edition 7) in the lymph nodes and the effect of the adjuvant treatment was more significant in the patients with ulcerated primary melanoma. Grade 3–4 adverse events occurred in 54% of patients in the ipilimumab arm versus 25% of the placebo arm. Five patients (1%) died due to treatment-related toxicity. Adverse events led to permanent discontinuation of the therapy in 52% of patients who had started treatment with ipilimumab [17]. The median follow-up period in this study was 5.3 years. The results indicated a significant benefit with ipilimumab in terms of RFS, metastasis-free survival (DMFS), and OS. The rate of the 5-year OS in the group receiving ipilimumab was 65.4% in comparison with 54.4% in the group with the placebo, the hazard ratio (HR) for death was 0.72 [23]. The EORTC 18071 study resulted in the registration of ipilimumab in the United States, but not in Europe. Hence, the implementation of this therapy is limited because of its high toxicity and the fact that the trials with the anti-PD-1 antibodies (nivolumab and pembrolizumab) and BRAF and MEK inhibitors gave more beneficial results (Table 20.2).

The results of another study (E1609) showed a similar efficacy of a lower dose of ipilimumab (3 mg/kg) with lower toxicity. This was a phase III trial in patients with resected high-risk cutaneous melanoma (AJCC seventh edition stage IIIB, IIIC, M1a, or M1b) with 2 coprimary end points: OS and RFS. In this study, a 2-step hierarchic approach was designed: ipilimumab 3 mg/kg versus high-dose IFN alfa-2b followed by ipilimumab 10 mg/kg versus high-dose IFN alfa-2b (HDI). One thousand six hundred seventy adult patients were randomized (1:1:1) to ipilimumab 3 mg/kg ($n = 523$), HDI ($n = 636$), or ipilimumab 10 mg/kg ($n = 511$). Treatment-related adverse events grade ≥ 3 occurred in 37% of patients receiving ipilimumab 3 mg/kg, in 79% in HDI arm and in 58% in ipilimumab 10 mg/kg arm, discontinuation due to adverse events occurred in 35%, 20%, and 54%, respectively. Based on comparison of ipilimumab 3 mg/kg versus HDI significant OS and RFS differences in favor of ipilimumab 3 mg/kg (hazard ratio [HR], 0.78; 95.6% CI, 0.61 to 0.99; P =0.044; RFS: HR, 0.85; 99.4% CI, 0.66 to 1.09; $P = 0.065$) were reported. In the second step trends in favor of ipilimumab 10 mg/kg versus HDI did not achieve statistical significance [31].

The randomized study CheckMate 238 in group of patients in clinical IIIB, IIIC, and IV stages after resection of metastases, showed that after 1 year of treatment with nivolumab, RFS was improved by 10% in comparison to treatment with ipilimumab, nivolumab showed also a lower toxicity than ipilimumab (18-month RFS: 65% vs. 53%) [23]. This was the only phase III study where patients after the resection of distant metastases were included. Moreover, there was an improvement in DMFS (HR 0.73). Treatment-related grade 3 or 4 adverse events were observed in 14.4% of patients receiving nivolumab in comparison with 45.9% in the group treated with ipilimumab [27]. The update of the data from 2018 with the 3-year

Table 20.2 The summary of major contemporary clinical trials with adjuvant therapy after resection of high-risk melanoma

	EORTC 18071 Ipilimumab vs placebo	BRIM-8 Vemurafenib vs placebo	COMBI-AD Dabrafenib + trametinib vs placebo	Checkmate 238 Ipilimumab vs nivolumab	EORTC 1325/ Keynote 054 Pembrolizumab vs placebo
Author	Eggermont 2015 [17] Eggermont 2016 [23]	Maio 2018 [24]	Long 2017 [25] Hauschild 2018 [26]	Weber 2017 [27–29] Ascierto 2020 [41]	Eggermont 2018 [30] Eggermont 2020 [42]
Population	IIIA (>1 mm), IIIB, IIIC	IIC, IIIA, IIIB, IIIC	IIIA (>1 mm), IIIB, IIIC	IIIB, IIIC, IV	IIIA (>1 mm), IIIB, IIIC
BRAF mutations	?	100%	100%	41%/43%	
RFS	41% vs 30% (5y)	82% vs 63% (12 m); 62% vs 53% (24 m) 79% vs 58% (12 m) 46% vs 47% (24 m) IIIC 84% vs 66% (12 m) 72% vs 56% (24 m) IIC–IIIB	67% vs 44% (2y) HR = 0.47 58% vs 39% (3y) 54% vs 38% (4y) HR 0.49 52% vs 36% (5y)	66% vs 53% (18 m) HR 0.66; 62.6% vs 50.2% (24 m) HR 0.65; 58% vs 45% (36 m) HR 0.68; 52% vs 41% (48 m)	HR 0,57; 18-month difference 18.2%: 71.4% vs 53.2%; 36-month difference 20%: 64% vs 44%
OS	65% vs 54% (5y) HR = 0.72	BD	91% vs 83% (2l) 86% vs 77% (3l) HR=0.57	NA	NA

OS overall survival, *RFS* relapse-free survival, *NA* not available

follow-up period confirmed the beneficial effects of nivolumab irrespective of the PD-L1 expression status and BRAF mutation in terms of RFS (HR 0.66) and DMFS (HR 0.76) [28]. At a median follow-up of 36 months patients receiving nivolumab had superior RFS compared with patients in ipilimumab arm (HR 0.68; 95% CI, 0.56–0.82; $p < 0.0001$) [29]. In the nivolumab versus ipilimumab treatment arms, 3-year RFS rates were 58% versus 45%; DMFS was also improved with nivolumab compared with ipilimumab, HR 0.78 (95% CI, 0.62–0.99). Superior recurrence-free survival was consistently seen across subgroups according to stage, PD-L1 expression, and *BRAF* status 8% of patients had to stop treatment in the nivolumab arm because of toxicity and between 10% and 15% of patients has grade 3/4 immune-related adverse events.

The Keynote-054/EORTC 1325 was a randomized phase III study, which included 1019 patients and resulted in a decrease of the risk of recurrence (HR for RFS 0.57) and DMFS after 1 year of adjuvant treatment with pembrolizumab in comparison with the placebo in the group of patients in stage III, characterized by a higher risk (i.e., stage IIIA with the micro-metastasis size >1 mm, IIIB and IIIC) [30]. A reclassification with reference to a new classification of stage III according to AJCC (eighth edition) confirmed the benefits in terms of RFS (test for interaction: $p = 0.68$) after 1 year of treatment with pembrolizumab in comparison with the placebo (excluding IIIA stage), respectively:

- IIIB stage (79.0% vs. 65.5%; HR 0.59 [99% CI 0.35–0.99])
- IIIC stage (73.6% vs. 53.9%; HR 0.48 [99% CI 0.33–0.70])
- IIID stage (50.0% vs. 33.3%; HR 0.69 [0.24–2.00]) [32]

Moreover, further analysis demonstrated that the occurrence of immune-related adverse events was associated with a longer RFS in the pembrolizumab arm (HR, 0.61; 95% CI, 0.39–0.95; $P = 0.03$), but in the placebo arm. When compared to the placebo arm, the reduction in the hazard of recurrence or death in the group of patients receiving adjuvant pembrolizumab was greater after the onset of an irAE than without or before an irAE (HR, 0.37; 95% CI, 0.24–0.57 vs. HR, 0.61; 95% CI, 0.49–0.77, respectively; $P = 0.03$) [33]. Longer follow-up confirmed RFS and DMFS benefits for adjuvant pembrolizumab when compared with placebo: 3-year RFS rate 63.7% versus 44.1% for pembrolizumab versus placebo (HR 0.56) and 3.5-year DMFS rate 65.3% versus 49.4% (HR 0.60, $p < 0.0001$), respectively.

Nivolumab and pembrolizumab are currently registered for adjuvant treatment in the United States and the European Union.

For nivolumab and pembrolizumab, treatment-related adverse events (AEs) tended to be mild and manageable, and occurred in 85% and 78% of patients, respectively, with the most common being fatigue, skin reactions (rash, pruritus), diarrhea, nausea, and endocrine disorders. Rates of grade 3+ treatment-related adverse events (14.4% and 14.7%) resulting in treatment discontinuation (9.7% vs. 13.8%) were similar.

Currently, the results of an ongoing phase III study comparing the use of nivolumab and the combination of nivolumab with ipilimumab in adjuvant treatment (CheckMate 915) are awaited, although press release data did not show the additional benefit from adding of ipilimumab to nivolumab in adjuvant setting. The randomized phase II trial on adjuvant therapy in high-risk stage IV melanoma (IMMUMED) after complete resection or radiotherapy conducted within 8 weeks prior to enrollment compared three different strategies: 1-year nivolumab monotherapy, nivolumab plus ipilimumab combination, and placebo [34]. With a minimum follow-up of 6 months after the end of treatment, the superiority of combination of nivolumab and ipilimumab was demonstrated in terms of RFS (HR vs. nivolumab 0.40 and HR vs. placebo 0.23) with greater impact in *BRAF* mutated population; 12 month (24 month) RFS rates were 75% (70%) for nivolumab plus ipilimumab, 52% (42%) for nivolumab, and 32% (14%) for placebo arms. However, the combination was highly toxic with grade 3/4 treatment-related adverse events occurring in 71% of patients. Clinical benefit of nivolumab plus ipilimumab was reported despite a treatment discontinuation rate of more than 79% and a maximum dose of 2 infusions for 50% of the patients treated with the combination.

Moreover, the adjuvant immunotherapy trials with pembrolizumab (KEYNOTE-716; NCT03553836) [35]; or nivolumab (CheckMate76K; NCT04099251) in patients with surgically resected high-risk stage II melanoma are currently ongoing.

Molecularly Targeted Therapy

Adjuvant therapy with the use of dabrafenib with trametinib in the group of high-risk stage III patients with *BRAF* mutation demonstrated an improvement of RFS (HR 0.47), DMFS (HR 0.51; 91% vs. 70% after 1 year, 77% vs. 60% after 2 years and 71% vs. 57% after 3 years) and OS (HR 0.57) in comparison with the placebo. In this study (COMBI-AD), dabrafenib in combination with trametinib were used for 12 months in comparison with placebo (in a population of patients after radical lymph node dissection in IIIA stage with the metastasis size >1 mm, IIIB/C) [29]. The benefits in treatment with dabrafenib in combination with trametinib were observed in all the analyzed subgroups. The updated data from the 4-year follow-up periods confirmed the benefits of treatment with dabrafenib in combination with trametinib (RFS: 54%; HR: 0.49; DFS: 67%; HR: 0.53) [25]. With 5 year follow-up, the percentage of relapse-free patients was 52% for dabrafenib plus trametinib arm as compared to 36% with placebo arm (HR for relapse or death, 0.51; 95% CI, 0.42 to 0.61).

Moreover, the mathematical model was developed to evaluate the cure rate of patients treated with adjuvant therapy and in this case the cure rate makes up as much as 17% [26]. The safety profile of dabrafenib in combination with trametinib was compliant with the profile observed in the studies in metastatic setting and the treatment was relatively well tolerated (although 26% of patients discontinued treatment) [36].

Formally, positive clinical study BRIM-8 [24] also concerned the application of vemurafenib in monotherapy in adjuvant treatment (in comparison with the placebo) in stage IIC–III melanoma *BRAF* mutated patients after complete resection (this has so far been the only study comprising patients with stage II melanoma). The median disease-free survival (DFS) was 23.1 months in the group treated with vemurafenib, in comparison with 15.4 months in the group with the placebo (HR 0.8; $p = 0.026$), yet this effect was limited solely to the subgroup with tumor stage IIC–IIIA–IIIB, and was not observed in patients with more advanced melanomas (IIIC). Currently, it is obvious that the monotherapy with BRAF inhibitors is not the optimal treatment method in comparison with the combined treatment with BRAF and MEK inhibitors for these patients.

Conclusions

The summary of the results of systemic adjuvant treatment after the resection of high-risk melanoma is presented in Table 20.2. Other methods of immunotherapy (e.g. interleukin 2), vaccinations, or cytotoxic drugs do not have any applications in post-operative adjuvant treatment [1, 2, 37].

To sum up, in accordance with the European and American recommendations [1–3, 38], adjuvant treatment with anti-PD-1 immunotherapy with (nivolumab or pembrolizumab) or combined treatment of BRAF and MEK inhibitors (dabrafenib in combination with trametinib for the patient population with *BRAF* mutation) has become a new therapeutic standard for patients after resection of melanomas with a high risk of recurrence (stage IIIA–IIID after complete resection and additionally nivolumab in resected stage IV). This, in turn, leads to the fact that all patients with melanomas in stages from IIIA to IV should be discussed at multidisciplinary team meetings so as to guarantee patients' optimal, modern, and as effective as possible treatment options. Additionally, it must be remembered that high-risk melanomas (also these without nodal metastases) should be included in prospective clinical trials concerning new methods of adjuvant treatment. Moreover, there is large complexity for treatment choice in adjuvant therapy of melanoma for three reasons: (1) as new AJCC classification (edition 8) has been effective since 2018 (and the trials were conducted according to AJCC edition 7 staging system); (1a) patients with stage IIIA have an excellent prognosis even better than those with stage IIB and stage IIC; (1b) patients with stage IIID have a poor prognosis and deserve different strategies in clinical trials, (2) completion lymph node dissection is not further the standard approach after positive sentinel lymph node due to lack of benefit for melanoma-specific survival according to MSLT-II and DeCOG trials (and currently adjuvant therapy can be started immediately after positive sentinel node biopsy) [39, 40], and finally, (3) clinical trials in adjuvant setting included different populations and comparators (Table 20.2).

Treatment in the adjuvant setting is with curative intent. The time to relapse after the failure of adjuvant treatment may reflect different mechanisms of resistance, treatment with the same therapy for first-line metastatic disease as that received in the adjuvant setting is unlikely to be curative. There are very limited data available to guide optimal sequence selection of BRAF-targeted therapy and immunotherapies in the metastatic setting after failure of adjuvant therapy [43]. The choice of first-line treatment for disease recurrence after adjuvant treatment failure should therefore be influenced by several factors including the treatment received in the adjuvant setting, the time until relapse, the type of recurrence (symptomatic or not), the molecular profile.

References

1. Michielin O, van Akkooi ACJ, Ascierto PA, Dummer R, Keilholz U, ESMO Guidelines Committee. Cutaneous melanoma: ESMO Clinical Practice Guidelines for diagnosis, treatment and follow-up. Ann Oncol. 2019;30(12):1884–901. https://doi.org/10.1093/annonc/mdz411.
2. Rutkowski P, Wysocki PJ, Nasierowska-Guttmejer A, et al. Cutaneous melanomas. Oncol Clin Pract. 2019;15:1–19. https://doi.org/10.5603/OCP.2018.0055.
3. NCCN Guidelines. Cutaneous melanoma version 2.2020.
4. Gershenwald JE, Scolyer RA, Hess KR, Sondak VK, Long GV, Ross MI, Lazar AJ, Faries MB, Kirkwood JM, McArthur GA, Haydu LE, Eggermont AMM, Flaherty KT, Balch CM, Thompson JF, for members of the American Joint Committee on Cancer Melanoma Expert Panel and the International Melanoma Database and Discovery Platform. Melanoma staging: evidence-based changes in the American Joint Committee on Cancer eighth edition cancer staging manual. CA Cancer J Clin. 2017;67(6):472–92. https://doi.org/10.3322/caac.21409.
5. Eggermont AMM, Dummer R. The 2017 complete overhaul of adjuvant therapies for high-risk melanoma and its consequences for staging and management of melanoma patients. Eur J Cancer. 2017;86:101–5. https://doi.org/10.1016/j.ejca.2017.09.014.
6. Amaria RN, Prieto PA, Tetzlaff MT, Reuben A, Andrews MC, Ross MI, Glitza IC, Cormier J, Hwu W-J, Tawbi HA, Patel SP, Lee JE, Gershenwald JE, Spencer CN, Gopalakrishnan V, Bassett R, Simpson L, Mouton R, Hudgens CW, Li Z, Zhu H, Cooper ZA, Wani K, Lazar A, Hwu P, Diab A, Wong MK, McQuade JL, Royal R, Lucci A, Burton EM, Reddy S, Sharma P, Allison J, Futreal PA, Woodman SE, Davies† MA, Wargo† JA. Neoadjuvant plus adjuvant dabrafenib and trametinib versus standard of care in patients with high-risk, surgically resectable melanoma: a single-centre, open-label, randomised, phase 2 trial. Lancet Oncol. 2018;19:181–93.
7. Long GV, Saw RPM, Lo S, Nieweg OE, Shannon KF, Gonzalez M, Guminski A, Lee JH, Lee H, Ferguson PM, Rawson RV, Wilmott JS, Thompson JF, Kefford RF, Ch'ng S, Stretch JR, Emmett L, Kapoor R, Rizos H, Spillane AJ, Scolyer RA, Menzies AM. Neoadjuvant dabrafenib combined with trametinib for resectable, stage IIIB–C, BRAFV600 mutation-positive melanoma (NeoCombi): a single-arm, open-label, single-centre, phase 2 trial. Lancet Oncol. 2019;20(7):961–71.
8. Amaria RN, Reddy SM, Tawbi HA, Davies MA, Ross MI, Glitza IC, Cormier JN, Lewis C, Hwu WJ, Hanna E, Diab A, Wong MK, Royal R, Gross N, Weber R, Lai SY, Ehlers R, Blando J, Milton DR, Woodman S, Kageyama R, Wells DK, Hwu P, Patel SP, Lucci A, Hessel A, Lee JE, Gershenwald J, Simpson L, Burton EM, Posada L, Haydu L, Wang L, Zhang S, Lazar AJ, Hudgens CW, Gopalakrishnan V, Reuben A, Andrews MC, Spencer CN, Prieto V, Sharma P, Allison J, Tetzlaff MT, Wargo JA. Neoadjuvant immune checkpoint blockade in high-risk resectable melanoma. Nat Med. 2018;24(11):1649–54.
9. Blank CU, Rozeman E, Fanchi LF, Sikorska K, van de Wiel B, Kvistborg P, Krijgsman O, van den Braber M, Philips D, Broeks A, van Thienen JV, Mallo HA, Adriaansz S, Ter Meulen S, Pronk LM, Grijpink-Ongering LG, Bruining A, Gittelman RM, Warren S, van Tinteren H, Peeper DS, Haanen JBAG, van Akkooi ACJ, Schumacher TN. Neoadjuvant versus adjuvant ipilimumab plus nivolumab in macroscopic stage III melanoma. Nat Med. 2018;24(11):1655–61. https://doi.org/10.1038/s41591-018-0198-0.
10. Blank CU, Versluis JM, ILM R, Sikorska K, van Houdt WJ, van Thienen JV, Adriaansz S, Mallo HA, van Tinteren H, van de Wiel BA, Grijpink-Ongering LG, Bruining A, JBAG H, van Akkooi ACJ, Schumacher TN, Rozeman EA. 3-year relapse-free survival (RFS), overall survival (OS) and long-term toxicity of (neo)adjuvant ipilimumab (IPI) + nivolumab (NIVO) in macroscopic stage III melanoma (OpACIN trial). Ann Oncol. 2019;30(Suppl_5):mdz255.003. https://doi.org/10.1093/annonc/mdz255.003.
11. Rozeman EA, Menzies AM, van Akkooi ACJ, Adhikari C, Bierman C, van de Wiel BA, Scolyer RA, Krijgsman O, Sikorska K, Eriksson H, Broeks A, van Thienen JV, Guminski AD, Acosta AT, Ter Meulen S, Koenen AM, LJW B, Shannon K, Pronk LM, Gonzalez M,

Ch'ng S, Grijpink-Ongering LG, Stretch J, Heijmink S, van Tinteren H, JBAG H, Nieweg OE, WMC K, Zuur CL, RPM S, van Houdt WJ, Peeper DS, Spillane AJ, Hansson J, Schumacher TN, Long GV, Blank CU. Identification of the optimal combination dosing schedule of neoadjuvant ipilimumab plus nivolumab in macroscopic stage III melanoma (OpACIN-neo): a multicentre, phase 2, randomised, controlled trial. Lancet Oncol. 2019;20(7):948–60. https://doi.org/10.1016/S1470-2045(19)30151-2.

12. Rozeman EA, Menzies AM, Krijgsman O, Hoefsmit EP, van de Wiel BA, Sikorska K, Van TM, Eriksson H, Bierman C, Gonzalez M, Shannon K, Broeks A, Kerkhoven R, Spillane AJ, Saw RP, van Akkooi ACJ, Scolyer RA, Hansson J, Long GV, Blank CU. 18-months relapse-free survival (RFS) and biomarker analyses of OpACIN-neo: A study to identify the optimal dosing schedule of neoadjuvant (neoadj) ipilimumab (IPI) + nivolumab (NIVO) in stage III melanoma. Ann Oncol. 2019;30(Suppl_5):mdz394.072. https://doi.org/10.1093/annonc/mdz394.072.

13. Huang AC, Orlowski RJ, Xu X, Mick R, George SM, Yan PK, Manne S, Kraya AA, Wubbenhorst B, Dorfman L, D'Andrea K, Wenz BM, Liu S, Chilukuri L, Kozlov A, Carberry M, Giles L, Kier MW, Quagliarello F, McGettigan S, Kreider K, Annamalai L, Zhao Q, Mogg R, Xu W, Blumenschein WM, Yearley JH, Linette GP, Amaravadi RK, Schuchter LM, Herati RS, Bengsch B, Nathanson KL, Farwell MD, Karakousis GC, Wherry EJ, Mitchell TC. A single dose of neoadjuvant PD-1 blockade predicts clinical outcomes in resectable melanoma. Nat Med. 2019;25(3):454–61. https://doi.org/10.1038/s41591-019-0357-y.

14. Dummer R, Gyorki DE, Hyngstrom J, Berger A, Conry R, Demidov L, Sharma A, Treichel SA, Gorski K, Anderson A, Faries M, Ross MI. Primary 2-year results of the phase 2, multicenter, randomized, open-label trial of efficacy and safety for talimogene laherparepvec (T-VEC) neoadjuvant treatment plus surgery vs surgery in patients with resectable stage IIIB–IVM1a melanoma. Ann Oncol. 2019;30(Suppl_5):v851–934. https://doi.org/10.1093/annonc/mdz394.

15. Amaria RN, Menzies AM, Burton EM, Scolyer RA, Tetzlaff MT, Antdbacka R, Ariyan C, Bassett R, Carter B, Daud A, Faries M, Fecher LA, Flaherty KT, Gershenwald JE, Hamid O, Hong A, Kirkwood JM, Lo S, Margolin K, Messina J, Postow MA, Rizos H, Ross M, Rozeman EA, Saw RPM, Sondak V, Sullivan RJ, Taube JM, Thompson JF, van de Wiel BA, Eggermont AM, Davies MA, International Neoadjuvant Melanoma Consortium Members, Ascierto PA, Spillane A, van Akkooi AC, Wargo J, Blank CU, Tawbi HA, Long GV. Neoadjuvant systemic therapy in melanoma: recommendations of the International Neoadjuvant Melanoma Consortium. Lancet Oncol. 2019;20(7):e378–89. https://doi.org/10.1016/S1470-2045(19)30332-8.

16. Menzies AM, Rozeman EA, Amaria RN, Chan Chi Huang A, Scolyer RA, Tetzlaff MT, Van De Wiel BA, Lo S, Tarhini AA, Tawbi HA-H, Burton EM, Karakousis G, Ascierto PA, Spillane A, Davies MA, Van Akkooi ACJ, Mitchell TC, Long GV, Wargo JA, Blank CU, and International Neoadjuvant Melanoma Consortium (INMC). Pathological response and survival with neoadjuvant therapy in melanoma: A pooled analysis from the International Neoadjuvant Melanoma Consortium (INMC). J Clin Oncol. 2019;37(15_Suppl):9503.

17. Eggermont AM, Chiarion-Sileni V, Grob JJ, Dummer R, Wolchok JD, Schmidt H, Hamid O, Robert C, Ascierto PA, Richards JM, Lebbé C, Ferraresi V, Smylie M, Weber JS, Maio M, Konto C, Hoos A, de Pril V, Gurunath RK, de Schaetzen G, Suciu S, Testori A. Adjuvant ipilimumab versus placebo after complete resection of high-risk stage III melanoma (EORTC 18071): a randomised, double-blind, phase 3 trial. Lancet Oncol. 2015;16(5):522–30.

18. Eggermont AMM, Gore M. Randomized adjuvant therapy trials in melanoma: surgical and systemic. Sem Oncol. 2007;34:509–15.

19. Sondak VK, Gonzalez RJ, Kudchadkar R. Adjuvant therapy for melanoma: a surgical perspective. Surg Oncol Clin N Am. 2011;20:105–14.

20. Eggermont AM, Suciu S, Testori A, Kruit WH, Marsden J, Punt CJ, Santinami M, Salès F, Schadendorf D, Patel P, Dummer R, Robert C, Keilholz U, Yver A, Spatz A. Ulceration and stage are predictive of interferon efficacy in melanoma: results of the phase III adjuvant trials EORTC 18952 and EORTC 18991. Eur J Cancer. 2012;48(2):218–25.

21. Ives NJ, Suciu S, Eggermont AMM, Kirkwood J, Lorigan P, Markovic SN, Garbe C, Wheatley K, International Melanoma Meta-Analysis Collaborative Group (IMMCG). Adjuvant interferon-α for the treatment of high-risk melanoma: an individual patient data meta-analysis. Eur J Cancer. 2017;82:171–83. https://doi.org/10.1016/j.ejca.2017.06.006.

22. Eggermont AMM, Rutkowski P, Dutriaux C, Hofman-Wellenhof R, Dziewulski P, Marples M, Grange F, Lok C, Pennachioli E, Robert C, van Akkooi ACJ, Bastholt L, Minisini A, Marshall E, Salès F, Grob JJ, Bechter O, Schadendorf D, Marreaud S, Kicinski M, Suciu S, Testori AAE. Adjuvant therapy with pegylated interferon-alfa2b vs observation in stage II B/C patients with ulcerated primary: Results of the European Organisation for Research and Treatment of Cancer 18081 randomised trial. Eur J Cancer. 2020;133:94–103. https://doi.org/10.1016/j.ejca.2020.04.015. Epub 2020 May 26. PMID: 32470710.
23. Eggermont AM, Chiarion-Sileni V, Grob JJ, Dummer R, Wolchok JD, Schmidt H, Hamid O, Robert C, Ascierto PA, Richards JM, Lebbé C, Ferraresi V, Smylie M, Weber JS, Maio M, Bastholt L, Mortier L, Thomas L, Tahir S, Hauschild A, Hassel JC, Hodi FS, Taitt C, de Pril V, de Schaetzen G, Suciu S, Testori A. Prolonged survival in stage III melanoma with ipilimumab adjuvant therapy. N Engl J Med. 2016;375(19):1845–55.
24. Maio M, Lewis K, Demidov L, Mandalà M, Bondarenko I, Ascierto PA, Herbert C, Mackiewicz A, Rutkowski P, Guminski A, Goodman GR, Simmons B, Ye C, Yan Y, Schadendorf D, BRIM8 Investigators. Adjuvant vemurafenib in resected, BRAFV600 mutation-positive melanoma (BRIM8): a randomised, double-blind, placebo-controlled, multicentre, phase 3 trial. Lancet Oncol. 2018;19(4):510–20. https://doi.org/10.1016/S1470-2045(18)30106-2.
25. Long GV, Hauschild A, Santinami M, Atkinson V, Mandalà M, Chiarion-Sileni V, Larkin J, Nyakas M, Dutriaux C, Haydon A, Robert C, Mortier L, Schachter J, Schadendorf D, Lesimple T, Plummer R, Ji R, Zhang P, Mookerjee B, Legos J, Kefford R, Dummer R, Kirkwood JM. Adjuvant dabrafenib plus trametinib in stage III BRAF-mutated melanoma. N Engl J Med. 2017;377(19):1813–23. https://doi.org/10.1056/NEJMoa1708539.
26. Hauschild A, Dummer R, et al. Longer follow-up confirms relapse-free survival benefit with adjuvant dabrafenib plus trametinib in patients with resected BRAF V600–mutant stage III melanoma. J Clin Oncol. 2018;36(35):3441–9. https://doi.org/10.1200/JCO.18.01219.
27. Weber J, Mandala M, Del Vecchio M, Gogas HJ, Arance AM, Cowey CL, Dalle S, Schenker M, Chiarion-Sileni V, Marquez-Rodas I, Grob JJ, Butler MO, Middleton MR, Maio M, Atkinson V, Queirolo P, Gonzalez R, Kudchadkar RR, Smylie M, Meyer N, Mortier L, Atkins MB, Long GV, Bhatia S, Lebbé C, Rutkowski P, Yokota K, Yamazaki N, Kim TM, de Pril V, Sabater J, Qureshi A, Larkin J, Ascierto PA, CheckMate 238 Collaborators. Adjuvant nivolumab versus ipilimumab in resected stage III or IV melanoma. N Engl J Med. 2017;377(19):1824–35.
28. Weber JS, Mandalà M, Del Vecchio M, Gogas H, Arance AM, Cowey CL, Dalle S, Schenker M, Chiarion-Sileni V, Rodas IM, Grob J-J, Butler M, Middleton MR, Maio M, Atkinson V, Dummer R, de Pril V, Qureshi AH, Larkin JMG, Ascierto PA. Adjuvant therapy with nivolumab (NIVO) versus ipilimumab (IPI) after complete resection of stage III/IV melanoma: Updated results from a phase III trial (CheckMate 238). J Clin Oncol. 2018;36 (Suppl; abstr 9502) 2018 ASCO Annual Meeting.
29. Weber JS, Del Vecchio M, Mandala M, Gogas H, Arance AM, Dalle S, Cowey CL, Schenker M, Grob JJ, Chiarion-Sileni V, Marquez-Rodas I, Butler MO, Maio M, Middleton MR, Tang T, Saci A, De Pril V, Lobo M, Larkin JMG, Ascierto PA. Adjuvant nivolumab (NIVO) versus ipilimumab (IPI) in resected stage III/IV melanoma: 3-year efficacy and biomarker results from the phase 3 CheckMate 238 trial. Ann Oncol. 2019;30(Suppl_5):v533–63. https://doi.org/10.1093/annonc/mdz255.
30. Eggermont AMM, Blank CU, Mandala M, Long GV, Atkinson V, Dalle S, Haydon A, Lichinitser M, Khattak A, Carlino MS, Sandhu S, Larkin J, Puig S, Ascierto PA, Rutkowski P, Schadendorf D, Koornstra R, Hernandez-Aya L, Maio M, van den Eertwegh AJM, Grob JJ, Gutzmer R, Jamal R, Lorigan P, Ibrahim N, Marreaud S, van Akkooi ACJ, Suciu S, Robert C. Adjuvant Pembrolizumab versus Placebo in Resected Stage III Melanoma. N Engl J Med. 2018 May 10;378(19):1789–801. https://doi.org/10.1056/NEJMoa1802357.
31. Tarhini AA, Lee SJ, Hodi FS, Rao UNM, Cohen GI, Hamid O, Hutchins LF, Sosman JA, Kluger HM, Eroglu Z, Koon HB, Lawrence DP, Kendra KL, Minor DR, Lee CB, Albertini MR, Flaherty LE, Petrella TM, Streicher H, Sondak VK, Kirkwood JM. Phase III study of adjuvant ipilimumab (3 or 10 mg/kg) versus high-dose interferon Alfa-2b for resected high-risk melanoma: North American Intergroup E1609. J Clin Oncol. 2019;27:JCO1901381. https://doi.org/10.1200/JCO.19.01381.

32. Eggermont AMM, Blank CU, Mandala M, Long GV, Atkinson VG, Dalle S, Haydon A, Lichinitser M, Khattak A, Carlino MS, Sandhu S, Larkin J, Puig S, Ascierto PA, Rutkowski P, Schadendorf D, Koornstra R, Hernandez-Aya L, Di Giacomo AM, van den Eertwegh AJ, Grob JJ, Gutzmer R, Jamal R, Lorigan PC, Lupinacci R, Krepler C, Ibrahim N, Kicinski M, Marreaud S, van Akkooi AC, Suciu S, Robert C. Prognostic and predictive value of AJCC-8 staging in the phase III EORTC1325/KEYNOTE-054 trial of pembrolizumab vs placebo in resected high-risk stage III melanoma. Eur J Cancer. 2019;116:148–57. https://doi.org/10.1016/j.ejca.2019.05.020.
33. Eggermont AMM, Kicinski M, Blank CU, Mandala M, Long GV, Atkinson V, Dalle S, Haydon A, Khattak A, Carlino MS, Sandhu S, Larkin J, Puig S, Ascierto PA, Rutkowski P, Schadendorf D, Koornstra R, Hernandez-Aya L, Di Giacomo AM, van den Eertwegh AJM, Grob JJ, Gutzmer R, Jamal R, Lorigan PC, Krepler C, Ibrahim N, Marreaud S, van Akkooi A, Robert C, Suciu S. Association between immune-related adverse events and recurrence-free survival among patients with stage III melanoma randomized to receive pembrolizumab or placebo: a secondary analysis of a randomized clinical trial. JAMA Oncol. 2020;6(4):519–27. https://doi.org/10.1001/jamaoncol.2019.5570.
34. Schadendorf D, Hassel JC, Fluck M, Eigentler T, Loquai C, Berneburg M, Gutzmer R, Meier F, Mohr P, Hauschild A, Becker JC, Menzer C, Kiecker C, Dippel E, Simon J, Conrad B, Garbe C, Körner S, Livingstone E, Zimmer L. Adjuvant IMMUnotherapy with nivolumab (NIVO) alone or in combination with ipilimumab (IPI) vs. placebo in stage IV melanoma patients with no evidence of disease (NED): A randomized, double-blind, phase II trial (IMMUNED) on behalf of DeCOG. Ann Oncol. 2019;30(Suppl_5):v851–934. https://doi.org/10.1093/annonc/mdz394.
35. Luke JJ, Ascierto PA, Carlino MS, Gershenwald JE, Grob JJ, Hauschild A, Kirkwood JM, Long GV, Mohr P, Robert C, Ross M, Scolyer RA, Yoon CH, Poklepovic A, Rutkowski P, Anderson JR, Ahsan S, Ibrahim N, M Eggermont AM. KEYNOTE-716: phase III study of adjuvant pembrolizumab versus placebo in resected high-risk stage II melanoma. Future Oncol. 2020;16(3):4429–38. https://doi.org/10.2217/fon-2019-0666.
36. Schadendorf D, Hauschild A, Santinami M, Atkinson V, Mandalà M, Chiarion-Sileni V, Larkin J, Nyakas M, Dutriaux C, Haydon A, Robert C, Mortier L, Lesimple T, Plummer R, Schachter J, Dasgupta K, Manson S, Koruth R, Mookerjee B, Kefford R, Dummer R, Kirkwood JM, Long GV. Patient-reported outcomes in patients with resected, high-risk melanoma with BRAFV600E or BRAFV600K mutations treated with adjuvant dabrafenib plus trametinib (COMBI-AD): a randomised, placebo-controlled, phase 3 trial. Lancet Oncol. 2019;20(5):701–10. https://doi.org/10.1016/S1470-2045(18)30940-9.
37. Dreno B, Thompson JF, Smithers BM, Santinami M, Jouary T, Gutzmer R, Levchenko E, Rutkowski P, Grob JJ, Korovin S, Drucis K, Grange F, Machet L, Hersey P, Krajsova I, Testori A, Conry R, Guillot B, WHJ K, Demidov L, Thompson JA, Bondarenko I, Jaroszek J, Puig S, Cinat G, Hauschild A, Goeman JJ, van Houwelingen HC, Ulloa-Montoya F, Callegaro A, Dizier B, Spiessens B, Debois M, Brichard VG, Louahed J, Therasse P, Debruyne C, Kirkwood JM. MAGE-A3 immunotherapeutic as adjuvant therapy for patients with resected, MAGE-A3-positive, stage III melanoma (DERMA): a double-blind, randomised, placebo-controlled, phase 3 trial. Lancet Oncol. 2018;19(7):916–29. https://doi.org/10.1016/S1470-2045(18)30254-7.
38. Bello DM, Ariyan CE. Adjuvant therapy in the treatment of melanoma. Ann Surg Oncol. 2018;25(7):1807–13.
39. Faries M, Thompson J, Cochran A, et al. Completion dissection or observation for sentinel-node metastasis in melanoma. N Engl J Med. 2017;376(23):2211–22. https://doi.org/10.1056/nejmoa1613210.
40. Leiter U, Stadler R, Mauch C, et al. German Dermatologic Cooperative Oncology Group (DeCOG). Complete lymph node dissection versus no dissection in patients with sentinel lymph node biopsy positive melanoma (DeCOG-SLT): a multicentre, randomised, phase 3 trial. Lancet Oncol. 2016;17(6):757–67. https://doi.org/10.1016/S1470-2045(16)00141-8.
41. Ascierto PA, Del Vecchio M, Mandalá M. i wsp. Adjuvant nivolumab versus ipilimumab in resected stage IIIB-C and stage IV melanoma (CheckMate 238): 4-year results from a multicen-

tre, double-blind, randomised, controlled, phase 3 trial. Lancet Oncol. 2020;21(11):1465–77. https://doi.org/10.1016/S1470-2045(20)30494-0. Epub 2020 Sep 19. PMID: 32961119.

42. Eggermont AMM, Blank CU, Mandala M. i wsp. Longer follow-up confirms recurrence-free survival benefit of adjuvant pembrolizumab in high-risk stage III melanoma: updated results from the EORTC 1325-MG/KEYNOTE-054 Trial. J Clin Oncol. 2020: JCO2002110.

43. Keilholz U, Ascierto PA, Dummer R, Robert C, Lorigan P, van Akkooi A, Arance A, Blank CU, Chiarion Sileni V, Donia M, Faries MB, Gaudy-Marqueste C, Gogas H, Grob JJ, Guckenberger M, Haanen J, Hayes AJ, Hoeller C, Lebbé C, Lugowska I, Mandalà M, Márquez-Rodas I, Nathan P, Neyns B, Olofsson Bagge R, Puig S, Rutkowski P, Schilling B, Sondak VK, Tawbi H, Testori A, Michielin O. ESMO consensus conference recommendations on the management of metastatic melanoma: under the auspices of the ESMO Guidelines Committee. Ann Oncol. 2020;31(11):1435–48. https://doi.org/10.1016/j.annonc.2020.07.004. Epub 2020 Aug 4. PMID:32763453.

Part VIII
Special Techniques and Populations

Chapter 21
Adoptive Cell Therapy

Guy Ben-Betzalel

Introduction

The current landscape in the treatment of metastatic and advanced cancers has undergone dramatic changes in the past years. Chemotherapy has been replaced and supplanted by biological agents—tyrosine-kinase inhibitors, targeted antibodies, and immunotherapy. Immunotherapy has revolutionized cancer therapy in a few cancer types—mainly melanoma, Merkel cell carcinoma, non-small cell lung cancer, and renal cell carcinoma. In melanoma, median overall survival has rocketed from 8 months (ref) to more than 5 years [1]. Immunotherapy in oncology is currently based on antibodies that inhibit two checkpoints in the lymphocyte—antigen-presenting cells interface and in the lymphocyte—tumor interface. The two most commonly used antibodies are directed against the Cytotoxic T-cell Lymphocyte Antigen-4 (CTLA-4) receptor and the Programmed cell Death 1 (PD-1) receptor [2].

Adoptive Cell Therapy is a different class of immunotherapy. Rather than using antibodies to drive or suppress immune response, ACT uses autologous T-cells that are either unchanged from the donor T-cells or are genetically modified to recognize and act upon specific antigens on the target cells. ACT has yet to find a significant role in the therapy of solid tumors, however, it has dramatically changed the outcome of advanced line therapy for hematological malignancies [3].

There are three classes of adoptive cell therapy technologies: Tumor Infiltrating Lymphocytes (TIL) therapy, T-cell Receptor (TCR) therapy, and Chimeric-Antigen Receptor (CAR)—T cells (see Table 21.1). All these technologies share a common initial step—the harvesting of peripheral lymphocytes from the patient. In TIL

G. Ben-Betzalel (✉)
Ella Lemelbaum Institute for Immuno-Oncology and Melanoma, Sheba Medical Center, Ramat Gan, Israel
e-mail: Guy.Ben-Betzalel@sheba.health.gov.il

P. Rutkowski, M. Mandalà (eds.), *New Therapies in Advanced Cutaneous Malignancies*, https://doi.org/10.1007/978-3-030-64009-5_21

Table 21.1 Comparison of ACT

	TIL	TCR	CAR-T
Production	Ex vivo expansion of T-cell obtained from resected tumor	Apheresis of peripheral T-cells, transduction with TCR directed against tumor	Apheresis of peripheral T-cells, transduction with CAR against tumor
Obligatory lymphodepleting protocol	Yes	Yes	Yes
MHC dependent	Yes	Yes	No
Il-2 support	Yes	Variable	No
Toxicity	Mainly due to preparatory lymphodepleting protocol; High-dose IL-2-mediated toxicity—SIRS, pulmonary edema, capillary leak	Adverse events second preparatory lymphodepleting protocol; CRS	Preparatory lymphodepleting protocol, CRS, ICANS(neurological toxicity)
Disadvantages	Benefit not known after failure of checkpoint blockade, requires surgical resection of tumor	Difficulty in finding the right target antigen; toxicity	Only approved for CD19+ hematological malignancies; toxicity

therapy these lymphocytes are harvested from an active tumor site. In TCR and CAR-T therapy, the lymphocytes are harvested from the peripheral blood of the patient. In addition these technologies differ greatly in the active end-product which is returned to the patient. This will be further reviewed in the following pages.

Tumor-Infiltrating Lymphocytes

Adoptive cell therapy with Tumor-Infiltrating Lymphocytes (TILs) was the earliest technique of treating patients with T-cells active against the tumor, first developed in murine models by Steve Rosenberg at the surgical branch in the National Institute of Health [4]. In TIL therapy, unlike more modern ACT with TCR and CAR-T cells, the T cells are resident in the metastatic deposits and are harvested by removing a metastatic lesion. The resected tumor is digested and cultured with IL2 to allow for T-cell proliferation. The T cells then undergo a Rapid Expansion (REP) phase during which the cells are with an anti CD-3 antibody, IL2, and allogeneic feeder cells to allow for a 1000–2000 fold expansion to a total of 5×1010–1×1011. The expanded T-cells are then infused to the patient and repeated doses of high-dose IL2 infusions (720,000 IU/kg) are given every 8 hours per tolerance to allow for expansion and activation of the cells in vivo.

Initial attempts at TIL therapy used T-cells selected by IFN-gamma reactivity assay, however, later studies showed using young, unselected TIL resulted in comparable results [5] and were abandoned.

Like more modern adoptive cell therapy techniques, treatment with TILs require a preparatory chemodepleting regimen. Chemodepletion that is clinically evident usually as deep lymphopenia results in less competition with pre-existing T-cells, removal of lymphoid and myeloid-derived suppressor cells, and higher levels of IL-7 and IL-15 [6]. Bone marrow recovery is usually evident within 2 weeks of the therapy. This is usually a combination of high-dose chemotherapy with Fludarabine (25 mg/m^2) and Cyclophosphamide (60 mg/kg) with some series also attempting a combination of high-dose chemotherapy and total body irradiation [7].

Most of the clinical efficacy data regarding TIL therapy comes from a large series of metastatic melanoma patients. The largest series was published in early 2020 by the group of the Ella Lemelbaum Institute at Sheba Medical Center in Israel [8]. In an intent-to-treat population of 179 metastatic melanoma patients refractory to standard therapy 107 were treated and evaluable. The patients had highly advanced disease with 81% having visceral metastases and 22% having CNS metastases. Objective responses were seen in 28% with an additional 15% achieving showing stabilization of their disease. About 69% of responding patients had significant visceral disease and 24% had CNS disease showing that responses can be achieved even in very advanced disease stages.

In a long median follow-up of 7.2 years, responses appear to be durable with median progression-free survival (PFS) of responders of 15.4 months and median overall survival (OS) of more than 58 months. Nonresponders achieved a PFS of 2.6 months and OS of 6.3 months.

Toxicities were either chemotherapy-related or secondary to therapy with high dose IL2. Grade 3–4 febrile neutropenia secondary to preparatory chemodepletion was seen in 91% of patients. Two patients developed late toxicity deemed related to the high-dose chemotherapy regimen; one patient developed thyroid cancer and the other developed myelodysplastic syndrome. Three patients developed fatal acute cardiomyopathy most likely related to high-dose cyclophosphamide. Fatal cardiomyopathy had not been previously reported in ACT TIL trials. Median number of high-dose IL2 doses was 6.5. The most common adverse events related to IL2 were pulmonary congestion (38%), hypotension (20%), diarrhea (13%), hyperbilirubinemia (13%), and renal failure (13%). Most of these adverse events were transient and resolved with follow-up.

Absolute lymphocyte count (ALC) dropped to a median of 0.027 K/μL with levels starting to rise at day 5 after TIL transfusion. Of note, ALC measured at day 7 and day 14 post TIL administration showed a statistically significant increase in the group of patients who responded to therapy compared to the nonresponders. Responding patients had an average of 1.64 K/μL at day 7 post TIL transfusion compared to 0.46 K/μL in non-responding patients ($p \leq 0.0005$). Other parameters shown to be associated with response to therapy were a total number of cells infused (61 × 109 in responders vs. 44 × 109 in non-responders, $p = 0.002$), CD8 cells frequency, and total CD8 number.

Multivariate analysis for a response to therapy revealed that ECOG performance status and ALC at day 7 were independent predictors of response with ALC being the strongest predictor.

TIL therapy is now being commercialized with the product "Lifiluecel" (Iovance Biotherapeutics) under development for patients with metastatic melanoma who had progressed on immunotherapy. Data of 68 patients from the phase II trial were presented at ASCO 2020 conference and showed an objective response in 36.4% of patients. It should be noted that these patients did not receive prior anti PD-1 + anti CDTLA-4 combination therapy and it is still unknown whether the patients who have failed anti PD-1–Anti CTLA-4 therapy can still respond well to TIL therapy.

In addition, it seems that TIL therapy may have a role in treating metastatic uveal melanoma, a rare form of melanoma that is generally thought of as resistant to current immunotherapy with checkpoint blockade. Preliminary data from small series show promising results with 35% response rates [9].

TIL isolation and production has been proven to be possible not only from melanoma metastatic lesions but also from breast cancer [10], cervical cancer [11], renal cell carcinoma [12], non-small cell lung cancer [13], and types of solid tumors. However, clinical data is sparse. Therapy in solid tumors outside of melanoma is now being expanded in clinical trials.

T-Cell Receptor Therapy

T-Cell Receptor (TCR) gene therapy begins with the harvesting of peripheral lymphocytes from the blood of the patient in a process known as leukapheresis. These peripheral T-cells are then transduced with retroviral vectors that lead to incorporation of encoding the TCR alpha and beta chains thus creating a new, modified, TCR in these T-cells [14]. These TCR-modified T-cells can be directed against tumor-specific antigens, cancer-testis antigens, or other antigens that are overexpressed on tumor cells. It is important to note that TCR-modified T-cells act upon their targets in an MHC-dependent fashion.

Much like TIL therapy, before transfusion of the TCR modified T-cells, a preparative lymphodepleting chemotherapy regimen is administered to the patient. Also in similarity to TIL therapy, IL-2 infusions are given to the patient after the TCR product transfusion in order to facilitate expansion and activation of the T-cells.

TCR therapy first trials were performed in Melanoma, directed against the melanoma-specific antigens MART-1 and gp-100. MART-1 and gp-100 are overexpressed in the majority of melanoma cells and are thus a favorable target for T-cell recognition [15]. The first clinical trials were published in 2009 and demonstrated responses in up to 30% of patients in a cohort of 32 patients [16].

Cancer-testis antigens derive from genes that are expressed in cells during embryogenesis and are silenced in normal somatic cells. During dedifferentiation process of cancer cells, aberrant expression of these genes tends to occur—providing rather specific targets for immune activation with minimal activity against normal cells. Notable examples are NY-ESO which is significantly expressed in synovial sarcoma and MAGE-A3 which is expressed in more than 60% of melanoma patients [17]. In a 2013 phase I/II study [18], 7 metastatic melanoma patients and 1 synovial sarcoma patient were treated with anti-MAGE-A3 TCR therapy. Objective responses were seen in 4 melanoma patients and in the single sarcoma patient.

Interesting to note that the target for modified TCR can also rely on viral antigens. TCR modified to recognize Human Papilloma Virus (HPV)-16 E6 epitope has been shown [19] to have clinical activity in a single patient treated with TILs modified to contain TCR against the E6 epitope. This may lead to a way of treating HPV-related cancers in the future with TCR therapy.

Toxicities from therapy with TCR are mostly three. First, bone marrow suppression secondary to the preparative high-dose chemotherapy [20] (usually Cyclophosphamide and Fludarabine) may manifest as pancytopenia with resultant neutropenic fever and sepsis. This neutropenia is transient and reversible. The second main toxicity is cytokine-release syndrome from activation of the modified T-cells in vivo [21]. These cause an array of cytokine-mediated changes leading to a SIRS-like scenario with fever progressing to shock, multiorgan failure, and in extreme cases—death. Treatment for cytokine-release syndrome is supportive as this is usually a transient complication of therapy. The last common complication arises from on and off-target effect of the T-cells as these modified TCRs can be present on normal tissue [16]. An example of off-target effect can be seen in melanoma patients treated with MART-1 TCR leading to uveitis due to injury of uveal melanocytes. Activity against skin melanocytes resulted in rashes and development of vitiligo.

TCR therapy is an intriguing future immunotherapeutic option. However, as current strategies use antigens which are, on one hand, not solely expressed on tumor cells and on the other hand not constitutively expressed on tumor cells finding an effective target with acceptable toxicity may prove to be difficult.

Chimeric-Antigen Receptor T-Cell Therapy

Chimeric-Antigen Receptors (CARs) are hybrid receptors which are genetically engineered to allow recognition and activation of T-cells against specific targets in a non-MHC-dependent fashion. As with TCR therapy, T-cells are transfected with the CAR via a viral vector. The CAR itself is composed of an scFv of an antibody as the extracellular binding domain, an intracellular CD3Zeta chain for downstream signaling and a costimulatory molecule—mostly CD28 and CD137.

Current CAR T cell therapy focuses mainly on hematological malignancies with CD19 as the target [22]. CD19 is an effective target as it appears early in the differentiation of B cells and remains expressed until plasma cell differentiation. CD19 is also highly expressed on B cells in comparison to CD20 and CD22.

As said, unlike TCR modified T-cells CARs act in an MHC-independent fashion. This was first shown by Eshhar in 1989 [23]. Since then CARs have seen dramatic changes in recent years leading to the establishment of four different generations:

- First-generation CARs were engineered to contain the intracellular CD3zeta domain only. This led to limited signaling ability and inability to prime resting T-cells leading to limited response.
- In second-generation CARs, the addition of a second costimulatory molecule (either CD28 or CD137, 4-1BB) lead to an improved activation and expansion of the T cells. These second-generation CAR T cells are the basis for currently approved CAR T cell therapy.
- Third-generation CARs combine the potential of the two costimulatory domains noted above to induce a stronger and prolonged T-cell activation and expansion.
- Fourth-generation CAR T cells, also known as TRUCKs(T-cells Redirected for Universal Cytokine-mediated Killing) carry additional genes to potentiate even further the T cell response. These can take the form of genes allowing for enhanced cytokine secretion or of genes encoding other costimulatory ligands.

CAR T-cell therapy requires a preparatory lymphodepleting protocol using high-dose chemotherapy similar to those used in TIL and TCR therapy.

Toxicity from CAR-T cell therapy is diverse and is categorized into three main categories—Cytokine Release Syndrome (CRS, cytokine storm), Immune Effector Cell-Associated Neurotoxicity Syndrome (ICANS), and on-target off-tumor effects.

Cytokine storm relates to a spectrum of symptoms occurring due to activation of high numbers of T-cells leading to significantly elevated levels of cytokines. The main cytokine mediating this inflammatory response is IL-6; however, this is preceded by elevation of TNFα and IFN$_\gamma$. Other cytokines involved are IL-2, IL-8, and IL-10 [24]. The incidence and severity of CRS have been linked to the disease burden before initiation of therapy [25].

Clinically CRS peaks 1–2 weeks post T cells product transfusion. It presents as a nonspecific SIRS-like state that includes fever, fatigue, nausea, weakness, and myalgia and can involve any system in the body including but not limited to hepatic, renal, cardiovascular, and the respiratory system. Management of severe CRS is accomplished by supportive therapy and treatment with anti-IL-6-R antibody Tocilizumab or Siltuximab [26], which binds soluble IL-6. Tocilizumab has been granted approval by both FDA and EMA. Treatment is guided by the American Society for Bone-Marrow Transplant (ASBMT) grading system [27].

ICANS is a severe neurotoxicity syndrome that occurs following therapy with CAR-T cell therapy. It is often a combination of encephalopathy including but limited to delerium, aphasia, ataxia, and seizures. Usually, brain MRI is normal; however, it is possible patients who develop ICANS may have abnormal findings on brain MRI done prior to therapy [28]. In severe cases, the clinical presentation can include cerebral edema that can be life-threatening. The underlying pathophysiology is not completely understood and is possibly related to increased permeability of the blood–brain barrier during therapy [29]. ICANS can occur with or without concomitant CRS, however, its severity does not seem to correlate with that of the cytokine storm. Some cases of ICANS appear in a biphasic fashion—appearing alongside the CRS symptoms, within 5 days of therapy and a second later phase after CRS has subsided. Treatment of ICANS is usually with corticosteroids or with anti IL-6, which is usually more effective in the first phase of the syndrome. As in the case of CRS, the treatment of ICANS is guided by the severity grading of the ASBMT guidelines.

On-target off-tumor toxicity occurs when the modified receptor on the infused T-cells recognizes a similar epitope in an antigen other than the one it was designed to recognize. This leads to an attack of those T-cells on an unintended target causing unexpected adverse events.

Approved Indications in CAR-T Cell Therapy

Tisagenlecleucel (Kymriah) is a CAR-T cell therapy directed against CD19 and was studied in refractory childhood/young adult B-cell ALL. It was the first CAR-T cell therapy to be approved after studies showed an overall remission rate of 81% at 1-year median follow-up with 6 months overall survival of 90% [30]. Tisagenlecleucel was further studied in large B-cell lymphomas including Diffuse Large B-Cell Lymphoma (DLBCL), high-grade B-cell lymphoma, and DLBCL arising from follicular lymphoma. It was approved for these indications after a large phase II study showed a response rate of 52% with a median duration of response not reached after 14 months follow-up.

The second available CAR-T cell therapy, Axicabtagene ciloleucel (Yescarta) is a second-generation CAR-T agent, similar to Tisagenlecleuce. It differs from the latter by the fact that it uses a retroviral vector and a CD28 co-stimulatory domain while the former uses a lentivirus and 4-1BB as the co-stimulatory domain. Axicabtagene ciloleucel was approved for the same indications as Tisagenlecleuce was after a phase II study showed 72% response rate with 51% complete remission rate. At 1-year follow-up overall survival was 60% with median overall survival not-reached [31].

Unlike CAR-T cell therapy in hematological malignancies, the pace forward in solid tumors has still not reached maturity. Unlike CD-19, solid tumors usually lack a specific suitable target antigen that would allow responses in the tumor without affecting healthy tissue. In addition, solid tumors are complicated in that they reside in an elaborate microenvironment, which may hinder the capacity of T-cells to infiltrate the tumor and attack the tumor cells, even if they do recognize them.

To summarize, adoptive T-cell therapy has undergone a vast and exciting way since its early days starting with Steve Rosenberg's studies with TILs. Today, TIL therapy and TCR are used to treat patients daily, although still in clinical trials settings. CAR-T cell therapy has made the leap forward and evolved from clinical trials into the next generation therapy for patients with CD19+ hematological malignancies with high success rates.

It remains to be seen whether the success seen today with CAR-T cell therapy leads to sustained and prolonged remissions. It also remains to be seen whether the success in hematological malignancies can be expanded to solid tumors. Finding the right target that would allow for effective and safe CAR-T therapy in solid tumors is a challenge, but when that is accomplished it would mark the next step in the continued revolution of immunotherapy in cancer.

References

1. Larkin J, et al. Five-year survival with combined nivolumab and ipilimumab in advanced melanoma. N Engl J Med. 2019;381:1535–46.
2. Ribas A, Wolchok JD. Cancer immunotherapy using checkpoint blockade. Science. 2018;359:1350–5.
3. Rohaan MW, Wilgenhof S, Haanen JBAG. Adoptive cellular therapies: the current landscape. Virchows Arch Int J Pathol. 2019;474:449–61.
4. Rosenberg SA, et al. Use of tumor-infiltrating lymphocytes and interleukin-2 in the immunotherapy of patients with metastatic melanoma. A preliminary report. N Engl J Med. 1988;319:1676–80.
5. Itzhaki O, et al. Establishment and large-scale expansion of minimally cultured 'young' tumor infiltrating lymphocytes for adoptive transfer therapy. J Immunother Hagerstown Md. 2011;1997(34):212–20.
6. Gattinoni L, et al. Removal of homeostatic cytokine sinks by lymphodepletion enhances the efficacy of adoptively transferred tumor-specific CD8+ T cells. J Exp Med. 2005;202:907–12.
7. Goff SL, et al. Randomized, prospective evaluation comparing intensity of lymphodepletion before adoptive transfer of tumor-infiltrating lymphocytes for patients with metastatic melanoma. J Clin Oncol Off J Am Soc Clin Oncol. 2016;34:2389–97.
8. Besser MJ, et al. Comprehensive single institute experience with melanoma TIL: long term clinical results, toxicity profile, and prognostic factors of response. Mol Carcinog. 2020;59:736–44.
9. Chandran SS, et al. Treatment of metastatic uveal melanoma with adoptive transfer of tumour-infiltrating lymphocytes: a single-centre, two-stage, single-arm, phase 2 study. Lancet Oncol. 2017;18:792–802.
10. Lee HJ, et al. Expansion of tumor-infiltrating lymphocytes and their potential for application as adoptive cell transfer therapy in human breast cancer. Oncotarget. 2017;8:113345–59.
11. Stevanović S, et al. Complete regression of metastatic cervical cancer after treatment with human papillomavirus-targeted tumor-infiltrating T cells. J Clin Oncol Off J Am Soc Clin Oncol. 2015;33:1543–50.
12. Andersen R, et al. T-cell responses in the microenvironment of primary renal cell carcinoma-implications for adoptive cell therapy. Cancer Immunol Res. 2018;6:222–35.
13. Ben-Avi R, et al. Establishment of adoptive cell therapy with tumor infiltrating lymphocytes for non-small cell lung cancer patients. Cancer Immunol Immunother CII. 2018;67:1221–30.
14. Rosenberg SA, Restifo NP. Adoptive cell transfer as personalized immunotherapy for human cancer. Science. 2015;348:62–8.
15. Chen YT, et al. Serological analysis of Melan-A(MART-1), a melanocyte-specific protein homogeneously expressed in human melanomas. Proc Natl Acad Sci U S A. 1996;93:5915–9.
16. Johnson LA, et al. Gene therapy with human and mouse T-cell receptors mediates cancer regression and targets normal tissues expressing cognate antigen. Blood. 2009;114:535–46.
17. Roeder C, et al. MAGE-A3 is a frequent tumor antigen of metastasized melanoma. Arch Dermatol Res. 2005;296:314–9.

18. Morgan RA, et al. Cancer regression and neurological toxicity following anti-MAGE-A3 TCR gene therapy. J Immunother Hagerstown Md. 2013;1997(36):133–51.
19. Draper LM, et al. Targeting of HPV-16+ epithelial cancer cells by TCR gene engineered T cells directed against E6. Clin Cancer Res Off J Am Assoc Cancer Res. 2015;21:4431–9.
20. Robbins PF, et al. Tumor regression in patients with metastatic synovial cell sarcoma and melanoma using genetically engineered lymphocytes reactive with NY-ESO-1. J Clin Oncol Off J Am Soc Clin Oncol. 2011;29:917–24.
21. Lee DW, et al. Current concepts in the diagnosis and management of cytokine release syndrome. Blood. 2014;124:188–95.
22. Grupp SA, et al. Chimeric antigen receptor-modified T cells for acute lymphoid leukemia. N Engl J Med. 2013;368:1509–18.
23. Gross G, Gorochov G, Waks T, Eshhar Z. Generation of effector T cells expressing chimeric T cell receptor with antibody type-specificity. Transplant Proc. 1989;21:127–30.
24. Brudno JN, Kochenderfer JN. Toxicities of chimeric antigen receptor T cells: recognition and management. Blood. 2016;127:3321–30.
25. Shimabukuro-Vornhagen A, et al. Cytokine release syndrome. J Immunother Cancer. 2018;6:56.
26. Neelapu SS, et al. Chimeric antigen receptor T-cell therapy - assessment and management of toxicities. Nat Rev Clin Oncol. 2018;15:47–62.
27. Kansagra AJ, et al. Clinical utilization of chimeric antigen receptor T-cells (CAR-T) in B-cell acute lymphoblastic leukemia (ALL)–an expert opinion from the European Society for Blood and Marrow Transplantation (EBMT) and the American Society for Blood and Marrow Transplantation (ASBMT). Bone Marrow Transplant. 2019;54:1868–80.
28. Gust J, et al. Glial injury in neurotoxicity after pediatric CD19-directed chimeric antigen receptor T cell therapy. Ann Neurol. 2019;86:42–54.
29. Rice J, Nagle S, Randall J, Hinson HE. Chimeric antigen receptor T cell-related neurotoxicity: mechanisms, clinical presentation, and approach to treatment. Curr Treat Options Neurol. 2019;21:40.
30. Maude SL, et al. Tisagenlecleucel in children and young adults with B-cell lymphoblastic leukemia. N Engl J Med. 2018;378:439–48.
31. Neelapu SS, et al. Axicabtagene ciloleucel CAR T-cell therapy in refractory large B-cell lymphoma. N Engl J Med. 2017;377:2531–44.

Chapter 22
Immunotherapy in Immunosuppressed Patients

H. K. Oberoi and S. Valpione

Immunotherapy Overview

Over the past two decades, several antibodies targeting immune checkpoint proteins or their ligands have demonstrated high activity across different tumour types such as melanoma [1, 2], non-small cell lung cancer [3], Merkel cell carcinoma [4], Hodgkin lymphoma [5], head and neck tumours [6], renal cancer [7], bladder cancer [8], and several tumours with microsatellite instability [9]. The first fully humanised monoclonal antibodies (mAbs) approved in clinical practice targeted the Cytotoxic T-Lymphocyte Antigen 4 (CTLA-4, ipilimumab, and tremelimumab), the programmed cell death 1 (PD-1) receptor (nivolumab and pembrolizumab) and its ligand PD-L1 (durvalumab, atezolizumab, and avelumab). These novel therapies achieved an unprecedented survival improvement in patients with advanced tumours that, until now, had a very short life expectancy.

H. K. Oberoi
Vall d'Hebron Institute of Oncology (VHIO), Vall d'Hebron University Hospital, Barcelona, Spain
e-mail: hoberoi@vhio.net

S. Valpione (✉)
Cancer Research UK Manchester Institute, The University of Manchester, Manchester, UK

The Christie NHS Foundation Trust, Manchester, UK

P. Rutkowski, M. Mandalà (eds.), *New Therapies in Advanced Cutaneous Malignancies*, https://doi.org/10.1007/978-3-030-64009-5_22

Selected Patient Populations: HIV and Immunotherapy

Epidemiology

Patients affected by Human Immunodeficiency Virus (HIV) chronic infection present a higher risk of tumour development including skin cancers [10, 11]. Currently, there are 38 million people living with HIV (PLHIV) worldwide [UNAIDS, 2020]. Antiretroviral therapy (ART) largely slowed down disease progression and terminal stage immune-failure, leading to a significant improvement of PLHIV life expectancy [12]. Thus, non-AIDS-defining malignancies (NADMs) are nowadays one of the leading causes of death of PLHIV, accounting for up to 70% of all tumours [13].

In addition to the direct carcinogenic effect coming from coinfections with oncogenic viruses such as herpesvirus 8 (HHV8), papillomavirus (HPV), Epstein–Barr virus (EBV), hepatitis B (HBV) and C viruses (HCV), PLHIV might also experience, along with a reduction of helper T cells, a chronic inflammation status that can induce immune checkpoint molecules upregulation on immune cells and a dysregulation of the anticancer immune surveillance.

Non-melanoma Skin Cancer (NMSC)

The HIV-infected population has an increased risk two- and fivefold of developing basal cell carcinoma (BCC) and squamous cell carcinoma (SCC), respectively, in regard to general population [14]. Incidence of Kaposi Sarcoma (KS) has decreased significantly with the introduction of antiretroviral therapy, but remains a common diagnosis in HIV-infected patients with a prevalence of 6% [10]. Merkel Cell Carcinoma (MCC) also presents a 2 threefold increased risk in PLHIV [15].

Melanoma

The incidence of melanoma in HIV infected patients is 2.6 times higher as compared to non-HIV patients [16], reflecting both a decreased efficiency of the host immune response in eliminating potentially malignant cells and the development of effective anti-HIV therapy which prolongs survival, arising the possibility of tumour development. In addition, melanoma shows a more aggressive phenotype and poorer survival outcomes in PLHIV, possibly as consequence of the immuno-suppressive status of these patients. Access to standard cancer treatment continues to be low for PLHIV due to concerns about the safety of cancer drugs and life expectancy in the context of HIV infection [17].

Immune Checkpoints (ICP) in HIV Infection and Skin Cancer

In cancer patients and patients with chronic viral infections, upregulation of checkpoint inhibitory molecules on immune cells leads to the inhibition of antitumour and antiviral responses and thus to a reduced tumour or virus surveillance [18, 19]. Patients with both cancer and HIV infection should, theoretically, benefit from the immunotherapy with anti-checkpoint antibodies.

The administration of mAbs targeting immune checkpoint molecules such as CTLA-4 and PD-1 significantly improves overall survival (OS) of metastatic melanoma patients and, although immune-related adverse events (irAEs) may infrequently cause substantial morbidity and even mortality, in particular with CTLA-4 blockade, many patients experience excellent quality of life while they are on therapy [1].

In vitro and in vivo data suggest a major role of immune checkpoint molecules in the pathogenesis and progression of HIV infection. PD-1/PD-L1, CTLA-4, TIM-3, LAG-3, and TIGIT are highly expressed on the lymphocytes of HIV-positive as compared to HIV-negative patients [20–23]. These immune checkpoint molecules have been involved in chronic viral persistence, usually define exhausted T cells during HIV infection and together with impaired CD8 T cell function, cause systemic immune dysfunction and dysregulation, a key mechanism in HIV-associated oncogenesis [20–23]. However, due to their immunodeficient status, HIV infected melanoma patients are generally excluded from novel clinical trials. As a consequence, scarce information is available about the efficacy and safety of these therapeutic strategies in HIV infected melanoma patients, and the potential drug interactions with ART.

Few experimental evidences have tested immune checkpoint blockade applicability in HIV infection and contrasting results are reported in the literature. Wightman et al. have shown that treatment with anti-CTLA-4 mAb in metastatic melanoma could reactivate HIV from latency [24], and multiple case reports and prospective studies have documented transient increases in HIV transcription in CD4 cells in PLHIV and HIV-associated malignancies on ART who are treated with anti-PD-(L)1 drugs, although many of these participants later experienced decreases in plasma HIV RNA.

However, the evidence towards a safe and advantageous immune checkpoint blockade in PLHIV with cancer seems to outweigh the reports against this approach. Immunotherapy appears feasible in this specific population, with no deleterious effects on HIV infection and tolerability; on the contrary, since checkpoint inhibitors can bring back antigen-specific effector functions hampered by T cell exhaustion under chronic human infections with HIV, HBV or HCV, these therapies could possibly improve antiviral responses as well.

A potential therapeutic benefit was first suggested after observing benefits of anti-PD1 administration to simian Immunodeficiency virus (SIV)-infected monkeys, an animal model that closely resembles HIV infection in humans. In SIV-infected macaques, blockade of PD-1 by an anti-PD-1 mAb increased the number of virus-specific CD4+ T cells and memory B cells as well as the levels of envelope-specific antibodies. These immunological effects are associated with the lack of side effects and a significant increase of survival [25–27]. Sabbatino et al. have reported a melanoma tumour response associated with a decreased viral replication and an increased number of CD4$^+$ T cells in a patient with both HIV infection and metastatic melanoma during treatment with ART and an anti-CTLA-4 mAb [28]. Moreover, Trautmann et al. reported that PD-1 blockade enhances the survival and proliferation of HIV-specific cytotoxic T cells, also associated with an increased cytotoxicity and production of cytokines in response to antigen challenge in vitro [29]. Moreover, in vitro PD-1 blockade plus a CD28 agonist synergistically increased HIV-specific CD4$^+$ helper T cell proliferation [22]. Also, the study of the immunophenotype of 24 cancer samples of PLHIV with non-small cell lung cancer (NSCLC) showed that, although no significant difference in PD-L1 expression within the tumours vs controls was found, there was a positive correlation between PD-L1 expression and the density of tumour-infiltrating lymphocytes (TIL) [30]. Moreover, RNA Sequencing study of tumour tissue from five PLHIV cases and three controls demonstrated an enrichment of chemotaxis (CCL18), antigen presentation (HLA-A, HLA-DRA), T cell cytotoxicity (LAMP-1), and macrophage activation (SPP1) pathways. These data suggest that cancers in PLHIV may have a more favourable the tumour microenvironment immunophenotype, and therefore should respond better to anti-PD-1/PD-L1 antibody therapy than those from non-HIV infected patients [30]. However, despite these encouraging preclinical findings, clinical evidences are still scarce.

Clinical Experience

Case reports and retrospective cohort studies from the US and European collaborative groups (Table 22.1) have described an acceptable safety profile with the use of nivolumab, pembrolizumab, and ipilimumab in PLHIV, with reported tumour responses in Hodgkin lymphoma, melanoma, and lung cancer. A systematic review of immune checkpoint inhibitors (ICPI) in PLHIV noted overall response and toxicity that were similar to the general population. In the subset of patients in whom viral load was measured, HIV remained suppressed in almost all patients, thus excluding a detrimental reactivation of viral replication. The response of PLHIV treated with ICPI is very heterogeneous, and not necessarily linked to the antitumour activity. Notably, ICPI use in KS was associated with an overall response rate of 63%.

Table 22.1 Clinical reports of PLHIV with skin cancer treated with checkpoint inhibitors

Clinical cases + series	Disease type	Treatment	BOR
Heppt et al.	9 MM + 1 MCC	Nivolumab (3), Pembrolizumab (3), Ipilimumab (3), Ipilimumab-Nivolumab (1)	2 CR, 1 PR, 6 PD, 1 NR
Linge et al.	1 MCC	Sequential Pembrolizumab and Avelumab	CR
Davar et al.	2 MM	Pembrolizumab	1 PR, 1 PD
Spano et al.	1 MM	Nivolumab	PR
Tio et al.	9 MM	Pembrolizumab (4), Sequential Pembrolizumab—Ipilimumab (2), Ipilumumab-Nivolumab (2), Sequential Ipilimumab-Nivolumab (1)	1 CR, 2 PR, 3 SD, 3 PD
Galanine et al.	8 KS	Nivolumab	1 CR, 2 PR, 3 SD
Park et al.	2 MM + 1 cSCC	NR	NR
Al Homsi et al.	MCC	Avelumab	PR
Burke et al.	MM	Ipilimumab	CR
Ruzewick et al.	MM	Ipilimumab	PR
Tomsitz et al.	MM	Sequential Ipilimumab—Nivolumab	PD
Scully et al.	cSCC	Pembrolizumab	NR
	$N = 31$ (exc. KS)		ORR (12/26) = 46%

MM metastatic melanoma, *KS* Kaposi sarcoma, *cSCC* cutaneous squamous cell carcinoma, *MCC* Merkel cell carcinoma, *CR* complete response, *PR* partial response, *SD* stable disease, *BOR* best overall response, *ORR* overall response rate, *NR* not reported

Ongoing Trials

Supported by this retrospective evidence, the first clinical trials of anticancer immunotherapy in PLHIV have been designed. The earliest prospective study of durvalumab in ART-treated PLHIV with solid tumours (DURVAST trial) showed ~50% (9/16 patients) disease control rate, with stability of $CD4^+$ and $CD8^+$ T cell counts and plasma HIV-1 viremia during the study [31]. Other clinical trials addressing the unmet need of immunotherapy in PLHIV with cancer are ongoing: a phase II trial of second-line pembrolizumab for NSCLC in PLHIV (NCT03304093) was started in November 2017 by the Intergroupe Francophone de Cancerologie Thoracique (IFCT-CHIVA2), other two prospective studies are testing the tolerability and activity of nivolumab plus ipilimumab (NCT02408861) and pembrolizumab (NCT02595866) in HIV-infected patients with solid tumours, and a phase IV trial studying the combination of ipilimumab and nivolumab in NSCLC includes a cohort of HIV-infected patients (CheckMate 817, NCT02869789).

Checkpoint inhibition with new experimental drugs also seems promising, since in vitro TIM-3 signalling pathway blockade enhances the cytotoxicity of HIV-specific CD8[+] T cells and ameliorates the effect if HIV on CD4[+] T cells [32]. Furthermore, the ex vivo blockade of LAG-3 significantly augments both cytotoxic and helper HIV-specific T cell responses [33]. Lastly, in vivo dual PD-L1 and TIGIT blockade restores HIV-specific CD8[+] T cell responses [34].

Selected Patient Populations: Solid Organ Transplant and Immunotherapy

Epidemiology

There are 100,000 solid organ transplants (SOT) performed worldwide each year [35]. Increasing post-transplantation survival in SOT recipients (SOTR), accompanied by higher doses and longer duration of immunosuppression, often with multidrug regimens, have been linked to an increased risk and incidence of cancers, in particular skin malignancies [36]. As consequence, cancer has been reported as the second leading cause of death in these patients [37], presumably because of the chronic immunosuppressive therapy is necessary to maintain allograft tolerance as well as less aggressive cancer treatments imposed by comorbidities [38].

Different types of organ transplants are also associated with higher risk of cancer, in particular skin cancer, with heart transplants carrying the highest risk, followed by lung, kidney, and liver transplants [36]. These disparities are currently explained by the different levels of immunosuppression required according to organ transplants.

Skin cancer diagnosis is typically 3–8 years after transplantation, with more than 90% of tumours being BCC or SCC. SCC, the most common type of skin cancer in SOTRs, has a 65–250 fold increased incidence over the general population, whereas BCC, the second most common type, has an incidence 10 times higher and many SOTRs are diagnosed with multiple tumours, which also tend to be more aggressive [36, 39]. Melanoma has a 2–5 fold increased incidence in SOTRs, higher in African Americans (17-fold) [40]. Risk factors for melanoma include less than 18 years at the time of transplant and a pre-transplant history of melanoma, in addition to the common risk factors for melanoma such as age more than 50-years, white race, family history of melanoma, high levels of UV exposure, and high numbers of nevi [39, 41]. Melanoma in the transplant population has been shown to be more aggressive and, when matched for Breslow thickness and Clark level, has been associated with worse outcomes [36]. Among other rare skin cancers subtypes, MCC has a 5–50 times higher incidence [36] whereas the risk of KS is associate with an 80 to 500 fold increase [39]. Similarly to HPHIV, SOTS immunosuppressed patients were excluded from the pivotal immunotherapy studies.

Role of Immune Checkpoints in SOTRs

The PD-1/PD-L1 axis plays an important role in organ transplant tolerance. PD-1 upregulation and associated T cell exhaustion phenotypes in multiple animal models indicate that an intact PD-1/PD-L1 axis is required for transplant tolerance [42]. Anti-PD-1 treatment not only directly interferes with the tolerogenic PD-1/PD-L1 pathways, but has also been described to impair the forkhead box P3 (FoxP3) regulatory T cell-mediated graft tolerance in the tubular cells of the kidney [43]. These preclinical evidences make use of PD-1/PD-L1 blockade particularly controversial in SOTSs due to the risk of graft rejection, which has been documented. Graft rejection has also been reported with older immunostimulatory therapies, such as interferon; however, mouse models show that immunecheckpoint blockade of CTLA-4 can be associated with graft survival if administered once transplant tolerance has been established [44, 45].

Clinical Evidence for Immune Checkpoints in SOTRs

Due to the immunosuppressant anti-rejection therapies that could impair responses to checkpoint inhibitors and the risk of transplant rejection, SOTR patients were excluded from immunotherapy clinical trials. Moreover, there are only few reports regarding the safety and activity/efficacy of modern immunotherapies in this population. As consequence, given the lack of data on the use of immune checkpoint inhibitors in SOTRs, clinical guidance is an unmet need. Moreover, as seen above, cancer has been reported as the second leading cause of death in these patients, making the therapeutic decisions for oncologists not infrequent, and particularly difficult.

The largest retrospective study, published by Abdel-Wahab et al. [46] analyzed patients treated at MD Anderson plus a systematic review and included 39 patients with a history of SOTR treated with checkpoint inhibitors. Of these, 24 patients had advanced melanoma and 6 cSCC. Overall, allograft rejection rate was 41%, after a median time of 21 days, and 81% of the rejections lead to graft loss. The most frequent transplant was renal (48%), followed by hepatic (36%) and cardiac transplants (21%). Patients receiving single-agent calcineurin inhibitors seemed to have the lower rejection rate against those with single-agent prednisone (78% compared with 11%), with no differences in survival. Immuno-related toxicity was observed in 21% of patients and did not correlate with tolerance loss (none experienced allograft rejection and all improved with corticosteroids). Eighteen patients (46%) died, mainly because of allograft rejection or rejection complications. No difference in the frequency of allograft rejection between anti-PD-1 and anti-CTLA-4 was observed. Median overall survival in patients who had allograft rejection was 5 months vs. 12 months in patients who did not ($p = 0.03$). Of the 22 melanoma cases reported in the study, eight (36%) showed tumour responses: seven had complete or partial response and one had stable disease. Responses were more frequent in patients without allograft rejection (6/14, 43%) than among patients with allograft rejection (2/8, 25%). Median overall survival in the 22 melanoma patients was 10.4 months (95% CI 2.6–18 months). All five patients with cSCC achieved complete or partial tumour response.

Other previous case reports included 13 kidney, 14 liver, and 2 heart transplant recipients receiving anti-PD-1/CTLA-4-based immunotherapy. Together with the MD Anderson series, the data suggest a rejection rate of 50% in kidney transplant and 36% in liver transplant. Another series of 6 patients with kidney transplant treated with ipilimumab showed 1/6 allograft rejection, with survival ranging 3–26 months [47].

Overall, the available data suggest that the use of checkpoint inhibitors in prior SOTRs may lead to relatively rapid allograft rejection, often be accompanied by high mortality rates. The rate of rejection may be higher with PD-1/L1 blockade because allo-immunity largely relies on an alloantigen-mediated response that resembles the mechanism of tumour immune rejection with acute T lymphocyte infiltration and positive expression of PD-1 and PD-L1 proteins in transplantation biopsies [46]. Renal transplant patients may be better candidates for these medications given the possibility of returning to dialysis if rejection does occur, although rejection rates in kidney transplants can reach as high as 50% of cases.

Although there is evidence suggesting that CTLA-4-based immunotherapy is associated with a lower risk of rejection and therefore perhaps could be considered in the first instance, the activity of CTLA-4 immunotherapy is low.

Considering the available evidence, immunotherapy with checkpoint inhibitors should be reserved to patients with no other therapeutic options due to the high risk of allograft rejection, patient counselling must be performed stressing the high risks and within multidisciplinary teams prepared to manage transplant rejections. Prospective studies are needed to establish the best treatment regimen for transplant patients with advanced cancers to optimize the antitumour response and minimize the risk of allograft loss.

Selected Patient Populations: Cirrhosis and Immunotherapy

Epidemiology

Liver cirrhosis (LC), the end stage of chronic liver disease, affects 0.1% of the European population and this condition negatively affects life expectancy. LC is a limiting factor for anticancer therapy of liver and non-hepatic malignancies: it may limit surgical and interventional approaches to cancer treatment, influence pharmacokinetics of anticancer drugs, increase side effects of chemotherapy, render patients susceptible for hepatotoxicity, and ultimately result in high risk scores for morbidity and mortality.

Role of Immune Checkpoints in LC

In LC, the chronic active immune-mediated inflammatory processes cause structural and immune-microenvironment alterations that compromise reticuloendothelial function and lead to impaired immune surveillance [48]. Hepatocellular carcinoma (HCC), the most common primary liver cancer, can develop at any stage of LC and can be a result of the carcinogenic effect of chronic tissue damage and inflammation or of the direct tumorigenic effect of hepatitis viruses that sustain the liver disease. Approximately 25% of HCC have high inflammatory scores, with abundant or moderate tumour infiltrating lymphocytes (TILs) [49]. This cellular infiltrate is often dysfunctional, with a higher proportion of CD4$^+$ helper/Tregs to cytotoxic T cells and is accompanied by an immunosuppressive immune environment rich in transforming growth factor (TGF-β), interleukin-10 (IL-10), myeloid-derived suppressor cells (MDSCs) as well as Tregs and expression of lymphocyte inhibitory ligands that enable escape of tumour cells from immune surveillance [50, 51]. In non-hepatic cancer, preclinical and retrospective data have shown an increased risk for liver metastases with underlying LC.

For the reasons seen above, in HCC, unlike in most other solid malignancies, the prognosis is also determined by the degree of LC and its complications including portal hypertension, ascites, and life-threatening bleeding events from gastro-oesophageal varices. Thus, patients with compensated LC might clinically benefit from anticancer treatment, and systemic therapies might be preferable to surgical interventions in selected cases due to the high risks of complications. However, since clinical studies usually exclude patients with underlying liver cirrhosis, only little is known about anticancer treatment in patients with non-hepatic cancer and concomitant LC.

Clinical Evidence for Immune Checkpoints in LC

Most data available in this cancer patient population were derived from trials with small patient numbers and the study design was mostly retrospective and prospective evidence from dedicated clinical trials with checkpoint inhibitors is scarce. Nivolumab (anti-PD1) has recently been approved as a second-line therapy for HCC, supported by the results of the phase I/II CheckMate 040 trial [52]. An acceptable safety profile and responses to treatment up to 20% were observed in non-infected and infected patients with hepatitis B and C viruses. Preliminary results of the phase III CheckMate 459 trial that compared sorafenib and nivolumab failed to demonstrate overall survival improvement in the whole population, although further subgroup analyses are yet to be presented. In these trials, patients with Child Pugh class A to B7 were included, and as for the CheckMate 040 trial, no specific safety concerns were reported.

Additionally, a large number of phase I/II clinical trials, which include compensated cirrhosis patients, are currently ongoing in advanced HCC testing other ICPI as well as oncolytic viruses, vaccines, and adoptive cell therapy, but results are not available as yet.

Overall, the recommendations available indicate that patients with compensated LC, whose prognosis is mostly determined by the cancer, should be considered for antitumour treatment. On the contrary, the management of patients with decompensated liver function should instead focus on LC and its complications since life expectancy is mainly influenced by the liver disease and antitumour treatment itself can accelerate liver failure.

References

1. Postow MA, Chesney J, Pavlick AC, et al. Nivolumab and Ipilimumab versus Ipilimumab in untreated melanoma. N Engl J Med. 2015;372:2006–17.
2. Robert C, Schachter J, Long GV, et al. Pembrolizumab versus Ipilimumab in advanced melanoma. N Engl J Med. 2015;372:2521–32.
3. Reck M, Rodríguez-Abreu D, Robinson AG, et al. Pembrolizumab versus chemotherapy for PD-L1–positive non–small-cell lung cancer. N Engl J Med. 2016;375:1823–33.
4. Nghiem PT, Bhatia S, Lipson EJ, et al. PD-1 blockade with pembrolizumab in advanced merkel-cell carcinoma. N Engl J Med. 2016;374:2542–52.
5. Killock D. Haematological cancer: anti-PD-1 therapy with nivolumab after allo-HSCT for Hodgkin lymphoma. Nat Rev Clin Oncol. 2017;14:261.
6. Burtness B, Harrington KJ, Greil R, et al. Pembrolizumab alone or with chemotherapy versus cetuximab with chemotherapy for recurrent or metastatic squamous cell carcinoma of the head and neck (KEYNOTE-048): a randomised, open-label, phase 3 study. Lancet. 2019;394:1915–28.
7. Motzer RJ, Tannir NM, McDermott DF, et al. Nivolumab plus Ipilimumab versus sunitinib in advanced renal-cell carcinoma. N Engl J Med. 2018;378:1277–90.
8. Bellmunt J, De Wit R, Vaughn DJ, et al. Pembrolizumab as second-line therapy for advanced urothelial carcinoma. N Engl J Med. 2017;376:1015–26.
9. Dudley JC, Lin M-T, Le DT, Eshleman JR. Microsatellite Instability as a biomarker for PD-1 blockade. Clin Cancer Res. 2016;22:813 LP–820.
10. Yarchoan R, Uldrick TS. HIV-associated cancers and related diseases. N Engl J Med. 2018;378:1029–41.
11. Asgari MM, Ray GT, Quesenberry CP, Katz KA, Silverberg MJ. Association of multiple primary skin cancers with human immunodeficiency virus infection, CD4 count, and viral load. JAMA Dermatol. 2017;153:892–6.
12. Trickey A, May MT, Vehreschild J-J, et al. Survival of HIV-positive patients starting antiretroviral therapy between 1996 and 2013: a collaborative analysis of cohort studies. Lancet HIV. 2017;4:e349–56.
13. Bonnet F, Burty C, Lewden C, et al. Changes in cancer mortality among HIV-infected patients: the mortalité 2005 survey. Clin Infect Dis. 2009;48:633–9.

14. Silverberg MJ, Leyden W, Warton EM, Quesenberry CP Jr, Engels EA, Asgari MM. HIV infection status, immunodeficiency, and the incidence of non-melanoma skin cancer. J Natl Cancer Inst. 2013;105:350–60.
15. Lanoy E, Costagliola D, Engels EA. Skin cancers associated with HIV infection and solid-organ transplantation among elderly adults. Int J Cancer. 2010;126:1724–31.
16. Patel P, Hanson DL, Sullivan PS, Novak RM, Moorman AC, Tong TC, Holmberg SD, Brooks JT. Incidence of types of cancer among HIV-infected persons compared with the general population in the United States, 1992–2003. Ann Intern Med. 2008;148:728–36.
17. Suneja G, Lin CC, Simard EP, Han X, Engels EA, Jemal A. Disparities in cancer treatment among patients infected with the human immunodeficiency virus. Cancer. 2016;122:2399–407.
18. Moskophidis D, Lechner F, Pircher H, Zinkernagel RM. Virus persistence in acutely infected immunocompetent mice by exhaustion of antiviral cytotoxic effector T cells. Nature. 1993;362:758–61.
19. Barber DL, Wherry EJ, Masopust D, Zhu B, Allison JP, Sharpe AH, Freeman GJ, Ahmed R. Restoring function in exhausted CD8 T cells during chronic viral infection. Nature. 2006;439:682–7.
20. Blackburn SD, Shin H, Haining WN, Zou T, Workman CJ, Polley A, Betts MR, Freeman GJ, Vignali DAA, Wherry EJ. Coregulation of CD8+ T cell exhaustion by multiple inhibitory receptors during chronic viral infection. Nat Immunol. 2009;10:29–37.
21. Kaufmann DE, Walker BD. PD-1 and CTLA-4 inhibitory cosignaling pathways in HIV infection and the potential for therapeutic intervention. J Immunol. 2009;182:5891 LP–5897.
22. Kassu A, Marcus RA, D'Souza MB, Kelly-McKnight EA, Golden-Mason L, Akkina R, Fontenot AP, Wilson CC, Palmer BE. Regulation of virus-specific CD4+ T cell function by multiple costimulatory receptors during chronic HIV infection. J Immunol. 2010;185:3007–18.
23. Fromentin R, Bakeman W, Lawani MB, et al. CD4+ T cells expressing PD-1, TIGIT and LAG-3 contribute to HIV persistence during ART. PLoS Pathog. 2016;12:e1005761.
24. Wightman F, Solomon A, Kumar SS, Urriola N, Gallagher K, Hiener B, Palmer S, Mcneil C, Garsia R, Lewin SR. Effect of ipilimumab on the HIV reservoir in an HIV-infected individual with metastatic melanoma. AIDS. 2015;29.
25. Hryniewicz A, Boasso A, Edghill-Smith Y, et al. CTLA-4 blockade decreases TGF-β, IDO, and viral RNA expression in tissues of SIVmac251-infected macaques. Blood. 2006;108:3834–42.
26. Linge A, Rauschenberg R, Blum S, Spornraft-Ragaller P, Meier F, Troost EGC. Successful immunotherapy and irradiation in a HIV-positive patient with metastatic Merkel cell carcinoma. Clin Transl Radiat Oncol. 2019;15:42–5.
27. Cecchinato V, Tryniszewska E, Ma ZM, et al. Immune activation driven by CTLA-4 blockade augments viral replication at mucosal sites in simian immunodeficiency virus infection. J Immunol. 2008;180:5439–47.
28. Marra A, Scognamiglio G, Peluso I, Botti G, Fusciello C, Filippelli A, Ascierto PA, Pepe S, Sabbatino F. Immune checkpoint inhibitors in melanoma and HIV infection. Open AIDS J. 2017;11:91–100.
29. Trautmann L, Janbazian L, Chomont N, et al. Upregulation of PD-1 expression on HIV-specific CD8+ T cells leads to reversible immune dysfunction. Nat Med. 2006;12:1198–202.
30. Pinato DJ, Kythreotou A, Mauri FA, et al. Functional immune characterization of HIV-associated non-small-cell lung cancer. Ann Oncol Off J Eur Soc Med Oncol. 2018;29:1486–8.
31. Gonzalez-Cao M, Morán T, Dalmau J, et al. Assessment of the feasibility and safety of durvalumab for treatment of solid tumors in patients with HIV-1 infection: the phase 2 DURVAST study. JAMA Oncol. 2020;6(7):1063–7.
32. Sakhdari A, Mujib S, Vali B, et al. Tim-3 negatively regulates cytotoxicity in exhausted CD8+ T cells in HIV infection. PLoS One. 2012;7:e40146.
33. Tian X, Zhang A, Qiu C, et al. The upregulation of LAG-3 on T cells defines a subpopulation with functional exhaustion and correlates with disease progression in HIV-infected subjects. J Immunol. 2015;194:3873–82.

34. Chew GM, Fujita T, Webb GM, et al. TIGIT marks exhausted T cells, correlates with disease progression, and serves as a target for immune restoration in HIV and SIV infection. PLoS Pathog. 2016;12:e1005349.
35. Matesanz R, Mahillo B, Alvarez M, Carmona M. Global observatory and database on donation and transplantation: world overview on transplantation activities. Transplant Proc. 2009;41:2297–301.
36. Howard MD, Su JC, Chong AH. Skin cancer following solid organ transplantation: a review of risk factors and models of care. Am J Clin Dermatol. 2018;19:585–97.
37. Acuna SA, Fernandes KA, Daly C, Hicks LK, Sutradhar R, Kim SJ, Baxter NN. Cancer mortality among recipients of solid-organ transplantation in Ontario, Canada. JAMA Oncol. 2016;2:463–9.
38. Ajithkumar TV, Parkinson CA, Butler A, Hatcher HM. Management of solid tumours in organ-transplant recipients. Lancet Oncol. 2007;8:921–32.
39. Euvrard S, Kanitakis J, Claudy A. Skin cancers after organ transplantation. N Engl J Med. 2003;348:1681–91.
40. Fattouh K, Ducroux E, Decullier E, Kanitakis J, Morelon E, Boissonnat P, Sebbag L, Jullien D, Euvrard S. Increasing incidence of melanoma after solid organ transplantation: a retrospective epidemiological study. Transpl Int. 2017;30:1172–80.
41. Robbins HA, Clarke CA, Arron ST, et al. Melanoma risk and survival among organ transplant recipients. J Invest Dermatol. 2015;135:2657–65.
42. Wang L, Han R, Hancock WW. Programmed cell death 1 (PD-1) and its ligand PD-L1 are required for allograft tolerance. Eur J Immunol. 2007;37:2983–90.
43. Riella LV, Paterson AM, Sharpe AH, Chandraker A. Role of the PD-1 pathway in the immune response. Am J Transplant. 2012;12:2575–87.
44. Cecchini M, Sznol M, Seropian S. Immune therapy of metastatic melanoma developing after allogeneic bone marrow transplant. J Immunother Cancer. 2015;3:10.
45. Greenberg JN, Zwald FO. Management of skin cancer in solid-organ transplant recipients: a multidisciplinary approach. Dermatol Clin. 2011;29:231–41.
46. Abdel-Wahab N, Safa H, Abudayyeh A, et al. Checkpoint inhibitor therapy for cancer in solid organ transplantation recipients: an institutional experience and a systematic review of the literature. J Immunother Cancer. 2019;7:106.
47. Zehou O, Leibler C, Arnault J-P, Sayegh J, Montaudié H, Rémy P, Glotz D, Cordonnier C, Martin L, Lebbé C. Ipilimumab for the treatment of advanced melanoma in six kidney transplant patients. Am J Transplant. 2018;18:3065–71.
48. Jenne CN, Kubes P. Immune surveillance by the liver. Nat Immunol. 2013;14:996–1006.
49. Sia D, Jiao Y, Martinez-Quetglas I, et al. Identification of an immune-specific class of hepatocellular carcinoma, based on molecular features. Gastroenterology. 2017;153:812–26.
50. Hoechst B, Ormandy LA, Ballmaier M, Lehner F, Krüger C, Manns MP, Greten TF, Korangy F. A new population of myeloid-derived suppressor cells in hepatocellular carcinoma patients induces CD4$^+$CD25$^+$Foxp3$^+$ T cells. Gastroenterology. 2008;135:234–43.
51. Makarova-Rusher OV, Medina-Echeverz J, Duffy AG, Greten TF. The yin and yang of evasion and immune activation in HCC. J Hepatol. 2015;62:1420–9.
52. El-Khoueiry AB, Sangro B, Yau T, et al. Nivolumab in patients with advanced hepatocellular carcinoma (CheckMate 040): an open-label, non-comparative, phase 1/2 dose escalation and expansion trial. Lancet. 2017;389:2492–502.

Chapter 23
New Therapies in Advanced Cutaneous Malignancies: Conclusions

Piotr Rutkowski and Mario Mandalà

Skin cancers, mostly basal cell carcinoma (BCC) and squamous cell carcinoma (SCC), are responsible for about 98% of all skin cancers, and they are the most common malignancies in the Caucasian population. Skin carcinomas, also defined as non-melanoma skin cancers (NMSC), are responsible for about 1/3 of all new cancer cases diagnosed in humans. On the other hand, melanoma accounts for a small percentage of all skin malignancies, but it is responsible for the majority of deaths due to cutaneous cancers. Although majority of patients with skin cancer are diagnosed in early-stage disease and cured surgically, still there is a worldwide significant number of patients at stage III–IV disease, where other treatment modalities may be necessary. Recent developments and approvals of targeted agents and immunotherapy significantly changed the landscape of cutaneous malignancies therapy in the metastatic setting and they have lately translated into progress in adjuvant treatment in high-risk locoregional disease.

In this comprehensive book, we have focused on new therapies in advanced cutaneous malignancies and we provide the practicing oncologist a wide overview on state-of-the-art contemporary systemic therapy of melanoma, SCC, BCC, and Merkel cell carcinoma relevant in everyday practice. Furthermore, we present molecular and immunological landscape of these malignancies navigating twenty-first-century treatment with the help of worldwide renowned experts.

P. Rutkowski (✉)
Department of Soft Tissue/Bone Sarcoma and Melanoma, Maria Sklodowska-Curie National Research Institute of Oncology, Warsaw, Poland
e-mail: piotr.rutkowski@pib-nio.pl

M. Mandalà
University of Perugia, Unit of Medical Oncology, Ospedale Santa Maria Misericordia, Perugia, Italy
e-mail: mario.mandala@unipg.it

P. Rutkowski, M. Mandalà (eds.), *New Therapies in Advanced Cutaneous Malignancies*, https://doi.org/10.1007/978-3-030-64009-5_23

The survival of advanced, unresectable metastatic melanoma and skin carcinomas has been greatly improved within the last few years. This unprecedented development is mainly related to the introduction of two different therapeutic strategies: nonspecific immunotherapy with use of monoclonal antibodies anti-CTLA4 or anti-PD1 (immune checkpoint inhibitors) in melanoma, SCC, and Merkel cell carcinoma and targeted therapy with hedgehog inhibitors and serine-threonine kinase inhibitors (BRAF and MEK) in BCC and melanoma, respectively [1–7]. Targeted therapy and immunotherapy have different benefits and weaknesses with more rapid and larger response rates but shorter durability with targeted agents, and slightly lower and later responses but more durable control of disease with immunotherapy. In Table 23.1, we summarized the comparison of targeted and immunotherapy in melanoma. In Table 23.2, we have listed all new systemic therapies available in advanced cutaneous malignancies.

The constitutive hyperactivation of the RAS/RAF/MEK/ERK pathway (termed also as the Mitogen-Activated Protein Kinase—MAPK pathway) has been identified in the majority of sporadic melanomas as the critical player in the regulation of cell proliferation, invasion, and survival. Current standard treatment of *BRAF*-mutated melanomas with a combination of BRAF and MEK inhibitors (dabrafenib and trametinib, vemurafenib and cobimetinib, or encorafenib and binimetinib) led to impressive prolongation of median overall survival exceeding 2 years. The summary of outcomes of pivotal randomized studies with BRAF+MEK inhibitors is presented in Table 23.3 [8–18].

Table 23.1 Comparison of targeted therapy and checkpoint immunotherapies in melanoma

Feature	Targeted therapy	Immunotherapy (anti-PD-1 +/- anti-CTLA-4)
Schedule	Administered continuously every day orally	Administered IV every 2–6 weeks
Safety (AEs)	Acute Grade 3/4 AEs in 35–65% of patients Dose reductions required in approximately 25% of patients and discontinuation in about 10% No long-term toxicities	Grade 3/4 AEs in 8–20% of patients, drug discontinuation due to AEs in 2–10% on anti-PD-1 monotherapy Grade 3/4 AEs in >50% of patients and drug discontinuation >35% due to AEs on anti-CTLA-4 and anti-PD-1 combination
Objective response rate (ORR)	ORR 64–70% of patients	ORR: 30–40% on anti-PD-1; ORR: 57–62% on combination anti-PD-1/anti-CTLA-4 (38–52% on *BRAF+*)
Overall survival (OS)	Median OS: 25–34 months and 2-year OS rate: 52%; 3-year OS: 44%, 5-year OS: 34%, disease progression usually occurs after stopping treatment	Median OS 17–31 months; 2-year OS rate 55–60%; 3-year OS 45%, 5-year OS 43–44% for treatment-naive patients with anti-PD-1 monotherapy; 5-year OS rate for anti-PD-1/anti-CTLA-4—52% Responses are durable; responses are maintained even after stopping treatment

AE adverse events, *IV* intravenous, *ORR* objective response rate, *OS* overall survival, *Anti-PD-1* anti-programmed death-1, *Anti-CTLA-4* anti-cytotoxic T lymphocyte antigen-4

Table 23.2 New systemic therapies available in advanced cutaneous malignancies

Diagnosis	Molecular target	Therapy
Melanoma	*BRAFV600* mutation	BRAF + MEK inhibitors (vemurafenib + cobimetinib, dabrafenib + trametinib[a], encorafenib + binimetinib)
	PD-1/PD-L1/ anti-CTLA-4 Oncolytic viruses	Nivolumab[a/b], pembrolizumab[a], atezolizumab[c], ipilimumab T-VEC
	KIT	Different tyrosine kinase inhibitors (imatinib, nilotinib[d])
BCC	Hedgehog	Vismodegib, sonidegib
Dermatofibrosarcoma protuberans	PDGFR-β	Imatinib
Merkel cell carcinoma	PD-1/PD-L1	Avelumab, pembrolizumab, nivolumab[d]
SCC	PD-1	Cemiplimab, pembrolizumab

[a]Registered also for adjuvant therapy
[b]Nivolumab is also approved in combination with ipilimumab for unresectable/metastatic melanoma
[c]Atezolizumab approved in the United States in combination with vemurafenib and cobimetinib for *BRAF V600* mutated advanced melanoma
[d]Not formally approved

The current results of anti-PD-1 therapy with pembrolizumab or nivolumab monotherapy indicate median overall survival of approximately 2 years, but a combination of anti-PD-1 and anti-CTLA-4 (nivolumab with ipilimumab) was shown to be superior in terms of progression-free and overall survival (OS) with recent data confirming for the first time in metastatic melanoma median OS more than 5 years. Due to sustained activity of these drugs even after stopping therapy, they are often considered as the first-line therapy of choice independently of *BRAF* mutation status. The outcomes of phase III trials with anti-PD-1 +/− anti-CTLA-4 immune checkpoint inhibitors are summarized in Table 23.4 [19–29]. The current efforts are underway to determine how best to integrate combination immunotherapy with other treatment modalities as well as to establish the correct choice of sequence of therapy in *BRAF*-mutated cases. The first such trial was reported with positive results on combination of atezolizumab (Tecentriq) plus cobimetinib (Cotellic) and vemurafenib (Zelboraf) for the treatment of patients with *BRAF V600* mutation-positive advanced melanoma leading to approval of this combination by the FDA in July 2020. The approval was based on results from the multicenter, double-blind, placebo-controlled, randomized, phase 3 IMspire150 study evaluating patients with previously untreated *BRAF V600* mutation-positive metastatic or unresectable locally advanced melanoma [30]. The study compared the efficacy and safety of atezolizumab plus cobimetinib and vemurafenib to the combination of placebo plus cobimetinib and vemurafenib. The primary end point of the study was investigator-assessed progression-free survival (PFS). Overall, the addition of atezolizumab to

Table 23.3 Advanced BRAFV600 mutated melanoma. The summary of results of phase III trials with BRAF + MEK inhibitors

Authors	Long 2015 [8] Flaherty 2016 [9] Robert 2019 [10, 11]		Robert 2014 [12] Robert 2015 [13] Robert 2019 [11]		Larkin2014/2015[14, 15] Atkinson 2015 [16]		Dummer 2018 [17], Ascierto 2020 [18]	
Drug(s)	Dabrafenib	Dabrafenib + Trametinib	Vemurafenib	Dabrafenib + Trametinib	Vemurafenib	Vemurafenib + cobimetinib	Vemurafenib	Encorafenib + Binimetinib
ORR	53%	69%	51%	64%	50%	70%	66	63%
Median PFS (months)	8.8	11	7.3	12.6	7.2	12.3	7.3	14.9
Median OS (months)	18.7	25.1	18.0	25.6	17	23	16.9	33.6
2-year OS rate	42.1%	51.4%	37.8%	54.2%	38.0%	48.3%	43.2%	57.6%
5-year OS rate	NR	34% (pooled from COMBI-V and COMBI-D trials)	NR	34% (pooled from COMBI-V and COMBI-D trials)	26%	31%	NR	NR

NR not reported

Table 23.4 Selected clinical trials investigating immunotherapy in advanced melanoma

	Pembrolizumab 10 mg/kg q2w	Pembrolizumab 10 mg/kg q3w	Nivolumab in BRAF-wt melanomas	Ipilimumab + Nivolumab
Study	KEYNOTE-006	KEYNOTE- 006	Checkmate 066	Checkmate 067
Authors	Robert 2015 [19] Schachter 2016, 2017 [20, 21] Robert 2019 [22] Long 2020 [23]	Robert 2015 [19] Schachter 2016,2017 [20, 21] Robert 2019 [22] Long 2020 [23]	Robert 2015 [24] Ascierto 2019 [25]	Larkin 2015 [26] Wolchok 2016 [27] Wolchok 2017 [28] Larkin 2019 [29]
N (% 1st line)	279 (65.6%)	277 (66.8%)	210 (100%)	314 (100%)
BRAF-mutated	35.1%	35.0%	0%	32.%
ORR	33.7%	32.9%	40%	57.6%
Median PFS	5.6 months	4.1 months	5.4 months	11.5 months
1-year OS rate	74.1%	68.4%	72.9%	NR
2-year OS rate	55%	55%	57.7%	NR
3-year OS rate	51%		51%	58%
5-year OS rate	43% (first line)		NR	52%

NR not reported

cobimetinib and vemurafenib led to a longer PFS, compared to placebo plus cobimetinib and vemurafenib (median PFS, 15.1 months vs. 10.6 months, respectively; HR, 0.78; 95% CI, 0.63–0.97; $P = 0.025$).

The results of next such trial on combination of spartalizumab (anti-PD-1 drug) with dabrafenib and trametinib in *BRAF*-mutated melanoma patients did not confirmed benefit from adding immunotherapy to targeted therapy in triplet combination and therefore studies on combination of less toxic immunotherapies (e.g., anti-PD-1 + T-VEC or anti-PD-1 and LAG3 inhibitors) are eagerly awaited.

BRAF+MEK inhibitors induce a prompt response and tumor control in the majority of patients with *BRAF-V600* mutated advanced melanomas. However, the response duration is usually limited due to activation of mechanisms of resistance. Due to these features, this therapy should be considered as a treatment of choice in patients with symptomatic disease and/or high tumor burden [31, 32]. There are no final data concerning the optimal sequence of immunotherapy and molecularly targeted therapy in patients with melanomas with *BRAF-V600* mutated melanoma, as well as the choice of adjuvant systemic therapy in *BRAF-V600* mutated high-risk melanomas. However, the activity of BRAF inhibitor is maintained after immunotherapy and immunotherapy may also show activity (anti-PD-L1 +/−anti-CTLA-4) after progression to BRAF inhibitors. In rare cases of patients with melanomas harboring *KIT* gene mutations, the activity of KIT kinase inhibitors has been observed [33].

To summarize, cutaneous malignancies as related to potent UV carcinogenic factor, present the highest tumor mutation burden (TMB) values among all human cancers, what makes them all ideal targeted for further development in immunotherapy [34] and combined therapy.

In the end, we would like to express my sincerest gratitude to all of those at Springer who have guided us, especially Mr. Prakash Jagannathan as a Project Coordinator for this challenging book.

References

1. Michielin O, Akkooi AV, Ascierto PA, et al. Cutaneous melanoma: ESMO Clinical Practice Guidelines for diagnosis, treatment and follow-up. Ann Oncol. 2019;30(12):1884–901. https://doi.org/10.1093/annonc/mdz4.
2. NCCN Guidelines. Cutaneous melanoma version 1.2020.
3. Rutkowski P, Wysocki PJ, Nasierowska-Guttmejer A, et al. Cutaneous melanomas. Oncol Clin Pract. 2020;16:163–82. https://doi.org/10.5603/OCP.2020.0021.
4. Rutkowski P, Owczarek W, Nejc D, et al. Skin carcinomas. Oncol Clin Pract. 2020;16:143–62. https://doi.org/10.5603/OCP.2020.0018.
5. NCCN Guidelines. Basal Cell Skin Cancer version 1.2020.
6. NCCN Guidelines. Squamous Cell Skin Cancer version 2.2020.
7. NCCN Guidelines. Merkel Cell Carcinoma version 1.2020.
8. Long GV, Stroyakovskiy D, Gogas H, et al. Dabrafenib and trametinib versus dabrafenib and placebo for Val600 BRAF-mutant melanoma: a multicentre, double-blind, phase 3 randomised controlled trial. Lancet. 2015;386:444–51.
9. Flaherty K, Davies MA, Grob JJ, et al. Genomic analysis and 3-y efficacy and safety update of COMBI-d: A phase 3 study of dabrafenib (D) + trametinib (T) vs D monotherapy in patients (pts) with unresectable or metastatic BRAF V600E/K-mutant cutaneous melanoma. J Clin Oncol. 2016; 34 (suppl; abstr 9502).
10. Long GV, Flaherty KT, Stroyakovskiy D, et al. Dabrafenib plus trametinib versus dabrafenib monotherapy in patients with metastatic BRAF V600E/K-mutant melanoma: long-term survival and safety analysis of a phase 3 study [published correction appears in Ann Oncol. 2019 Nov 1;30(11):1848]. Ann Oncol. 2017;28(7):1631–9. https://doi.org/10.1093/annonc/mdx176.
11. Robert C, Grob JJ, Stroyakovskiy D, et al. Five-year outcomes with dabrafenib plus trametinib in metastatic melanoma. N Engl J Med. 2019;381(7):626–36. https://doi.org/10.1056/NEJMoa1904059.
12. Robert C, Karaszewska B, Schachter J, et al. Improved overall survival in melanoma with combined dabrafenib and trametinib. N Engl J Med. 2015;372:30–9.
13. Robert C, Karaszewska B, Schachter J, et al. Two year estimate of overall survival in COMBI-v, a randomized, open-label, phase III study comparing the combination of dabrafenib and trametinib with vemurafenib as fist-line therapy in patients with unresectable or metastatic BRAF V600E/K mutation-positive cutaneous melanoma. European Cancer Congress 2015, abstract 3301.
14. Larkin J, Ascierto PA, Dréno B, Atkinson V, Liszkay G, Maio M, Mandalà M, Demidov L, Stroyakovskiy D, Thomas L, de la Cruz-Merino L, Dutriaux C, Garbe C, Sovak MA, Chang

I, Choong N, Hack SP, McArthur GA, Ribas A. Combined vemurafenib and cobimetinib in BRAF-mutated melanoma. N Engl J Med. 2014;371(20):1867–76.

15. Larkin JMG, Yan Y, McArthur GA, et al. Update of progression-free survival (PFS) and correlative biomarker analysis from coBRIM: phase III study of cobimetinib (cobi) plus vemurafenib (vem) in advanced BRAF-mutated melanoma. J Clin Oncol. 2015;33 (Suppl): abstract 9006.

16. Atkinson V, Larkin J, McArthur G, et al. Improved overall survival (OS) with cobimetinib (COBI) + vemurafenib (V) in advanced BRAF-mutated melanoma and biomarker correlates of efficacy. Society for Melanoma Research 2015. LBA 1.

17. Dummer R, Ascierto PA, Gogas HJ, et al. Overall survival in patients with BRAF-mutant melanoma receiving encorafenib plus binimetinib versus vemurafenib or encorafenib (COLUMBUS): a multicentre, open-label, randomised, phase 3 trial [published correction appears in Lancet Oncol. 2018 Oct;19(10):e509]. Lancet Oncol. 2018;19(10):1315–27. https://doi.org/10.1016/S1470-2045(18)30497-2.

18. Ascierto PA, Dummer R, Gogas HJ, et al. Update on tolerability and overall survival in COLUMBUS: landmark analysis of a randomised phase 3 trial of encorafenib plus binimetinib vs vemurafenib or encorafenib in patients with BRAF V600-mutant melanoma. Eur J Cancer. 2020;126:33–44. https://doi.org/10.1016/j.ejca.2019.11.016.

19. Robert C, Schachter J, Long GV, Arance A, Grob JJ, Mortier L, Daud A, Carlino MS, McNeil C, Lotem M, Larkin J, Lorigan P, Neyns B, Blank CU, Hamid O, Mateus C, Shapira-Frommer R, Kosh M, Zhou H, Ibrahim N, Ebbinghaus S, Ribas A, KEYNOTE-006 Investigators. Pembrolizumab versus ipilimumab in advanced melanoma. N Engl J Med. 2015;372(26):2521–32.

20. Schachter J, Ribas A, Long GV, et al. Pembrolizumab versus ipilimumab for advanced melanoma: Final overall survival analysis of KEYNOTE-006. J Clin Oncol. 2016;34 (suppl; abstr 9504).

21. Schachter J, Ribas A, Long GV, et al. Pembrolizumab versus ipilimumab for advanced melanoma: final overall survival results of a multicentre, randomised, open-label phase 3 study (KEYNOTE-006). Lancet. 2017;390(10105):1853–62. https://doi.org/10.1016/S0140-6736(17)31601-X.

22. Robert C, Ribas A, Schachter J, et al. Pembrolizumab versus ipilimumab in advanced melanoma (KEYNOTE-006): post-hoc 5-year results from an open-label, multicentre, randomised, controlled, phase 3 study. Lancet Oncol. 2019;20(9):1239–51. https://doi.org/10.1016/S1470-2045(19)30388-2.

23. Long GV, Schachter J, Arance A, Grob J-J, Mortier L, Daud A, Carlino MS, Ribas A, McNeil CM, Lotem M, Larkin JMG, Lorigan P, Neyns B, Blank CU, Petrella TM, Hamid O, Jensen E, Krepler C, Diede SJ, Robert C. Long-term survival from pembrolizumab (pembro) completion and pembro retreatment: Phase III KEYNOTE-006 in advanced melanoma. J Clin Oncol. 2020;38(15_Suppl):10013.

24. Robert C, Long GV, Brady B, et al. Nivolumab in previously untreated melanoma without BRAF mutation. N Engl J Med. 2015;372(4):320–30.

25. Ascierto PA, Long GV, Robert C, et al. Survival outcomes in patients with previously untreated BRAF wild-type advanced melanoma treated with nivolumab therapy: three-year follow-up of a randomized phase 3 trial [published correction appears in JAMA Oncol. 2019 Feb 1;5(2):271]. JAMA Oncol. 2019;5(2):187–94. https://doi.org/10.1001/jamaoncol.2018.4514.

26. Larkin J, Chiarion-Sileni V, Gonzalez R, Grob JJ, Cowey CL, Lao CD, Schadendorf D, Dummer R, Smylie M, Rutkowski P, Ferrucci PF, Hill A, Wagstaff J, Carlino MS, Haanen JB, Maio M, Marquez-Rodas I, McArthur GA, Ascierto PA, Long GV, Callahan MK, Postow MA, Grossmann K, Sznol M, Dreno B, Bastholt L, Yang A, Rollin LM, Horak C, Hodi FS, Wolchok JD. Combined nivolumab and ipilimumab or monotherapy in untreated melanoma. N Engl J Med. 2015;373(1):23–34.

27. Wolchok JD, Chiarion-Sileni V, Gonzalez R, Rutkowski P, Grob JJ, Cowey CL, Lao C, Schadendorf D, Ferrucci PF, Smylie M, Dummer R, Hill A, Haanen JBAG, Maio M, McArthur GA, Walker D, Jiang J, Horak CE, Larkin CMG, Hodi FS. Updated results from a phase III

trial of nivolumab (NIVO) combined with ipilimumab (IPI) in treatment-naive patients (pts) with advanced melanoma (MEL) (CheckMate 067). J Clin Oncol. 2016;34 (suppl; abstr 9505).

28. Wolchok JD, Chiarion-Sileni V, Gonzalez R, et al. Overall survival with combined nivolumab and ipilimumab in advanced melanoma [published correction appears in N Engl J Med. 2018 Nov 29;379(22):2185]. N Engl J Med. 2017;377(14):1345–56. https://doi.org/10.1056/NEJMoa1709684.

29. Larkin J, Chiarion-Sileni V, Gonzalez R, et al. Five-Year Survival with Combined Nivolumab and Ipilimumab in Advanced Melanoma. N Engl J Med. 2019;381(16):1535–46. https://doi.org/10.1056/NEJMoa1910836.

30. Gutzmer R, Stroyakovskiy D, Gogas H, et al. Atezolizumab, vemurafenib, and cobimetinib as first-line treatment for unresectable advanced BRAFV600 mutation-positive melanoma (IMspire150): primary analysis of the randomised, double-blind, placebo-controlled, phase 3 trial. Lancet. 2020;395(10240):1835–44. https://doi.org/10.1016/S0140-6736(20)30934-X.

31. Michielin O, van Akkooi A, Lorigan P, et al. ESMO consensus conference recommendations on the management of locoregional melanoma: the ESMO Guidelines Committee [published online ahead of print, 2020 Jul 22]. Ann Oncol. 2020;31(11):1449–61. https://doi.org/10.1016/j.annonc.2020.07.005.

32. Keilholz U, Ascierto PA, Dummer R, et al. ESMO consensus conference recommendations on the management of metastatic melanoma: the ESMO Guidelines Committee [published online ahead of print, 2020 Jul 22]. Ann Oncol. 2020;31(11):1435–48. https://doi.org/10.1016/j.annonc.2020.07.004.

33. Guo J, Si L, Kong Y, et al. Phase II, open-label, single-arm trial of imatinib mesylate in patients with metastatic melanoma harboring c-Kit mutation or amplification. J Clin Oncol. 2011;29(21):2904–9. https://doi.org/10.1200/JCO.2010.33.9275.

34. Chan TA, Yarchoan M, Jaffee E, et al. Development of tumor mutation burden as an immunotherapy biomarker: utility for the oncology clinic. Ann Oncol. 2019;30(1):44–56. https://doi.org/10.1093/annonc/mdy495.

Index

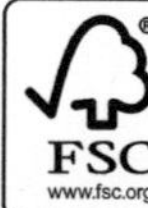